YALE UNIVERSITY
SCHOOL OF MEDICINE
HEART BOOK

YALE
UNIVERSITY
School of Medicine
HEART
BOOK

MEDICAL EDITORS

Barry L. Zaret, M.D.

Robert W. Berliner Professor of Medicine
Professor of Diagnostic Radiology
Chief, Section of Cardiovascular Medicine
Yale University School of Medicine

Marvin Moser, M.D.

Clinical Professor of Medicine
Yale University School of Medicine

Lawrence S. Cohen, M.D.

Ebenezer K. Hunt Professor of Medicine
Yale University School of Medicine

EDITORIAL DIRECTOR
Genell J. Subak-Sharpe, M.S.

MANAGING EDITOR
Diane M. Goetz

ILLUSTRATIONS
Briar Lee Mitchell

HEARST BOOKS
New York

This book is based on current medical research, knowledge, and understanding, and to the best of the editors' ability, the material is accurate and valid. Even so, any individual reader should not use the information to alter a prescribed regimen or in any form of self-treatment without first seeking the advice of his or her personal physician. The editors do not bear any responsibility or liability for the information or for any uses to which it may be put.

The following are reproduced with permission:

From the American Heart Association,

From *Risk Factor Prediction Kit*, 1990:
P. 26, "Coronary Heart Disease Risk Factor Prediction Chart—Framingham Heart Study"
From *1991 Heart and Stroke Facts*, 1990:
P. 27, "Danger of Heart Attack by Risk Factors Present"
P. 34, "Age-Adjusted Death Rates for Major Cardiovascular Diseases"
P. 145, "What You Can Do (Heart Attack—Signals and Actions)"
P. 238, "Estimated Annual Number of Americans, by Age and Sex, Experiencing Heart Attack"
P. 272, "Estimated Percent of Population with Hypertension by Race and Sex, U.S. Adults Age 18–74"
From *Cardiovascular and Risk Factor Evaluation of Healthy American Adults*, 1987:
P. 33, "The American Heart Association's Recommendations for Periodic Health Examinations"
From *Silent Epidemic: The Truth About Women and Heart Disease*, 1989:
P. 238, "The American Heart Association's Check-up Checklist for Women: Items to Discuss with a Doctor"
Copyright © American Heart Association.

•

The American Cancer Society, Inc: Adapted from "7-Day Plan to Help You Stop Smoking Cigarettes":
P. 75, "Interpreting Your Score," and p. 79, "Reasons to Quit Smoking"

•

Adapted from *The American Medical Association Family Medical Guide*, by the American Medical Association. Copyright © 1982 by the American Medical Association. Reprinted by permission of Random House, Inc:
P. 80, "Alcohol Content By the Drink," and p. 81, "Beyond the Legal Limit: The Possible Cumulative Effects of Drinking"

•

Modified from American College of Sports Medicine: *Resource Manual for Guidelines for Exercise Testing and Prescription*, 4th ed., Philadelphia, Lea & Febiger, 1991:
P. 89, "Sample Exercise Prescriptions"
Modified from American College of Sports Medicine: *Resource Manual for Guidelines for Exercise Testing and Prescription*. Philadelphia, Lea & Febiger, 1988:
P. 91, "Signs of Excessive Effort" and "When to Defer Exercise"

•

From Nordic Press, 104 Peavey Road, Chaska, Minn. 55318. From *Nordic Tracks*, vol. 2, issue 1, 1990:
P. 90, "Recommended Heart Rate Ranges for Cardiovascular Fitness"

•

From *Journal of Chronic Diseases*, vol. 22, Bortner, "A Short Rate Scale as a Potential Measure of Pattern A Behavior," 1969, Pergamon Press plc:
P. 100, "The Bortner Type A Rating Scale"

•

From *The Relaxation Response* by Herbert Benson with Miriam Z. Klipper. Copyright © 1975 by William Morrow & Co., Inc.:
P. 102, "The Relaxation Response"

•

From *Journal of the American Medical Association*, 1990, 264: 2919–2922, Copyright © 1990, American Medical Association:
P. 169, "Typical Prophylactic Antibiotic Schedule"

•

Library of Congress Cataloging-in-Publication Data

Yale University School of Medicine heart book / Medical editors, Barry L. Zaret, Marvin Moser, Lawrence S. Cohen. Editorial director, Genell J. Subak-Sharpe.
    p. cm.
Includes bibliographical references and index.

ISBN 0-688-09719-7
1. Heart—Diseases—Popular works. I. Zaret, Barry L.
II. Moser,   Marvin. III. Cohen,   Lawrence
S. IV. Subak-Sharpe, Genell J. V. Yale University. School of
Medicine.   VI. Title: Yale university school of medicine heart book
    [DNLM: 1. Heart Diseases. 2. Heart Diseases—prevention &
control.   WG 200 Y18]
RC672.Y35 1992
616.1'2—dc20
DNLM/DLC
for Library of Congress   91-28057
                                                            CIP

Printed in the United States of America

First Edition

1 2 3 4 5 6 7 8 9 10

BOOK DESIGN BY MICHAEL MENDELSOHN / M′N O PRODUCTION SERVICES, INC.

This book is dedicated to our patients,
students, and colleagues,
with gratitude for all that they have taught us.

FOREWORD

During the germination of this book, a fellow Yale faculty member posed a most provocative question: "Why should we devote so much of our time and effort to do this book at this time?" Why indeed? The question forced us to stop for a moment, to focus on our objectives, and to analyze just why we were so convinced that there really was a need for this particular book.

First, there's the pervasive public preoccupation with the subject. Go to a cocktail party and the conversation invariably turns to cholesterol or exercise. Dinner party hostesses proudly introduce dishes by announcing: "This is absolutely free of animal fat and we've cut the calories in half!" Four-star restaurants and company cafeterias alike offer "heart healthy" selections. And it seems that every other item in the supermarket is labeled either "lite" or cholesterol-free.

Why this sudden emphasis on cardiovascular health? For the answer, we need only to look at mortality statistics of recent decades. In the 1950s, cardiovascular diseases claimed about one million American lives each year. In the 1960s, the cardiovascular death rate began a precipitous decline. By 1990, the death rate from heart attacks was about half of what it was in 1950, with an even more dramatic reduction in stroke mortality.

Many factors have contributed to these tremendous gains, especially the advances in medical technology. Of all the medical disciplines affected by the technological revolution, cardiovascular medicine has reaped the most dramatic benefits. Today, we routinely treat many conditions that were once invariably fatal; many others can be prevented, either by medical intervention or by life-style changes. In short, we have advanced from a state in which there was little that either physician or patient could do to challenge fate to one in which we all can be active participants in the prevention and treatment of cardiovascular diseases.

In order to fully benefit from modern cardiovascular medicine, however, each individual needs a basic level of knowledge and understanding. What steps can I take to prevent or delay heart disease? When is it appropriate to seek medical help? And what should I expect? Simply lacking such basic information can add to the worry and anxiety generated by illness. Indeed, the stress of going to a doctor or entering a hospital without knowing what to expect can exacerbate the underlying problem.

Unfortunately, the public's need for basic knowledge in cardiovascular medicine has not been matched by reliable sources of comprehensive and understandable information. Thus, this book was conceived to fill this information gap. In clear, simple language, this book covers the entire spectrum of cardiovascular disease. It begins with the basics by describing the heart and circulation, and providing an overview of what can go wrong. The next section tells how you can reduce your risk of a heart attack by eliminating or modifying detrimental life-style factors. This is followed by a discussion of symptoms and diagnosis, which serves as an introduction to an encyclopedia of common heart disorders and more detailed chapters on categories of cardiovascular diseases.

In the section on special situations, you will find chapters on heart disease in women, children, and the elderly, as well as a discussion of racial and ethnic factors. Five chapters are devoted to the major modalities of treatment: drugs, angioplasty and interventional cardiology, surgery, pacemakers, and emergency treatments. The chapter on cardiac rehabilitation outlines how to resume an active, productive life following a heart attack or heart surgery. Finally, the chapter on the patient as a consumer offers practical guidelines on dealing with today's health-care system.

A concluding word of caution: This book should not be used to alter a regimen prescribed by your physician or to devise your own treatment program —this should be entrusted only to a physician who knows your medical history. Instead, the information in this book is intended to improve your role as an informed partner in maintaining or achieving cardiovascular health.

ACKNOWLEDGMENTS

The creation of a book of this scope inevitably involves scores of dedicated people. While it is impossible to cite all of the people who have made this book possible, there are some whose efforts deserve special mention.

Above all, we are indebted to the dozens of Yale officials, physicians, researchers, and other staff members who have made this book possible. We are grateful to Dean Leon E. Rosenberg, M.D., for his support in allowing this book to go forward.

A team of skilled medical writers and editors have worked diligently to make the manuscript readable and understandable. They include Brenda Becker, Diana Benzaia, Gail Bronson, Monty Brower, Diane Debrovner, Tony Eprile, Tim Friend, Rebecca Hughes, Joan Lippert, Ruth Hedrick Livingston, Ruth Papazian, Joan Reisman, Caroline Tapley, and Luba Vikhanski.

Hope Subak-Sharpe has pitched in to check facts and type manuscripts; Everton Lopez has also spent long hours doing typing duty. Allison Handler, R.N., provided much useful patient care information. Catherine Caruthers has been instrumental in putting the manuscript together, editing and writing when necessary, and keeping track of myriad details. We also acknowledge the talent, diligence, and patience of our illustrator, Briar Lee Mitchell. Joanne Mayfield, Astrid Swanson, and June Coons have spent many hours arranging meetings, tracking down manuscripts, and helping coordinate efforts of the Yale and New York editors.

We also want to thank Ann Bramson, our editor at William Morrow, for her insightful handling of this book. Edward D. Johnson, the copy editor, has done a marvelous job in catching all those inconsistencies and "gremlins" that somehow creep into this kind of manuscript. Ann Cahn helped to take the project from manuscript to book. Finally, we thank the many spouses who have done everything from critiquing chapters to baby-sitting.

THE EDITORS

CONTENTS

CONTENTS

LIST OF CONTRIBUTORS

John C. Baldwin, M.D.
Professor and Chief,
Cardiothoracic Surgery

William Batsford, M.D.
Professor of Medicine
Director, Electrophysiology Laboratory

Jeffrey R. Bender, M.D.
Assistant Professor of Medicine
Director, Cardiovascular Immunology Laboratory

Henry R. Black, M.D.
Professor of Internal Medicine
Director, Preventive Cardiology Service
Co-Director, Yale Vascular Center

Lawrence M. Brass, M.D.
Associate Professor of Neurology
Director, Yale Stroke Program

Matthew M. Burg, Ph.D.
Assistant Clinical Professor of Psychology in Psychiatry

Henry S. Cabin, M.D.
Associate Professor of Medicine and Pathology
University Director, Coronary Care Unit
Associate Director, Cardiac Catheterization Laboratory

Michael W. Cleman, M.D.
Associate Professor of Medicine
Director, Cardiac Catheterization Laboratory
    and PTCA Services

Lawrence S. Cohen, M.D.
Ebenezer K. Hunt Professor of Medicine

Lawrence Deckelbaum, M.D.
Professor of Medicine
Director, Cardiac Catheterization Laboratory
West Haven V.A. Medical Center

John A. Elefteriades, M.D.
Associate Professor of Cardiothoracic Surgery
Director, Adult Cardiac Procedures

Michael D. Ezekowitz, M.D., Ph.D.
Professor of Medicine
Director, Cardiovascular Division
West Haven V.A. Medical Center

Michele Fairchild, M.A., R.D.
Associate Director of Clinical Nutrition
Yale–New Haven Hospital

Jonathan Isaacsohn, M.D.
Assistant Professor of Medicine
Director, Yale Lipid Service
Associate Director, Christ Hospital Cardiovascular
    Research Center

Charles S. Kleinman, M.D.
Professor of Pediatrics, Obstetrics, and Gynecology
    and Diagnostic Imaging
Chief, Section of Pediatric Cardiology

Gary S. Kopf, M.D.
Professor of Cardiothoracic Surgery

Forrester A. Lee, M.D.
Assistant Professor of Medicine
Co-Director, Cardiopulmonary Transplant Program

Craig A. McPherson, M.D.
Associate Professor of Medicine
Director, Coronary Care Unit and Arrythmia Clinic
West Haven V.A. Medical Center

Marvin Moser, M.D.
Clinical Professor of Medicine

Adrian Ostfeld, M.D.
Anna M.R. Lauder Professor of Epidemiology
    and Public Health
Professor of Medicine

Caroline Piselli, R.N., M.B.A.
Manager, Center for Health Promotion
Yale–New Haven Hospital

Michael Remetz, M.D.
Assistant Professor of Medicine

Lynda E. Rosenfeld, M.D.
Associate Professor of Medicine and Pediatrics
Co-Director, Electrophysiology Laboratory

Robert Soufer, M.D.
Director, V.A. PET Center
Associate Professor of Diagnostic Radiology
    and Medicine

Virginia Utermohlen, M.D.
Assistant Professor of Nutrition
Cornell University

Frans J. Th. Wackers, M.D.
Professor, Diagnostic Radiology and Medicine
Director, Cardiovascular Nuclear Imaging
    and Stress Laboratories

Lawrence H. Young, M.D.
Associate Professor of Medicine

Raphael Zahler, M.D., Ph.D.
Assistant Professor of Medicine

Barry L. Zaret, M.D.
Robert W. Berliner Professor of Medicine
Professor of Diagnostic Radiology
Chief, Section of Cardiovascular Medicine

COLOR ATLAS

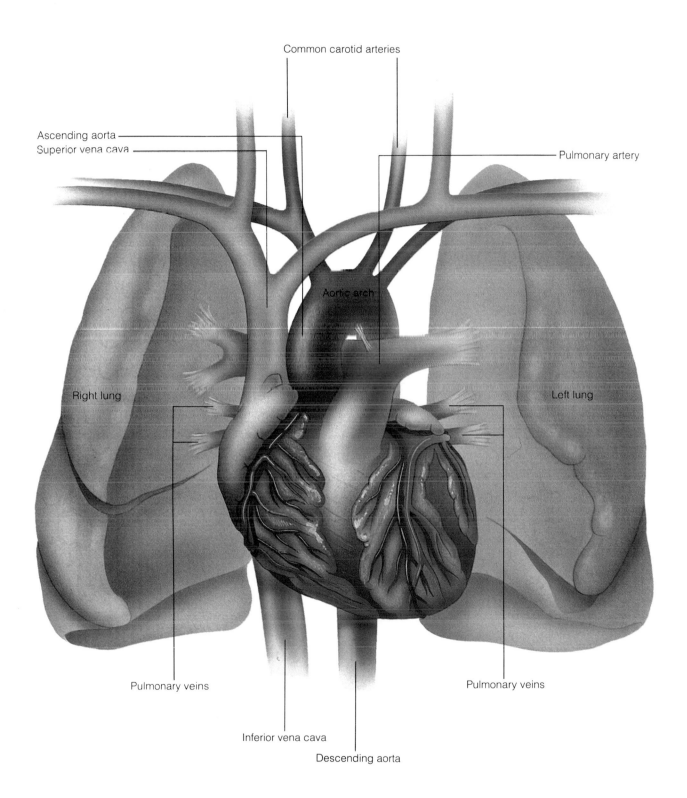

Common carotid arteries

Ascending aorta
Superior vena cava

Pulmonary artery

Aortic arch

Right lung

Left lung

Pulmonary veins

Pulmonary veins

Inferior vena cava

Descending aorta

A normal heart with the lungs and major vessels

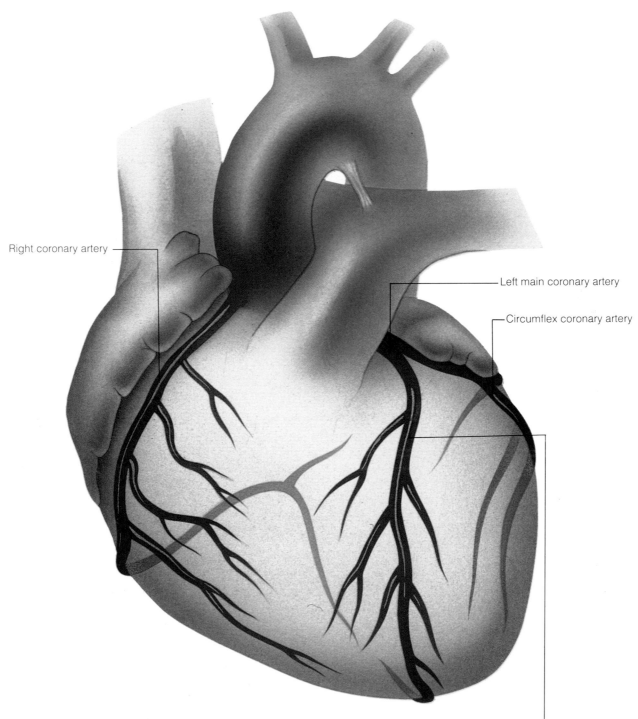

Right coronary artery

Left main coronary artery

Circumflex coronary artery

Left anterior descending coronary artery

A normal heart showing the coronary arteries

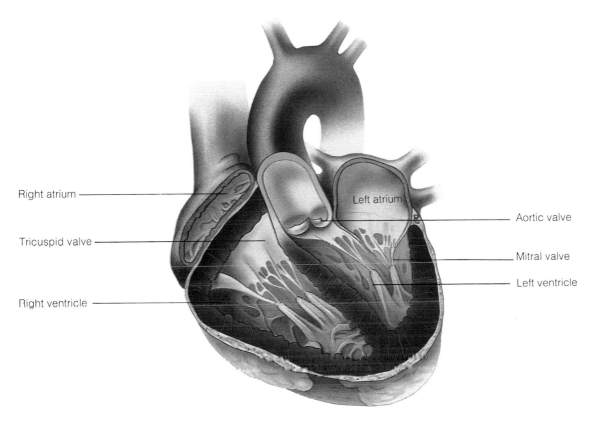

Right atrium

Tricuspid valve

Right ventricle

Left atrium

Aortic valve

Mitral valve

Left ventricle

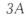

Cross section of a normal heart showing all four chambers

3A

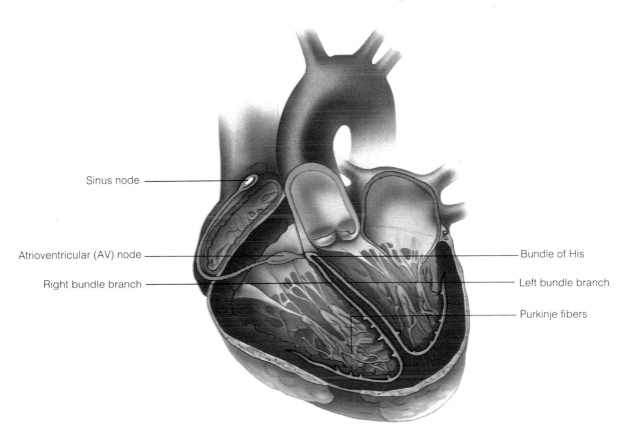

Sinus node

Atrioventricular (AV) node

Right bundle branch

Bundle of His

Left bundle branch

Purkinje fibers

The heart's electrical conduction system

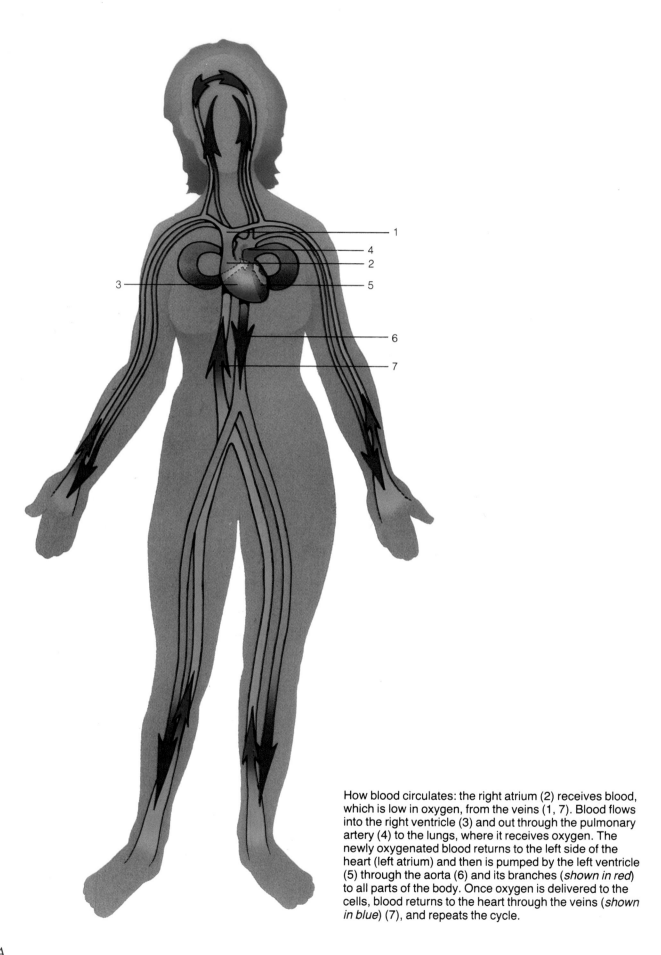

How blood circulates: the right atrium (2) receives blood, which is low in oxygen, from the veins (1, 7). Blood flows into the right ventricle (3) and out through the pulmonary artery (4) to the lungs, where it receives oxygen. The newly oxygenated blood returns to the left side of the heart (left atrium) and then is pumped by the left ventricle (5) through the aorta (6) and its branches (*shown in red*) to all parts of the body. Once oxygen is delivered to the cells, blood returns to the heart through the veins (*shown in blue*) (7), and repeats the cycle.

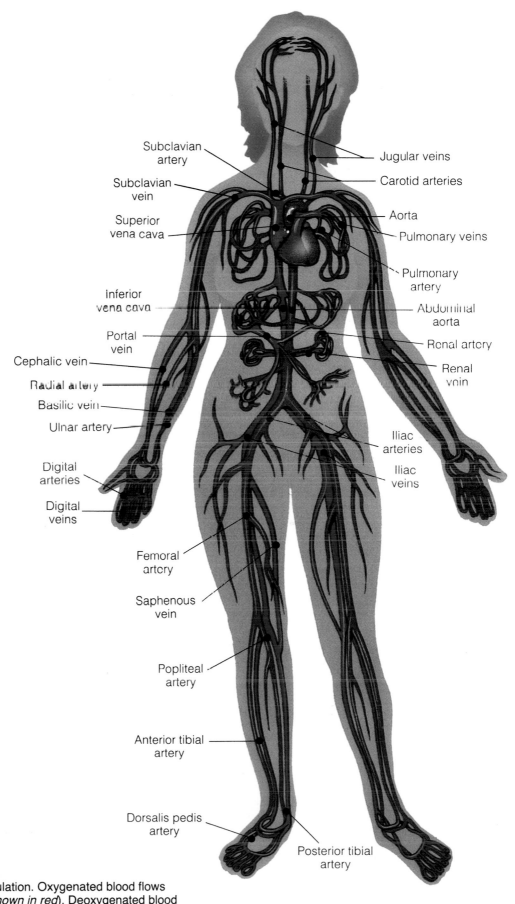

Subclavian artery

Subclavian vein

Superior vena cava

Inferior vena cava

Portal vein

Cephalic vein

Radial artery

Basilic vein

Ulnar artery

Digital arteries

Digital veins

Jugular veins

Carotid arteries

Aorta

Pulmonary veins

Pulmonary artery

Abdominal aorta

Renal artery

Renal vein

Iliac arteries

Iliac veins

Femoral artery

Saphenous vein

Popliteal artery

Anterior tibial artery

Dorsalis pedis artery

Posterior tibial artery

Full body showing circulation. Oxygenated blood flows through the arteries (*shown in red*). Deoxygenated blood flows through the veins (*shown in blue*).

HOW BLOOD CIRCULATES THROUGH THE HEART

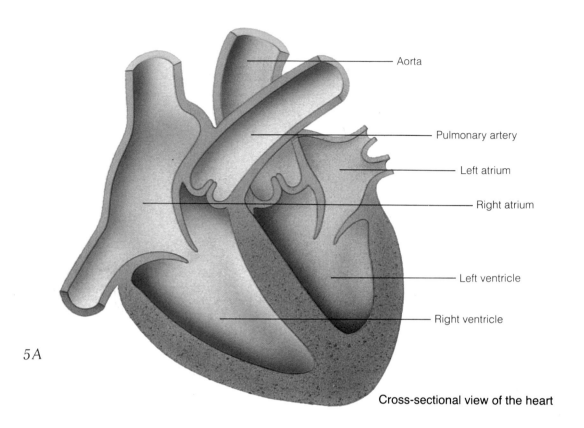

Aorta

Pulmonary artery

Left atrium

Right atrium

Left ventricle

Right ventricle

5A

Cross-sectional view of the heart

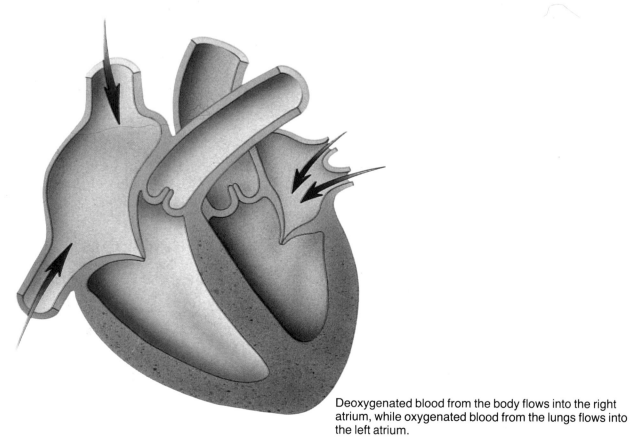

Deoxygenated blood from the body flows into the right atrium, while oxygenated blood from the lungs flows into the left atrium.

5B

HOW BLOOD CIRCULATES THROUGH THE HEART

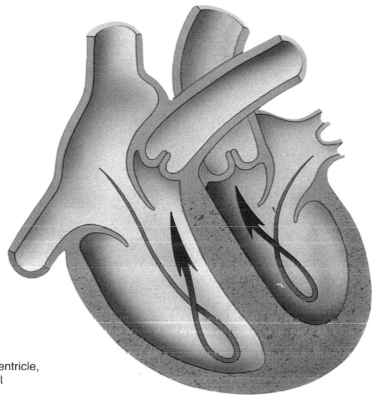

5C

Blood from the right atrium flows into the right ventricle, while blood from the left atrium flows into the left ventricle.

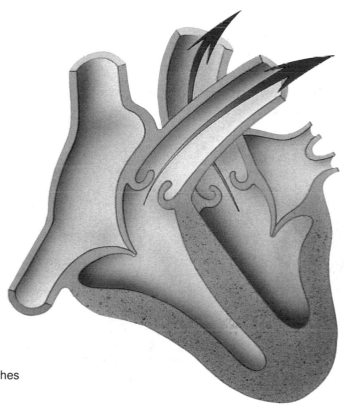

Blood is then pumped through the aorta and its branches to the various parts of the body, and through the pulmonary artery to the lungs.

5D

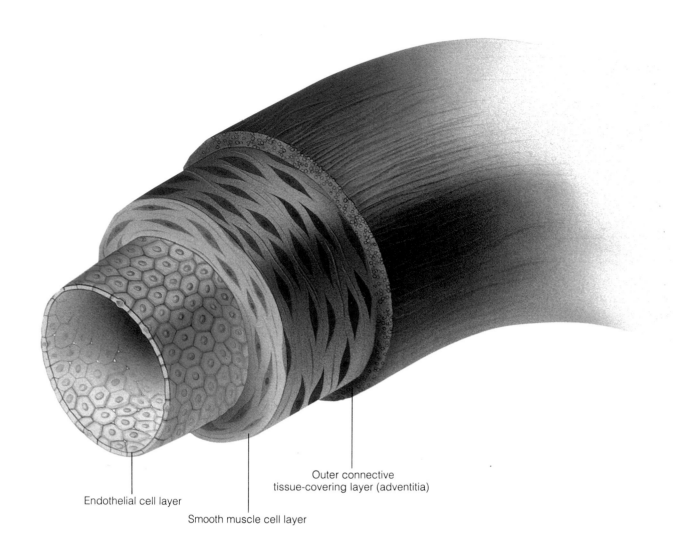

Endothelial cell layer

Smooth muscle cell layer

Outer connective
tissue-covering layer (adventitia)

Cross section of an artery

PART I

THE HEART AND HOW IT WORKS

THE HEART AND CIRCULATION

HENRY S. CABIN, M.D.

INTRODUCTION

The cardiovascular system is an elaborate network that performs two major tasks: It delivers oxygen and nutrients to body organs and removes waste products of metabolism from tissue cells. Its major components are the heart—a hollow muscular pump—and a circulatory system of large and small elastic vessels or conduits that transport blood throughout the body. In the course of one day, the amount of blood pumped through the heart of a normal healthy adult at rest reaches approximately 2,100 gallons. (See box, "The Amazing Heart and Blood Vessels.")

THE HEART

The heart, the central organ of the cardiovascular system, is located between the two lungs in the middle of the chest. (See color atlas, #1.) Two-thirds of the heart lies to the left of the breastbone and one-third to the right. Placing a hand on the chest, we can feel the heartbeat on the left side of the rib cage because in that spot, the bottom left corner of the heart, which is somewhat tilted forward, comes closest to

the surface of the body. The adult heart is about the size of two clenched fists. It is shaped like a cone and weighs about 7 to 15 ounces, depending on the size and weight of the individual.

THE HEART CHAMBERS

The human heart is divided into four chambers—the right atrium and right ventricle and the left atrium and left ventricle. (See color atlas, #3A.) The walls of the chambers are made of a special muscle, the myocardium, that contracts rhythmically under the stimulation of electrical currents. The left and right atria and the left and right ventricles are separated from each other by a wall of muscle called the septum (atrial septum for the atria and ventricular septum for the ventricles).

The circulation system is described in greater detail later in this chapter, but basically it works as follows. (See color atlas, #5A to 5D.) Blood returning from the body through the venous system enters the heart through the right atrium, where it collects and is then pumped to the right ventricle. Each time the right ventricle contracts, it propels this blood, which is low in oxygen content, into the lungs, where it is enriched with oxygen. Pulmonary veins return the blood to the left atrium, which contracts and sends it to the left ventricle. The left ventricle, the main pumping chamber of the heart, ejects the blood

The Amazing Heart and Blood Vessels

- The adult human heart is about the size of two clenched fists.

- In an average lifetime, the heart pumps 1 million barrels of blood—enough blood to fill 3.3 supertankers. This only takes into account its work at rest. During exercise or stress, the heart may pump ten times as much blood as it does at rest.

- In one year, the human heart beats 3 million times. The heart of a 70-year-old has beaten more than 2.5 billion times.

- Even when a person is at rest, the muscles of the heart work twice as hard as the leg muscles of a person running at top speed.

- The amount of energy expended by the heart in 50 years is enough to lift a battleship out of the water.

- The electrical signal produced by the sinus node travels over the entire surface of the heart in only 21/100 to 26/100 of a second.

- Stretched end to end, the vessels of the circulatory system—arteries, arterioles, capillaries, venules, and veins—would measure about 60,000 miles.

- The oxygen and nutrients transported in the bloodstream and delivered with each beat of the heart nourish 300 trillion cells.

- The capillaries, the smallest blood vessels in the body, are so tiny that ten of them together are only as thick as a human hair.

- In total area, the capillary walls are equal to about 60,000 to 70,000 square feet, or roughly the area of one and a half football fields.

through the aorta into the major circulatory network. Because it delivers blood to the entire body, this ventricle works harder than all other chambers; as a result, its walls can be more than ½ inch thick—two to three times thicker than the walls of the right ventricle.

THE VALVES

Blood in the heart is kept flowing in a forward direction by a system of four one-way valves, each closing off one of the heart's chambers at the appropriate time in the cardiac cycle. The valves open to let the blood through when the chambers contract, and snap shut to prevent it from flowing backward as the chambers relax. The valve system also helps maintain different pressures on the right and left sides of the heart.

The valves differ significantly in structure. The two valves separating the ventricles from the circulatory system are called semilunar because of their crescent-shaped cusps. At the juncture of the right ventricle and the pulmonary artery lies the pulmonary valve. It consists of three cusps, or flaps of tissue, that open freely when the right ventricle contracts and blood is ejected into the lungs, and then fall back as the ventricle relaxes. The other semilunar valve, the aortic valve, lies between the left ventricle and the aorta and also has three cusps. It is flung open when the left ventricle squeezes down to propel blood into the main circulation. When the left ventricle relaxes, the pressure in the aorta pushes the valve closed.

The ventricles are separated from the atria by valves that, in addition to the cusps, have thin but strong cords of fibrous tissue. Called chordae tendineae, these cords tether the valves to the ventricular walls. When the ventricles contract, small muscles in their walls, called papillary muscles, pull the cords, which act as guide wires, and control the closure of the valve leaflets, preventing them from flapping too far backward.

The valve located between the left ventricle and left atrium is a cone-shaped funnel that resembles a miter—a triangular head dress worn by bishops and abbots—and is therefore called the mitral valve. It has two leaflets that are remarkably mobile and can open and close rapidly. The corresponding valve between the right ventricle and right atrium is called the tricuspid valve. As its name suggests, it has three cusps, or leaflets, that are thinner than those of the mitral valve and just as mobile.

ENDOCARDIUM AND PERICARDIUM

On the inside, the heart is lined with a protective layer of cells that form a smooth membrane called the endocardium. On the outside, the heart is encased in a two-layered fibrous sac (like a cellophane casing) called the pericardium, which extends to cover the roots of the major blood vessels. The inner layer of the pericardium is attached to the heart muscle, while the outer layer, connected by ligaments to the vertebral column, the diaphragm, and other body structures, holds the heart firmly in place. The layers are separated by a thin film of lubricating fluid that allows the heart to move freely within the outer pericardium.

CORONARY ARTERIES AND VEINS

Because the heart never rests while it supplies blood to the rest of the body, it actually works harder than any other muscle in the body and needs a much richer blood supply than other muscles. The heart supplies blood to itself through two coronary arteries, the right and the left, which leave the aorta about ½ inch above the aortic valve and run around the outside of the heart. Both arteries lie in grooves on the outside of the heart muscle and branch off into a system of smaller vessels and capillaries that supply the muscle fibers. After giving off its oxygen in the capillaries, the blood travels through coronary veins and drains directly into the right atrium, where it joins the venous blood from the rest of the body.

When the heart is working harder than usual, the coronary arteries dilate to increase oxygen supply to the heart muscle. During extreme physical exertion, flow in these arteries may increase by five to six times.

The better an individual's physical condition, the more efficient is his or her heart in using the blood supply available. When blood supply is insufficient to meet the increased requirements in oxygen and nutrients and to wash away waste materials, the heart aches, just as other muscles might ache from an excessive workload. The lack of oxygen stimulates nerve cells, and chest pain, or angina pectoris, is noted. In contrast to other muscles of the body, however, the heart cannot stop for rest without devastating consequences.

THE CONDUCTION SYSTEM

Electrical currents that regulate the heart rhythm originate in cells of the heart muscle (myocardium) and travel through a network of specialized fibers referred to as the heart's conduction system. Its major elements include the sinus or sinoatrial node, the atrioventricular or AV node, the bundle of His, and the Purkinje fibers. (See color atlas, #3B.)

The sinus node, known as the heart's pacemaker, is a microscopic bundle of specialized cells located in the top right corner of the heart. Any portion of the heart muscle can generate electrical impulses, but in normal function, the impulses originate in this pacemaker. If the pacemaker's function is disrupted, another part of the conduction system can take over the impulse-firing task.

Impulses are transmitted through muscle fibers of the two atria to the atrioventricular node, located on the juncture between the right and left sides of the heart, in the area where the right atrium and right ventricle meet. From the atrioventricular node, they travel along the bundle of His and the Purkinje fibers—fibrous pathways named after the scientists who first described them—through the muscles of the right and left ventricles.

THE CARDIAC CYCLE

Electrical activity coordinates the rhythmic contraction and relaxation of the heart's chambers known as the cardiac cycle. Most currents in the heart are less than a millionth of an ampere (the current running through a 100-watt bulb is approximately 1 ampere), but they exert a powerful influence on the heart muscle.

The cardiac cycle consists of two phases, called diastole and systole. Diastole, during which the heart's ventricles are relaxed, is the longer phase, taking up approximately two-thirds of the cycle. Systole, the phase during which blood is ejected from the ventricles, takes up the remaining one-third.

During diastole, the sinus node generates an impulse that forces the two atria to contract. In this phase, the tricuspid and mitral valves are open, and blood is propelled from the atria into the relaxed jventricles. By the end of diastole, the electric impulse reaches the ventricles, causing them to contract.

During systole, the contracting ventricles close the tricuspid and mitral valves. Shortly afterward, the pressure of the blood inside the ventricles rises sufficiently to force the pulmonary and aortic valves to open, and blood is ejected into the pulmonary artery and the aorta. As the ventricles relax again, blood backs up from the pulmonary artery and the aorta, closing down the pulmonary and aortic valves. The pressure in the relaxed ventricles is now lower than in the atria, the tricuspid and mitral valves open again, and the cardiac cycle starts anew.

This seemingly lengthy sequence of events in fact takes approximately a second. The familiar double throb (lub dub) of the beating heart corresponds to the two sets of synchronized contractions that occur during the cardiac cycle: The throbbing sound we hear comes not only from the snapping of the valves, but also from the accompanying vibrations of other heart structures and from the turbulence produced by the flow of blood.

HEART RATE AND CARDIAC OUTPUT

In an average adult, the pacemaker fires approximately 70 impulses a minute at rest, which means that in one minute the heart goes through a full cardiac cycle 70 times. Athletes have larger and stronger hearts that can deliver an adequate supply of blood while beating slower than the hearts of untrained individuals. Generally, the greater the physical fitness of an individual, the slower the heart rate at rest. Some well-trained athletes, for example, are known to have a pulse rate of 35 beats per minute—half the average figure for the general population. For them, the slow heart rate is efficient and does not pose a danger. For a 75-year-old untrained individual, however, a rate of 35 to 40 might be inadequate to pump sufficient blood to the brain or other vital organs. Fatigue or even fainting might result.

Because the lungs are so close to the heart and the walls of the pulmonary vessels are thinner and thus offer less resistance, the right ventricle does not have to exert nearly as much energy to do its job of supplying blood to the lungs as the left ventricle does in supplying the rest of the body.

The amount of blood pumped by the heart in one minute is called the cardiac output. When there is a need for an increased blood supply, as during physical exertion, the heart most commonly increases its output by beating faster—for example, up to 140 or 150 beats per minute. This mechanism, however, has its limits: Above a certain rate, the heart's chambers do not have time to fill properly and fail to pump efficiently.

STROKE VOLUME

The cardiac output is determined not only by the heart rate but also by the amount of blood the ventricles eject or pump out with each contraction. This amount is called the stroke volume. Usually the ventricles expel about half the blood they contain, which corresponds to about 3 ounces in an average person at rest. A decrease in the stroke volume is one of the first signs of a failing heart. While both ventricles pump out the same amount of blood in each stroke, cardiologists usually measure only the stroke volume of the left ventricle, because it is the one that pumps blood to all of the body's organs except the lungs.

The Major Arteries

Name	Origin	Supplies
Abdominal aorta	Thoracic aorta	Stomach, liver, kidneys, intestinal tract
Aortic arch	Left ventricle	Head, neck, arms
Brachial	Base of neck	Shoulders and arms
Carotid, common	Aorta	Neck and head
Carotid, external	Common carotid	Front part of neck, face, ear and scalp
Carotid, internal	Common carotid	Front part of brain, eye, nose and forehead
Celiac	Abdominal aorta	Esophagus, stomach, duodenum, gallbladder, pancreas, spleen, etc.
Coronary, left	Aorta	Left atrium, left ventricle
Coronary, right	Aorta	Right atrium, parts of both ventricles
Femoral	Iliae	Lower extremities
Hepatic	Celiac	Liver, gallbladder, stomach, pancreas
Iliac	Abdominal aorta	Pelvis, legs
Popliteal	Femoral	Thigh, lower legs
Pulmonary	Right ventricle	Lungs
Radial	Brachial artery	Forearms, hands
Renal	Abdominal aorta	Kidneys, adrenal glands
Subclavian	Aorta	Neck, arms, brain, skull, lining of heart and lungs
Tibial, anterior	Popliteal	Front of leg, ankle
Tibial, posterior	Popliteal	Back of leg, knee, sole and back of foot
Ulnar	Brachial	Forearm and part of hand

The Major Veins

Name	Drains from	Carries blood to
Hepatic	Liver	Inferior vena cava
Jugular, external	Side of neck	Subclavian vein
Jugular, internal	Neck, face, brain	Innominate vein
Portal vein	Abdominal organs, intestines	Liver
Pulmonary	Lungs	Left atrium
Vena cava, inferior	Abdomen, thighs, legs	Right atrium
Vena cava, superior	Head, neck, chest wall, arms	Right atrium

Note: Many veins are paired with, and have the same name as, major arteries. These veins return to the heart the blood that the arteries deliver to the tissues.

THE CIRCULATION

The circulatory system is an intricate network of vessels that supplies blood to all body organs and tissues. The part of the network that delivers blood to all parts of the body except the lungs is called the systemic circulation, while the flow of blood through the lungs is referred to as the pulmonary circulation. Placed end to end, all the blood vessels of the body would stretch some 60,000 miles in length.

THE SYSTEMIC CIRCULATION: THE ARTERIES AND CAPILLARIES

Blood that has been oxygenated in the lungs—bright red in color—is pumped out of the heart through the aorta, the body's largest artery, which measures approximately 1 inch in diameter. The coronary arteries, which provide the heart's own blood supply, branch out from the aorta just above the aortic valve. The aorta arches upward from the left ventricle to the upper chest, then runs down the chest into the abdomen. It forms the main trunk of the arterial part of the circulation, which branches off into numerous arteries that deliver oxygen-rich blood to various tissues. (See box, "The Major Arteries.")

The arteries are further subdivided into smaller tubes, the arterioles, which in turn branch off into even smaller vessels, the capillaries. While the walls of larger and medium-sized blood vessels are made of a layer of connective tissue and muscle cells with a very thin inner lining called the endothelium (see color atlas, #6), the walls of the capillaries consist of endothelium alone.

Most capillary walls are only one cell thick, and sometimes the blood flow through these vessels consists of a single red blood cell at a time. It is in the capillaries that the exchange of substances between the blood and the tissues takes place. Through the walls of the capillaries, the blood gives off its oxygen and nutrients and picks up carbon dioxide and waste products.

A large part of the waste is extracted from blood as it flows through the kidneys, where the plasma—the fluid component of blood—seeps through the capillary walls of the kidney's excreting mechanism. Most of the fluid is reabsorbed into the bloodstream; a fraction of a percent, together with the waste, is removed from the body as urine, which accumulates at a rate of about a quart a day in a healthy adult.

The blood pressure on the arterial side of the circulatory system is relatively high, but it decreases as the arteries branch off into arterioles and capillaries. On the venous side, the blood pressure is relatively low. The difference in pressure contributes to the driving force that propels the blood through the circulatory system.

THE VEINS

The capillaries carrying blood that now has a lower oxygen content merge to form the venules, which in turn converge into successively larger veins. (See box, "The Major Veins.") Venous blood, sometimes referred to as blue, is in fact a purplish or dark red color.

Venous blood enters the right atrium through two major vessels: the superior vena cava, which brings blood from the upper part of the body, including the brain; and the inferior vena cava, which brings blood from the lower part. Since the pressure in the veins is normally significantly lower than in the arteries, the walls of the veins are considerably thinner than arterial walls.

The larger veins have a system of internal one-way valves that prevents the blood from flowing downward under the pull of gravity when an individual stands up. When he or she moves, the veins are squeezed by the surrounding muscle, which helps propel more blood toward the heart. Without valves in the veins, blood would pool in the legs, which would then be perpetually swollen.

THE PULMONARY CIRCULATION

The main function of the pulmonary circulation is to deliver oxygen to the blood and free it of carbon dioxide. This goal is accomplished as the blood flows through the lungs. The pressure in this part of the system is only about one-sixth as great as in the systemic circulation, and the walls of pulmonary arteries and veins are significantly thinner than the walls of corresponding vessels in the rest of the body.

In the pulmonary circulation, the roles of arteries and veins are the opposite of what they are in the systemic circulation: Blood in the arteries has less oxygen, while blood in the veins is oxygen-rich. The circuit starts with the pulmonary artery, which extends from the right ventricle and carries blood with a low oxygen content to the lungs. In the lungs, it branches off into the two arteries, one for each lung, and then into arterioles and capillaries.

The gas exchange between the air we breathe in and the blood takes place in the pulmonary capillaries. Their walls act like filters by allowing molecules of gas but not molecules of fluid to pass through. The total surface area of the capillaries in the lungs ranges from 500 to 1,000 square feet.

The carbon dioxide and waste products are removed from the blood in the pulmonary arteries across capillary walls and leave the body through the mouth and nose. The blood that has picked up oxygen returns to the heart through four pulmonary veins and into the left atrium.

THE BLOOD

Blood is a life-sustaining fluid that helps maintain an optimum environment within the body by providing a constant supply of nutrients from the outside world and removing waste products from the tissues. Its cells are produced in the marrow of bones, primarily the flat bones such as the ribs and the breastbone. The volume of blood in an average adult amounts to approximately 10.5 pints.

TYPES OF BLOOD CELLS

The blood has two main components: cells of several types and a solution called plasma, in which the cells are suspended. The vast majority of blood cells are erythrocytes, or red blood cells, which outnumber white blood cells by about 700 to 1 in the healthy adult. The major function of the red blood cells, of which there are about 25 trillion, is to transport oxygen. They contain the red pigment hemoglobin, a complex protein arranged around iron that carries oxygen and releases it whenever needed. Red cells are smaller than white cells and live three to four months. They are created at a rate of approximately 8 million a second to keep the supply constant.

The white blood cells are called leukocytes. There are several types, which vary in size and shape, but all share the function of defending the body against a wide variety of invading organisms. They are produced in increased amounts in response to infection.

The platelets are plate-shaped disks that, together with special substances in the plasma, trigger the blood-clotting mechanism and prevent an uncontrollable loss of blood when the vessels are damaged.

THE PLASMA

Plasma is a yellowish fluid that consists of 90 percent water and various salts, glucose, cholesterol, proteins, etc. Proteins in the plasma perform a wide variety of functions, from transporting molecules of nutrients to acting as antibodies in the immune response.

CONTROL OF CARDIO-VASCULAR FUNCTION

The cardiovascular system plays an important role in maintaining homeostasis—that is, a stable environment—inside the body. It can carry out, or signal other systems to carry out, rapid short-term adjustments in response to demands placed on the body by various human activities and changing external conditions. For example, when blood supply to one area is increased, the flow to other organs must be reduced, or else the cardiac output has to be increased. Throughout these adaptations, blood pressure must remain constant to maintain the vital functions of all body tissues.

To perform the adjustments, the cardiovascular system communicates with other organs through a complex network of monitoring and signaling mechanisms. It sends out signals about its condition and, in turn, receives messages that control its performance. The two main regulatory centers of cardiovascular function are the nervous system and the kidneys.

THE NERVOUS SYSTEM

The brain and other parts of the nervous system constantly monitor and control the heart and circulation. They receive information about the cardiovascular system through numerous receptors that generate coded impulses describing the body's internal environment. Different kinds of receptors transmit information about the stretching of the arterial walls and the resulting changes in blood pressure or about the stretching of the heart chambers and the chemical composition of blood. Little receptors in the carotid arteries in the neck, for example, help to adjust heart rate and the size of blood vessels in response to certain activities. When we stand up suddenly and blood pressure begins to decrease, these receptors sense a lack of pressure and send out signals to the heart to beat faster and the blood vessels to constrict or narrow down so that adequate blood pressure can be maintained.

In response to changes, the nervous system issues adjustment commands. Thus, if the receptors detect a decrease in oxygen and an increase in carbon dioxide in the blood, the brain sends a command to the respiratory center to increase the rate of respiration, which delivers more oxygen to the lungs. At the same time, the brain issues impulses that accelerate the heart rate and constrict the veins. This brings more blood to the lungs to be purified. As a result, an adequate supply of oxygen to body tissues is ensured.

Messages between the nervous and cardiovascular systems are relayed by chemicals called neurotransmitters. These are chemicals that travel between cells and can provoke a response in the target tissue. The neurotransmitter norepinephrine, an adrenaline-like substance, can increase the heart rate and force of contractions, as well as constrict the blood vessels. Thus, if we become frightened, more adrenaline is released, more blood is pumped out by the heart to muscles, and we become better able to run or react if necessary. (This is called the "flight or fight" reaction.) In contrast, other neurotransmitters, such as acetylcholine, slow down the heart.

THE KIDNEYS

The kidneys play an important role in regulating blood pressure. Because they influence the volume of fluids in the body, they can affect the pressure by changing the volume of circulating blood. They also release an enzyme called renin, which is converted into a powerful blood-pressure-elevating substance that constricts blood vessels and induces sodium and water retention. Delicate mechanisms allow the kidneys to adjust under a wide variety of situations. If we are deprived of water, for example, the kidneys stop putting out urine; if we eat a lot of salt, the kidneys respond by putting out more urine.

CHAPTER 2

WHAT CAN GO WRONG

LAWRENCE S. COHEN, M.D.

INTRODUCTION

The heart is one of the most efficient and durable pumps known to man. Hearts have been known to pump for more than 100 years without resting more than about a second at a time, a feat we have yet to equal with a man-made device. Like any other electromechanical device, however, the heart can become less efficient or break down. When something does go wrong, it can take many forms:

Arteriosclerotic disease occurs when fatty deposits block the inside of the coronary arteries, the blood vessels that supply blood to the heart muscle. *Angina* or a *heart attack* can occur when the heart's blood supply from the coronary arteries slows or stops.

High blood pressure results when the heart's efforts to pump blood meet with higher-than-normal resistance in the blood vessels outside the heart.

Heart failure occurs when the heart becomes excessively stiff or fatigued from working too hard—either because it must pump against too strong a resistance or because there has been a loss of heart muscle strength.

Arrhythmia (literally, "no rhythm") occurs when the heart's electrical system goes haywire. An arrhythmia can be anything from an innocuous extra beat in the atria (upper, receiving chambers) to a dangerous irregularity in the ventricles (lower, pumping chambers).

Valvular heart disease occurs when one or more of the heart's valves malfunctions because it has narrowed or fails to close properly. Heart failure is often the end result of valvular disease.

Heart muscle diseases of various kinds can rob the heart of its muscle tone and weaken it.

Congenital heart defects are faults in the anatomy of the heart that are present at birth.

The following sections describe what happens when something goes wrong with the heart or the circulatory system. (These conditions are covered in detail in other chapters.) Some cardiovascular conditions are preventable, many have symptoms that signal their presence, and many respond well to treatment. Anyone who suspects heart disease should see his or her physician promptly. If the symptoms are acute, early intervention in the nearest hospital emergency department may be lifesaving.

ARTERIOSCLEROTIC HEART DISEASE

Fats are essential to the functioning of many body organs, and it is normal to find fats in the bloodstream. In all people, starting very early in life, some fatty material begins to build up on the insides of the blood vessel walls, particularly in the medium and large arteries. Likewise, as people grow older, they experience some thickening and hardening of the arteries, a process known by the general name arteriosclerosis. In some people, the rate of deposit of fatty material on the artery walls is faster than in others. The result can be *atherosclerosis* (*athero* refers to the fatty substance). (See Chapter 11.) Although the two terms are often used interchangeably, atherosclerosis is a type of arteriosclerosis that is characterized by deposits of plaque—an amalgam of fatty substances, cholesterol, cellular wastes, calcium, and the blood clotting material fibrin—on the inner lining of the arteries.

Arteriosclerosis is particularly dangerous when the vessel that is involved is a coronary artery, one of those that supply the heart muscle with blood. This condition is called *coronary artery disease* (CAD). The inner opening, or lumen, of a coronary artery must be narrowed by 50 to 70 percent of its normal diameter before the reduction of blood flow to the heart is considered serious. Although sometimes the terms are used interchangeably, coronary heart disease (CHD) refers to the symptoms and features that can result from advanced CAD. Coronary heart disease causes almost 500,000 deaths every year and is the leading cause of death in Americans today. Fortunately, the number of deaths from CHD within the United States is decreasing rapidly. The death rate from this disease has declined by more than 45 percent since 1972–73.

Evidence of arteriosclerotic disease appears outside the heart as well. Besides angina pectoris and coronary heart disease, effects of arteriosclerosis can include a stroke or peripheral vascular disease (involvement of the vessels that supply blood to the legs). These complications occur when blood vessels become severely narrowed or occluded.

ANGINA

For most people, the pain of angina represents an imbalance between the heart muscle's need for oxygen and its supply via the coronary artery. Narrowing in one or more of the coronary arteries decreases the supply of oxygen, and such factors as exercise may increase the demand. Tissues deprived of oxygen release metabolites that activate pain fibers in the heart. Someone with angina feels an intense pain in the chest behind the breastbone, hence the term *angina pectoris*. Angina can be triggered by many different activities—exercise, emotional upset, exposure to cold, a heavy meal. In *stable angina*, the pain is brought on by a predictable amount of work and stops when there is reduced demand on the heart. In *unstable angina*, the pain comes on without a specific cause, and it may leave just as unpredictably.

Angina can be treated medically with a number of drugs that have various effects: They may dilate the blood vessels, lower blood pressure, slow the heart to reduce its need for oxygen, or reduce the likelihood of spasm. It is also treated by increasing the inner diameter of the blood vessels, using a procedure called percutaneous transluminal coronary angioplasty (PTCA), or simply balloon angioplasty. In severe cases, coronary artery bypass surgery may be needed to bypass narrowed or closed portions of the arteries. (See Chapters 24 and 25.)

About 2.5 million people in the United States today live with angina. In itself it is not fatal, but it is a warning sign or signal of underlying coronary artery disease. (See Chapter 11.)

HEART ATTACK

When a coronary artery is completely or almost completely blocked, either by an atherosclerotic plaque or by a blood clot, the result is a heart attack, or *myocardial infarction* (literally, death of heart muscle). Within minutes, the heart muscle begins to change. After about four to six hours, the portion of the affected muscle will have deteriorated to a nonfunctioning state. Because the damage occurs so swiftly, it is extremely important not to ignore the symptoms of a heart attack, which include chest pain, usually severe and persistent—lasting longer than two minutes; sweating; nausea; dizziness; and fainting. (Some heart attacks result from spasm of a coronary artery rather than from arteriosclerosis, but the symptoms are essentially the same.)

About 5 million Americans have a history of heart attack, angina pectoris, or both. As many as 1.5 million experience a heart attack each year, and about 500,000 will die. About 60 percent of these deaths occur within the first hour after the onset of symptoms (sudden death), often before the victim reaches the hospital.

The individual who sustains a heart attack and gets to the hospital quickly now has a much better chance of survival, thanks to a treatment known as thrombolysis, in which a clot-dissolving drug is injected into the bloodstream, where it can dissolve a clot in a coronary artery, restoring some blood flow. After receiving thrombolytic therapy, patients have several treatment options: continued medical therapy, balloon angioplasty, or a coronary artery bypass graft. Long-term medical treatment can involve any of the drugs used to treat angina, as well as aspirin, which causes the blood to be less susceptible to clotting.

VASCULAR DISEASES

Several types of disorders can affect the blood vessels that supply various parts of the body. The most common is peripheral vascular disease (PVD), which refers to disease in the vessels that supply blood to the arms and legs. (See Chapter 17.) It involves a progressive narrowing of these blood vessels—most often in the legs—because of atherosclerosis. Smoking is probably the biggest risk factor for peripheral vascular disease. Having diabetes also puts someone at increased risk for this type of vascular disease.

When atherosclerotic plaques form in the blood vessels of the legs, causing these vessels to narrow, the symptom that results is called *intermittent claudication*. This condition is usually felt as pain in the calves or thighs when walking or during other activities; the exercising leg muscles' need for blood exceeds their supply. Other symptoms of peripheral vascular disease include cold or painful toes (or, in some cases, fingers) or redness or bluish discoloration in the toes. This discoloration may be most marked after sitting for long periods of time. If the narrowed vessel is in the pelvic area, the pain may be felt in the buttocks; in severe cases, impotence can occur.

If an exercise treatment program fails to relieve the condition, further treatment may include bypass grafts or balloon angioplasty. Physicians can sometimes use lasers to vaporize plaques and thereby restore blood flow, although this treatment is not yet widely available.

OTHER VASCULAR DISORDERS

Vascular disease can also affect areas closer to the heart, such as the branches of the aorta. When the aorta or its branches are narrowed, organs and tissues throughout the body may be starved of oxygen. Symptoms can be dizziness, kidney impairment, intermittent claudication, pain when resting, paleness or redness of the feet, and changes in the skin or in some cases, there will be few if any symptoms.

Although technically not diseases of the peripheral arteries, some diseases of the branches of the aorta may cause a great deal of trouble. An *aneurysm*, for example, is a bulge in a major blood vessel at a point where there is a weakness in the vessel wall. Aneurysms in the ascending aorta (the portion of this major vessel after it leaves the heart) usually cause no symptoms but in some cases may cause chest pain, shortness of breath, difficulty in swallowing, and vocal cord paralysis.

Arteriosclerosis is the most common cause of an aneurysm of the descending aorta (the portion of the aorta below the diaphragm). This is usually asymptomatic and may not be detected unless a bulging or pulsation is felt by a physician during a routine examination of the abdomen. When pain occurs, it suggests that the vessel wall is being stretched or that there may be some tearing of the wall. Treatment involves surgical replacement of the diseased part of the aorta with a synthetic graft.

In a *dissecting aneurysm*, blood escapes through a tear in the wall of the aorta and the three layers of the aortic wall become separated; blood becomes trapped between them. X-rays typically will show this condition. When this type of aneurysm occurs in the ascending aorta or the aortic arch, surgery is necessary. A dissecting aneurysm in the descending thoracic aorta may wall off, and scar tissue may protect against further dissection. This can sometimes be handled by keeping blood pressure as low as possible with beta blockers and other medication, thus avoiding surgery.

HIGH BLOOD PRESSURE

Blood does not simply flow through the circulatory system like a lazy river. The heart pushes it, and the force with which it pushes is called blood pressure. The classic analogy used to explain this phenomenon is that of a garden hose: When the nozzle is open, the walls of the hose are under very little pressure and water pours out easily, but when the opening in the nozzle is narrowed, the pressure of the water against the walls of the hose is higher. If the body's blood vessels are narrowed, the heart must pump harder than normal against the resistance. This is called *high blood pressure*, or *hypertension*. (See Chapter 12.) Eventually the heart enlarges, the muscle thickens, the heart needs more oxygen to function, and it becomes less efficient. After many years, heart failure may result.

The high pressure of the blood within a blood vessel is a factor in driving blood fat or cholesterol into the vessel walls, speeding up the process of atherosclerosis. This increases the possibility of a stroke or heart attack occurring as a result of clot formation. A stroke is also more likely, because increased blood pressure over many years causes a ballooning of a blood vessel (aneurysm), and this may, under certain circumstances, burst. If an aneurysm involves blood vessels in the brain, a cerebral hemorrhage results. Over time, high pressure can also scar the body's arterioles (small arteries), reducing their ability to carry blood to specific areas of the body. An example of this is a progressive loss of kidney function as a result of damaged vessels.

Hypertension usually is present without any symptoms; hence it is sometimes called the silent killer. Once hypertension is advanced, symptoms include headaches, fainting, dizziness (sometimes), loss of renal (kidney) function, and, in late stages, convulsions and swelling of the brain. An estimated 50 million Americans have hypertension, and perhaps a third of them are unaware that they have it.

Although the origin of hypertension in about 90 percent of patients is unknown (this is called *primary hypertension*), it *is* known that the level at which blood pressure settles is controlled by a complex interaction of hormones, chemical cell receptors, sodium intake (in some people), and the nervous system. In the remaining 10 percent of patients, high blood pressure is a symptom of an underlying problem such as narrowing of the arteries supplying the kidneys, a kidney abnormality, tumor of the adrenal gland, or congenital defect of the aorta. This is called *secondary hypertension*.

Mild high blood pressure can sometimes be treated by restricting the amount of sodium (salt) in the diet and controlling weight. If these measures are not effective, there are several classes of medications that work to reduce the heart rate and thus the output of blood; cause the muscles in the blood vessel walls to relax; prevent the nerves from contracting the blood vessels; or interfere with the body's production of angiotensin, a chemical that causes the arteries to constrict. (See Chapter 23.)

STROKE

Like angina and heart attacks, strokes can be caused by a blockage in a blood vessel, only in this case the blockage is in one of the arteries that supply blood to the brain. (See Chapter 18.) In a *thrombotic stroke*, a blood clot (thrombus) forms in a carotid artery narrowed by arteriosclerosis. Four of every five strokes are of this type. In *hemorrhagic stroke*, the artery leaks or bursts, interrupting the brain's blood supply. The least common type of stroke is an *embolic stroke*, in which a blood clot travels to the brain from the heart or other vessels and lodges in a small vessel in the brain.

Symptoms of a stroke may include sudden weakness or numbness of the face, arm, and leg on one side of the body; loss of speech, or trouble talking or understanding speech; dimness or loss of vision, especially in one eye; and unexplained dizziness, unsteadiness, or sudden falls. These are all the result of a lack of oxygen in cells that make up various parts of the brain. About 10 percent of strokes are preceded by *transient ischemic attacks* (TIAs), sometimes called ministrokes. In these cases, blood vessels may go into spasm but are not usually closed off, or a small embolus may close off a small branch of a vessel. The symptoms may be similar to those of a stroke but last an average of only a few minutes or so. When the ministroke is over, the symptoms usually recede within 24 hours, whereas in a full-blown stroke they do not.

Intravenous anticoagulants can sometimes combat a stroke in progress, although this procedure is still somewhat experimental. Later, as with a blocked coronary artery, surgeons may be able to bypass a blocked carotid artery or remove a plaque under direct vision, in a procedure called a carotid endarterectomy, to prevent further strokes.

People who have had one stroke are at risk for having another; thus, preventing subsequent strokes is a major priority in treatment. Some of the preventive measures are the same as those recommended for preventing heart disease: use of aspirin or other anticoagulants, measures to keep blood pressure and cholesterol levels low, and smoke-free living.

About 500,000 Americans have strokes each year, and almost 3 million Americans alive today have had strokes in the past. Stroke is a major cause of disability and is the third leading cause of death in the United States—about 150,000 die of stroke each year. About 85,000 to 90,000 fewer stroke deaths are recorded each year than in the early 1970s—largely the result of earlier treatment of hypertension.

HEART FAILURE

Unlike a heart attack, heart failure is usually a slow process. (See Chapter 14.) There are several major causes of heart failure:

- *Long-standing hypertension.* As the heart strains under increased pressure, it begins to enlarge and weaken.
- *Narrowed exit valves in the heart (especially the aortic).* These increase the demand on the heart; the heart must pump harder to push the circulating blood.
- *Leaky heart valves.* Each time the heart pumps, some blood goes forward but some leaks back into its chamber. The heart must work harder to get adequate blood out to tissues.
- *Viral infections.* These may damage the heart muscle and weaken it to the point of heart failure.
- *Alcohol.* May cause similar damage to the heart.
- *Inefficiency.* Following a heart attack the heart muscle may not be able to pump efficiently, and blood backs up. This is the most common cause of heart failure.

About 50,000 Americans die annually of heart failure (sometimes called congestive heart failure). Although some 400,000 new cases are diagnosed each year, heart failure can be treated successfully in many cases, and more than 2 million Americans who have it are alive today.

When the heart can't do its job, blood flow slows. Blood returning to the heart from the veins backs up into the tissues, the way water builds up behind a dam. Sometimes fluid collects in the lungs and makes breathing more difficult, especially when lying down or during exercise. Other symptoms include easy fatigue, an inability to exercise, and, later, swelling in the ankles, legs, and abdomen.

Rest, a low-sodium diet, and a slower pace are nonmedical treatments for heart failure. Medical treatment may include the use of drugs that increase the pumping action of the heart, help the body elim-inate excess salt and water, or expand the blood vessels and decrease the resistance in those vessels, making the heart's work easier.

VALVULAR HEART DISEASE

The heart has four valves, two on the right (the pulmonic and tricuspid) and two on the left (the aortic and mitral), that control the flow of blood through the chambers of the heart and out to the body. Any of these valves may fail to function properly, but disease most commonly affects the valves on the left side of the heart. (See Chapter 13.) They may narrow (called *stenosis*), they may not close all the way (causing a backflow of blood called *regurgitation*), or they may close incorrectly (called *prolapse*). A *heart murmur* represents the sound that a leaky or narrowed heart valve makes as blood moves through it.

THE AORTIC AND MITRAL VALVES

Aortic stenosis is a narrowing of the aortic valve, through which blood flows from the left ventricle of the heart to the aorta, the major artery whose branches supply blood to various parts of the body. Sometimes this narrowness is a congenital (inborn) defect, but more often the valve narrows as a consequence of aging, or of infections, such as rheumatic fever. Aortic stenosis results in the left ventricle having to work harder and harder to push blood out. As this occurs, the muscular walls of the ventricle thicken, increasing their requirement for oxygen. Symptoms of aortic stenosis include chest pain when the oxygen needs exceed the supply from the coronary arteries; fainting (syncope), if the valve becomes very tight; and congestive heart failure, which usually does not occur unless the valve has been narrowed for many years. Valve replacement, either with a mechanical valve made of metal or plastic or with a valve from a pig, may help, although it does not provide a complete cure.

In *mitral stenosis*, the valve opening between the upper and lower chambers on the left side of the heart has become narrowed. The cause is almost always rheumatic fever, which is now rare in this country (although it is on the rise again in some communities) but is common in many parts of the world. When mitral stenosis occurs, the entry of blood into the left ventricle from the atrium is impeded by the narrow valve. Pressure builds up behind the valve, leading to an elevation of pressure in the lungs. This in turn may lead to shortness of breath (dyspnea), which is one of the major symptoms of mitral stenosis. Often, however, it occurs without any symptoms.

In *aortic regurgitation*, the aortic valve fails to close completely after the heart has pumped blood out into the aorta. Blood leaks back from the aorta into the left ventricle. In *mitral regurgitation*, improper closure causes blood to leak from the left ventricle back into the left atrium. In either case, the valve does not close properly because of a physical change in its shape or its support. This change may be the result of rheumatic fever; an infection (endocarditis), which may leave the valve scarred; or a heart attack, which causes loss of supporting muscle tissue. In the mitral valve, the change may be the result of a heart attack, which causes a loss of muscle tissue, or a spontaneous rupture of one of its muscular chords that normally act as guide wires to keep it in place.

Major symptoms include fatigue, shortness of breath, and edema. Medications such as digitalis, diuretics, and ACE inhibitors can help alleviate symptoms. (See Chapter 23.) Some defective mitral valves can be reconstructed or, failing that, replaced by an artificial valve.

Mitral valve prolapse is a congenital or developmental abnormality in which the leaflets, or flaps, of tissue that make up the valve are larger than normal. The valve fails to close properly; sometimes blood flows backward (regurgitates). The vast majority of individuals with mitral valve prolapse have no symptoms. If symptoms do occur, they may include chest pain, abnormal heart rhythms, dizziness, or palpitations. Severe mitral regurgitation is not common, and serious complications are extremely rare. Most cardiologists feel that the popular press makes too much of mitral valve prolapse. Although the condition is fairly common—it has been estimated to affect as many as 6 percent of the total population, and it occurs more often in women—it is not a problem for most of the people who have it.

A major problem with mitral prolapse is that its symptoms may mimic those of angina. A history of sticking pains occurring at rest or at odd times over various parts of the chest, rather than the pressure-type pains in the middle of the chest during exercise that are typical of angina, will help distinguish the two conditions. A typical murmur or clicking sound will help to make the diagnosis.

If treatment for mitral valve prolapse is necessary,

it may include the use of drugs to reduce the number of extra beats. Antibiotics at the time of dental work or other procedures are recommended to prevent infection.

THE PULMONIC AND TRICUSPID VALVES

In the pulmonic and tricuspid valves, any narrowing is rare and almost always congenital. Leakage (regurgitation) is unusual, but may occur when use of illicit intravenous drugs leads to infection that damages the valve. The infection, hallmarked by fever, often settles on these two valves because they are the first ones the bacteria come in contact with as they travel through the bloodstream. If the valve becomes leaky, swelling of the abdomen and legs may occur. As with other valves, treatment can include replacement, but this is rare and usually not as effective as it is when the aortic or mitral valve is involved.

RHEUMATIC HEART DISEASE

Years ago, before the antibiotic era, rheumatic heart disease was a major cause of valve disease. (See Chapter 13.) It started with a strep infection in the throat (which occasionally occurred without symptoms). Ten days to two weeks later, a bout of rheumatic fever would be noted. Inflammation of many of the body's connective tissues—not only in the heart, but in the joints and skin as well—would produce joint pain and swelling or a rash. A fever, arthritis-type pain, and, in children, the occurrence of a heart murmur or electrocardiographic (ECG) changes would indicate that the illness had affected the heart.

It is obviously important to treat strep throat with penicillin or another suitable antibiotic as soon as possible to prevent rheumatic fever and rheumatic heart disease. There is no treatment for rheumatic fever itself, but people who have already had it often take antibiotics daily or monthly to prevent streptococcal infections. Patients with any valve involvement must always take penicillin or some other appropriate antibiotic before dental work or other surgical procedures to prevent a heart valve infection. Fortunately, the wide use of antibiotics has almost eradicated rheumatic fever in this country, and many of those who have rheumatic fever do not end up with rheumatic heart disease or damaged heart valves.

CONGENITAL HEART DISEASE

The human heart develops between the eighth and tenth weeks after conception. When the heart is no larger than a small peanut, it is already fully developed and any congenital abnormalities are already present. (See Chapter 20.) Valve damage is not the only congenital condition that can affect the heart. Other forms of congenital heart disease include holes in the inner, separating walls of the heart that allow blood to leak or flow directly from one chamber or artery into another, rather than flowing in the proper sequence through the valves. A flow of blood from the left side of the heart directly into the right side is called a *left-to-right shunt*. The hole can be either between the two upper chambers of the heart (an *atrial-septal defect*) or between the two lower chambers (a *ventricular-septal defect*). In *patent ductus arteriosus*, a communication between the aorta and pulmonary artery remains, and blood flows directly between the two vessels.

In *coarctation of the aorta*, the aorta is pinched or narrowed after it leaves the heart. In *pulmonary stenosis* and *aortic stenosis*, the pulmonic or aortic valves are narrower than normal. *Congenital cyanotic defects* cause what are commonly called ''blue babies''—a term that comes from the fact that lack of oxygen causes the lips and fingernails to appear blue. Among the cyanotic heart defects are *tetralogy of Fallot*, which includes a ventricular-septal defect and a narrowing of the pulmonary valve, and *transposition of the great arteries*, in which the positions of the pulmonary artery and aorta are reversed. This means that part of the blood returning to the heart from the body is pumped back to the body without going back to the lungs for oxygen. Infants and children with these congenital defects often show such symptoms as shortness of breath, fainting, unusual color (blueness, most commonly), and heart murmurs that a physician can hear with a stethoscope.

All these congenital defects call for surgery, and almost all of them can be corrected successfully today.

About 25,000 babies with heart defects are born annually in this country, making congenital heart disease relatively uncommon. There are more than 500,000 who are living with congenital heart disease, but each year about 5,600 people, most of them infants, lose their lives to one of these conditions.

CARDIAC ARRHYTHMIAS: DISTURBANCES IN HEART RHYTHM

The heartbeat is regulated from centers within the heart and by nerve impulses from the brain and other parts of the nervous system. One group of cells at the top of the right atrium (the sinus node) emits electrical impulses that activate both atria. The current travels to another node (the atrioventricular node), which lies between the atria and ventricles, and from there, fibers activate the ventricular muscle.

Abnormalities in this sequence may cause *arrhythmias*, or may cause what are referred to as various degrees of heart block. (See Chapter 16.) Most irregularities of heartbeat are innocuous except when anatomic heart problems are also present, in which case an arrhythmia may have serious consequences. Ventricular arrhythmias are more serious than atrial arrhythmias, because the ventricles are the heart's pumping chambers. An arrhythmia is not necessarily an indication of underlying heart disease; sometimes the cause can be as simple as a poor night's sleep, smoking, or too much coffee, caffeinated cola, or alcohol.

Often an arrhythmia has no symptoms. Sometimes the patient can feel the irregular beating pattern, called a palpitation. Another sensation patients sometimes mention is a fluttering feeling in the chest or neck.

After a physician has used an electrocardiogram (ECG) or Holter monitor (see Chapter 10) to define the exact type of arrhythmia, the first step in treatment is to remove any of the environmental or self-imposed causes previously discussed. After that, the physician can prescribe a number of medications that usually can control the irregularity.

ATRIAL FIBRILLATION

In atrial fibrillation, the heart's two upper chambers, the atria, beat irregularly at about 400 to 600 times per minute. The ventricles do not respond to each of these beats; hence the pulse that reflects the actual pumping activity may only be about 100 to 150. Atrial fibrillation can be associated with several types of heart disease, including high blood pressure, coronary heart disease, and heart valve disease. It can also occur in persons with an overactive thyroid gland,

and occasionally it is noted in people without any evidence of heart disease.

A person with atrial fibrillation is at increased risk of embolic stroke, because the very rapid beats do not propel the blood through the heart efficiently. It begins to pool there, and, as a result, clots may form. One or more of these clots (emboli) can travel to the brain, or other parts of the body.

Atrial fibrillation responds to digitalis, which slows the ventricular rate. At times, medications such as quinidine or procainamide (Pronestyl) may stabilize the heart rhythm; beta blockers or calcium channel blockers are also helpful. (See Chapter 23.) Anticoagulants (blood thinners) reduce the risk of stroke. Aspirin has also been found to be useful in preventing clots from forming. If medications have been ineffective, a safe and effective technique called cardioversion may be used, where physicians administer an electric shock in order to convert the rhythm to normal.

VENTRICULAR TACHYCARDIA

Unlike the atrial arrhythmias, ventricular arrhythmias can be life-threatening. In ventricular tachycardia, the ventricle beats abnormally fast and inefficiently. This interferes with normal filling of the heart with blood and with ejection of the blood from the ventricle. It can lead to heart failure if prolonged, shock if severe or acute, or even death because the heart does not pump out sufficient blood to nourish vital organs. A wide variety of medications can treat ventricular tachycardia. Emergency personnel can sometimes normalize the heartbeat with electrical defibrillation, and cardiac researchers have developed automatic implantable cardiac defibrillators that correct ventricular tachycardia before it becomes dangerous. (See Chapters 26 and 27.)

VENTRICULAR FIBRILLATION

When a heart is in ventricular fibrillation, pumping action is almost nonexistent, and the heart merely quivers. If fibrillation is not stopped and normal rhythm restored in two to five minutes, death results. Ventricular fibrillation may occur in a heart attack victim. The primary symptom of ventricular fibrillation is loss of consciousness, which can rapidly lead to death. As with ventricular tachycardia, treatments include medications and electrical defibrillation.

BRADYARRHYTHMIA

Bradyarrhythmia means that the heart is beating more slowly than usual. There are two types of bradyarrhythmia. In *sinus bradycardia*, the sinus node, which initiates all the beats, may send out impulses at a slower than normal rate (for example, at 40 to 50 beats per minute). This may be due simply to aging or to damage to the heart caused by a heart attack, or it may be a side effect of medication. Trained athletes may also have a slow heartbeat that is not caused by any disease process.

In *heart block*, the sinus node may function properly, but there is an electrical blockage at the atrioventricular (AV) node. Some or all of the electrical impulses never reach the ventricle. A different group of cells below the atrioventricular node may take over, the way an emergency generator comes on in an electrical blackout. The heart beats, but slowly—there is too great a pause between impulses in the upper and lower chambers. Depending on the degree of heart block, the rate may be 50 or 60, or even as slow as 30 or 40. Heart block may be caused by a scar in the tissues that conduct the electrical impulses.

Some people can have periods of rapid heart rhythm alternating with periods of slow rhythm. The *brady-tachy syndrome* happens with aging, usually in people in their 60s. The sinus node beats more slowly than normal, but rapid rhythms, such as atrial fibrillation, periodically occur. In the course of a month, this may happen several times. Many people with this syndrome lead normal lives and, in fact, may be unaware that they have it. Existing medications can temporarily stabilize brady-tachy syndrome, but ultimately a pacemaker, as well as medication, may become necessary.

PREMATURE VENTRICULAR CONTRACTIONS

A premature ventricular contraction (PVC) is an early heartbeat. PVCs are usually benign. Common causes include caffeine, tobacco, alcohol, lack of sleep, and stimulant drugs such as epinephrine (adrenaline). The use of cocaine may cause frequent extra beats or even more serious abnormal heart rhythms. The patient may feel that the heart is skipping beats, stopping, or thumping in the chest. Treatment for premature ventricular contractions includes removal of the inciting event followed by antiarrhythmic medications if the skipped or extra beats cause symptoms. (Most of the time they do not.) If the cause of the contractions is underlying heart disease, that condition should be treated first, since the premature ventricular contraction may only be a symptom of an underlying problem.

OTHER DISORDERS

PERICARDITIS

Most often caused by a virus or other infection, pericarditis is an inflammation of the pericardium—the outer sac, or membrane, that surrounds the heart like a cellophane wrapping. In rare cases, pericarditis appears as part of a collagen vascular disease such as systemic lupus erythematosus, or as a complication of a tumor of the lung or of lymphoma (lymphatic cancer). It may also appear in the late stage of kidney disease, in patients having radiation therapy of the chest, or occasionally as a reaction to medications such as certain antiarrhythmic or antihypertensive drugs. Pericarditis caused by a viral infection tends to be less serious than pericarditis from other causes, because the viral infection usually runs its course and disappears. At times, however, viral pericarditis may be a recurrent illness.

Symptoms include variable types of chest pain, which often worsens when the individual lies down and improves when he or she sits up. In fact, any change of position may bring on pain. Sometimes pericarditis is accompanied by fever or shortness of breath. Treatments include bed rest, aspirin or nonsteroidal anti-inflammatory drugs (NSAIDs) for reducing inflammation, or, in persistent cases, cortisone. If pericarditis proves to be a relapsing condition, the pericardium may have to be removed surgically.

MYOCARDITIS

When the heart muscle itself becomes inflamed, the condition is known as myocarditis. Years ago, rheumatic fever was a common cause, but today, myocarditis is most often idiopathic—that is, no cause can be found, or it is secondary to a viral condition. In myocarditis, the heart muscle degenerates, becomes soft, and may no longer be able to function as an efficient pump. Patients who have it may develop heart failure or arrhythmias.

Cardiologists can sometimes control the symptoms of myocarditis with medication, and sometimes myocarditis goes away on its own. The patient recuperates and returns to a normal life. Sometimes, myocarditis is an inexorable progressive illness, and it is one of the reasons for cardiac transplants. This is not common, however. Researchers are now looking into treatment of some forms of myocarditis with immunosuppressive drugs, but this therapy is still considered experimental. (See Chapter 15.)

ENDOCARDITIS

Endocarditis is an infection of a heart valve or inner lining of the heart muscle. Because bacteria can destroy heart tissue, a valve can develop a leak if it is infected. Infection most often develops on a valve that was previously abnormal in some way, either scarred by rheumatic fever, congenitally abnormal, or prolapsed. Today, cardiologists are seeing endocarditis with increasing frequency in patients with normal valves who have used illicit intravenous drugs. Fever is the most common symptom; fatigue, weight loss, or heart failure may also be present.

About 19,000 cases of bacterial endocarditis, the most common type, are diagnosed each year; fewer than 2,000 of them are fatal. Many of the fatalities occur in intravenous drug abusers.

Antibiotics are usually effective against the bacteria that cause endocarditis. Anyone with a known heart valve problem should take antibiotics before having dental work, because bacteria from the mouth are capable of entering the bloodstream and causing endocarditis. This is true of any surgical procedure in which there is the possibility of bacterial contamination of the blood.

CARDIOMYOPATHIES

Cardiomyopathy is a term for a number of primary diseases of the heart muscle. In *hypertrophic cardiomyopathy*, the heart muscle, particularly the left ventricle, thickens. Sometimes the thickening of the heart muscle in the region directly below the aortic valve leads to a partial obstruction of blood leaving the left ventricle. *Restrictive cardiomyopathy* is characterized by the replacement of good heart muscle fibers with rigid, less elastic tissue, so that the heart (particularly the ventricles) cannot fill normally. *Amyloid heart disease* and *sarcoidosis* are rare types of restrictive cardiomyopathy in which proteins that the body manufactures infiltrate the heart muscle and cause symptoms of heart failure. Another rare type of restrictive cardiomyopathy is *hemochromatosis*, in which iron from the blood is deposited in the heart muscle. (See Chapter 15.)

Some of these heart problems can be controlled and treated. Increasingly, people who make the necessary life-style changes and receive proper medical care are able to keep their risks to a minimum.

PART II

HOW TO LOWER YOUR RISK OF HEART DISEASE

CHAPTER 3

CARDIOVASCULAR RISK FACTORS

HENRY R. BLACK, M.D.

INTRODUCTION

More than 68 million Americans currently have one or more forms of cardiovascular disease, according to the latest estimates from the federal government's National Center for Health Statistics. Many more are said to be *at risk* for developing one of these serious diseases. The concept of risk factors has evolved only over the past 45 years or so, and new factors are periodically added to the list as our comprehension of the disease process grows. To understand who is at risk and what risk actually means to an individual, one first needs to understand how diseases of the heart and circulatory system—particularly heart attacks—develop.

All heart attacks, with rare exceptions, are caused by atherosclerosis, or a narrowing and "hardening" of the coronary arteries resulting from fatty deposits called plaque. This process, by which the wall of the artery is infiltrated by deposits of cholesterol and calcium, narrows the lumen (the internal orifice) of the artery. When the degree of narrowing reaches a critical level, blood flow to the portion of the heart supplied by that artery is stopped and injury to the heart muscle—a heart attack—occurs. If the reduction in blood flow is not total and is only temporary, relative to muscle needs, permanent damage does not result but the individual may experience angina pectoris—

chest pain as a result of too little blood and oxygen to a portion of the heart in response to its needs (a process called ischemia). Atherosclerosis also occurs in other blood vessels, such as the carotid artery, which carries blood to the brain, or the arteries that provide blood to the legs, and can lead to similar problems. Significant atherosclerosis in the arteries supplying the brain may cause transient ischemic attacks (TIAs) or strokes, while peripheral arterial blood vessel disease, with intermittent claudication (pain on walking or similar activity), occurs when there is significant atherosclerosis in the arteries in the legs.

The fact that atherosclerotic plaque is largely made up of cholesterol has been known since the middle of the 19th century. Only in the 20th century, however, when general hygienic measures greatly reduced the toll from infectious diseases and allowed people to live considerably longer, did we realize the enormous impact of atherosclerosis on general health. By the 1930s and 1940s, the death rate in the United States from atherosclerotic heart disease was increasing at an alarming rate and it was clear that we were in the grips of a cardiovascular disease epidemic. The reasons for this epidemic were not entirely clear. Some scientists were convinced that there was a single cause for atherosclerosis—dietary fat and cholesterol—while others were more impressed by the association of high blood pressure or cigarette smoking with heart attacks. Most researchers favored the theory that there had to be multiple causes for atherosclerosis, although precisely what they were was debatable.

After World War II, the first large-scale, comprehensive study to determine the causes of atherosclerotic heart disease, the Framingham Heart Study, was begun. In 1948, researchers in the town of Framingham, Massachusetts, a suburb of Boston, enrolled 5,209 local residents, ranging in age from 30 to 62, in the study. They began examining the participants every two years, and they continue to do so. In the early 1970s, 5,135 adult offspring of the original participants joined the study.

Within a short time, the Framingham investigators established that there are, indeed, many factors that predispose an individual to the development of atherosclerosis. The list of these factors, now called cardiovascular risk factors (a term coined by Dr. William Kannel, the first director of the Framingham study), continues to grow as the information from Framingham and numerous other studies becomes available and we learn more about the possible causes of atherosclerotic disease.

This chapter defines cardiovascular risk factors, classifies them, briefly describes how they interact, and discusses what individuals and their physicians can do about them.

HOW RISK FACTORS ARE IDENTIFIED

A cardiovascular risk factor is a condition that is associated with an increased risk of developing cardiovascular disease. The association is almost always a statistical one, and so the fact that a particular person has a particular factor merely increases the *probability* of developing a certain type of cardiovascular disease; it does *not* mean that he or she is certain to develop heart or blood vessel disease. Conversely, the fact that an individual does not have a particular cardiovascular risk factor (or for that matter, *any* of the known cardiovascular risk factors) does not guarantee protection against heart disease. Even today, a number of individuals who have heart attacks or strokes have none of the identified risk factors.

The box "Cardiovascular Risk Factors" lists the currently accepted cardiovascular risk factors. To understand how this list was compiled, one must know a little about epidemiology and how its techniques have been applied to identify risk factors.

Cardiovascular Risk Factors

Risk Factors That Cannot Be Changed
Age
Gender
Heredity

Risk Factors That Can Be Changed
High blood pressure
Elevated serum cholesterol
Lipoprotein (a)
Cigarette smoking
Obesity
Glucose intolerance
Diabetes
Fibrinogen
Left ventricular hypertrophy
Cocaine
Behavioral factors (stress, Type A)

Protective Factors
HDL cholesterol
Exercise
Estrogen
Moderate alcohol intake

The epidemiologist studies populations. He or she begins by selecting a group that is representative of the population to which the information will later be applied. To examine the cause of atherosclerosis, for example, the study group selected should be largely composed of young and middle-aged adults who have no evidence of cardiovascular disease when the study begins. Because the differences between individuals will be small, the group must be large enough to allow the relationships between the factors being studied and the disease to become evident and to enable researchers to draw conclusions about these relationships. While earlier studies were limited to much smaller groups, the advent of computers has enabled epidemiologists to collect and analyze enormous amounts of data and to study very large groups or populations, sometimes numbering hundreds of thousands.

The study group must be followed for a considerable length of time. A chronic disease such as atherosclerosis, which has many causes and usually requires years for signs or symptoms of heart disease to develop, requires multiple observations over many years to determine how each potential risk factor is changing and interacting with the others.

For any epidemiological survey to be helpful, the appropriate factors must be studied. None of the risk factors on the currently accepted list got there by chance; each resulted from careful observations and educated guesses. For example, researchers knew that men had heart attacks more often than women. Likewise, older people have more vascular disease than children, while people with high blood pressure have more strokes than those with normal pressure.

And finally, for epidemiologic surveys to be valid, each factor studied and each clinical event (an objectively defined, observable disease process, such as a heart attack) that occurs during the study must be accurately and precisely measured. Epidemiologists have learned to standardize blood pressure and various laboratory measurements, for example, to ensure that study participants are evaluated equally. Early surveys relied upon information from death certificates, which were not always accurate. Contemporary studies have access to more detailed and accurate medical records, as well as to sophisticated laboratory tests and diagnostic equipment.

For a "candidate" cardiovascular risk factor to become a permanent member of the list, it must meet several criteria:

- The statistical association between the factor and cardiovascular disease must be strong. Generally, the presence of the factor should at least double the risk of disease. Epidemiologists consider anything less than this to be a weak association.

- The association should be consistent. The risk factor should produce disease regardless of gender, age, or race, and the association should be present in all or most of the studies in which it has been evaluated.

- The association must make biological sense. A factor may appear to be related statistically to a disease, but unless such a relationship is biologically plausible, the statistical association may have little meaning.

- The impact of the proposed risk factor should be able to be demonstrated experimentally in the laboratory. (This is usually, but not always, feasible.)

- Treatment that favorably changes the risk factor should reduce the incidence of disease. This has been achieved for some, but by no means all, of the factors listed in Table 3.1.

- The factor must make an independent contribution to increasing an individual's risk of developing disease. Some factors studied were found merely to occur together with another, genuine cardiovascular risk factor.

A statistical technique called multivariate analysis allows researchers to tease out true associations from those that appear to contribute but do not do so independently. A good example is coffee drinking, which seemed at first to be associated with an increased risk of heart disease. Multivariate analysis showed that the association was not independent, but rather due to the fact that many people smoke cigarettes when they drink coffee. When this fact was taken into account, it became clear that the real villain is the cigarette, not the caffeine.

Some cardiovascular risk factors are dichotomous; that is, they are either present or absent. Male gender and family history are two examples. Most risk factors, however, are continuous; that is, above a certain threshold level, risk rises as the strength or severity of the risk factor rises. For example, the more cigarettes smoked a day, the greater the risk of heart disease. This is also called a "dose-response."

The risk may rise dramatically when the strength of the risk factor exceeds a certain level. Blood pressure and blood cholesterol levels are typical of such risk factors. For both of these, there is a very small increase in risk as the level rises within the range considered "normal." This increased risk is so small that any attempt to lower it would not improve overall outlook. At the other end of the scale, there is a point (90 mm Hg for diastolic blood pressure and 240 mg/dl for serum cholesterol) above which risk increases substantially.

It is now possible to estimate quantitatively an individual's cardiovascular risk. This technique employs data gathered from epidemiologic surveys attributing varying levels of risk to such factors as blood pressure, serum cholesterol, age, and number of cigarettes smoked per day. (See Table 3.1.) Within seconds, an individual's probability of having a heart attack in a defined period of time can be calculated. This approach also shows that the impact of risk factors is at least additive and possibly multiplicative. What this means is that an individual's risk is determined in part by the *number* of risk factors present, as well as the level of each individual factor. (See Figure 3.1.) For example, someone who has mildly elevated blood pressure *and* serum cholesterol may be at greater risk of sustaining a heart attack or stroke than would an individual with even higher blood pressure whose serum cholesterol is normal.

This compounding effect has a number of important implications for individuals. First, it is not sensible to view the risk of having heart disease as great or small on the basis of a single risk factor. Second, a treatment program for risk factor reduction must

Table 3.1
Coronary Heart Disease Risk Factor Prediction Chart—Framingham Heart Study

1. Find Points for Each Risk Factor

Age (if female)				Age (if male)				HDL cholesterol		Total cholesterol		Systolic blood pressure			
Age	Pts.	Age	Pts.	Age	Pts.	Age	Pts.	HDL C	Pts.	Total C	Pts.	SBP	Pts.	Other	Pts.
30	-12	47–48	5	30	-2	57–59	13	25–26	7	139–151	-3	98–104	-2	Cigarettes	4
31	-11	49–50	6	31	-1	60–61	14	27–29	6	152–166	-2	105–112	-1	Diabetic—male	3
32	-9	51–52	7	32–33	0	62–64	15	30–32	5	167–182	-1	113–120	0	Diabetic—female	6
33	-8	53–55	8	34	1	65–67	16	33–35	4	183–199	0	121–129	1	ECG—LVH	9
34	-6	56–60	9	35–36	2	68–70	17	36–38	3	200–219	1	130–139	2		
35	-5	61–67	10	37–38	3	71–73	18	39–42	2	220–239	2	140–149	3	0 points for each no	
36	-4	68–74	11	39	4	74	19	43–46	1	240–262	3	150–160	4		
37	-3			40–41	5			47–50	0	263–288	4	161–172	5		
38	-2			42–43	6			51–55	-1	289–315	5	173–185	6		
39	-1			44–45	7			56–60	-2	316–330	6				
40	0			46–47	8			61–66	-3						
41	1			48–49	9			67–73	-4						
42–43	2			50–51	10			74–80	-5						
44	3			52–54	11			81–87	-6						
45–46	4			55–56	12			88–96	-7						

2. Sum Points For All Risk Factors—Framingham Heart Study

____ + ____ + ____ + ____ + ____ + ____ + ____ = ____

Age   HDL C   Total C   SBP   Smoker   Diabetes   ECG—LVH   Point total

Note: *Minus points subtract from total.*

3. Look Up Risk Corresponding to Point Total / 4. Compare to Average 10-Year Risk

Probability of CHD			Probability of CHD			Probability of CHD			Probability of CHD			Probability		
Pts.	5 Yr.	10 Yr.	Pts.	5 Yr.	10 Yr.	Pts.	5 Yr.	10 Yr.	Pts.	5 Yr.	10 Yr.	Age	Women	Men
≤1	<1%	<2%	10	2%	6%	19	8%	16%	28	19%	33%	30–34	<1%	3%
2	1%	2%	11	3%	6%	20	8%	18%	29	20%	36%	35–39	<1%	5%
3	1%	2%	12	3%	7%	21	9%	19%	30	22%	38%	40–44	2%	6%
4	1%	2%	13	3%	8%	22	11%	21%	31	24%	40%	45–49	5%	10%
5	1%	3%	14	4%	9%	23	12%	23%	32	25%	42%	50–54	8%	14%
6	1%	3%	15	5%	10%	24	13%	25%				55–59	12%	16%
7	1%	4%	16	5%	12%	25	14%	27%				60–64	13%	21%
8	2%	4%	17	6%	13%	26	16%	29%				65–69	9%	30%
9	2%	5%	18	7%	14%	27	17%	31%				70–74	12%	24%

Using Table 3.1

Table 3.1 was created using data from the Framingham Heart Study to help individuals determine their risk of developing coronary heart disease in five or ten years. It represents a first attempt at developing a data-based tool that patients and their physicians can use as a starting point for a discussion of modifying behavior.

Although the Framingham database is one of the most comprehensive available, it has some limitations. For example, it may be less accurate for African-Americans than for whites. The table has been criticized by some for its inclusion of both total cholesterol and HDL cholesterol, thereby perhaps giving extra weight to cholesterol as a risk factor. The table also indicates that an electrocardiogram is necessary to determine if left ventricular hypertrophy is present.

Nevertheless, the table is useful as a general tool for individuals to use in estimating their risk of developing coronary heart disease and comparing their risk to the average. They can also use it to see how changing a modifiable risk factor may affect their total risk. For example, a person who is a smoker can look at the difference in risk if smoking is stopped. Likewise, someone with elevated cholesterol can look at the effect of lowering it. Modifying a single risk factor may affect life expectancy by as much as eight years; when there are strong and multiple risk factors the effect can be substantial. Life expectancy is not the only reason to consider changing risk-prone behavior. Behavioral changes can also have a very positive effect on the quality of life.

Figure 3.1
Danger of Heart Attack By Risk Factors Present

This chart shows how a combination of three major risk factors can increase the likelihood of heart attack. For purposes of illustration, this chart uses an abnormal blood pressure level of 150 systolic and a cholesterol level of 260 in a 55-year-old male and female.

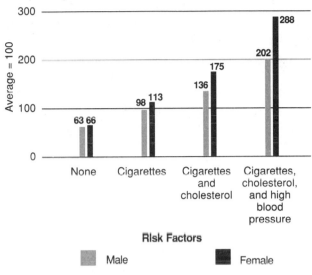

Example: 55-year-old male and female

Source: Framingham Heart Study, Section 37: The Probability of Developing Certain Cardiovascular Diseases in Eight Years at Specified Values of Some Characteristics (Aug. 1987).

be comprehensive. Third, it is likely that measures to prevent atherosclerotic heart disease and stroke will be most beneficial in those with the highest risk, and difficult to prove in those with only a minimally increased chance of developing these diseases.

THE EFFECT OF MODIFYING RISK FACTORS

Taking action that modifies a risk factor does not necessarily imply that the probability of a heart disease or stroke will be eliminated. Furthermore, when a strong risk factor is present, treating it—even if the treatment is very effective—does not necessarily mean that the risk is reduced. Fortunately, treatment

of the major risk factors—smoking, high blood pressure, and elevated cholesterol levels—has been shown to reduce the possibility of a heart attack.

In general, it is a monumental scientific undertaking to demonstrate that treatment or modification of a risk factor reduces the number of heart attacks, strokes, or other cardiovascular diseases. Because atherosclerosis has many causes and is almost always present in some degree in all of us, studies to show that a specific treatment works are difficult to design. Furthermore, the results may be hard to interpret and apply to the general population.

For a study of a proposed treatment (usually called a clinical trial) to be valid, it must have a control: The treatment must be tested against another treatment or against no treatment at all. ("Treatment" in a clinical trial might mean a drug or a modification in behavior such as exercising more or eating less saturated fat.) Volunteers enrolled in such a study must be representative of the patients in whom the treatment will be used. For example, if the subjects already have advanced atherosclerosis, the treatment used may appear ineffective, when in fact it might have been successful if started earlier in the course of the disease. If the subjects are at very low risk, the treatment may not appear to work because the likelihood that disease would develop is so small. It would be hard in this case to show a difference between the treatment and the control groups.

Investigators who conduct clinical trials must carefully define the population to be studied and the particular cardiovascular benefit they hope to achieve. Some treatments studied have mistakenly been judged ineffective when, in fact, the trial was simply too small or did not last long enough to show the benefit expected.

Unfortunately, too, clinical trials designed to evaluate the benefits or risks of therapy with respect to clinical events take a long time to complete. Because of the enormous effort and cost, it is impossible to devise ideal tests for every new and allegedly better approach to therapy. Physicians must analyze the findings from both epidemiologic surveys and clinical trials, synthesize the data, incorporate new information, and then apply it to individual patients. That is a difficult task.

RISK FACTORS THAT CANNOT BE CHANGED

AGE

The risk of cardiovascular events increases as we get older. In many epidemiologic surveys, age remains one of the strongest predictors of disease. More than half of those who have heart attacks are 65 or older, and about four out of five who die of such attacks are over age 65.

Of course, nothing can be done to reduce age. However, careful attention to diet and maintaining fitness may delay the degenerative changes associated with aging.

GENDER

Men are more likely than women to develop coronary heart disease, stroke, and other cardiovascular diseases that are manifestations of atherosclerosis. Whether this is because male hormones—androgens —increase risk or because female hormones— estrogens—protect against atherosclerosis is not completely understood. It is likely that both play a role, but that the protective role of estrogens is the predominant factor. This seems to be supported by the fact that heart disease risk for women rises dra- matically after menopause, when their bodies stop producing estrogen. Nevertheless, coronary heart disease is the number one cause of death among American women.

Women in the United States currently live an average of six years longer than men. Recently, some studies have suggested that much of the difference in life expectancy can be explained by the fact that more men than women smoke cigarettes. As more teenage girls are starting to smoke than are teenage boys, this advantage may disappear. Should this trend go unchecked, women may soon have as much coronary heart disease and other complications of cigarette smoking as do men, or more.

HEREDITY

There is no question that some people have a significantly greater likelihood of having a heart attack or stroke because they have inherited a tendency from their parents. In some instances, such as familial hypercholesterolemia (very high levels of cholesterol in the blood), the pattern of inheritance is well understood and the specific biochemical defects are well characterized. For most cardiovascular risk factors, however, the specific way in which inheritance plays a role is not at all clear. As in almost all situations in medicine, both heredity and environment play a role and it is often difficult to know where one stops and the other begins. Prior generations did not have the level of medical care we now enjoy, nor the general awareness about health; the details of the illness that one's grandparents or even parents had may not be precise. Prior to the 1960s, many more people smoked and little attention, if any, was paid to diet and fitness. So it is possible that environmental factors, not genes, were responsible for Grandpa's heart attack or stroke.

In practical terms, anyone who has a family history of heart disease that occurred at an early age (below 55) should be especially careful to reduce the impact of any risk that can be controlled. Even if one can successfully control known risk factors, there are, unfortunately, a number of inherited characteristics that we have not yet identified and so cannot favorably affect. Individuals with a history of atherosclerotic cardiovascular disease in the family simply have to be more vigilant if they wish to avoid heart attacks and strokes. We should remember, however, that almost every family has some member who died of a heart or blood vessel disease, since about half of all deaths are attributable to these diseases. If these episodes occurred in relatives who were 75 or 80, it may not be a major cause for concern.

Heredity also includes race. For reasons that are not completely understood, African-Americans have considerably higher rates of diabetes and both moderate and severe high blood pressure, adding to their overall risk of heart disease. (For more information, see below and Chapter 22.)

RISK FACTORS THAT CAN BE CHANGED

HIGH BLOOD PRESSURE

High blood pressure, or hypertension, is the risk factor that affects the greatest number of Americans and the one we know the most about. Estimates vary according to the source, but anywhere from 35 million to more than 60 million Americans have elevated blood pressure.

There are several ways to classify hypertension. It is generally agreed that high blood pressure is defined as readings that consistently exceed 140/90 mm Hg, when measured over a period of time with a blood pressure cuff (sphygmomanometer). Experts focused on diastolic blood pressure, the lower of the two numbers, which represents the resting pressure between heartbeats. Anyone with a reading equal to or greater than 90 mm Hg has *diastolic* hypertension, regardless of the level of the higher number, which represents the systolic, or pumping, pressure.

Some individuals, particularly those over 65 or 70 years of age, have what is called *isolated systolic hypertension*. The most recent expert committee defines this as a systolic blood pressure of 160 mm Hg or more, when the diastolic blood pressure is less than 90 mm Hg.

Actually, the levels of both systolic and diastolic blood pressures determine an individual's risk. In fact, of the two readings, the systolic blood pressure may be the superior predictor of all the complications we attribute to hypertension.

The most reliable early information on high blood pressure comes from the Framingham Heart Study, which showed early on that as both the systolic and diastolic blood pressure levels rise, the likelihood that an individual might develop coronary heart disease, stroke, congestive heart failure, peripheral vascular disease, and kidney problems rises as well. The association is strongest for stroke, although it is highly

significant for other cardiovascular diseases, too. The Framingham Heart Study also showed that people with hypertension had a higher death rate, when all causes were added together, than did those with normal readings. All of these findings have been amply confirmed by many other studies and apply to both men and women, as well as to people in their 60s and 70s and beyond.

Hypertension is a special problem for African-Americans. Overall, the percentage of blacks in the United States with hypertension is 50 percent greater than that of whites or Asians. Black men under the age of 45 are particularly prone to developing kidney failure from hypertension, eventually requiring dialysis or a kidney transplant. Blacks are also more likely than whites to have heart enlargement as a result of hypertension and ultimately to have congestive heart failure.

Hypertension often occurs together with other cardiovascular risk factors, particularly obesity, elevated levels of cholesterol and triglycerides, and diabetes mellitus. This suggests that there may be a common cause for these conditions, but it may simply be that an environmental factor, such as overeating, may lead to some or all of these problems.

There is a wealth of studies to show that successfully treating hypertension will substantially reduce the increased risk associated with it. Fortunately, too, we now have many well-tolerated antihypertensive medications that lower blood pressure and can be taken indefinitely. Although most of the treatment data are based on drugs, such measures as weight loss, salt restriction, and exercise may also lower blood pressure. As yet, however, no long-term studies have shown convincingly that these life-style changes are as successful as drugs in preventing strokes and other complications of hypertension. (For more information, see Chapter 12.)

HIGH BLOOD CHOLESTEROL AND RELATED LIPID PROBLEMS

Elevated levels of serum lipids (cholesterol and triglycerides) are extremely common and are one of the most important of the heart disease risk factors that can be changed. Yet, there is considerable confusion about the role of cholesterol as a cardiovascular risk factor. (See Chapter 4.)

Epidemiologic studies have shown that the level of total cholesterol in the blood is a strong predictor of the likelihood that an individual will develop coronary heart disease and, to a much lesser degree, a stroke. Most experts consider levels under 200 mg/dl to be normal and those between 200 and 239 mg/dl to be borderline high. Levels above 240 mg/dl present an increased risk for a heart attack—more than double the risk of levels below 200 mg/dl. About one out of four Americans falls into this latter category.

Total cholesterol levels are made up of several fractions. The most important and best studied are high-density lipoproteins (HDL cholesterol, or HDL-C) and low-density lipoproteins (LDL-C). These levels and their relationship to each other may be more important than total cholesterol levels in predicting heart disease risk. LDL levels over 160 mg/dl are definitely associated with increased risk, while values from 130 to 159 mg/dl are borderline. In contrast, HDL cholesterol is the fraction of cholesterol that appears to protect against coronary heart disease. The higher the level of HDL, the lower the risk. Ideally, it should be at least 35 mg/dl. A ratio of LDL to HDL greater than 3.5 or 4:1 is generally agreed to increase risk.

Many studies have failed to show an independent contribution to coronary heart disease risk from an elevation of triglycerides, another fatty component in the blood. Recent data, however, suggest that triglycerides may be an important predictor of risk, especially in women and those with diabetes mellitus.

While an individual's lipid profile is affected by age (total cholesterol rises with the years), gender (women tend to have higher levels of HDL), and heredity (elevated cholesterol and triglycerides tend to run in families, and certain families have extremely high levels), the picture can be significantly changed by life-style modifications. A diet low in saturated fat and cholesterol will lower serum cholesterol an average of 5 percent, but this diet may be more effective in some people. The general rule of thumb is that risk of coronary heart disease decreases by 2 percent for every 1 percent drop in total serum cholesterol.

Reducing alcohol intake in heavy drinkers and (for those who are overweight) body weight can significantly reduce triglyceride levels. Regular exercise will lower triglycerides and increase HDL cholesterol, and stopping smoking will also raise HDL cholesterol. For people with very high total cholesterol and LDL cholesterol levels, diet and exercise alone may not result in a great enough reduction, and these life-style measures may need to be combined with cholesterol-lowering drugs. (See Chapter 23.)

Lp(a)

Lipoprotein (a) or "Lp little a" was discovered in 1963, but its importance was not appreciated until recently.

Lp(a) is a molecule composed of the protein portion of low-density lipoprotein (LDL), which is called $apoB_{100}$, and another protein called apo(a). Apo(a) is very similar chemically to plasminogen, a naturally occurring substance that participates in dissolving clots that form in the bloodstream. Lp(a) has the opposite effect, however: It interferes with the normal process of clot lysis (dissolving) and thus may increase the likelihood that once a clot forms, a heart attack or stroke will occur.

Recent epidemiologic studies have shown that increased Lp(a) levels are associated with a greater frequency of coronary artery disease, increased clogging (stenosis) of coronary artery bypass grafts, and stroke (cerebrovascular disease). The impact of Lp(a) levels on the risk of coronary heart disease is as strong as that seen with total cholesterol levels or reduced high-density lipoprotein (HDL) levels, and the increase in risk attributable to high Lp(a) levels is independent of other risk factors. At this time, of the drugs available, only nicotinic acid seems to lower Lp(a) levels. Whether this reduction decreases the risk of developing disease is still unclear.

CIGARETTE SMOKING

Cigarette smoking is a major contributor to coronary heart disease, stroke, and peripheral vascular disease—even though smokers tend to be thinner and to have lower blood pressure than nonsmokers. Overall, it has been estimated that 30 to 40 percent of the approximately 500,000 deaths from coronary heart disease each year can be attributed to smoking. Individuals who smoke, regardless of their level of other risk factors or family history, are at significant risk of premature coronary disease and death. Smokers, for example, have less of a chance of surviving a heart attack than nonsmokers. Evidence from the Framingham Heart Study shows that the risk of sudden death increases more than tenfold in men and almost fivefold in women who smoke. Smoking is the number one risk factor for sudden cardiac death and for peripheral vascular disease.

Smoking cigarettes that are low in nicotine and tar does not decrease the risk of heart disease, which is increased by the effect of smoke on blood vessel walls. In fact, some people tend to smoke more and inhale deeply when they switch to this type of cigarette, increasing their exposure to the carbon monoxide in the smoke itself.

Fortunately, the risk of heart disease begins to decline rapidly as soon as smokers—even heavy, long-time smokers—stop. Ultimately, their level of risk is almost the same as that of people who have never smoked. (See Chapter 6.)

OBESITY

Any level of overweight appears to increase heart disease risk. Obesity can predispose the development of other risk factors, and the greater the degree of overweight, the greater the likelihood of developing other antecedants of atherosclerosis (such as high blood pressure and diabetes) that will increase the probability that heart disease will develop. Those who are obese (more than 30 percent over their ideal body weight) are the most likely to develop heart disease, even if they have no other risk factors. One recent study that examined more than 100,000 women age 30 to 55 showed that the risk for heart disease was more than three times higher among the most obese group than among the leanest group.

It also appears that how our weight is distributed may be even more important than exactly how much we weigh. There are two basic patterns of obesity: one in which excess fat is found primarily in the abdominal area (the "beer belly" or apple shape) and one in which excess fat deposits form around the hips and buttocks (the pear shape). The former type is called male-pattern obesity or android obesity; the latter, female-pattern or gynecoid obesity. Android obesity, which is also found in some women (especially after menopause), is associated with an increased risk of cardiovascular disease, specifically, coronary heart disease and stroke. A general rule of thumb is that a man's waist measurement should not exceed 90 percent of his hip measurement and that a woman's waist measurement should be no more than 80 percent of her hip measurement.

Android obesity appears to be most closely related not only to risk but also to other cardiovascular risk factors—namely hypertension, elevated triglycerides, low HDL cholesterol, elevated blood sugar levels, and diabetes mellitus. The common feature of all these conditions is an elevation in the level of insulin (the hormone that regulates the metabolism of sugar in the body) in the blood and a condition called insulin resistance, in which body tissues (especially the large muscles) do not respond normally to insulin. The likelihood that fat distribution and insulin resistance are related to genetics again points to the pivotal role of heredity in disease risk.

DIABETES MELLITUS AND INSULIN RESISTANCE

Individuals with diabetes mellitus, especially those whose diabetes occurs in adult life, have an increased incidence of coronary heart disease and stroke. Those who have slightly elevated blood sugar levels but do not have detectable diabetes also have an increased risk of developing these problems. Many individuals whose diabetes begins after age 40 or 50 (so-called adult-onset or Type II diabetes) often have higher than normal levels of circulating insulin. The primary role of insulin, a hormone produced by the pancreas, is to maintain blood sugar at normal levels and to assist this body fuel in entering each of the body's cells. For some reason, some individuals do not respond as readily to insulin, and more is required to do the job; they have insulin resistance. Elevated levels of insulin can raise blood pressure and assist in the deposition of and reduce the removal of cholesterol from plaques in the arteries. Both these actions increase the likelihood that atherosclerosis and its complications will develop.

Fortunately, weight reduction and exercise can improve the burning up of blood sugar (glucose) and prevent or slow down the onset of diabetes.

Individuals who develop diabetes in childhood (so-called juvenile-onset or Type I diabetes) are more likely to develop kidney and eye problems than coronary heart disease or strokes. In this type of diabetes, insulin is absent due to disease in the pancreas.

FIBRINOGEN

Serum fibrinogen is a component of the blood that plays a central role in the clotting process. Recent results from the Framingham Heart Study and elsewhere have shown that the level of fibrinogen is an independent cardiovascular factor. Why higher levels of this clotting factor increase risk is not yet known, but it is likely that individuals with higher levels may be more prone to develop clots in their arteries, thereby increasing the risk of a heart attack or stroke. Fibrinogen levels rise with age, and in that sense are not a risk factor that can be modified. However, fibrinogen levels are also adversely affected by cigarette smoking, which can be controlled.

BEHAVIORAL FACTORS

Coronary-prone behavior, sometimes referred to as "Type A" behavior, is felt by some, but not all, experts to be an important risk factor for coronary heart disease. Current definitions of Type A personality include a sense of time pressure and chronic impatience as well as excessive hostility. Contrary to popular belief, working hard or long hours is not necessarily a feature of the Type A or coronary-prone personality. Type A individuals tend to become upset easily, often for little cause, and are always in a hurry. They are constantly trying to do yet one more thing. Though many individuals who have heart attacks fit this personality description, current studies have not conclusively proved that a Type A personality is a true cardiovascular risk factor. (See Chapter 8.)

LEFT VENTRICULAR HYPERTROPHY (LVH)

The left ventricle is the chamber of the heart that pumps blood to all parts of the body except the lungs. Numerous studies show that individuals with left ventricular hypertrophy—an enlarged left ventricle in which the heart muscle has thickened—are prone to develop heart failure and are at greater risk of heart rhythm disturbances (arrhythmias) and sudden death. The majority of persons with an enlarged left ventricle either have hypertension or have already had a heart attack. Fortunately, we now know that successful treatment of hypertension will not only reduce blood pressure but will also reduce the size of the left ventricle and probably lower the risk associated with ventricular enlargement.

COCAINE

The escalating use of cocaine in the United States has resulted in angina, abnormal heart rhythms, high blood pressure, heart attacks, and death—even in healthy young adults. Cocaine constricts the coronary arteries, decreasing blood flow to the arteries of the heart, and reduces the amount of oxygen available to the heart while increasing the heart rate and its demand for oxygen. This combination of effects can precipitate a cardiac crisis and sometimes death, even upon the first use of the drug.

Cocaine is also a risk factor for congenital heart disease. Babies born to women who took cocaine during pregnancy are at increased risk of atrial-septal and ventricular-septal defects, as well as other congenital anomalies and adverse effects, such as low birth weight, that are directly related to the drug's action on the mother's cardiovascular system. (See Chapter 6.)

PROTECTIVE FACTORS

EXERCISE

While it is not clear that a sedentary life-style is a cardiovascular risk factor, the evidence is convincing that regular exercise will reduce the likelihood of a heart attack and may improve the chances of survival if one does occur. Exercise also seems to have a positive effect on a number of other risk factors. Whether its benefit lies in the fact that it helps control weight, improves the body's ability to use insulin, conditions the heart muscle, increases levels of protective HDL cholesterol, moderates stress, or lowers blood pressure—or a combination of these effects—is not clear. Whatever the reason, regular exercise can lower cardiovascular risk and it should be encouraged for everyone within the limits of each individual. (See Chapter 7.)

ESTROGEN

Estrogen (the major female sex hormone) protects against heart attacks and other forms of cardiovascular disease. Estrogen increases HDL cholesterol, which may explain how the hormone reduces the incidence of heart attacks in premenopausal women. It is now clear that once menopause occurs, women are at the same risk for heart attacks as are men. Thus, it is reasonable to advise that postmenopausal women receive estrogen replacement therapy unless it is medically contraindicated. Although it is likely that estrogen replacement therapy reduces the frequency of heart attacks, such therapy may increase the risk of cancer of the uterus. This risk can be reduced or eliminated by combining estrogen with progesterone, another female sex hormone. In fact, recent studies indicate that combined hormone therapy may actually reduce the possible risk of breast or uterine cancer. As an added advantage, postmenopausal estrogen replacement reduces the severity of osteoporosis—the bone thinning that is a leading cause of death and disability in older women. (See Chapter 19.)

ALCOHOL

In moderation—that is, no more than one or two drinks a day—alcohol may protect against coronary heart disease and atherosclerosis. Although the exact mechanism is not understood, it appears that alcohol raises HDL cholesterol. The association is certainly not strong enough to recommend that nondrinkers take up alcohol consumption. Furthermore, drinking four or more drinks per day can have deleterious effects. It raises blood pressure and puts the individual at significant risk of liver damage, central nervous system complications, and a number of other serious problems, some of which are cardiovascular. (See Chapter 6.)

A PROGRAM FOR CARDIOVASCULAR RISK FACTOR MODIFICATION

How should you use the information presented in this chapter to make certain that you are doing everything possible to avoid a heart attack, stroke, or other complication of atherosclerosis? The first step is to assess, with the help of a physician, whether or not you are a high- or low-risk individual.

For some answers, you do not need a doctor. Do you smoke cigarettes? Are you overweight? Do you drink too much? Is there heart disease or high blood pressure in the family? To fully assess risk, however, a physician is needed. He or she will measure blood pressure, send blood for serum cholesterol, triglyceride, and glucose measurements, and perform a history and physical examination. An electrocardiogram or more specialized procedures can be done to determine if the heart is enlarged. With this information, a table such as Table 3.1 may be helpful in assessing the interaction of various factors to determine total risk.

Once all of this information is collected and evaluated, a treatment program, directed at modifying risk factors, can be started. For those who are free of cardiovascular risk factors or clinical vascular disease, certain simple steps can always help, and will do little if any harm:

- *Eat a heart-healthy diet*—one low in saturated fats and cholesterol. Use monosaturated or polyunsaturated fat.
- *Reduce weight* if it is elevated. Even a small amount of weight loss can be helpful if you are overweight.
- *Moderate your salt intake.* Many people are not sensitive to salt and their blood pressure will not rise even if their intake of table salt and other forms of sodium is high. The problem is, we cannot distinguish who is and is not salt-sensitive without complex testing. Most of us eat more salt than we need. Many foods are naturally high in sodium and others have salt added in processing. Simple measures such as not adding salt to the food as it is cooked or at the table will reduce sodium intake to a reasonable amount. This degree of salt restriction

Table 3.2
The American Heart Association's Recommendations for Periodic Health Examinations

A (✔) indicates this test or medical procedure should occur at this age.

Age	Medical history	Physical exam	Blood pressure[1]	Plasma lipids[2]	Body weight	Fasting glucose	ECG	Baseline chest X-ray
20	✔	✔	✔	✔	✔	✔	✔	
25, 30, 35	✔	✔	✔	✔	✔	✔		
40	✔	✔	✔	✔	✔	✔	✔	✔
45, 50, 55	✔	✔	✔	✔	✔	✔		
60	✔	✔	✔	✔	✔	✔	✔	
61–75 (every 2½ years)	✔	✔	✔	Optional[3]	✔	✔		
75 and over (every year)	✔	✔	✔	Optional[3]	✔	Optional[3]		

[1]Blood pressure should be taken every 2½ years in normal patients.
[2]Plasma lipids include fasting cholesterol and triglycerides.
[3]Optional if baseline levels are well documented.
Note: These recommendations are reviewed periodically and are subject to change. They can, however, be used as a general guideline.

is absolutely safe and does not rob food of its taste, especially if herbs and spices are used as alternative flavorings.

- *Start a regular exercise program.* Virtually everyone can benefit from regular exercise. To be helpful, the program need not be too strenuous and can be tailored to an individual's preferences, schedule, and physical capabilities. Regular walking may be all that is necessary.

- *If you smoke, stop.* Nothing will be more beneficial!

- *If you drink alcohol, do so in moderation.*

- *Learn stress-reduction techniques* and avoid reacting to stressful situations in ways that will only serve to aggravate the problem.

- *Have your risk factor status assessed on a regular basis.* A clean bill of health on one occasion does not guarantee a lifetime of protection. Blood pressure, if normal, should be checked every two years or so, and cholesterol, if normal, should be checked every five years. (These recommendations are reviewed periodically as more is learned about risk. See Table 3.2 for current recommendations from the American Heart Association.)

What about individuals with definite hypertension or elevated cholesterol levels? The time to initiate therapy and the choice of therapy should be left to the physician, but always in consultation with the patient. In general, those who are at high risk because of very high blood pressure or cholesterol level or who have multiple risk factors require *drug* treatment, although a brief trial of diet, exercise, or other life-style changes may be appropriate first.

It is crucial to understand that treatment of cardiovascular risk factors is preventive medicine at its most challenging. After all, the physician is asked to select an effective and affordable regimen that does not make the patient sick and that can be useful for life. The irony is that in their early stages, neither hypertension nor high blood cholesterol produces symptoms, yet therapy for these conditions may interfere with enjoyment of life or, in some cases, actually cause symptoms.

Figure 3.2
Age-Adjusted Death Rates for Major Cardiovascular Diseases

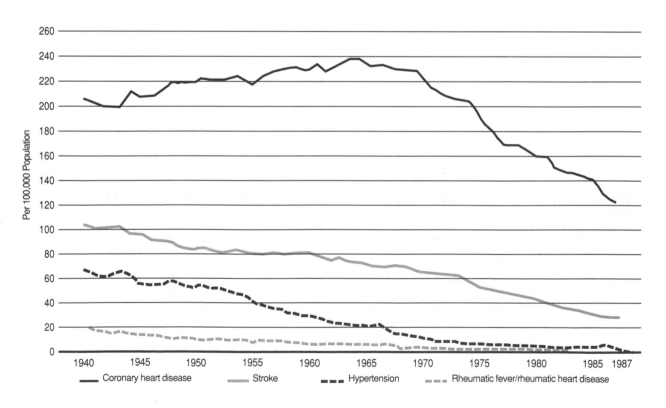

Source: National Center for Health Statistics, U.S. Public Health Service, DHHS and the American Heart Association.

Nevertheless, dietary or behavioral changes and drug therapy have proved worthwhile. It is clear that modifying cardiovascular risk factors is remarkably successful preventive medicine. In the United States, we have made considerable inroads against the epidemic of cardiovascular disease. Since 1972, we have reduced the death rate from strokes by more than 50 percent and deaths from coronary heart disease by more than 40 percent. (See Figure 3.2.) Other countries that have followed our lead are beginning to do as well. It is likely that with increased understanding and application of the principles discussed here, we can do even better.

CHAPTER 4

THE ROLE OF CHOLESTEROL

JONATHAN ISAACSOHN, M.D.

INTRODUCTION

Since the mid-1980s, when the National Cholesterol Education Program and the American Heart Association began a nationwide campaign to lower this country's average blood cholesterol level, the role of cholesterol in coronary heart disease (CHD) has come under scrutiny. In the public realm, manufacturers and advertisers played on consumer concerns by using oversimplified claims for products ranging from fish oil to breakfast cereals. Within the medical and scientific communities, the debate continues on what levels are truly "high" and on how best to approach the issue of controlling this major risk factor for cardiovascular disease.

One thing remains certain: A high level of cholesterol in the bloodstream is one of the major factors, along with smoking and high blood pressure, contributing to coronary heart disease, the nation's leading cause of death. How this risk factor relates to any one individual's health and life-style, however, is a far more complex matter. Cholesterol is not an immediate threat to the entire population, as some would claim; nor is it a "myth" generated by overzealous public health officials and medical experts, as others have contended.

In reality, elevated blood cholesterol does impart an increased risk for the development of coronary heart disease. The extent of this increase in risk depends on the degree of the cholesterol abnormality, together with other factors, including heredity, age, and gender. The presence of other coronary heart disease risk factors, such as high blood pressure, smoking, or diabetes, will also affect risk. The final determination of how to handle the cholesterol question rests with an individual and his or her physician.

In this chapter, we will examine the evidence that cholesterol does indeed pose a health risk and that control over cholesterol levels can lower that risk. The government's guidelines for cholesterol levels will be reviewed, and approaches to cholesterol control will be compared. First, however, it is essential to understand just what cholesterol is and what role it serves in the body.

THE NATURE OF CHOLESTEROL

Cholesterol has been portrayed by some as tantamount to a poison. In fact, cholesterol is a versatile compound that is vital (in small amounts) to the functioning of the human body. Only animals produce it; no plant product contains cholesterol unless an animal-based product, such as lard, has been added to

Triglycerides: What Is Their Role in Risk?

The exact role of triglycerides, or blood fats, in the development of coronary heart disease is uncertain. Unlike blood cholesterol, these fats must be measured after fasting, because the level of triglycerides in the blood goes up after a fatty meal. Whether a high level of fasting triglycerides in the blood is a definite risk factor for heart disease remains open to question. The international committee for the evaluation of hypertriglyceridemia as a vascular risk factor classified the hypertriglyceridemias into three groups: isolated moderate hypertriglyceridemia (triglycerides 200-400 mg/dl, total cholesterol <200 mg/dl); mixed hypertriglyceridemia (triglycerides 200-400 mg/dl, LDL cholesterol >130 mg/dl); and severe hypertriglyceridemia (triglycerides >400 mg/dl).

High triglycerides often appear along with other known risk factors, such as high blood cholesterol, obesity, and diabetes. But whether a high level of triglycerides is an *independent* risk factor is still being debated. Triglyceride level, unlike LDL cholesterol level, does not appear to have a continuous, graded relationship to coronary disease risk. There are subgroups of individuals with elevated triglycerides who are more susceptible to heart disease and others, with similar elevations, that are not. How to identify these subgroups is the subject of much research. An extremely high level of triglycerides—a relatively rare condition—poses an immediate risk to the pancreas and should be treated.

As it stands now, physicians tend to assess the risk of high triglycerides based on "the company they keep" in the bloodstream and on the rest of a patient's risk profile. Many lipid (blood fat) experts believe that a high level of triglycerides, along with a low level of HDL ("good") cholesterol, is a warning sign that merits further investigation and possible treatment. High triglycerides plus high LDL cholesterol is an important clue in diagnosing some inherited lipid disorders that carry a high risk of coronary heart disease. And high triglycerides in a person who already has coronary heart disease, or a family history of it, must be taken seriously. High triglycerides in a diabetic patient must be addressed. It is also possible that the testing of triglycerides only in a fasting state may present a deceptively low level and that an abnormally high increase in triglycerides after meals may pose risks of its own.

If treatment is deemed necessary, it will usually consist of dietary changes. Restriction of calories to reduce excess weight, a decrease in saturated fat and cholesterol, and reduced consumption of alcohol are the main dietary goals. Drug treatment is usually reserved for patients with high triglyceride levels, who have other risk factors and who do not respond to dietary changes.

---

it in processing. In humans, cholesterol serves three main functions. It is used by certain glands to manufacture steroid or cortisone-like hormones, including sex hormones; it helps the liver to produce bile acids, which are essential to the digestion of fats; and, most important, it is a main component of cell membranes and structures, a kind of building block for bodily tissues. Without it, mammalian life would not be possible.

The problem with cholesterol arises when the body has too much of it, or has deposits of it in the wrong places. Coronary heart disease results when cholesterol is deposited inside the walls of the heart's coronary arteries, the main suppliers of oxygen to the heart's own muscle tissue. There it contributes to the formation of fatty, toughened blockages called *plaque*. This buildup of plaque is variously called *arteriosclerosis*, *hardening of the arteries*, and *atherosclerosis*. Cholesterol can also be deposited within arteries elsewhere in the body, where it may contribute to the occurrence of stroke (from blocked arteries in the brain) and peripheral vascular disease (from arterial blockage in the legs).

How does cholesterol end up where it may do harm? Scientists have learned much about how it travels through the body and is deposited in the arterial walls. Cholesterol metabolism is based on the fact that oil and water don't mix. Cholesterol, a fatty or oily substance, cannot blend smoothly with blood, which is water-based. In order to travel throughout the body, cholesterol must be packaged in special molecules called *lipoproteins*. The lipids, or fatty cholesterol components, are wrapped inside a water-soluble protein coat. Different types of lipoproteins contain varying proportions of fat to protein.

The various lipoproteins form a dynamic economy within the body, transporting cholesterol to some tissues and removing it from others. The main cholesterol-carrying compound in the body is *low-density lipoprotein*, or LDL, cholesterol. LDL is often referred to as the "bad" cholesterol because it appears to play a key role in depositing cholesterol within arteries. (It's called low-density because it has very little protein, the densest substance in the molecule, and is composed mainly of fats.) High levels of LDL are linked to an increased risk of coronary heart disease.

High-density lipoprotein, or HDL, is termed "good" cholesterol because it appears to help remove cholesterol from artery walls and transport it to the liver for excretion. In contrast to LDL cholesterol, low levels of HDL are associated with an increased risk of coronary heart disease, while higher levels of HDL appear to protect against the disease.

Other subtypes of cholesterol particles include *chylomicrons*, which are produced by intestinal cells when fat is digested, and *very-low-density lipoprotein*, or VLDL, manufactured by the liver as an important precursor of LDL cholesterol production. VLDL is the major lipoprotein that transports the *triglycerides*, another type of fat, produced by the liver. (See box, "Triglycerides: What Is Their Role in Risk?")

For the purpose of determining heart disease risk, LDL and HDL are key. *Total blood cholesterol* is actually a composite number, made up of an individual's

Table 4.1

Average Total Serum Cholesterol Levels of U.S. Population Divided by Age and Sex

Race and age	Average	Race and age	Average
Men *All races*		**Women** *All races*	
20–74 years	211	20–74	215
20–24 years	180	20–24	184
25–34 years	199	25–34	192
35–44 years	217	35–44	207
45–54 years	227	45–54	232
55–64 years	229	55–64	249
65–74 years	221	65–74	246
White		*White*	
20–74 years	211	20–74 years	216
20–24 years	180	20–24 years	184
25–34 years	199	25–34 years	192
35–44 years	217	35–44 years	207
45–54 years	227	45–54 years	232
55–64 years	230	55–64 years	249
65–74 years	222	65–74 years	246
Black		*Black*	
20–74 years	208	20–74 years	212
20–24 years	171	20–24 years	185
25–34 years	199	25–34 years	191
35–44 years	218	35–44 years	206
45–54 years	229	45–54 years	230
55–64 years	223	55–64 years	251
65–74 years	217	65–74 years	243
Age-adjusted values: *All races,*		*Age-adjusted values:* *All races,*	
20–74 years White,	211	20–74 years White,	215
20–74 years Black,	211	20–74 years Black,	215
20–74 years	209	20–74 years	214

Sources: National Center for Health Statistics; R. Fulwood, W. Kalsbeck, B. Rifkind, et al., Total serum cholesterol levels of adults 20–74 years of age: United States, 1976–80. *Vital and Health Statistics*, Ser. II, No. 236. DHHS Pub. No. (PHS) 86-1686. Public Health Service. Washington, D.C.: U.S. Government Printing Office, May 1986.

Table 4.2
Mean Levels of Serum LDL Cholesterol

Sex and age	Mean
Male	
20–74 years	140
20–24 years	109
25–34 years	128
35–44 years	145
45–54 years	150
55–64 years	148
65–74 years	149
Female	
20–74 years	141
20–24 years	114
25–34 years	121
35–44 years	129
45–54 years	157
55–64 years	159
65–74 years	162

Source: National Center for Health Statistics, Division of Health Examination Statistics, unpublished data from the second National Health and Nutrition Examination Survey, 1976–80.

LDL cholesterol, HDL cholesterol, and VLDL cholesterol. (See Tables 4.1 and 4.2 for mean levels in the United States.) The ratio of LDL to HDL or total cholesterol to HDL may be as helpful as or more helpful than a simple measure of total cholesterol alone in estimating risk, a point that will be explored further in the section on cholesterol testing.

DIET, CHOLESTEROL, AND HEART RISK

Despite persistent doubts and controversy, there is overwhelming evidence that high blood cholesterol is associated with an increased risk of coronary heart disease, and furthermore, that the association is not merely coincidental but causative. Gaps remain, to be sure, in the understanding of how diet, cholesterol, and atherosclerosis interrelate, and research continues to fill those gaps. Meanwhile, ample data from vastly different types of research support the theory that high cholesterol levels in the blood are associated with increased risk. The most revealing avenues of research include the following.

STUDIES OF PLAQUE WITHIN ARTERIES

More than a century ago, pathologists in Russia analyzed the content of atherosclerotic plaque and discovered it to be composed of up to 70 percent cholesterol by weight. Since then, it has been determined that this cholesterol is brought to the arteries via the bloodstream and is not manufactured within the arteries themselves.

Inherited High Cholesterol: A Rare But Serious Risk

For many of the 25 percent or so of Americans who have high-risk levels of blood cholesterol, a high-fat, high-cholesterol diet is at least partially responsible. But for a small percentage, the cause is an inherited metabolic defect in the way their bodies clear cholesterol from the bloodstream. In individuals with normal cholesterol metabolism, special receptors on the surface of liver cells take up LDL cholesterol from the bloodstream. People with a disorder called *familial hypercholesterolemia* may lack some or almost all of these receptors entirely, or they may not function normally, causing extremely high levels of LDL cholesterol to circulate in the blood plasma.

This disorder causes elevated cholesterol levels (and thus higher-than-average heart disease risk) in about 1 out of every 500 Americans as the result of a gene inherited from one parent. A much more rare and more severe form of the disorder occurs when a child inherits the defective gene from both parents. This *homozygous* form of the disease, which occurs only once in a million births, causes coronary heart disease in childhood and adolescence and may require liver transplantation as a last treatment resort.

There are many other types of familial hyperlipidemia (inherited lipid disorders), causing abnormalities in various aspects of the blood lipid profile (LDL, HDL, triglycerides). People who are diagnosed with extremely high levels of cholesterol (above 300 mg/dl) or triglycerides (above 400 mg/dl) should encourage other members of their families, especially their children, to undergo testing. Patients with this disorder may be referred to a lipid clinic, a facility (usually in a major medical center) that specializes in treating blood cholesterol disorders. In cases of inherited cholesterol problems, diet therapy is usually necessary, but it may not be sufficient to bring cholesterol down to safe levels. Medication may be needed indefinitely to prevent premature coronary heart disease.

STUDIES OF LABORATORY ANIMALS

In most species of animals studied, atherosclerosis develops only when the animals' blood cholesterol levels are raised through a high-cholesterol, high-fat diet, no matter what other risk factors are present.

STUDIES OF HUMANS WITH INHERITED HIGH CHOLESTEROL

In a rare inherited disorder, the body accumulates extremely high levels of blood cholesterol from early childhood onward. People who have this condition develop coronary heart disease in youth, even when they have no other risk factors such as smoking or high blood pressure. (For more information on this rare disorder, called *familial hypercholesterolemia*, see box, "Inherited High Cholesterol: A Rare But Serious Risk.")

COMPARATIVE STUDIES OF HUMAN POPULATIONS

This type of research compares the rate of occurrence of various diseases among different populations. For decades, this epidemiologic research has shown a strong connection between a high-fat, high-chole-sterol diet, such as that consumed in most industrialized Western countries, and high levels of blood cholesterol and heart disease.

Some of these studies compare risk among different population groups. In the Seven-Countries Study (see Table 4.3), the dietary intake and heart disease rates of seven countries and 16 population subgroups were examined. A high correlation was found between the intake of dietary cholesterol and saturated fat and blood cholesterol levels (and, ultimately, heart disease rates). For example, the inhabitants of western Finland, who are active, outdoor people, not part of an industrialized society, have a high incidence of heart disease; their intake of dairy products is extremely high.

Other studies pinpoint the relationship of cholesterol to risk within a given population group. One famous example is the Framingham Heart Study, an ongoing research project that has tracked risk factors and heart disease occurrence among the residents of a small Massachusetts town for more than 40 years. Among the residents of Framingham, as cholesterol levels rose above 200 milligrams per deciliter (mg/dl), heart disease risk rose accordingly. This study showed that risk was essentially similar at all levels below 200 mg/dl. Another study, conducted on a far

Table 4.3
Results of Seven-Countries Study

Locality	Average serum cholesterol, mg per 100 ml	Coronary heart disease deaths, heart attacks, per 100	Locality	Percent calories saturated fatty acids	Coronary heart disease deaths, heart attacks, per 100
Velika Krsna (Yugoslavia)	156	0.2	Corfu	5.4	1.3
Dalmatia (Yugoslavia)	186	1.2	Crete	8.6	0.1
Montegiorgio (Italy)	196	1.7	Velika Krsna	8.8	0.2
Corfu (Greece)	198	1.3	Montegiorgio	8.9	1.7
Slavonia (Yugoslavia)	198	2.0	Dalmatia	9.5	1.1
Crevalcore (Italy)	200	1.8	Crevalcore	9.7	1.8
Crete (Greece)	203	0.1	Zrenjanin	10.0	0.3
Zrenjanin (Yugoslavia)	208	0.5	Belgrade Faculty	10.0	0.9
Belgrade Faculty (Yugoslavia)	216	0.9	Slavonia	13.0	2.0
Zutphen (Netherlands)	230	3.4	U.S. railroad workers	17.0	3.2
U.S. railroad workers	237	3.25	West Finland	18.8	2.2
West Finland	253	2.25	Zutphen	19.5	3.4
East Finland	264	2.4	East Finland	22.2	4.4

Note: Japan (Kyushu) was the seventh country studied. The diet here was lowest in total fat (9 percent) with only 3 percent from saturated fats. The Japanese also showed one of the lowest incidents of coronary events or deaths.

larger group of men for a research project called the Multiple-Risk Factor Intervention Trial (MRFIT), questioned whether even this "threshold" of risk exists. Among the 360,000 men screened for MRFIT, the relationship was simple and direct: The higher their blood cholesterol level, the higher their risk of coronary heart disease.

Finally, some researchers have tracked the patterns of blood cholesterol and coronary heart disease among groups of people who have migrated from countries or regions with low-fat diets to more developed areas with higher-fat eating patterns. For example, Japanese men living in Japan (where heart disease is rare despite a significant incidence of such risk factors as smoking and high blood pressure) were compared to Japanese men living in Honolulu and San Francisco. As these Japanese men moved eastward and adopted a progressively more American type of diet (and perhaps a different life-style), their blood cholesterol rates rose, as well as their rates of heart disease.

THE BENEFITS OF CONTROLLING CHOLESTEROL

Given all the evidence that high-fat, high-cholesterol diets contribute to elevated levels of cholesterol in the blood, and that high blood cholesterol is a definite risk factor for heart disease, it might seem natural to assume that lowering blood cholesterol, by diet or other means, would reduce that risk. To a scientist, however, this is nothing more than a hypothesis awaiting hard proof. Such proof has been time-consuming and expensive to gather. Not all subgroups of the population have been studied. Put into context, however, the evidence now points toward the conclusion that lowering cholesterol does have an impact on the process of plaque buildup in the blood vessels.

As such evidence continues to mount, it seems clear that lowering the average cholesterol level in Americans through moderate shifts in eating patterns may be an effective way to save thousands of lives over the next generation. At the very least, it is clear that people who already have coronary heart disease, or are at increased risk for developing it because of a poor family history, diabetes, high blood pressure, or a history of smoking, can benefit from lowering their blood cholesterol through diet and, if necessary, the use of cholesterol-controlling drugs.

A brief look at two landmark studies helps illustrate the scientific rationale for cholesterol control in healthy people. Both these studies are what scientists call *primary prevention trials*—studies of people who entered the research project without evidence of coronary heart disease. In the studies, one group of people was subject to a specific intervention, such as drug treatment or a special diet, and another group with similar characteristics to no intervention (in the case of drug treatment, members of the group were given a placebo, or sugar pill). Then, after a specified period of years, the groups were compared for their incidence of newly diagnosed heart disease or deaths.

In the Lipid Research Clinics Coronary Primary Prevention Trial, completed in the mid-1980s, two groups of middle-aged men with cholesterol levels above 265 mg/dl (average level of 290) were recruited from medical centers across the United States. These men were at the highest 5 percent of risk for a heart attack and probably are not representative of the entire population. Both groups were put on cholesterol-lowering diets. In addition, one group was given a cholesterol-lowering drug, cholestyramine, in high doses, while the others received a placebo. Despite the fact that many of the men treated with the drug took less of it than they were supposed to (because of its common side effects of gastrointestinal symptoms), this group showed a cholesterol level that was, on average, 9 percent lower—and a 19 percent reduction in risk of fatal and nonfatal heart attacks. Many other benchmarks of heart health were also better in this group, including lower rates of chest pain associated with heart disease, less need for bypass surgery, and fewer abnormal exercise stress tests. In general, the greater the cholesterol reduction achieved, the greater the risk reduction for coronary artery disease. Unfortunately, many of these patients were unable to tolerate the high doses of the drug used in this study.

Meanwhile, researchers in Finland—a nation with the highest rate of heart disease in the world—were reaching similar conclusions in a project called the Helsinki Heart Study. Again, middle-aged men at high risk were given medication, this time a drug called gemfibrozil, to lower their cholesterol levels, and compared over a five-year period with men on placebo. Drug treatment lowered cholesterol levels by about 8 percent, lowered triglyceride levels by 34 percent, and raised HDL cholesterol levels by 10 percent. The treated men had a 34 percent reduction in coronary heart disease rates.

Another kind of research, called *secondary prevention*, focuses on the question: If a person has already had a heart attack, can lowering cholesterol reduce the chances of another? The answer would appear to be yes. A study called the Coronary Drug Project compared the effect of several cholesterol-lowering drugs in people who had suffered a heart attack. The early results were encouraging, although hardly dramatic: After five years, the men receiving niacin (a B vitamin that lowers cholesterol when given in high doses) had a significantly lower rate of nonfatal heart attacks, but no difference in fatal cardiac problems. Interestingly, however, long-term follow-up of these men after 15 years has revealed that the treated group lived longer than those who were never treated—even though the treatment had been discontinued.

Perhaps the most compelling evidence that people with proven heart disease can benefit from lowered cholesterol levels comes from studies that use coronary angiography (X-ray pictures of the coronary arteries—those that supply blood to the heart muscle itself) to document the actual size and changes in the size of the fatty plaques. Several studies of people with known coronary artery disease, documented by angiography, have shown that a significant drop in blood cholesterol level can halt the growth of new coronary "lesions," as these blockages are called, and in some cases can cause some shrinkage of existing lesions. It appears from these studies that benefit can be demonstrated over a relatively short period of one to two years. However, in order to slow the progression of the disease, or better yet, try to reverse its effects, more extensive cholesterol lowering is necessary.

Does lowering cholesterol lengthen life? Critics of the cholesterol treatment recommendations have charged that the intervention studies failed to demonstrate a decrease in mortality. Indeed, in some major trials, *cardiovascular* death rates have been reduced, but overall death rates have been about the same for both the treated and the placebo group. However, none of these studies was designed to address the issue of total mortality. Such a study would have had to compare larger populations for longer periods.

A reduction in total mortality has, however, been demonstrated in some clinical trials. (The first was the Coronary Drug Project described above; the other two are Scandinavian projects called the Oslo Diet and Antismoking Study and the Stockholm Ischemic Heart Disease Study.) One more point deserves mention: Death rates are not the only issue in preventive health care. In all the intervention studies, the reduction in cardiac symptoms (such as angina)

and "events" (such as heart attacks) has contributed to an improved quality of life for the treated patients, regardless of overall death rates.

How well the conclusions from this research can be applied to the general population is not certain. None of the studies included women, children, elderly subjects, or persons who were at low risk. When the intervention consists only of such prudent health measures as eating a diet lower in saturated fat and cholesterol and getting more exercise, however, it seems clear to many experts that such changes can do no harm and may do much good. More data are obviously needed before definitive conclusions can be drawn.

In people with high risk, the primary benefit may be to delay the onset of so-called premature heart disease (that which occurs before age 65); in people at normal or low risk, such measures over a span of many years may help prevent cardiovascular disease in old age. To prove the benefits of cholesterol-lowering over a lifetime takes research so extensive that it is prohibitively expensive and difficult. According to many public health authorities, there is nothing to be gained by waiting 30 years to see the outcome of these measures; there is, however, ample evidence that lives may be saved by beginning such changes now.

MEASURING CHOLESTEROL

In 1987, an expert panel assembled by the U.S. government issued a set of guidelines for physicians in evaluating and treating patients for high blood cholesterol levels. (See box, "Cholesterol Testing and Treatment.") The purpose of such guidelines is to translate the vast accumulation of research data into relatively simple terms that busy doctors can use in practice.

Unfortunately, such guidelines can be easily presented to the public as a series of "magic numbers" determining one's medical fate. This is hardly the case. Throughout this discussion of risk evaluation and treatment, it is important to keep in mind that each person is treated as an individual, with a risk factor profile that may not easily fit a given mold. Treatment decisions, whether they relate to changing diet or taking medication, should be made in consultation with a physician and based on a thorough evaluation of an individual's total health profile.

Cholesterol Testing and Treatment

The following guidelines were issued in 1987 by the National Cholesterol Education Program of the National Heart, Lung, and Blood Institute to help physicians in making decisions on treatment for high blood cholesterol levels. Note that other coronary heart disease risk factors play a crucial role. These include male gender, a family history of coronary disease, cigarette smoking, high blood pressure, a low level of HDL cholesterol, diabetes, stroke or peripheral vascular disease, and obesity.

Blood cholesterol level	Treatment recommendations
Desirable (under 200 mg/dl)	Repeat test within five years; eat a prudent diet (low in total and saturated fat and cholesterol).
Borderline high risk (200 to 239 mg/dl)	No coronary disease and fewer than two other risk factors: Follow prudent diet and have cholesterol retested annually.
	Coronary disease or two other risk factors: Have LDL and HDL measured, and base further action on LDL level.
High risk (above 240 mg/dl)	Have LDL and HDL measured; further action based on LDL level.

Note: Some experts believe that HDL cholesterol should be tested along with total cholesterol as an initial test to screen for heart disease risk.

According to the government's guidelines, all adults should have their total blood cholesterol tested, or "screened" (a term that refers to widespread testing to uncover a hidden medical condition). A total blood cholesterol level of 200 mg/dl or below is considered "desirable." In this range, the only recommendation is for a repeat test every five years or so, along with ongoing health care as appropriate—including, ideally, a prudent diet that is lower in fat, cholesterol, and calories than the typical American diet.

Although this figure of 200 mg/dl has emerged in many studies as the point at which coronary risk starts to rise, as a cutoff point it is somewhat arbitrary. A person with a level of 195 and one with a level of 205 clearly have similar risks. Tests themselves have a margin of error; cholesterol values may vary by 15–20 mg/dl when determined by different tests on the same sample of blood. Similar variations are possible in blood samples taken from the same person over a period of weeks or months, even with no change in diet, medication, or activity. Thus, any test value should be understood as an indicator of possible risk, not an absolute determinant. Unfortunately, printouts of laboratory results may categorize a reading of 245 as "high risk," creating what is possibly unnecessary anxiety for a patient. This reading may be 20 or 25 points lower on a follow-up analysis.

For people with total blood cholesterol levels between 200 and 239 mg/dl, the expert panel recommended the same measures as for people under 200 mg/dl, provided they have no evidence of coronary disease and fewer than two other coronary risk factors. However, if they fall into this "borderline high" range and have two or more coronary risk factors, further testing is recommended. Those risk factors include being male; having a family history of coronary heart disease; cigarette smoking; diabetes; high blood pressure; and severe obesity. If total cholesterol is more than 240 mg/dl, further testing and possible treatment is definitely recommended, even if no other risk factors are present. (Incidentally, about 25 percent of adult Americans have cholesterol levels in this high-risk range.)

LIPOPROTEIN MEASUREMENT

It is recommended that patients with a total cholesterol in the borderline-high or high range have a second, more complete, test that measures high- and low-density lipoproteins. The measurement of HDL and LDL gives the physician a clearer picture of actual risk than does the total cholesterol level alone. In most cases, total cholesterol gives a fairly good picture of coronary risk, but not always.

For instance, it is possible that a somewhat high total cholesterol level may be due to a high proportion of protective HDL. For example, a cholesterol level of 250 may seem high, but if the HDL is 60 to 65 (a high level that is frequently seen in women), the risk of a heart attack may not be increased. High HDL levels are also seen in people who exercise a great deal. In this case, vigorous cholesterol control would be unjustified. In a number of cases, a desirable total cholesterol level can conceal an abnormally low level of HDL (below 30 to 35) and even occasionally a high level of LDL. For this reason, some experts have strongly contested the government's recommendation that total cholesterol alone be used as a screening test; they advocate the use of HDL testing in all people, especially those at high risk, as part of the initial testing. There are problems related to the measurement of HDL as well as conceptual problems of what to do with the isolated low HDL. Until these issues have been clarified, the decision to measure the lipoprotein tractions in someone with a total cholesterol in the "desirable" range rests with the individual and his or her physician.

Further decisions about how to treat elevated cholesterol are often based on the levels of LDL cholesterol, HDL cholesterol, and triglycerides in the blood. Triglycerides are often elevated to high levels in people with diabetes or in those who consume a great deal of alcohol. Ideally, LDL levels should be below 130 mg/dl, and HDL levels should be above 35 mg/dl. In patients with evidence of coronary heart disease, studies have demonstrated that reducing the LDL levels to around 100 mg/dl can slow the progression of the disease and even partially reverse its effects. If follow-up testing is needed to chart the progress of cholesterol control, the physician may just use total cholesterol testing for purposes of cost and convenience.

Can cholesterol be too low? Except in the case of some extremely rare inherited metabolic defects, it's unlikely. The body manufactures virtually all the cholesterol it needs, even on a low-fat, low-cholesterol diet. The suggestion has been made that low levels of cholesterol may be associated with certain types of cancer, based on limited evidence that people with unusually low cholesterol levels develop these cancers at higher than usual rates. There is little scientific proof for this assertion, however; in fact, populations that eat a lower-fat diet than North Americans also have lower rates of several types of cancer, including those of the breast and colon. If any relation is present between very low cholesterol levels and cancer, it may stem from the possibility that cancer changes many bodily components, including cholesterol, and may begin doing so even before the cancer is diagnosed. A marked weight loss may also result in low cholesterol levels. If cholesterol levels are 140 to 150, it is usually a good rather than a bad sign.

CONTROLLING CHOLESTEROL

If a person's cholesterol level is above the desirable range, the challenge for patient and doctor is to set a target for blood cholesterol that is both realistic and likely to provide benefit.

The cutoff points described above serve only as guidelines. Therapy must be planned in accordance with the entire lipid profile (total cholesterol, LDL, HDL, and triglycerides; personal and family medical history; life-style and dietary habits, including smoking, drinking, and exercise; and the person's own commitment to change).

Cholesterol can be lowered primarily through two approaches: diet and drugs. These modes of action are complementary, not mutually exclusive. As a rule, dietary change is recommended initially. (See box, "Strategies to Lower High Cholesterol," and see Chapter 5.) If cholesterol doesn't come down sufficiently, drug therapy may be added to—not substituted for—dietary modifications. The length of the trial period for diet alone depends on individual factors such as the presence of CHD and the person's responsiveness to dietary change.

Strategies to Lower High Cholesterol

- *Lose excess weight.* This is best accomplished by a modest reduction in caloric intake coupled with an increase in physical exercise. Avoid crash diets; instead, strive for a loss of 1 or 2 pounds a week until you achieve your desired weight goal. Then maintain that weight by a combination of exercise and moderate eating habits.

- *Increase intake of dietary fiber.* Studies show that soluble fibers help lower blood cholesterol. These fibers include pectin (found in apples and other fruits), guar (used in gum and as a thickener), and the fiber found in oats, corn, rice, and dried beans and other legumes. All types of dietary fiber have the added advantage of producing a feeling of satiety, thereby helping reduce total food intake.

- *Lower your total fat and cholesterol intake.* Use a cookbook that features low-fat, low-cholesterol recipes. Serve smaller portions of meat dishes and emphasize vegetables, pasta, and other low-fat, cholesterol-free foods. At the same time, reduce consumption of high-cholesterol foods like eggs, liver, and fatty meat.

- *Exercise regularly.* This helps in weight control and may also raise levels of HDL cholesterol.

(For more specific guidelines, see Chapter 5.)

DIET

Dietary therapy for elevated blood cholesterol consists of the same prudent eating habits recommended for the public at large (both adults and children over age 2): no more than 30 percent of total calories from fat, and no more than 10 percent from saturated fat, the kind found primarily in animal fats and in some vegetable oils such as coconut. The average American diet includes 37 percent of calories from fat. In addition, intake of dietary cholesterol (found in all animal products, including meat, poultry, egg yolks, and fish) should not exceed 300 milligrams per day. It is important to note that while fish contains cholesterol, it is low in saturated fat and may be eaten instead of certain cuts of beef, lamb, and other meats that are high in saturated fat. Poultry falls between fish and meat with respect to saturated fat content.

(See Tables 4.4 and 4.5.) One of the major sources of cholesterol is egg yolk. (See box, "Sources of Cholesterol in the American Diet.") One large egg yolk contains about 213 to 220 mg of cholesterol, almost 75 percent of a total day's ration.

If this level of dietary modification does not accomplish cholesterol control sufficiently, a "step two" diet that further restricts saturated fat to 7 percent of total calories may be recommended. At this level of restriction, the advice of a registered dietitian is usually needed to adopt eating patterns that are tasty, nutritious, and practical. (For a complete discussion of dietary goals, see Chapter 5.)

A key component of dietary therapy is the restriction of total calories to a level consistent with appropriate weight. Just losing excess pounds can help lower total cholesterol—and, as an added benefit, it can also help raise the level of protective HDL. For-

Table 4.4
Cholesterol/Fat/Calorie Content of Common Foods

Food	Calories	Cholesterol (mg)	Fats (gm) Polyunsaturated	Monounsaturated	Saturated*
Meat/fish/poultry:					
Beef, 1 oz lean chuck	71	26	0.1	0.8	0.9
Beef, 1 oz fatty	110	27	0.2	2.0	2.2
Beef liver, 1 oz	46	83	0	0	0.1
Chicken, 1 oz dark	58	26	0.6	1.0	0.6
Chicken, 1 oz white	47	22	0.2	0.3	0.3
Fish, 1 oz lean (sole)	40	27	0.1	0.1	0
Fish, 1 oz fatty (trout)	58	25	1.1	1.1	0.9
Lamb, 1 oz lean	53	17	0.2	0.2	0.1
Pork, 1 oz lean chop	60	28	0.1	0.8	0.9
Tuna, 1 oz water pack	45	11	0.1	0.1	0
Turkey, 1 oz white	48	22	0.2	0.3	0.3
Veal, 1 oz cutlet	51	28	0.1	0.8	2.2
Dairy products:					
Butter, 1 T	100	31	0.4	2.8	3.2
Cheese, 1 oz cheddar	115	28	0.3	3.0	6.0
Cheese, cottage (4% fat) ½ cup	110	16	0.1	1.0	1.6
Egg, 1 large	79	213	0.7	2.2	1.7
Ice cream, 1 cup (115 fat)	270	56	0.3	9.6	16.8
Milk, 1 cup whole	150	34	0.1	2.4	4.8
Milk, 1 cup 2% fat	120	22	0.1	2.0	2.4
Milk, 1 cup 1% fat	100	10	0.1	0.8	1.2
Milk, 1 cup skim	85	4	0	0.1	0.3
Yogurt, 1 cup plain, 1% fat	145	14	0.1	1.0	2.3

*Avoid foods with a high level of saturated fats.

YALE UNIVERSITY SCHOOL OF MEDICINE HEART BOOK

Table 4.5
Types of Fats According to Saturation

Type	% Polyunsaturated	% Monounsaturated	% Saturated
Mostly polyunsaturated:			
Corn oil	59	24	13
Cottonseed oil	52	18	26
Safflower oil	75	12	6
Soybean oil	59	23	14
Sunflower oil	66	20	10
Mostly monounsaturated:			
Canola oil	32	62	6
Chicken fat	22	47	31
Lard	12	47	41
Margarine, hard[1]	29	35–66	17–25
Margarine, soft[1]	61	14–36	10 17
Margarine, tub	46	22–48	15–23
Olive oil	9	72	14
Peanut oil	32	46	17
Sesame seed oil	40	40	18
Vegetable shortening, hydrogenated[1]	33	44–55	22–33
Mostly saturated:			
Beef fat	11	4	52
Butter	4	30	66
Coconut oil	2	6	87
Palm/palm kernel oil	2	10	80

[1]Ranges derived from manufacturers' data; check labeling.
Source: United States Department of Agriculture.
Note: In instances where total percentages are less than 100, water or other substances make up the difference.

tunately, a "fringe benefit" of prudent eating habits is that high-fat foods, the most concentrated source of calories, are replaced by lower-fat foods such as complex carbohydrates (found in grains, fruits, vegetables, and products made with them). Because gram for gram, fat contains more than twice as many calories as proteins or carbohydrates (9 calories versus 4), such dietary changes can facilitate weight loss without excessive deprivation. In addition, there is evidence that increasing dietary fiber intake also helps lower cholesterol. If obesity is one of a person's cardiovascular risk factors, an eating plan that com-

bines weight control and cholesterol control without "crash" diets or gimmicks can usually be devised.

How much can diet lower cholesterol? The answer varies from one individual to another. The amount of cholesterol and fat produced by the liver and how efficiently these substances are broken down depend not only on diet but also on other factors determined by heredity. The liver contains certain receptors that are capable of getting rid of LDL cholesterol. A person who has an adequate number of these receptors may have a normal cholesterol level despite a high-fat diet; if there is a deficiency in these receptors, high lipid levels may occur even on a moderately low-fat diet.

On average, dietary changes like those outlined tend to reduce total cholesterol some 5 to 10 percent, but this average figure does not predict how a given individual will respond to diet therapy. The only sensible course, then, is to give dietary modification a fair try, have cholesterol levels remeasured within six weeks to six months, and take it from there. It is important to remember that having a high cholesterol

Sources of Cholesterol in the American Diet

Meat, poultry, fish	38%
Eggs	36%
Dairy foods	15%
Animal fats	11%

level is not an emergency—there is almost always time to work on lowering it. If diet modification alone does not complete the task, and the physician believes that other factors point toward an increased risk, drug therapy may be the next step. But medication is not a panacea to counteract the effects of a high-fat diet. Continued dietary changes, in fact, can help the medication to do its job and may allow for the use of lower dosages, thus lessening the possibility of side effects.

OTHER LIFE-STYLE MEASURES

In addition to diet changes, other changes can have a positive impact on cholesterol levels and on the proportion of "good" to "bad" lipoproteins. One important step is for cigarette smokers to quit smoking; in addition to causing injury to blood vessel walls, smoking appears to lower the level of HDL ("good") cholesterol. (See Chapter 6.) If triglycerides are elevated, alcohol intake should be curtailed. While one or two drinks a day may indeed raise HDL levels, as has been reported, this is not a justification for excessive drinking, which has severe negative effects on the cardiovascular system, brain, and liver. (See Chapter 6.)

Finally, there is some evidence that regular exercise has a beneficial effect on HDL cholesterol levels. Just how much exercise is needed to achieve this effect is uncertain, but given the other benefits of moderate exercise on the heart, it certainly cannot hurt. Exercise can help keep weight down, and weight reduction can certainly help maintain a "desirable" lipid profile. (See Chapter 7.)

MEDICATION

The decision to prescribe a cholesterol-lowering drug should not be taken lightly. For one thing, such drugs may need to be taken indefinitely in order to maintain their benefits. For another, no drug is without risk, particularly when taken over the long term. The benefits of drug treatment must be weighed against its cost, inconvenience, and potential side effects.

The types of medication in longest use (and thus with the longest record of safety and effectiveness) have tended to produce a fairly high rate of inconvenient, if usually harmless, side effects. Recently, newer drugs have been developed that may produce similar benefits with a lower rate of side effects. Choosing a type of medication also depends on the composition of a person's lipoprotein profile, because various agents have differing impacts on total cholesterol, LDL, HDL, and triglycerides. The major drugs are summarized in Table 4.6. (For a more detailed discussion of cholesterol-lowering medications, see Chapter 23.)

In deciding whether or not to put a patient on cholesterol-lowering drugs, a doctor must consider, first and foremost, whether the patient already has heart disease, and if not, what his or her risk is of getting it, and what factors might complicate drug treatment (for example, other health problems, other medications, difficulty in remembering to take medication). More vigorous therapy is recommended in patients who have heart disease and whose cholesterol levels are high. On the other hand, a non-smoking, thin, active woman with normal blood pressure may not derive much benefit from lowering a mildly elevated cholesterol level. In this case, the possible risk of drug treatment may outweigh the potential benefit.

The person who takes cholesterol-lowering medications should be a partner with his or her physician, reporting any side effects or other problems. Often a change in dosage or a different type of medication may be able to solve the problem. It is usually possible to establish a regimen using a single drug or a combination of drugs that will improve the lipid profile with minimal side effects.

CHOLESTEROL, RISK, AND COMMON SENSE

If cholesterol control is to be a rational part of preventive health care, it must be treated as one element in the entire risk factor profile. Smoking, for example, raises the coronary heart disease risk of a person with a cholesterol level of 200 mg/dl to that of a person with 250 to 300 mg/dl. To focus exclusively on cholesterol reduction while continuing to smoke, then, would be poor judgment. Age, sex, family history, blood pressure, weight, presence or absence of diabetes, and amount of regular exercise are other risk factors that must, to varying degrees, be taken into account. (See Chapter 3.)

Unanswered questions remain. For example, should cholesterol control be pursued as aggressively in women as in men, and should treatment for both sexes be the same? Women have not been included in any of the major cholesterol intervention studies. Before menopause, they have lower heart disease rates than men do, apparently because of the protection of female hormones. After menopause, however, they catch up quickly: Cardiovascular disease

Table 4.6
Major Cholesterol-Lowering Drugs

Drugs	Long-term safety	LDL-cholesterol lowering	Special precautions
Cholestyramine (Questran, Colestid, Questran Light, Cholybar)	Yes	10%–25%	Can alter absorption of other drugs. Can increase triglyceride levels and should not be used by people with an excess of triglycerides in the blood. May cause constipation.
Gemfibrozil (Lopid)	Preliminary evidence	5%–15%	Should be used with caution by people with gallbladder or kidney disease.
Lovastatin (Mevacor)	Not established	25%–50%	Monitor for liver function and muscle enzyme abnormalities.
Nicotinic acid or niacin (Nia-Bid, Nicolar, and others)	Yes	15%–30%	Monitor liver function abnormalities and uric acid and blood sugar levels.
Probucol (Lorelco)	Not established	10%–15%	Lowers HDL-cholesterol; significance of this has not been established.

is the biggest killer of American women as well as of American men, albeit some eight to ten years later. Major, long-term studies of the effects of hormone therapy after menopause are now under way to answer some of these gender-related questions. (See Chapter 19.)

Age is another variable in need of further study. What does elevated cholesterol mean for the elderly? The relative risk of a high cholesterol level declines as an individual gets older. However, the absolute death rate from coronary heart disease increases with advancing age, so that treatment may have an impact on death rates in the elderly. But how much should we disturb the life-style of a 75- or 80-year-old person for a benefit that is possible but has not been proved for those of advanced age? There are as yet no answers; common sense and good science suggest that a modified diet that does not prove too burdensome to an elderly person is a reasonable approach to therapy. A more aggressive approach, using drug therapy, may be appropriate in an older individual with heart disease or one who has very high cholesterol levels, is unresponsive to dietary intervention, and is otherwise healthy. Although we do not have specific intervention data in the elderly, a case can be made for giving these individuals the benefit of the doubt, assuming they will behave like

a middle-aged population, until it is proven that they do not. (See Chapter 21.)

At what age should we start intervening? Cholesterol levels are lower in children than in adults, but tend to rise with age—at least in societies with high-fat diets. The benefits of preventing this rise may not be evident for a generation. But here, too, are there some dangers in rigidly restricting cholesterol intake in younger children? We have no answers, but an across-the-board restriction of high-fat junk foods and bacon-and-egg breakfasts probably will not hurt and may do some good. (See Chapter 20.)

In many respects, the American diet is more healthful than it was several decades ago. Consumption of red meat, whole milk, and eggs is down (by about 40 percent); people are eating more fish, poultry, fruits, vegetables, and low-fat dairy products. Most sectors of American society are also smoking less. The results, whether direct or indirect, can be seen in our gradually receding rate of coronary heart disease deaths, even when adjusted for the aging of the population. Dietary changes, along with better control of hypertension, have probably played a major role in the decrease in heart disease. Based upon the evidence, it is reasonable to assume that even better results may be expected if we adjust our dietary patterns even further to control cholesterol levels.

CHAPTER 5

ADOPTING A HEALTHFUL DIET

MICHELE FAIRCHILD, M.A., R.D.
VIRGINIA UTERMOHLEN, M.D.

INTRODUCTION

Americans know much more—and seem to care much more—about having a healthy diet than ever before. A number of surveys have shown that we are cutting our consumption of high-fat meats and whole-milk dairy products, while increasing the amount of fish, chicken, pasta, grains, and fresh fruits and vegetables we eat. Food manufacturers are beginning to respond: the array of low-fat, or even non-fat, and low-sodium products has burgeoned; what's more, many have been reformulated as food science has become more sophisticated. So-called "healthy" foods now taste better than they did as recently as a year or two ago. Even fast-food restaurant chains have reacted, replacing animal fats with vegetable fats in some of their fried foods, cutting the percentage of fat in their hamburgers, offering grilled as well as deep-fried chicken, and opening salad bars.

As a result, the average amount of fat in the typical American diet has dropped from a high of 42 percent of calories in 1960 to its current level of about 37 percent. Animal products, which were the source of 70 percent of fat consumed in 1960, were only 57 percent in 1982, a reflection in part of the public's switch to margarine in place of butter and the disappearance of lard in many commercial and home-made baked goods.

Even so, those who follow food trends note that sales of premium ice creams and high-fat cheeses have increased exponentially, as has consumption of soft drinks and sweets. Restaurateurs find that even those who conscientiously order fish and steamed vegetables for dinner "reward" themselves by having the fudge pie for dessert. About half of all Americans are overweight. There are vast numbers of people who haven't yet been persuaded to change their eating habits, and legions more who are confused by seemingly conflicting claims ("Oat bran lowers cholesterol" vs. "Oat bran is no better than other fibers"), or who want to change but don't know how to begin. Average intake of saturated fat is at least 50 percent higher than most experts believe it should be, while cholesterol and sodium intake levels are twice the recommended levels.

THE TYPICAL AMERICAN DIET AS A RISK FACTOR

At the center of this concern about the foods we eat is strong evidence implicating diet in the development of coronary artery disease, high blood pressure, stroke, and other vascular diseases, with additional evidence suggesting linkage to obesity, breast cancer, colon cancer, adult (Type II) diabetes, and diseases of the liver, kidneys, and gallbladder.

Of greatest concern are diseases of the heart and blood vessels, which together account for almost half of all deaths in this country. The common denominator for most of these diseases is atherosclerosis, which is caused by the buildup of plaque—deposits of fatty substances, cholesterol, fibrous tissue, and calcium—in the inner lining of the arteries. This buildup may be fueled by an excess of cholesterol and other fats circulating in the blood (serum cholesterol and triglycerides). The main contributor to this excess is a diet high in fat—especially saturated fat—as well as dietary cholesterol. This relationship is explained later in this chapter and in greater detail in Chapter 4, which also makes the case for decreasing serum cholesterol levels in order to lower the risk of coronary heart disease.

The risk of high blood pressure is also affected by diet. Chapter 12 explains how excess sodium may, in susceptible individuals, increase this risk and gives practical advice for decreasing sodium as a possible means of preventing or treating high blood pressure. Although the dietary recommendations in this chapter are not specifically meant for people with hypertension, the emphasis on fresh fruits, vegetables, and meats, rather than on canned or highly processed ones, automatically reduces the daily consumption of sodium. About one-third of sodium in the average diet comes from processing, while another third is added in cooking or at the table. The remaining third is found naturally in foods.

The total number of calories in the diet, as well as the proportion of those calories that comes from fat, has been associated with coronary artery disease. Caloric intake that exceeds the amount needed to fuel the body's activities results in excess weight. An individual whose weight exceeds the desirable level by 20 percent or more is considered obese, and obesity is an independent risk factor for heart disease. In addition, it affects blood pressure and blood cholesterol and triglyceride levels and contributes to the development of diabetes.

For most adults, the body's need for calories declines with age. Following the section on implementing the dietary recommendations in this chapter is a section designed to help people achieve and maintain a desirable weight.

Although the main concern here is to help readers lower their risk of heart disease and stroke, the prudent diet that is recommended is basically the same one endorsed not only by the American Heart As-

sociation and the National Heart, Lung, and Blood Institute but also by the American Academy of Pediatrics, American Dietetic Association, American Cancer Society, National Cancer Institute, American Diabetes Association, the Centers for Disease Control, and the U.S. Departments of Agriculture and Health and Social Services. The dietary recommendations are appropriate for all healthy Americans over the age of two. (See box, "Low-Fat Diets and Children.")

These same dietary changes are appropriate for people who already have elevated blood cholesterol (above 200 mg/dl), coronary heart disease, or cerebrovascular disease. They are important as well for people who have had coronary artery bypass grafts, which are as subject to atherosclerosis as the arteries they replace. At Yale, our emphasis is on the gradual introduction of changes. (See box, "Magic Bullets.") In treating most heart disease patients we begin with

Low-Fat Diets and Children

The American Academy of Pediatrics and the American Heart Association recommend the same low-fat diet for children over age 2 that is recommended for adults. Before age 2, children need a higher percentage of fat for proper growth and organ development. There have been disturbing cases of failure to thrive (slowed growth and development) in children of middle-class families in which having sufficient food to eat should not be a problem. Unfortunately, in their desire to protect their children against future disease, parents have sometimes gone overboard in restricting food intake.

Children need sufficient calories to fuel growth and provide energy for their daily activities. Because they cannot eat large quantities of food at any one time, they need a certain amount of food that is calorically dense—in other words, fat. After children reach 24 months, parents can gradually introduce low-fat dairy products and make other sensible changes. A good place to curb fat intake is in snack food, by offering fruit, raw vegetables, rice cakes, and ginger snaps, for example, in place of potato chips and cream-filled cupcakes.

While it is important to guard against obesity, children need to develop a healthy attitude toward food. It is better to encourage regular exercise in place of watching television than to make dieting an obsession.

A parent who is considering making changes in a child's diet should consult the child's pediatrician to be sure that the changes are appropriate and will still provide sufficient fat and calories to promote proper growth.

diet and other life-style measures. If the diet recommended in this chapter does not produce significant reductions in levels of serum cholesterol in six to nine months, medical intervention may be necessary. This should be individualized for each patient and done in consultation with a physician and a registered dietitian. It may take the form of further reductions in dietary cholesterol and saturated fat, and it may include simultaneous introduction of drug therapy.

This chapter provides practical guidelines for shifting diet in a healthier direction: eating more whole, or unprocessed, grains, cereals, legumes, fruits, and vegetables, for example. At the same time, the emphasis is on eating smaller portions, consuming fewer calories, and consuming less fat (especially saturated fat), cholesterol, sodium, and alcohol. To understand how to translate all these recommendations into everyday menus, it is helpful to have a brief introduction to the main elements of a balanced diet.

DIETARY COMPONENTS

The energy the body needs to carry out its basic functions comes from three sources: carbohydrates, proteins, and fats. Most foods are a mixture of more than one energy source. Meat and cheese, for example, are considered protein foods, but can have large amounts of fat. Except for processed meats, such as luncheon meats, these animal products have no carbohydrates. (Milk is the only animal product that contains a significant amount of carbohydrates, in the form of lactose, a type of sugar.) Foods generally classified as carbohydrate foods, which are plant products, can have high amounts of protein, are usually very low in fat, and rarely contain saturated fats. Fats, while found in other foods, are most familiar in their pure forms, such as butter, margarine, and oil. When foods containing these three basic elements are combined in appropriate proportions and in a variety of

"Magic Bullets"

Every few years another quick dietary fix seems to capture the attention of people who are looking for ways to have their cake and eat it too. In the mid-1980s, reports of a lower incidence of coronary heart disease among Greenland Eskimos, who eat a diet high in oily varieties of fish, intrigued nutrition researchers. The key element seemed to be omega-3 fatty acids, a type of polyunsaturated oil found in these fish and to a lesser degree in other types of fish and in plants. Using concentrated sources of omega-3 in small, controlled clinical trials involving heart disease patients, the researchers confirmed that the oil could lower blood levels of very-low-density cholesterol and triglycerides. They also found that at certain doses the oil tended to thin the blood. In some patients, it actually caused gastrointestinal bleeding.

Unfortunately, this did not deter some manufacturers from marketing fish-oil capsules to people looking for a magic bullet. The American Heart Association and others recommend that the public get fish oil from fish rather than from capsules.

In the late 1980s, oat bran replaced fish oil as a painless way to lower serum cholesterol without resorting to more major dietary changes. Within months, supermarket shelves were stocked with everything from oat bran beer to oat bran potato chips. What was ignored was research indicating that the oat bran was effective *in conjunction with a low-fat diet*. Just as quickly as oat bran was embraced, it was discarded after the publication in

the *New England Journal of Medicine* of research —later criticized as poorly designed—showing that oat bran is not effective. Many members of the public missed the point on both counts: Oat bran alone—or in high-fat products such as potato chips —is not the answer, but as part of a low-fat diet it can be another way to help control serum cholesterol. Oat bran is still available as it was before—plain, in rolled oats, and in some oat-based cold cereals (those with no more than 1 to 2 grams of fat per serving are best).

What will be the magic bullet of the 1990s? Some nutrition watchers think garlic—touted as a cure for everything from constipation to the common cold—may be next in line. Epidemiologic studies show that populations that eat large amounts of garlic have a lower incidence of coronary heart disease. These populations, it should be noted, also eat large quantities of onions, which confounds the data. Although some researchers feel there may be a place for garlic as there is for oat bran, it is far too early to make recommendations. Further research is under way to document preliminary studies from Germany showing a 10 to 12 percent reduction in serum cholesterol attributed to garlic intake.

The point of all this is that decisions about diet, either positive or negative, are complex and should never be made on the basis of one study. There are no magic bullets! Dietary change is a gradual process that requires thought and effort.

forms, they make up a balanced diet that provides the body with all the vitamins and minerals it needs and a sufficient amount of energy to function.

CARBOHYDRATES

Carbohydrates are the body's major energy source, fueling the activities of the brain, central nervous system, and muscles. What the body doesn't use immediately as glucose, it converts and stores as glycogen and fat. Glycogen, which is stored in the liver and the muscles, can be broken down quickly to restore blood glucose levels rapidly when they drop or to provide fuel for exercise. The amount of glycogen that can be stored is limited; the amount of fat, unfortunately, is not.

There are three main types of carbohydrates: starches (also called complex carbohydrates), which are found primarily in cereals, grains, and starchy vegetables; sugars (also called simple carbohydrates), which occur naturally in fruits, berries, and some vegetables, and are also found in refined form as table sugar and syrup and in processed foods; and fibers, which are found in whole grains, beans, legumes, fruits, and vegetables.

Sugar is best obtained from fruits and certain vegetables, because they provide vitamins, minerals, and fiber, rather than from foods high in refined sugars (such as commercial baked goods), which add nothing but calories and may also be high in fat. While there is no evidence that too much sugar, refined or otherwise, will lead to high blood sugar (hyperglycemia), glucose intolerance, or diabetes, it may contribute to obesity, which is a risk factor for diabetes and heart disease.

Starches, having suffered for many years from an image problem, are finally being recognized as mainstays of a healthy diet. No longer considered lowly peasant food (or worse, fattening!), they now appear in the trendiest restaurants in innovative dishes drawn from a multitude of cuisines. The public is coming to recognize that potatoes, breads, beans, rice dishes, and pastas are actually relatively low in calories for the amount of satiety (the feeling of fullness) they offer. Their poor reputation has come from the fact that we have traditionally prepared and eaten them with butter, cream sauces, and cheese.

Complex carbohydrates should be represented in the diet in more servings per day—6 to 11—than any other category of food. Fortunately, they come in great variety and tend to be delicate in taste, so they lend themselves to the addition of herbs, spices, and other ingredients that heighten flavor and texture.

Fiber, or roughage, is a type of carbohydrate that is not broken down by the body during digestion. It can be divided into two types, soluble and insoluble, and a healthy diet should have some of each. (See box, "Sources of Dietary Fiber.") Soluble fibers—such as pectin, guar (a common thickening agent), and the fibers found in barley, oat bran, legumes, and dried beans—are those that mix with water to become a gummy gel. (Oatmeal is a good example of a soluble fiber.) Research suggests that soluble fiber may help lower the level of cholesterol, especially low-density-lipoprotein (LDL) cholesterol, in the blood. A diet that is high in complex carbohydrates and fiber and in which about one-third of the fiber is soluble has been shown in several studies to lower insulin requirements and improve blood-sugar control in some diabetics.

Insoluble fibers are the parts of plants that do not dissolve in water, but pass through the digestive system essentially intact. In fact, they absorb water and thus produce a soft, bulky stool. These fibers (cellulose is the most common kind) are found in most grains and seeds and in the skins of fruits and vegetables. High-fiber foods typically are low in calories and fat and thus beneficial to people trying to control their weight or their blood cholesterol levels.

Noting that populations that eat a diet high in insoluble fiber have low rates of colon cancer, some scientists believe that insoluble fiber may play a role in reducing the risk of this type of cancer. Although there is no consensus on this, there is agreement that

---

Sources of Dietary Fiber

High in soluble fiber	High in insoluble fiber
Apples	Blackberries
Barley	Graham crackers
Beans	Kidney beans
Broccoli	Lima beans
Cabbage	Parsnips
Carrots	Pears
Corn	Pinto beans
Oat bran	Strawberries
Oats	Wheat bran
Peas	White beans
Plums	Whole grain bread
Potatoes	
Psyllium	
Rice bran	
Tangerines	
Unprocessed wheat bran	

insoluble fiber helps prevent constipation and, by promoting a feeling of fullness, may aid in weight control.

PROTEIN

Protein is the key element in the body's metabolic processes. It is vital to the growth and maintenance of tissues that make up the brain, muscles, connective tissue, skin, hair, blood, and organs, and to the production of infection-fighting cells and antibodies.

Because protein is so essential to life, the body has developed a unique system for recycling it. The proteins in the body are constantly being turned over and broken down, and the end products excreted. When protein is consumed in the proper amounts it is broken down by the body to provide new building blocks, called amino acids, for the body's own proteins. However, when more protein is eaten than is necessary for this replacement process, the excess amino acids are used as fuel or stored as fat.

There are 20 kinds of amino acids, and the body can produce 11 of them. The remaining nine, known as the "essential" amino acids, must be obtained from food. Most of the protein from animal sources—meat, poultry, fish, and diary products—is "complete"—that is, it contains all nine essential amino acids in the proper proportions. In contrast, vegetable sources of protein are incomplete—they lack certain essential amino acids. Strict vegetarians can nevertheless get the full complement of amino acids by combining legumes with grains, nuts, or seeds. Rice with beans and pasta with peas are good combinations.

It was once assumed that because protein is so vital to supporting the maintenance of the body, the higher the protein content, the better the diet. Now, however, it is recognized that excess protein is not risk-free. A high-protein diet makes the kidney work harder to excrete urea, the end product of protein-amino-acid breakdown. The kidneys work at full capacity after a high-protein meal, which a normal kidney can handle without difficulty. People with diabetes mellitus, especially insulin-dependent diabetics, are prone to kidney disease, and the progression of this disease may be slowed by a diet very low in protein.

FAT

Although fats have taken on a villainous role in the minds of many people, they are essential in small amounts to promote growth in children, for energy reserves, to carry vitamins A, D, E, and K in the blood-stream, and to manufacture prostaglandins, sex hormones, and cell membranes. They also keep skin from getting too dry, and in food they add flavor, texture, and aroma. They help promote a feeling of fullness (although the reason for this is not clearly understood) and keep the feeling of hunger from returning as quickly as it does after protein and carbohydrate meals.

Fats are part of the broad category of lipids, which includes fatty acids, triglycerides, sterols, cholesterol, and other substances not soluble in water. Dietary fats, as well as oils (which are a form of fat), can be classified as saturated, nonsaturated, or polyunsaturated. Most fat-containing foods, even those such as oil that are 100 percent fat, contain a mixture of these three types.

Saturated fat interferes with the removal of cholesterol from the blood and thus has the effect of raising the levels of serum cholesterol—the cholesterol circulating in the bloodstream. This happens because saturated fat appears to curtail the entry of the cholesterol-carrying low-density lipoproteins (LDLs) into the cells. When they do not get enough LDL cholesterol, the cells (especially those in the liver) make their own. The excess production is returned to the bloodstream, raising serum cholesterol levels.

Saturated fats, which can also serve as a precursor to cholesterol, have a greater effect on raising serum cholesterol than dietary cholesterol itself. In contrast, monounsaturated and polyunsaturated fats help lower the amount of total cholesterol in the blood by lowering LDL-cholesterol, although polyunsaturates also seem to lower HDL (the good cholesterol).

With the exception of the tropical oils—palm, palm kernel, and coconut—saturated fats come from animal sources and tend to be solid at room temperature. The most familiar sources are butter, cheese, and the fat found in red meats. Monounsaturated oils are liquid at room temperature, although they may become solid in the refrigerator. Major sources of monounsaturates include canola, olive, peanut and cashew oils, as well as olives, cashews, peanuts, and peanut products. Polyunsaturated oils, which are liquid even at cold temperatures, include cottonseed, safflower, sunflower, soybean, and corn oil, as well as the oils found in almonds, filberts, and pecans. (See box, "Sources of Fats and Oils.")

Hydrogenation, commonly used in the manufacture of margarine, is a chemical process used to make liquid fats more solid. In doing so, it makes them more saturated. For this reason, scientists once believed that margarines containing large amounts of hydrogenated oils were not as beneficial as softer margar-

YALE UNIVERSITY SCHOOL OF MEDICINE HEART BOOK

Sources of Fats and Oils

Saturated	Mono-unsaturated	Poly-unsaturated
Butter	Avocado	Almonds
Cheese	Canola oil	Corn oil
Chocolate	Cashews	Cottonseed oil
Cocoa butter	Olives	Filbert nuts
Coconut	Olive oil	Fish
Coconut oil	Peanuts	Margarine (most)
Cream	Peanut oil	Mayonnaise
Egg yolk	Peanut butter	(commercially
Hydrogenated		made)
oil		Pecans
Lard		Safflower oil
Meat		Salad dressing
Milk		Soybean oil
Palm oil		Sunflower oil
Poultry		Walnuts
Vegetable		
shortening		

ines. As analysis of fatty acids has become more sophisticated, researchers have come to realize that hydrogenation changes some oils, such as corn oil, to stearic acid, the one form of saturated fat that does not raise serum cholesterol. Thus, the type of oil used in margarine has become more important than the relative hardness or softness of the margarine. Corn, safflower, and soybean oil margarines are all good choices.

In recent years, Americans have been eating less saturated fat, but they are also consuming an unprecedented amount of polyunsaturated oils. Few populations have ever eaten as much polyunsaturated oil as we currently do. Some studies have raised concern that excessive consumption of polyunsaturates could suppress the immune system and raise the risks of cancer and gallstones, but this has not been proved. At present, the benefits of a diet higher in polyunsaturated fats than in saturated fats seem clearly to outweigh the risks. Nevertheless, other research has shown that monounsaturates may be better than polyunsaturates in conserving "good" high-density-lipoprotein (HDL) cholesterol while lowering low-density-lipoprotein (LDL) cholesterol. Olive oil has traditionally been consumed in large quantities, without any known adverse effects, in Italy, Spain, and Greece, where death rates from coronary artery disease are lower than in the United States. However, that does not mean that oils high in monounsaturates should be used to excess. Because high total fat intake—not just excessive saturated fat—is a risk factor for coronary artery disease, the goal is to lower the total intake of fat, not simply to replace saturated fat with other forms of fat. Instead, complex carbohydrates are the best substitution for saturated fat in the diet.

Finally, fat seems to play a unique role in weight maintenance, regardless of calorie level. It was once believed that "a calorie is a calorie" and that the most important factor in weight reduction was the total amount of calories consumed. A number of studies now show that not all calories are created equal, at least as far as fat calories are concerned. A person will lose weight faster on a low-fat, high-carbohydrate diet than on a high-fat diet of the same number of calories. This seems to be because the body metabolizes fat differently from protein and carbohydrates. Some studies, for example, have shown that about 25 percent of calories from carbohydrates are burned by the body in the process of converting them for storage as fat tissue. Only about 3 percent of fat calories are burned in the metabolic process that converts them to body fat, so more is left to store.

YALE DIETARY RECOMMENDATIONS

The Yale Nutrition Services recommendations are based on the principles of variety, balance, and moderation. No individual food is prohibited, but some categories of food are stressed over others. By choosing a variety of foods in each category, individuals will be able to meet the recommended dietary allowances (RDAs) for vitamins and minerals without the need for supplements. Compared to the typical American intake, the recommended diet contains fewer calories and less total fat, saturated fat, cholesterol, salt, and alcohol, and slightly less protein. The percentage of complex carbohydrates and fiber is increased, with the addition of more fruits, vegetables, cereals, grains, and legumes.

The recommendations call for an overall daily intake measured in percentages of total calories as follows:

- At least 55 percent carbohydrates
- Less than 30 percent fat, including:
  less than 10 percent saturated fat
  10–15 percent monounsaturated fat
  up to 10 percent polyunsaturated fat
- 15–20 percent protein

In addition:

- Cholesterol intake should be no more than 250 milligrams a day.

- Sodium intake should be 1,000 to 3,000 milligrams a day.

IMPLEMENTING THE DIET

DETERMINING CALORIE NEEDS

Implementing the diet requires doing some calculations. Although this may seem a complex process, it only has to be done once. Once the daily fat grams are determined, it's only a matter of keeping track of these. And after a short while on a low-fat diet, as an individual begins to develop a sense of how many grams are in various foods, even counting the grams becomes unnecessary.

Since the recommendations listed above are based on total calorie intake, the first task is to figure out how many calories are needed daily. This number depends on height, weight, gender, age, activity level, and whether the goal is to maintain or lose weight. The first task is to calculate ideal body weight using Table 5.1 or part A of the box "Calculate Your Calorie Quota." The reason for the gender difference is that men tend to have a lower percentage of body fat (up to 20 percent is considered acceptable) than women (up to 25 percent is acceptable) and so have a greater percentage of muscle. Since muscle weighs more than fat, men tend to weigh more, inch for inch.

Once a desirable weight level is determined, calorie needs can be figured by calculating the basal metabolic rate (the amount of energy needed just to breathe and carry out bodily functions such as digestion) and then adding calories according to a daily activity level. An easier way is to use the formula in part C of the box "Calculate Your Calorie Quota." Individuals who need to lose or gain weight should also use part D. (Additional information on weight loss appears at the end of this section.)

Table 5.1
Ideal (Desirable) Weight

| Height[1] | | MEN Weight (lb)[1] | | | WOMEN Weight (lb)[1] | | |
Feet	Inches	Average	Acceptable weight		Average	Acceptable weight	
4	10				102	92	119
4	11				104	94	122
5	0				107	96	125
5	1				110	99	128
5	2	123	112	141	113	102	131
5	3	127	115	144	116	105	134
5	4	130	118	148	120	108	138
5	5	133	121	152	123	111	142
5	6	136	124	156	128	114	146
5	7	140	128	161	132	118	150
5	8	145	132	166	136	122	154
5	9	149	136	170	140	126	158
5	10	153	140	174	144	130	163
5	11	158	144	179	148	134	168
6	0	162	148	184	152	138	173
6	1	166	152	189			
6	2	171	156	194			
6	3	176	160	199			
6	4	181	164	204			

Sources: Obesity in America, Guidelines for Body Weight. Public Health Service, NIH 79-359. Dept. of Health, Education, and Welfare, 1979.
[1]Height without shoes, weight without clothes.

Calculate Your Calorie Quota

Determining Your Caloric Needs

The following is a method of roughly estimating caloric needs for healthy, nonpregnant adults 18–50 years old.

A. Calculate your ideal body weight.

Height: _____ feet _____ inches

Women: Allow 100 pounds for first 5 feet of height
      plus 5 pounds for each additional inch

Ideal body weight _____

Men: Allow 106 pounds for first 5 feet of height
      plus 6 pounds for each additional inch

Ideal body weight _____

Example:

Woman 5'2"

        100

+ _____   +10

        110

Man 5'7"

        106

        +42

        148

B. Classify yourself by life-style and activity level.

Sedentary _____   Active _____   Very Active _____

C. Determine your energy needs.

Multiply your ideal body weight by your activity level:

Sedentary = 13   Active = 15   Very Active = 17

_____ X _____ = _____ calories/day
   (Ideal body weight)   (Activity level)

D. Adjust for weight gain or weight loss.

_____ − 500   = _____ To LOSE 1 pound a week
   (Calories from section C)

_____ + 500   = _____ To GAIN 1 pound a week

E. DAILY CALORIC GOAL = _____ Calories

FIGURING FAT GRAMS

Once caloric intake has been determined, the next step is to figure the appropriate number of grams of fat to average per day. Fats, as well as proteins and carbohydrates, are usually listed in grams on packaged foods (there are about 28 grams to 1 ounce). There are about 4 calories in every gram of protein or carbohydrate, 7 in each gram of alcohol, and 9 in each gram of fat. So gram for gram, fats have more than twice the calories of carbohydrates or proteins.

The percentage figures in the dietary recommendations are based solely on the caloric contributions of various foods, not their weight or volume. To understand the difference, consider a certain type of ham that claims to be 95 percent fat-free and has 128 calories in a serving of 100 grams (3.5 ounces). That means that in 100 grams it has 5 grams of fat and 95 grams of other ingredients (water, protein, carbohydrates). Thus the claim is true—only 5 percent of the weight comes from fat. But since each gram of fat is 9 calories, 45 of the 128 calories—or 35 percent—comes from fat. Table 5.2 shows how many total grams of fat and grams of saturated fat are appropriate for a given calorie level. Alternatively, take the number of daily calories, drop the final zero, and divide by 3 to get total fat grams; divide by 3 again to get saturated fat.

RECOMMENDED SERVINGS AND PORTION SIZES

Although ultimately individuals will need to consider their average fat-gram allowance in choosing what to eat, most people find it difficult to make the leap from fat grams to menus. An easier way to develop an eating plan is to think in terms of servings per day. Generally, to follow a low-fat, high-carbohydrate diet and still get sufficient calories and nutrients (vitamins

Table 5.2
Maximum Daily Fat Intake by Calorie Level

Total calorie level (calories/day)	Maximum total fat (grams/day)	Maximum saturated fat (grams/day)
1,000	33	11
1,200	40	13
1,400	47	15
1,600	53	17
1,800	60	20
2,000	67	22
2,200	73	24
2,400	80	26
2,600	87	28
2,800	93	30
3,000	100	32

and minerals) an individual should have the following each day:

- Three to five servings of vegetables, including at least one leafy green vegetable and one yellow or orange one. (One serving is 1 cup raw or ½ cup cooked.)

- Two to four servings of fruit. (One serving equals one piece of medium-sized fresh fruit or ½ cup juice or canned fruit.)

- Six to 11 servings of breads, cereals, pasta, rice, dried peas or beans. (One serving equals a slice of bread, 1 cup dry cereal or popcorn, or ½ cup cooked cereal, pasta, rice, dried peas, or beans.)

- Two servings (three for pregnant or breast-feeding women) of skim or 1 percent fat milk and low-fat or nonfat dairy products. (One serving equals 8 ounces of milk or yogurt, 1 ounce of a hard cheese containing less than 5 grams of fat, ⅓ cup of cottage cheese.)

- Two servings or less of lean, well-trimmed beef, veal, lamb, pork, skinless poultry, or fish; poultry and fish should be favored over meat. (One serving equals 3 ounces cooked weight.) Or substitute nuts, dried peas, beans, lentils (1 cup serving equals 2 to 3 ounces of meat, fish, or poultry) or peanut butter (4 tablespoons equal 2 ounces of meat, fish, or poultry).

- Five to eight servings of margarine or polyunsaturated or monounsaturated oils (one serving equals 1 *teaspoon*).

The following are exceptions:

- Egg whites are unlimited; egg yolks should be limited to three or four a week, including those used in cooking and baking.

- Shrimp and lobster are low in fat, but somewhat higher in cholesterol than other fish and shellfish, and should be limited to one serving a week.

- Organ meats are high in cholesterol and should be eaten only occasionally. Liver, however, is an excellent source of vitamins and iron (especially important for premenopausal women) and is recommended about once a month.

The spread in the number of servings accounts for a difference in total caloric intake. Thus, while everyone should have at least six servings from the bread and cereal group, 11 servings may only be appropriate for a 6-foot male in his 20s who is not obese. Some people, once they recognize that fish and chicken are more healthful than fatty red meat and that olive oil is better than butter, go overboard and begin to eat the "good" foods in unlimited quantities. Paying attention to the number of servings and portion sizes is crucial to having a healthful diet.

The sizes of standard portions—particularly the meat servings—may come as a surprise to some people. Three ounces (cooked weight) of meat is about the size of one's palm or a deck of playing cards, a good deal smaller than the T-bone steaks some restaurants routinely serve. On the other hand, some individuals may be daunted by the idea of three to five servings of vegetables. These add up quickly, however, as most people serve more than half a cup of an individual vegetable. The book *Sample Heart-Healthy Menus* gives examples of daily menus ranging from approximately 1,100 to 1,800 calories.

FOODS TO EMPHASIZE

The recommended diet emphasizes complex carbohydrates, fruits, and vegetables, which are rich in vitamins and minerals and high in fiber. Complex carbohydrates come in great variety and include starchy vegetables (potatoes, corn, and green peas), legumes, grains, and nuts and seeds. Legumes, in turn, consist of beans (black, cranberry, fava, kidney, lima, pinto, mung, navy, pea, and soy, among others), peas (black-eyed, chick, cow, field, and split), peanuts, and lentils. Grains include barley, corn, oats, rice, rye, wheat (including bulgur, wheat germ, and sprouts), as well as

Sample Heart-Healthy Menus

DAY 1

Breakfast
4 oz fresh squeezed orange juice
1 banana
1 cup 40% bran flakes
4 oz 1% milk
coffee

Lunch
1 cup vegetable medley soup
3 oz lean hamburger on whole wheat bun with lettuce, tomato, Bermuda onion slices and ketchup
1 medium baked apple with cinnamon
8 oz sparkling water with slice of lime

Snack
3 vanilla wafers
club soda with lemon

Dinner
½ cup fresh garden salad with 1 tablespoon Dijon vinaigrette dressing
3 oz chicken piccata
1 medium baked potato with fresh chives and 1 tsp margarine
½ cup steamed fresh green beans with dill
1 peach half with 2 tbsp raspberries

Day's total:

Calories	1521	% of calories
Carbohydrates	222 gm	56
Protein	74 gm	19
Fat	44 gm	25

DAY 2

Breakfast
4 oz fresh apple juice
1 cup raisin bran cereal
8 oz 1% milk
herbal tea with 1 tbsp honey

Lunch
2 oz tuna fish salad
2 slices whole grain bread
4 carrot sticks
4 celery sticks
2 tbsp herb-vegetable yogurt dip
3 fig bars
1 cup 1% milk

Snack
1 oz pretzel sticks
8 oz lemon/lime seltzer

Dinner
¾ cup linguini
3 shrimp Fra Diavolo
1 slice Italian bread
½ cup steamed broccoli with lemon
poached pear half with orange sauce

Day's total:

Calories	1720	% of calories
Carbohydrates	278 gm	63
Protein	67 gm	15
Fat	42 gm	22

DAY 3

Breakfast
1 cup oatmeal
1 tbsp raisins
1 tbsp brown sugar
½ whole grain English muffin
1 tbsp raspberry preserves
1 cup 1% milk
coffee

Lunch
1 cup hearty minestrone soup
2 oz honey roasted turkey
1 slice rye bread
2 tsp mayonnaise
¼ cup bean sprouts
4 celery sticks
¾ cup orange sherbet
iced tea with lemon

Dinner
3 oz poached salmon with lemon and dill marinade
¾ cup brown rice
¾ cup baked hubbard squash
1 tsp brown sugar
2 tsp margarine
½ cup fresh hot strawberry and rhubarb compote
1 cup 1% milk

Day's total:

Calories	1843	% of calories
Carbohydrates	271 gm	58
Protein	77 gm	16
Fat	55 gm	26

DAY 4 (Weekend)

Brunch
8 oz fresh squeezed orange juice
1 Belgian waffle
2 tbsp boysenberry syrup
1 poached egg
1 cup fresh fruit medley
coffee with 1% milk

Snack
3 oat-bran graham crackers
1 medium fresh peach
8 oz sparkling water with lime

Dinner
2 oz chicken stir-fried with
1¾ cup carrots, broccoli, snow peas, water chestnuts, and scallions
¾ cup whole wheat angel hair pasta
1 cup watercress and cherry tomato salad
1 tbsp herbed vinaigrette dressing
½ cup mandarin orange sections
iced tea with lemon

Day's total:

Calories	1137	% of calories
Carbohydrates	168 gm	57
Protein	48 gm	16
Fat	35 gm	27

flours and cereals made from these grains. Nuts (almonds, Brazil nuts, cashews, filberts, pecans, and walnuts, among others) and seeds (pumpkin, sunflower, and sesame) are carbohydrates that, like legumes and grains, are high in protein. Because they contain more fat, nuts and seeds should be used in smaller quantities than the other complex carbohydrates.

Combining any of the legumes with any of the grains, nuts, or seeds produces the complete array of essential amino acids and thus provides all the protein necessary for a healthful diet. Alternatively, grains can be combined with nuts or seeds. Adding a small amount of a nonfat or low-fat dairy product (such as milk, cheese, or yogurt) to legumes, grains, nuts, or seeds will also satisfy protein requirements.

Other good, relatively low-fat sources of protein include fish, poultry (except duck and goose) without its skin and fat, lean red meat (beef, veal, lamb, and pork), and low-fat or nonfat dairy products. Fish, poultry, or meatless meals should be substituted for meat several times a week. The growing consumer market for fish has made it possible to find fresh or flash-frozen fish thousands of miles from their source. If possible, a variety of fish should be chosen. The more fatty fish, such as salmon, mackerel, herring, rainbow trout, whitefish, and striped bass, are high in omega-3 fatty acids, a form of polyunsaturated fat that is chemically different from the omega-6 fatty acids predominant in vegetable oils. Omega-3 fatty acids may lower blood levels of triglycerides and very-low density lipoproteins (VLDLs). Less oily, milder-tasting fish such as flounder, haddock, cod, and sole are much lower in omega-3 fatty acids, but they are still beneficial, because they are low in fat and cholesterol. Like oily fish, they are also high in protein, zinc, and B vitamins, especially niacin and B_6. Shellfish, while somewhat higher in cholesterol than fin fish, are still moderate in cholesterol and low in fat and can be eaten once a week.

Although there are other arguments for eliminating meat from the diet, it is not necessary to give up red meat completely to maintain a low-fat eating plan. It is particularly important for children, teenagers, and women of child-bearing age to consume foods that are good sources of iron. These include fish, leafy green vegetables, and iron-enriched breads and cereals, but the most concentrated source is still lean red meat. It is possible, although it sometimes requires the use of supplements, to get sufficient iron without red meat, but even a few ounces of meat a week provide enough to meet iron requirements for these groups.

For those who want to continue eating meat, the best way to use it is as a side dish, rather than as the main component of a meal. For example, dinner might be couscous (a Middle Eastern pasta whose grains are very fine, smaller than grains of rice) tossed with herbs, carrots, broccoli, zucchini, and mushroom and some julienned strips of lean beef.

Lean cuts of beef include round tip, top loin, top round, eye of round, tenderloin, top sirloin, rump, and flank (trimmed). Lean pork cuts include tenderloin, sirloin roast, and loin chops. The leg is the leanest cut of lamb, and all cuts of veal are low in fat except the breast.

Skim or 1 percent fat milk, buttermilk, skim milk cheeses and yogurt, and margarine should be used in place of whole milk, high-fat cheeses, cream, and butter. The number of new *nonfat* products—cottage cheese, yogurt, frozen yogurt, mock sour cream, and mozzarella and ricotta cheeses, among others—seems to grow by the month. These dairy products are also high in calcium, which is important for children, teenagers, pregnant and nursing women, and premenopausal women in general (to help prevent the bone-thinning disease osteoporosis).

FOODS AND BEVERAGES TO USE IN MODERATION

Caffeine-containing beverages, especially coffee, have been the object of much study, and the results have been conflicting and confusing. Some of the studies showing that coffee drinking increases the risk of heart disease have turned out to be poorly designed (they didn't consider the effects of tobacco in coffee drinkers who also smoke, for example, or they used boiled coffee, not generally drunk by Americans). A careful, large-scale study of more than 45,500 men reported in the *New England Journal of Medicine* in 1990 now seems to have satisfied the critics. It found that coffee drinking, even at levels of 6 or more cups a day, was not associated with an increased risk of heart disease or stroke. In fact, the only increased risk seemed to be with 4 or more cups a day of *decaffeinated* coffee. In any case, most experts feel that the key for healthy adults without symptoms is still moderation—no more than 5 cups a day. For those in whom caffeine increases anxiety, exacerbates arrhythmias, or produces other undesirable symptoms, even 1 or 2 cups may be too many.

Moderation is also the watchword for adults who drink alcoholic beverages. While *light* drinking may raise protective HDL cholesterol levels, excessive alcohol consumption can raise blood pressure and triglyceride levels. It can also cause a type of heart disease known as alcoholic cardiomyopathy. The generally accepted recommendation for those who drink is no more than 1 to 2 ounces of ethanol a day. This translates into about 2 glasses of beer or wine or 2 ounces of hard liquor. (For additional information, see Chapter 6.)

The other important reason to limit alcohol consumption is weight control. Each gram of alcohol has 7 calories (there are about 200 calories in an ounce), compared to 4 in carbohydrates or protein. More important, calories from alcohol are considered "empty calories," since they add no nutritive value to the diet. When alcohol is served in a mixed drink, such as a Manhattan or a whiskey sour, the calorie count is even higher.

Foods to use less frequently are those high in cholesterol, such as egg yolks and organ meats, and those high in saturated fat. The list of high-saturated-fat foods is long, but several categories stand out: fried foods, luncheon meats (bologna, salami, liverwurst, etc.), rich, creamy desserts, and many commercial baked goods. Careful shoppers can now find some of the more traditional luncheon meats such as pastrami that are made with turkey instead of pork or beef, but some of these substitutes and virtually all of the originals are high in sodium. (See box, "Smart Substitutions.") Also available are nonfat coffee cakes, nonfat frozen yogurts and low-fat versions of other creamy desserts, and cookies made with unsaturated oils. Many manufacturers have responded to public demand by dropping tropical oils, such as coconut and palm, from their desserts. Food labels that merely say "vegetable oils," however, are suspect, since this broad category includes tropical oils.

Smart Substitutions

	Instead of	Try
Breakfast	Two scrambled eggs	Egg substitute or one whole egg scrambled with one egg white
	Croissant	Bagel
	White toast with butter	Whole-grain toast with margarine or jelly
	Danish pastry	Small bran or blueberry muffin
Lunch	Turkey roll sandwich	Fresh turkey breast sandwich
	Pastrami sandwich	Turkey pastrami or lean roast beef sandwich
	Pepperoni pizza	Plain or vegetable (except eggplant parmesan) pizza
	Oil-packed tuna	Water-packed tuna
	New England clam chowder	Manhattan clam chowder
Dinner	Deep-fried chicken	Oven-crisped chicken
	Roast duck	Roast turkey
	French fries	Baked or boiled potato or rice
	Garlic bread	Bread sticks
Beverages	Whole milk	Skim or 1% milk
	Soft drinks	Seltzer or sparkling water with fruit juice
	Chocolate malted	Chocolate milk shake with skim milk
Snacks	Potato chips	Pretzels
	Oil-popped popcorn	Air-popped popcorn
	Molasses cookies	Ginger snaps
Dessert	Devil's food cake	Angel food cake
	Ice cream pop	Fudge pop
	Ice cream	Ice milk
	Frozen yogurt	Frozen nonfat yogurt
	Sherbet	Fruit ice or sorbet
	Apple pie	Baked apple

MAINTAINING DESIRABLE WEIGHT

According to the 1988 Report of the Surgeon General, the more overweight a person is (up to 19 percent above desirable weight), the greater the risk of premature death. Obesity (20 percent or more above ideal weight for a year or more) is a significant risk factor for coronary artery disease. It also raises the risk of a variety of other health problems, including diabetes, hypertension, and even arthritis and back pain. Table 5.1 can be used as a guide for determining whether a person's weight is within, above, or below the desirable range for his or her height. This will help in setting individually tailored weight goals. Particularly for those with known heart disease or any other serious medical problem, it is a good idea to consult a doctor and registered dietitian before beginning a weight loss program.

When weight control experts talk about overweight, they are really talking about "overfat." Because muscle weighs more than fat, a physically fit person who has a greater percentage of body weight as muscle than a sedentary person does can actually weigh more but not be overweight. For this reason, weight tables, while convenient, are not as accurate an indication of whether a person is at his or her ideal weight as are other methods. The simplest of these is the mirror test—if the person looks flabby and fat, chances are he or she is overweight. More elaborate tests include skinfold thickness (measuring body fat with calipers) and underwater weighing.

Individuals can get a general sense of whether they are carrying excess body fat by measuring the fat on the upper arm. Hold the arm out at shoulder level, bend the elbow, and use the thumb and finger of the other hand to gently pinch the flesh on the underside of the upper arm midway between the shoulder and elbow. Remove finger and thumb, keeping them the same distance apart, and measure; anything more than an inch between them is too much.

How excess fat is distributed may also affect the risk of coronary heart disease and other obesity-related diseases. The risk seems to be higher among those who have what is referred to as a male fat-distribution pattern, or an apple, rather than a pear, shape. Apple-shaped people (primarily men and postmenopausal women) tend to carry their excess weight around their waist (the potbelly), while pear-shaped people (primarily premenopausal women) carry their excess weight on the hips, buttocks, and thighs. One explanation for this may be that fat in the abdomen is metabolically more active than fat in other parts of the body. Fatty acids released into the bloodstream when abdominal fat is metabolized find their way into the nearby portal vein, through which they are transported directly to the liver. This in turn stimulates increased cholesterol output.

Hormones seem to control fat distribution, although the tendency toward one pattern or the other is inherited. When estrogen production declines after menopause, women tend to accumulate more abdominal fat and their risk of heart disease rises. A man is at increased risk of heart disease if his waist size exceeds his hip size; for a woman, risk increases if her waist measurement is more than 80 percent of her hip measurement. For example, a woman who has 40-inch hips should not have a waist measurement of more than 32 inches in order to be in the low-risk category. Although nothing can be done to change the inherited fat-distribution pattern, the weight itself can be lost through diet and exercise.

Body weight is governed by a simple equation. The excess calories in the food eaten, minus the calories burned during exercise, equal the extra weight that the body will accumulate. (See box, "The Caloric Equation.") It is best to tackle both sides of the equation at the same time, eating the same varied, healthful diet advocated in the previous section, but using smaller portions, while exercising with more regularity and vigor. Exercise not only consumes calories in and of itself, it also revs up the body's metabolic rate so that calories are expended ("burned") at a higher rate, even at rest. This helps reverse the slowdown in the body's metabolic "burn rate" that can result from eating less. Not only does exercise aid in losing extra pounds and maintaining ideal weight, it also may be an independent protective factor against coronary artery disease. (See Chapter 7.)

People who are overweight despite eating a healthful, low-fat diet can achieve and maintain an appropriate weight level simply by exercising more and eating less of each food group, without eliminating anything. They can continue to eat the variety of foods they favored all along, but in smaller amounts. The majority of people who are overweight, however, are still eating a diet with excess fat—especially saturated fat. Simply by concentrating on eating less fat, they will consume fewer total calories.

Losing weight is easier than keeping the weight off. All too often, people resort to their old behavior (overeating and inactivity) and gain back their weight—and then some—after "dieting." The regained weight tends to represent excess body fat rather than muscle. When people allow their weight

The Caloric Equation

You gain one pound of body fat if you consume 3,500 calories more than you expend. If you eat all of the following, you will consume 3,500 calories: a Big Mac, large order of french fries, a small Coca-Cola, 1 cup Häagen-Dazs ice cream, 1 cup honey-roasted cashews and peanuts, and 3 beers.

Conversely, you can lose a pound of body fat by walking 5 miles each day for a week, provided you do not increase your food intake.

to go up and down like a yo-yo, they end up flabbier than when they started. Even people who are not chronic dieters may fall victim to this yo-yo syndrome, as winter inactivity and overeating often cause yearly weight cycling: up in the fall, down in the spring.

To lose weight and maintain an ideal level, individuals have to concentrate on the long haul. The most important factor in effecting a permanent change is changing behavior with respect to food as well as activity. Favorite foods do not have to be eliminated entirely, even if they are high in fat. In fact, cutting out these foods entirely leads to cravings and often results in binges. Instead, the goal is to learn to enjoy them sparingly—for instance, savoring one chocolate chip cookie instead of devouring an entire jar of them at one sitting.

Although all the information needed for successful weight loss is contained here, some people find they do better in a structured program where they get peer support or are accountable to a health professional or group leader. In choosing such a program there are two red flags to watch for. One is a diet program that does not emphasize the crucial role of regular exercise in weight control. The other is any regimen that seems monotonous and does not allow a variety of foods. Drastic, formula-type or short-term diets that are restricted to a narrow range of foods may produce immediate weight loss, but they are rarely successful in long-term weight management. In addition, such regimens promote the breakdown of lean muscle tissue, including heart muscle, at least for the first few days of the diet. This happens because it takes the body longer to mobilize its fat stores for energy than it does to cannibalize its own protein.

In addition, the body tries to compensate for a starvation diet by lowering its metabolic rate. Thus, after a low-calorie diet, the body can get by on fewer calories than before. For example, a person who previously needed 1,800 calories a day to maintain normal weight may now need only 1,500 calories after a short–term drastic diet. Consequently, this person will gain weight even if he or she consumes only 1,800 calories.

These low-calorie diets also provoke a feeling of deprivation, and for that reason they almost invariably backfire. Even if people manage to take off their unwanted weight using such diets, they often reward themselves after the diet is over by overindulging in the formerly forbidden foods and regaining the shed pounds. Furthermore, many of these diets are so low in calories (below 1,200) that they cannot be nutritionally complete.

A slow, steady weight loss—no more than 1 or 2 pounds a week—is easiest to maintain. In fact, we feel so strongly about this that when participants in our diet groups consistently lose more than 2 pounds a week, they are dropped from the program because they are merely perpetuating unproductive behavior.

The best diet, then, for losing weight and maintaining the loss is one that can be enjoyed indefinitely. Like a successful exercise program, a healthier diet should be built into each individual's daily routine. The following section gives tips for translating the dietary recommendations into a daily routine.

PRACTICAL TIPS

SHOPPING FOR FOOD

It remains generally true that people can achieve a healthier diet by buying fresh food, preparing it themselves, and avoiding prepackaged foods. However, by shopping carefully and especially by reading labels, consumers can find healthful prepared foods. While some manufacturers have responded to public demand with excellent low-fat, nonfat, and low-salt products, others have attempted to exploit consumer interest with deceptive labeling practices. One common ploy, for example, is used by producers of some vegetable oils and peanut butters who proclaim that the products contain no cholesterol. The claim ignores the fact that cholesterol is found only in animal foods, not in vegetable products. The unwary consumer may be led to believe that cholesterol has been specially eliminated from these particular products. The problem is that health claims have become so widespread on product packaging that the uninformed consumer can easily be confused.

New regulations from the Food and Drug Administration (FDA), which take effect in 1993, should end many of these practices. Nutrition labeling will be required for most foods under the jurisdiction of the FDA, although not for foods, notably meat and poultry, that come under the jurisdiction of the U.S. Department of Agriculture. At present the FDA is still developing exact definitions for certain descriptive phrases such as "light" or "lite" (see box, "Food Label Definitions"), setting standards for how nutrition information will be visually interpreted (such as in a bar graph or a pie chart), and making decisions on other issues such as state and federal overlap of regulations.

There are certain standards that manufacturers must follow even now. All canned, frozen, and packaged products (except fresh foods) must list ingredients in descending order according to volume. The only exceptions are certain standardized products, such as ketchup, that meet "standards of identity" set by the FDA. All products containing fat must list the kind of animal or vegetable fat used. Finally, all enriched or fortified foods and those for which the manufacturer makes nutritional claims must carry a nutrition label containing certain facts about the product. These include serving size, number of servings per container, and the amount of carbohydrates, protein, fat, calories, and sodium per serving. In addition, the label must give the percentage of the U.S. Recommended Daily Allowance (more general than the Recommended Dietary Allowance) for protein, vitamin A, vitamin C, thiamin, niacin, riboflavin, calcium, and iron contained in one serving. Saturated fat, polyunsaturated fat, cholesterol, and other items are optional unless the manufacturer makes a specific claim about them (such as that a product is low in cholesterol). Beginning in 1993, saturated fat, cholesterol, sodium, total carbohydrates, complex carbohydrates and sugar, total protein, and dietary fiber must also appear on the food labels. The serving size must be expressed in common household terms (such as ½ cup).

The key items to pay attention to are the serving size, calories, and grams of fat. Some serving sizes listed on labels are unrealistically small in order to make the fat or calories appear low; most are correct, but some are smaller than many people are used to eating (2 teaspoons of peanut butter, for example). Consumers need to keep the serving size in mind when eating, but the purchase decision can be made on the basis of a simple rule of thumb: 3 grams of fat

Food Label Definitions

reduced-calorie Must be one-third lower in calories than the nonmodified food product that it resembles (e.g., reduced-calorie vanilla pudding, 85 calories, versus regular vanilla pudding, 177 calories).

low-calorie One serving supplies no more than 40 calories and contains no more than 4 calories per gram (e.g., low-calorie French dressing, 22 calories, versus regular French dressing, 67 calories).

less or lower cholesterol Cholesterol reduced, but by less than 75 percent (e.g., Butter Blend, 10 mg cholesterol, versus butter, 33 mg cholesterol).

low-cholesterol Less than 20 mg per serving (low-cholesterol gravy, 1 mg cholesterol, versus gravy, 5 mg cholesterol).

no cholesterol Less than 2 mg per serving (egg substitute, 0 mg cholesterol, versus one egg, 274 mg cholesterol).

leaner At least 25 percent less fat than the standard product (e.g., leaner sausage, 12 gm fat, versus regular sausage, 23 gm fat).

extra-lean No more than 5 percent fat (e.g., extra-lean ham, 116 calories, versus regular ham, 192 calories).

light or lite No standardized definition. May refer to color, calories, fat, sodium, or density (light-batter fish fillet, 310 calories, versus crispy fish fillets, 290 calories). Exceptions include light cream, which must contain between 18 and 30 percent fat; fruit canned in light syrup, which is lower in sugar; lite beer, which generally has about ⅓ fewer calories than the regular version of the same brand; and lite salt, which is made with potassium rather than sodium.

natural A food that has been altered as little as possible from the original farm-grown state.

low-sodium Containing 140 mg sodium or less per serving (low-sodium soup, 85 mg, versus regular soup, 920 mg).

very-low-sodium Containing 35 mg sodium or less per serving (e.g., Diet Sprite, 35 mg, versus Diet Pepsi, 67 mg).

sugarless/sugar-free Food does not contain sucrose, but may contain other sugars such as corn syrup, dextrose, levulose, sorbitol, mannitol, maltitol, xylitol, or natural sweeteners (e.g., sugar-free cookies, 25 calories, versus regular cookies, 50 calories).

per 100 calories a serving. At 9 calories a gram, 3 grams would be about 27 calories, or 27 percent of the 100 calories, within the guidelines for total fat. The guidelines are for the entire diet, not each individual food. Nevertheless, it is easy to see that a ½ cup serving of a premium ice cream that can contain 24 grams of fat (depending on brand and flavor) will have to be offset by a lot of steamed vegetables and other low-calorie foods.

When reading labels it may also be helpful to visualize the fat. For example, 5 grams of fat is approximately equal to a pat of butter or margarine or a teaspoon of oil.

PREPARING FOOD

Filling the cupboards and refrigerator with low-fat, low-cholesterol foods is half the battle. The other half is getting them on the table without adding too much fat, while still presenting them in a way the family will enjoy. The first step is to trim any excess fat before cooking. Even lean cuts of meat have exterior fat that can easily be trimmed. With poultry, removing the skin and the fat attached to it cuts the amount of fat to a little less than half. This is fine for most chicken and turkey dishes, but not practical for roasting, as the result is much too dry. In this case, removing the skin before eating is sufficient.

Fat that can't be eliminated before cooking can be drained off afterward. Be sure to drain the excess fat off ground meat before adding other ingredients. Refrigerate soups and stews until the fat congeals on top to make the removal of fat easy before reheating. If time does not allow preparing ahead, use a paper towel to soak up the surface oil or a skimmer to pour it off. A gravy separator (a pitcher with a spout that comes from the bottom) is another handy gadget for removing excess fat.

The second major way to control fat is via the method of cooking. Deep-frying, sautéing, breading and frying, basting with oil, and, with some exceptions, cooking in a casserole are methods that add unnecessary fat. Instead, try broiling, roasting, baking, steaming, poaching, and stir-frying. With stir-frying, use only a little oil and be sure it is very hot, since foods soak up more oil when it is only warm. Blanching vegetables first cuts frying time and thus the amount of oil absorbed. Sautéing is acceptable if a nonstick pan or nonstick vegetable spray is used.

Steaming isn't only for vegetables. Fish lends itself to steaming (a wok with a plate balanced above water level on overturned coffee cups makes an inexpensive

fish steamer). Chicken or fish can be baked in a foil package in the oven, which produces the same effect as steaming. For example, place pieces of chicken breast, seasoned with herbs and spices, in foil along with a selection of vegetables such as onions, mushrooms and zucchini, and perhaps a little white wine, and steam-bake for 20 minutes at 375° F.

Although many cooks like to experiment from time to time, most find that they develop a repertoire of 10 to 20 dishes that are repeated over and over. Perhaps the best way to ease gradually into low-fat eating is to work with family favorites and learn how to modify these recipes rather than to learn a whole new way of cooking.

The three main principles of adapting recipes are reduction, substitution, and modification. Below are some tips for accomplishing this in some American standbys, but any recipe can be modified with a little analysis of its ingredients. Learn to determine why an ingredient is included in a recipe, and it will be easier to find an appropriate substitution or to decide whether it can be reduced or even eliminated. An ingredient may be there primarily to add flavor, or for bulk, texture, moisture, or eye appeal. Crunchy nuts, for example, could be replaced by crunchy celery, jicama, or water chestnuts. Parmesan cheese topping on a casserole gives a flavorful browned appearance, but it can be mixed half and half with nonfat bread crumbs for the same effect. Or eliminate it entirely and mix the bread crumbs with herbs. (Homemade breadcrumbs made in seconds in the blender or food processor are better than commercial ones, which sometimes have fat and sodium added.) Here are some other modifications and cooking tips:

- Steam vegetables with herbs, such as green beans with dill or carrots with basil, rather than adding butter.

- Use puréed potatoes or other vegetables instead of cream to thicken soups and stews. Barley, rice, and orzo can also add thickness to soup. In cream soups, use nonfat dry milk or evaporated skim milk instead of cream.

- Although its primary contribution is flavor, fat is sometimes added for moisture. In this case, fruit or vegetable juice, low-sodium broth, vinegar, wine, or beer can be used instead, depending on the dish.

- Tenderize lean meat by marinating it in herbs mixed with something acidic: tomato juice, citrus juice, vinegar, yogurt, or wine.

- Sugar can be reduced by at least one-third in

baked goods without affecting the final product. Experiment to see if more can be removed.

- Dishes other than baked goods can be sweetened with undiluted frozen apple juice or puréed bananas or pears. Spices such as cinnamon add a sweet taste without calories. Although honey has a few more calories than sugar, it is much sweeter, so less is needed.

- Make mashed potatoes with skim milk or whip them with butter-substitute granules or some of the water in which they were cooked.

- Substitute ground turkey for ground beef and turkey or chicken cutlets for veal.

- Use 3 tablespoons of cocoa powder and 1 tablespoon of polyunsaturated oil in place of each ounce of baking chocolate.

- Try whipping very cold or partially frozen evaporated skim milk in place of heavy cream. (Chill the beaters and bowl in the freezer first.)

- Experiment with nonfat yogurt and light sour cream in place of traditional sour cream. In hot dishes, add 1 teaspoon of cornstarch for every cup of yogurt to keep it from separating on heating. Another sour cream substitute can be made from 1 cup of low-fat cottage cheese beaten with 1 tablespoon of lemon juice and 2 tablespoons of skim milk.

- Use one whole egg plus one white in place of two whole eggs, or use ¼ cup of egg substitute. In some recipes, two egg whites can substitute for a whole egg.

- Cut the amount of meat and increase the amount and variety of vegetables in stews.

- Salt can be eliminated from virtually any dish except yeast breads, in which it is needed to control rising. Since salt is an acquired taste, by gradually restricting it in the diet, it is possible to get used to tasting less and less of it. Herbs, spices, garlic, onions, citrus juices, and vinegars such as fruit or rice vinegars can be used instead to enhance the flavor of many foods. (See Chapter 12 for additional tips.)

- Instead of using a ham bone to add a smoky flavor to pea soup, add a sweet red pepper that has been roasted, slightly charred, and peeled.

For those looking for inspiration, there are a number of good low-fat cookbooks on the market. Ethnic cookbooks, particularly the dozen or so cuisines of the Mediterranean area, offer some excellent choices as well. (See box, "Recommended Cookbooks.")

Recommended Cookbooks

The American Heart Association Cookbook, 5th ed. Times Books, 1991.

The American Heart Association Low-Fat, Low-Cholesterol Cookbook. Times Books, 1989.

Choice for a Healthy Heart by J. C. Piscatella. Workman Publishing, 1987.

Cooking À La Heart by L. Hachfeld, B. Eykyn, and the Mankato Heart Health Program, revised ed. Appletree Press, 1992.

The Fischer/Brown Low Cholesterol Gourmet by L. Fischer and V. Brown. Acropolis Books, 1988.

Fresh Ways with Fish and Shellfish, Pasta, Poultry and Vegetables. Time-Life Healthy Home Cooking Series, 1986.

Jane Brody's Good Food Book. W. W. Norton, 1985.

The Living Heart Diet by M. E. DeBakey, A. M. Gotto, L. W. Scott, and J. P. Foreyt. Raven Press, 1984.

Low Calorie Cooking by J. Shaper. Longmeadow Press, 1987.

Mediterranean Light by M. R. Shulman. Bantam Books, 1989.

EATING AWAY FROM HOME

For more than a decade, Americans have been eating one out of three meals away from home—in restaurants, school or company cafeterias, and fast food outlets. With more and more women joining the work force, this trend can only grow stronger. Those for whom dining out still means a special occasion generally can celebrate without concern about diet. Those who find themselves regularly relying on someone else's menus will need to devise a strategy to stay in control of what they eat.

The strategy starts with choosing a restaurant. It will be easier to find low-fat entrées in a seafood restaurant than in one that specializes in continental cuisine (read heavily sauced). Restaurateurs who pride themselves on offering "family-style service," "overstuffed sandwiches," "he-man portions," or "all you can eat" are less likely to be concerned about nutritional balance. Generally speaking, restaurants that offer mostly freshly prepared dishes rather than mass-precooked, flash-frozen portions can be more flexible. These restaurants are often recognizable by their limited menus. Even if their cuisine tends toward butter and sauces, they are usually willing to offer plain broiled fish, chicken, or lean steak with the sauce served on the side or not at all. If the choice of restaurants is limited by budget, convenience, or dining companions, it is still possible to put together an acceptable meal. The box "Heart-Healthy Selections from Restaurant Menus" suggests dishes to choose and avoid. These tips may also be helpful:

- Do not arrive at the restaurant famished, or virtually everything on the menu will be appealing, making it easy to overorder. Have a small salad, a piece of fruit, soda crackers, or bouillon first.

- It is also a good idea not to arrive early, which increases the temptation to have a drink or a snack while waiting for companions.

- Those who drink alcohol should decide beforehand to skip it, limit it to one drink (perhaps a white wine spritzer or light beer), or have an after-dinner drink in place of dessert. Besides adding empty calories, alcohol may increase appetite or affect the resolve to use moderation in the rest of the meal. Sipping a spicy Bloody Mary mix without the vodka, a fruit juice spritzer, nonalcoholic beer, or sparkling water with a slice of lime will still provide the opportunity to relax and ease into the meal.

- If nuts or chips are provided with cocktails, ask the waiter or waitress to stand by, remove one or two, and then have the dish taken away.

- If possible, decide what to order before arriving at the restaurant. When this is not possible—or for diners who prefer to remain flexible—à la carte choices are best. Complete dinners and fixed-price offerings usually have more courses than are necessary.

- Be the first in the group to order to avoid the temptation to be influenced by the choices of others.

- Skip the appetizer or look for fruit or vegetable juice, clear soup or consommé, or fruit. (Vegetable juice, broth, bouillon, and consommé are somewhat high in sodium, which may be a problem for some people with heart failure or uncontrolled high blood pressure.) If fruit isn't offered as an appetizer, check the dessert column.

- Do not make assumptions about unfamiliar dishes, but ask how they are made. Fish stew may conjure up a picture of bouillabaisse in a tomato-flecked broth, but turn out to be more like lobster Newburg, with a thick creamy sauce.

- Be creative with the menu categories. In place of an entrée, have two appetizers, or an appetizer, soup, and salad, or an appetizer and a side dish, or soup and a half order (pasta is often available in half orders), or have an appetizer and split an entrée.

- Do not be afraid to ask for a special order. Many restaurants are happy to honor requests such as to broil rather than fry, to serve the sauce on the side, and to use margarine rather than butter. Even better, ask what the chef can do for someone who prefers a low-fat dinner. Often there are some excellent choices that don't appear on the menu, and some chefs take it as a challenge to come up with something appetizing and nutritious. Nevertheless, find out what the "something" is, because chefs do not necessarily know about nutrition.

- The endless bread basket (or more specifically, the butter dish) is a common problem. If the bread is robust and crusty, learn to savor its flavor alone. If it is cottony and tasteless, it is better skipped than slathered with butter. In any case, have the basket removed when everyone has been served.

- Ask to have a sprinkle of lemon juice on the salad or bottles of vinegar and oil put on the table. If the house dressing is really tempting, order it on the side. Then try this trick: Dip the fork in the dressing, then spear the lettuce.

- Learn to eyeball appropriate portion sizes and do not feel obliged to finish everything. The palm of the hand or a deck of playing cards approximates 3 ounces of meat. If the portion is too large, share it, leave half of it, or ask for the rest in a doggy bag. (Put the leftovers in the freezer at home immediately to avoid the temptation to snack later.)

- To slow down eating, choose foods that require work—unfilleted fish, crab legs, artichokes. If chopsticks are available, use them.

- If a rich dessert is an absolute must, split it with a companion or plan for it by keeping the rest of the meal light.

- Relax and savor every bite of the food—its sight, smell, texture, and taste.

Heart-Healthy Selections from Restaurant Menus

CHINESE

Choose	Limit
Steamed dumplings	Spare ribs
Hot and sour soup[1]	Egg rolls
Wonton soup[1]	Fried noodles or wonton
Stir-fried seafood, chicken, or bean curd with vegetables	Lobster sauce (contains egg yolk)
Steamed whole fish	Sweet and sour pork
Moo goo gai pan (chicken)	Egg foo yung
	Cold noodles in sesame sauce

FAST FOOD

Choose	Limit
Salad bar (dressing on side)	French fries
Regular single hamburger	Double hamburgers, cheeseburgers
Rare roast beef	Fried fish
Grilled chicken sandwich	Chicken nuggets
Baked potato (1 T. topping)	Fried chicken
	Ham and egg sandwich
	Thick shakes
Hot cakes or waffle (syrup, no butter)	
Coffee, tea, or diet drinks	

FRENCH

Choose	Limit
Bouillabaisse	Pâté
Coq au vin	Béchamel sauce
Steamed mussels	Béarnaise sauce
Fish en papillote	Au gratin dishes
Ratatouille	

GREEK

Choose	Limit
Tzatziki (cucumbers and yogurt)	Taramasalata
Greek salad[1]	Lamb (unless made from the leg)
Plaki (fish with tomatoes, onions, and garlic)	Dishes made with phyllo dough
Shish kebab	

INDIAN

Choose	Limit
Naan and chapati (breads)	Paratha and poori (breads)
Vegetable curry	Ghee (clarified butter)
Biryani and pilaf (rice dishes)	
Tandoori fish or chicken	
Raita	

ITALIAN

Choose	Limit
Minestrone[1]	Fettucine Alfredo or Carbonara
Escarole soup[1]	Tuna in oil
Linguine with red clam sauce	Veal scallopine
Pasta primavera	Veal parmigiana
Veal marsala	Zabaglione
Chicken or fish in wine or tomato sauce	Cream-filled desserts

JAPANESE

Choose	Limit
Sushi	Tempura
Sashimi	
Miso[1]	
Pickled vegetables[1]	
Chicken teriyaki[1]	
Yakimono (broiled)[1]	
Sukiyaki[1]	

MEXICAN

Choose	Limit
Salsa	Flour tortillas (made with lard)
Guacamole (without sour cream)	Refried beans (usually made with lard)
Black bean soup	Nachos topped with cheese
Beef, seafood, or chicken	Tacos, chimichangas, and other fried tortillas
Tostados or fajitas	Nachos topped with cheese
Tamales	
Seviche	
Rice and beans	
Fish Veracruzana (with tomatoes, peppers, and olives)[1]	

MIDDLE EASTERN

Choose	Limit
Mussels or grape leaves stuffed with rice	Fatty lamb or beef casseroles
Couscous with chicken or vegetables	
Hot bulgur or tabouli	
Shish kabob	
Imam bayildi (eggplant and tomato casserole)	

(continued)

[1]Moderate to high in sodium.

Heart-Healthy Selections from Restaurant Menus (continued)

SMORGASBORD (BUFFET)		STEAKHOUSES	
Choose	**Limit**	**Choose**	**Limit**
Tossed salad (dressing on side)	Mayonnaise-based salads	Steamed or broiled fish, if available	T-bone steak
Fruit salad	Cheese platter	London broil	Surf and turf
Vinegar-based coleslaw	Potatoes au gratin	Filet mignon	Porterhouse steak
Pickled fish[1]	Casseroles	Baked potato (limit butter)	Fried potatoes
Roast turkey breast	Stews		Onion rings
Lean roast beef	Pies and pastries		
Baked or boiled potato			
Steamed vegetables			

[1]Moderate to high in sodium.

CHAPTER 6

SMOKING, ALCOHOL, AND DRUGS

RAPHAEL ZAHLER, M.D., Ph.D.
CAROLINE PISELLI, R.N., M.B.A.

INTRODUCTION

Of all the risk factors for heart disease, the ones over which an individual has the most control are those related to "bad habits," namely the use or abuse of tobacco (especially cigarettes), alcohol, and illicit drugs. Numerous studies show that people who use these substances have a marked increase in risk of developing heart disease. Still, there is heartening news for longtime smokers, drug users, and heavy drinkers who quit: The increased risks can be lowered and even eliminated.

The benefits of controlling or, better still, eliminating these risk factors can be dramatic. In fact, smoking cessation is the single most effective step that smokers can take to lower their risk of heart disease. Former smokers live significantly longer than do continuing smokers, and their reduced incidence of heart disease is one of the major reasons.

This chapter reviews the dangers of smoking, drinking, and using illicit drugs. The ways in which these habits raise the risk of heart disease and methods for quitting or moderating consumption are also discussed. The chapter also reiterates a key theme, namely, that quitting can lower the risk of the development and progression of heart disease, even after decades of use.

SMOKING

Cigarette smoking is by far the leading cause of premature or preventable deaths in the United States. And cancer is not, as many people believe, the only risk of smoking. According to a 1990 report by the Surgeon General, tobacco use is responsible for more than 350,000 deaths a year from heart disease. Cigarettes hold the dubious distinction of being the only mass-marketed product that when used as directed actually *causes* disease and death. If cigarettes were invented now, health officials would no doubt ban their sale. Unfortunately, for a variety of reasons, appropriate restrictions on smoking are often difficult to implement.

SMOKING AND LUNG DISEASE

Since the first Surgeon General's Report on Smoking and Health in 1964, lung cancer has been recognized as one of the long-term dangers of smoking. However, lung cancer is not the only pulmonary disease caused by tobacco. Smoking is also the most important risk factor for developing chronic bronchitis and emphysema, a chronic pulmonary disease in which the lungs gradually lose their normal elasticity. A person with emphysema is often short of breath, and persons with chronic bronchitis frequently cough up thick phlegm. Emphysema also makes the heart (particularly the right side) work harder. This strain on the heart can lead to a debilitating disease called cor pulmonale, in which the right atrium and ventricle enlarge and fail to function adequately.

SMOKING AND HEART DISEASE

Smoking by itself greatly increases the risk of heart disease, but there is a synergistic effect when cigarette smoking is combined with other cardiovascular risk factors, such as high blood pressure, high serum cholesterol (or low HDL) levels, obesity, and a family history of heart disease. When smoking is combined with these factors, the increased risk is not simply additive; instead, the risks are compounded, with the total risk exceeding the sum of the individual risks. Thus, even moderate smoking can triple a person's risk of heart disease.

The increased cardiovascular risk from smoking is significantly lower among pipe and cigar smokers than among cigarette smokers, probably because they are less likely to inhale. However, when smokers switch from cigarettes to pipes or cigars, they may continue to inhale, and their risk may not be reduced. Likewise, changing to low-tar, low-nicotine, or filtered cigarettes has not been shown to lower and may even increase the risk of heart disease. Nicotine is only one of about 4,000 potentially harmful substances in cigarettes, and some of these other compounds may affect the heart. There is also evidence that people who switch to low-nicotine, low-tar cigarettes inhale more deeply, thereby increasing the amount of harmful substances entering the body.

The heart disease risk in users of smokeless tobacco (chewing tobacco and snuff) has not been thoroughly studied. However, the nicotine from smokeless tobacco has been shown to have the same adverse effect on the heart and blood vessels as that from cigarettes.

Fortunately, cigarette smoking has become less popular in the United States, particularly among people with more than a high school education and in the group at highest risk of heart disease: middle-aged men. Unfortunately, there has also been a dramatic rise in smoking among teenagers, especially teenage girls. If this trend continues, the number of female smokers is expected to equal the number of male smokers by the mid-1990s and then surpass it.

As a consequence of increased smoking by women, lung cancer has replaced breast cancer as the number one cause of cancer death among women. In recent decades, the risk of heart disease has also risen among women smokers. Since smoking interferes with estrogen production and metabolism, it lowers the natural protection against premature atherosclerosis conferred by estrogen. Taking certain oral contraceptives (especially those with high levels of estrogen) raises the smoking-related risk of vascular disease even higher, especially in women over age 35.

HOW SMOKING RAISES CARDIOVASCULAR RISK

ATHEROSCLEROSIS

Research has shown conclusively that smoking accelerates arteriosclerosis (hardening of the arteries) and atherosclerosis (a type of arteriosclerosis characterized by fatty deposits in the artery walls), increasing the risk of heart disease, stroke, and peripheral vascular disease. Consequently, smokers have a higher risk of cardiovascular disease in general, and heart attacks in particular, than nonsmokers.

Cigarettes may promote atherosclerosis by a variety of mechanisms. Smoking increases the levels of carbon monoxide, a poisonous gas that is inhaled in smoke. Over the long term, this increased level of carbon monoxide from the inhaled smoke itself contributes to damaging the lining of the blood vessels and accelerates the process of atherosclerosis.

Smoking also affects serum cholesterol. Smokers tend to have decreased levels of high-density lipoproteins (HDL—the "good" cholesterol) and increased levels of low-density lipoproteins (LDL—the "bad" cholesterol) and triglycerides (a blood fat), thereby raising the risk and severity of atherosclerosis.

Blood levels of fibrinogen, a component of blood necessary for clotting, are raised by smoking. This may increase the likelihood of blood clots forming and blocking the coronary arteries, leading to a heart attack or stroke. Such clots are most likely to form on areas of the endothelium (the inner lining of blood vessel walls) that are clogged by atherosclerotic plaque and have been roughened by prior damage, rather than on those that remain smooth and intact. Smoking may also cause blood platelets to clump abnormally, adding to the risk of clotting.

Stopping smoking results in an increase in the ratio of HDL to LDL cholesterol and lowers the level of fibrinogen in the blood. Both of these changes help reduce the risk of a heart attack.

SHORT-TERM EFFECTS

Smoking causes surges in the concentrations of catecholamines (the stimulatory chemical messengers of the autonomic nervous system) as well as increases in carbon monoxide in the blood. Both of these short-term effects can exacerbate *existing* heart disease, resulting, for instance, in attacks of angina (chest pain). Nicotine raises blood pressure and heart rate, requiring the heart to work harder. It also constricts the coronary arteries, thereby lessening the supply of blood and oxygen to the heart muscle. It also promotes irregular heartbeats (cardiac arrhythmias).

HOW SMOKING CESSATION LOWERS RISK

The increased cardiovascular risk from smoking can actually be reversed simply by stopping smoking. Even smoking fewer cigarettes or switching to a pipe or cigars has been shown to lower the risk, but stopping all tobacco use is much more effective in eliminating the increased risk. Not surprisingly, the greatest benefits are to heavy smokers, those who smoke more than two packs a day. (See Figure 6.1.)

Some smokers are reluctant to quit smoking for fear of gaining weight. Still, the health benefits of quitting far outweigh any increased health risks from the average 5-pound weight gain that may follow smoking cessation. (Even this minor weight gain can be avoided or reversed with careful planning prior to quitting and behavior modification.)

Quitting lowers the risk of heart disease for people who have never had any symptoms, as well as those who have suffered extensive heart disease. Often a heart attack or a coronary artery bypass graft operation compels individuals to stop smoking, and it

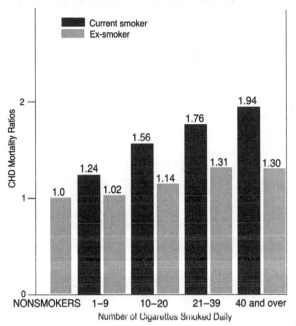

Figure 6.1
Cessation of Smoking and Coronary Heart Disease (CHD): Mortality Ratios of Current Smokers Versus Ex-smokers

Source: E. Rogot and J. L. Murray, *Smoking and causes of death among U.S. veterans. 16 years of observation. Public Health Reports* 95(3). 213–222, May–June 1980.

is certainly true that they will be better off if they quit. However, a heart attack does irreversible damage to part of the muscle of the heart. Therefore, it is much better to stop smoking whether or not heart disease may be present—or, better yet, never start. After a heart attack, quitting smoking may be the most effective single risk factor intervention. It can lower the risk of developing a second heart attack and of dying of a future heart attack if it does occur.

Even for people who have been smoking for decades, the cardiac benefits of quitting are great—and they start the moment a person quits. Within 20 minutes after the last puff, nicotine-induced constriction of the peripheral blood vessels lessens, decreasing the coldness of the hands and feet that troubles some smokers. Eight hours later, the blood's oxygen level returns to normal, and its carbon monoxide level lessens.

Perhaps most important, the risk of having a heart attack starts to decline *within the first day* after stopping smoking. According to the 1990 Surgeon General's Report on the Health Benefit of Smoking Cessation, the smoking-related excess risk of heart disease is cut in half within one year of quitting. Within 5 to 10 years after stopping, the average ex-smoker's risk of heart disease is the same as that of someone who has never smoked. This is true for both men and women.

In contrast to the heart, the lungs take somewhat longer to show the beneficial effects of quitting. But there, too, the rewards of stopping smoking are great: Ten years after quitting, a former pack-a-day smoker has nearly the same chance of avoiding fatal lung cancer and other smoking-linked cancers as does a lifetime nonsmoker.

SMOKING CESSATION METHODS

Quitting "cold turkey," rather than tapering off gradually, seems to be the best method for most people, although it is not successful for everyone. It helps if friends, relatives, or coworkers who smoke can stop on the same day—or at least not smoke in front of the new ex-smoker. Many smokers who want to stop can do it on their own, while others may need the help of individual or group counseling, relaxation training, hypnosis, or behavior modification to ease withdrawal symptoms.

Among structured programs, the best success rates have been reported for those that provide the quitter with a support system and that include counseling and education on behavior modification, stress management, and nutrition. Behavior modification is the most important component. It makes people confront the reasons why they smoke and assists them in finding the path that will help each one individually achieve success in quitting. (See the "Why Do You Smoke?" self-assessment quiz.) Most smokers are accustomed to lighting up in response to stress. By learning better techniques for managing stress, they can prevent themselves from starting to smoke again.

Sometimes weight gain accompanies smoking cessation. Part of the reason is that, with quitting, taste buds regain their keenness, so food tastes better. Eating also provides something to do with the hands and mouth, which want a cigarette. Finally, it appears that metabolism (the rate at which the body expends calories) is speeded up by nicotine and tends to slow down with quitting. Exercise can help boost metabolism again, while nutritional counseling can teach quitters how to choose healthy, low-fat snacks and structure their regular meals to compensate for extra nibbling. With these changes, most weight gain is not significant.

Smokers who want to quit and fear weight gain should keep in mind that although true obesity is also a risk factor for heart disease, a few extra pounds are not nearly as detrimental as smoking. It would take an additional 75 pounds to offset the benefit the average smoker gains from quitting. Furthermore, most ex-smokers find that once they have completely stopped smoking, it is easier to lose the few extra pounds than it was to give up smoking.

Yale–New Haven Hospital's Center for Health Promotion offers a smoking cessation program called Smoke Stoppers, developed by the National Center for Health Promotion, to its employees and patients, as well as corporate and community participants. The program features behavior modification, stress management, and nutritional counseling, and has a success rate of 50 percent to 70 percent at the end of one year. On average, program participants gain approximately 2 pounds. The program's success is largely attributed to carefully trained and certified instructors. All are ex-smokers who can empathize with the participants—and see through their defenses and denial.

At the first group session, smokers in the Yale program learn about the benefits of smoking cessation and methods of treatment. They do not quit at that meeting, but set a "quit date" within the next week. In the interim, they are encouraged to start keeping a diary of their activities, including smoking. (See box, "Daily Cigarette Count.") This diary-keeping helps them identify the individual behavior that has chained them to the smoking habit. Such analysis, in itself, often results in a curtailment of smoking, which lowers the body's dependence on nicotine, thus easing the next step: quitting cold turkey.

At the next meeting, the program participants throw out their cigarettes and learn survival techniques for their first day of "staying quit." Daily meetings over the next three weeks then reinforce this support, with nutritional counseling and extensive training in stress management techniques. Those participants who are found to be highly nicotine dependent and those in whom withdrawal symptoms pose a particular problem can consult their doctors about nicotine-replacement therapy. The instructors follow up with the quitters at intervals of six, 12, and 18 months after the quit date. Participants who begin to smoke again are invited to repeat the program at no charge.

Some other programs and individuals have reported success with the "wrap" method. During the period before the quit date, the smoker wraps each pack of cigarettes with paper and rubber bands (a variation calls for wrapping each individual cigarette in aluminum foil). Whenever there is an urge to smoke, the automatic response is broken by the chore

Why Do You Smoke? A Self-Assessment Quiz

Here are some statements made by people to describe what they get out of smoking cigarettes. How often do you feel this way when smoking? Choose one number for each statement.

5 = always   4 = frequently   3 = occasionally   2 = seldom   1 = never

A. I smoke cigarettes in order to keep myself from slowing down. _____
B. Handling a cigarette is part of the enjoyment of smoking. _____
C. Smoking cigarettes is pleasant and relaxing. _____
D. I light up a cigarette when I feel angry about something. _____
E. When I have run out of cigarettes, I find it almost unbearable until I can get more. _____
F. I smoke cigarettes automatically without even being aware of it. _____
G. I smoke cigarettes to stimulate me, to perk myself up. _____
H. Part of the enjoyment of smoking a cigarette comes from the steps I take to light up. _____
I. I find cigarettes pleasurable. _____
J. When I feel uncomfortable or upset about something, I light up a cigarette. _____
K. I am very much aware of the fact when I am not smoking a cigarette. _____
L. I light up a cigarette without realizing I still have one burning in the ashtray. _____
M. I smoke cigarettes to give me a "lift." _____
N. When I smoke a cigarette, part of the enjoyment is watching the smoke as I exhale it. _____
O. I want a cigarette most when I am comfortable and relaxed. _____
P. When I feel "blue" or want to take my mind off cares and worries, I smoke cigarettes. _____
Q. I get a real gnawing for a cigarette when I haven't smoked for a while. _____
R. I've found a cigarette in my mouth and didn't remember putting it there. _____

How to Score

1. Enter the numbers you have selected for the test questions in the spaces below, putting the number you have selected for question A over line A, for question B over line B, etc.
2. Total the 3 scores on each line to get your totals. For example, the sum of scores over lines A, G, and M gives you your score on Stimulation. Scores over 11 or above indicate that this factor is an important source of satisfaction for the smoker. Scores of 7 or less are low and probably indicate that this factor does not apply to you. Scores in between are marginal.

_____ (A)		_____ (G)		_____ (M)	=	Stimulation
_____ (B)	+	_____ (H)	+	_____ (N)	=	Handling
_____ (C)	+	_____ (I)	+	_____ (O)	=	Relaxation
_____ (D)	+	_____ (J)	+	_____ (P)	=	Crutch
_____ (E)	+	_____ (K)	+	_____ (Q)	=	Craving
_____ (F)	+	_____ (L)	+	_____ (R)	=	Habit

Source: Adapted from "Smoker's Self Test" by Daniel Horn, Ph.D., Director of the National Clearinghouse for Smoking and Health, Public Health Service.

Interpreting Your Score

- Stimulation. You smoke because it gives you a lift. Substitute a brisk walk or a few simple exercises.
- Handling. You like the ritual and trappings of smoking. Find other ways to keep your hands busy.
- Relaxation. You get a real sense of pleasure out of smoking. An honest consideration of the harmful effects may help kill the "pleasure."
- Crutch (or negative feelings). If you mostly light up when you're angry or depressed, you're using smoking as a tranquilizer. In a tough situation, take a deep breath to relax, call a friend, and talk over your feelings. If you can learn new ways to cope, you're on your way to quitting.
- Craving. Quitting smoking is difficult for you if you feel you're psychologically dependent, but once you've stopped, it will be possible to resist the temptation to smoke because the withdrawal effort is too tough to face again.
- Habit. If you usually smoke without even realizing you're doing it, you should find it easy to break the habit pattern. Start by asking, "Do I really want this cigarette?" Change smoking patterns and make cigarettes hard to get at.

Source: Adapted from "7-Day Plan to Help You Stop Smoking Cigarettes," American Cancer Society, 1978.

Daily Cigarette Count

Instructions: Attach a copy of this table to a pack of cigarettes. Complete the information each time you smoke a cigarette (those from someone else as well as your own). Note the time and evaluate the need for the cigarette (1 is for a cigarette you feel you could not do without; 2 is a less necessary one; 3 is one you could really go without). Make any other additional comments about the situation or your feelings. This record helps you understand when and why you smoke.

Time	Need	Feelings/Situation
6 AM		
6:30		
7		
7:30		
8		
8:30		
9		
9:30		
10		
10:30		
11		
11:30		
12 PM		
12:30		
1		
1:30		
2		
2:30		
3		
3:30		
4		
4:30		
5		
5:30		
6		
6:30		
7		
7:30		
8		
8:30		
9		
9:30		
10		
10:30		
11		
11:30		
12 AM		
12:30		
1		
1:30		

of having to unwrap and rewrap the pack. For each cigarette, the smoker must write down the time and his or her mood and current activity, and then rate the importance of the cigarette. Like the diary, this helps potential quitters start to think about why they smoke.

A program of this type requires a time and financial commitment that may be difficult or unnecessary for some people. On the other hand, some smokers find that the financial commitment is an added incentive to quit.

A number of government and voluntary health agencies offer free or nominally priced self-help materials for smokers who want to quit on their own. (See box, "Smoking Cessation Resources.") The American Cancer Society and the American Lung Association run relatively inexpensive smoking-cessation programs, as do the Seventh Day Adventists and some hospitals. At the same time that they introduce workplace no-smoking policies, many employers are offering such programs as well.

SECONDHAND SMOKE

Smokers are not the only people harmed by tobacco. Toxic fumes from cigarettes pose a health threat to all those around smokers—family, friends, and co-workers. Because the organic material in tobacco does not burn completely, smoke contains many toxic chemicals, including carbon monoxide, nicotine, and tar. Cotinine, a breakdown product of nicotine in the body, can be detected even in infants of smoking parents, as well as in nonsmoking adults who were unaware that they had been passively exposed to smoking.

As a result of this exposure, smokers' children have more colds and flu, and they are more likely to take up smoking themselves when they grow up. Women who smoke increase the risk of miscarriage, delivering an underweight baby, and other health problems during delivery and infancy. There seems to be an increased incidence of sudden infant death syndrome (SIDS) among babies whose mothers smoke. Otherwise, most of the effects of passive smoking appear to be reversible. For instance, women who quit smoking before becoming pregnant or during their first four months of pregnancy eliminate their risk (unless other factors are present) of bearing a baby of low birth weight.

Smoking Cessation Resources

Local offices of the American Cancer Society, the American Heart Association, and the American Lung Association can provide pamphlets on smoking cessation and resources for low-cost cessation programs. To find the office in your area, check your local telephone book or contact:

American Cancer Society
1599 Clifton Road NE
Atlanta, GA 30329

American Heart Association
7320 Greenville Avenue
Dallas, TX 75231

American Lung Association
1740 Broadway
New York, NY 10019

A "Quit Kit" of smoking cessation information, lists of local stop-smoking programs, and over the phone counseling is available from:

The National Cancer Institute
Cancer Information Clearinghouse
Office of Cancer Communication
Building 31, Room 10A18
9000 Rockville Pike
Bethesda, MD 20205
1-800-4-CANCER for all areas of the U.S. except:
Alaska (800) 638-6070
Oahu, HI (800) 524-1234

National Center for Health Promotion
Smoker Stoppers Program
3920 Varsity Drive
Ann Arbor, MI 48108
(313) 971-6077

For several years, secondhand smoke (passive smoking) has been implicated as potentially raising the risk of lung cancer. Evidence linking passive smoking to heart disease has been documented. New estimates released recently by the Surgeon General's office indicate that passive smoking may cause ten times as much heart disease as lung disease. Accordingly, passive smoking is now ranked as the third leading cause of preventable death, after active smoking and alcohol abuse.

Researchers suggest that nonsmokers who live with smokers have a 30 percent higher risk of dying from heart disease than do other nonsmokers. Since the U.S. Environmental Protection Agency estimates that exposure to secondhand smoke in the workplace is about four times that of a typical household, the problem may be even worse for employees.

Not only can passive smoking contribute to the development of heart disease, but it also has been shown to worsen the condition of people with existing heart disease. The transportation of oxygen to the heart via red blood cells is hampered by the carbon monoxide in secondhand smoke. In people whose oxygen supply is already hampered by coronary artery disease, this places an excess burden on the heart. There is also evidence that passive smoking makes blood platelets abnormally sticky and more likely to form clots; these effects play a role in the development of atherosclerotic plaques on the artery walls.

The exposure of nonsmokers to environmental tobacco smoke is reduced—but not eliminated—when smokers and nonsmokers are placed in separate rooms that are ventilated by the same system. Since it is not practical to remove all tobacco smoke through air filters in ventilation systems, many municipalities and employers have now instituted no-smoking policies, either prohibiting all cigarette smoking within their buildings and certain public places or confining it to areas that are ventilated separately, with exhaust channeled directly outdoors.

QUITTING TIPS

- Make a list of all the possible reasons to quit and the benefits you'll receive from doing so. Mark those that are most important to *you*, such as "so my children won't breathe my smoke or mimic my smoking." Read over the list at least once a day and try to add to it.

- Think about your smoking patterns—when and why you have each cigarette. This analysis alone can help taper off the habit, lower your body's dependence on nicotine, and help you get a head start on actually quitting.

- Choose a date, in advance, to give up smoking completely. One popular day is the Great American Smokeout sponsored each November by the American Cancer Society, but it can be your birthday, the anniversary of a special day, or *any* day.

- Share your plan with a friend, coworker, or spouse. If your confidant is a smoker, ask him

or her to quit with you. If not, ask for understanding and support or make it a challenge and propose a bet that you can do it.

- Start getting ready to quit by changing the type of cigarette you smoke (such as from regular to menthol) and the brand. Buy only one pack at a time and switch each time. Stop carrying matches or a lighter, and keep your cigarettes in an unhandy place.

- Get a large jar and start collecting all your butts in it.

- In another large jar start collecting the money you would normally spend on cigarettes each time you forgo buying a pack. Set aside the saved money as a reward for yourself.

- Remember, the first days are the hardest, so do whatever is needed to get through them. At first, it may be necessary to avoid activities that trigger the urge to smoke, such as socializing with other smokers. Try to spend as much time as possible in places where smoking is prohibited (or at least awkward).

- Brush your teeth or use mouthwash or spray several times a day. Enjoy the clean taste in your mouth.

- Change the behavior associated with your strongest urges. For example, if you always have a cigarette with your coffee during your morning break, have tea or juice or go for a quick walk instead.

- Keep your mouth and hands busy. Especially during the difficult early days, eat plenty of healthful snacks (such as fresh vegetables or fruits), chew gum (or consider a nicotine-containing gum available by prescription), and try holding a pencil between your fingers, doodling, or whittling. Suck on a toothpick or a straw.

- Enjoy not smoking: Think of the healthy returns of quitting; savor the taste of food, now that tobacco is no longer dulling the taste buds.

HELPING OTHERS TO QUIT

Smoking is psychologically and physically addictive, making it difficult for most people to quit. By keeping

Reasons to Quit Smoking

1. Add years to your life.
2. Help avoid lung cancer, emphysema, bronchitis, and heart attacks.
3. Give heart and circulatory system a break.
4. Get rid of smoker's cough.
5. Feel more vigorous in sports.
6. Improve stamina.
7. Stop smoke-related head and stomach aches.
8. Regain sense of smell and taste.
9. Have smoke-free rooms and closets.
10. End cigarette breath.
11. Save money.
12. Eliminate yellow stains on teeth and fingers.
13. Stop burning holes in clothes or furniture.
14. Get rid of messy ashtrays, ashes on carpets.
15. Set good example for others.
16. Prove self-control.
17. _____.
18. _____.
19. _____.
20. _____.

Source: Adapted from "7-Day Plan to Help You Stop Smoking Cigarettes," American Cancer Society, 1978.

these tips in mind, a supportive nonsmoker can make a decisive difference for a friend, family member, or coworker who is trying to stop smoking:

- Do not nag or preach.
- Praise the smoker's efforts to stop, no matter how tentative or small.
- Show confidence in the smoker's ability to quit.
- Invite the smoker to share pleasurable activities in places where smoking is prohibited. For example, go to the movies, visit a museum, attend a concert, or have dinner in a restaurant with a nonsmoking section.
- Offer healthful snacks to keep the quitter's mouth and hands busy while keeping weight gain to a minimum.
- Encourage the smoker to call you for help in "getting through" a sudden urge for a cigarette.
- Most important, be patient.

ALCOHOL

After smoking, excess alcohol is the second most common cause of preventable death. Alcohol is toxic to virtually every organ in the human body, but when consumed in moderate amounts, it is detoxified by the liver and does little or no harm. Alcoholic beverages contain ethyl alcohol (ethanol), which is metabolized in the body to acetaldehyde. In large amounts, both ethanol and acetaldehyde interfere with normal functions of organs throughout the body, including the heart.

There is a significantly higher incidence of high blood pressure among those who consume more than 2 ounces of ethanol a day (which translates into 4 ounces of 100-proof whiskey, 16 ounces of wine, or 48 ounces of beer). Abrupt withdrawal of alcohol from those consuming large amounts on a regular basis may cause the condition known as delirium tremens (DTs), which is associated with a significant risk of cardiac arrest.

Binge drinking can provoke arrhythmias (irregular heart rhythms)—frequently in the form of atrial fibrillation—in people with no previous symptoms of heart disease. This alcohol-induced rhythm disturbance is most common among people who have chronically abused alcohol. It is sometimes called "holiday heart" because it often occurs over the holidays or on weekends, after consumption of more alcohol than usual. People who are deprived of sleep are susceptible to developing "holiday heart" from drinking too much at one time, even if they do not regularly abuse alcohol.

Alcohol is thought to provoke arrhythmias by stimulating the sympathetic nervous system. Alcoholics tend to have higher blood levels of the chemical messengers of this system such as epinephrine (adrenaline). Deficiency of the trace mineral magnesium, which often occurs with chronic alcohol abuse, may also play a role.

Up to a third of all cases of a type of heart disease called cardiomyopathy are attributed to excessive drinking. Alcoholic cardiomyopathy occurs most often in middle-aged men. In this disorder, the heart muscle (myocardium)—particularly the right and left ventricles—enlarges and becomes flabby. (See Chapter 15.) As the working cells deteriorate, they become more sparse, and are replaced by fibers of connective tissue in the spaces between the cells (interstitial fibrosis). Eventually, alcoholic cardiomyopathy can result in heart failure, in which the heart does not pump blood efficiently to all parts of the body. Fatigue, shortness of breath during exercise, and swelling in the ankles are its most common symptoms. The heart's inability to send blood efficiently to the kidneys, where excess salt and water are normally filtered out, means the body begins to retain salt, and thus water. This in turn raises blood volume and causes a backup of fluid into tissues such as the lungs (hence the breathing difficulty).

When individuals with congestive heart failure caused by alcoholic consumption continue to drink, their prognosis is poor. In contrast, those who abstain from alcohol raise their chances of reversing the progress of alcoholic cardiomyopathy, especially if the problem is detected early: Their hearts may return to normal size, and they can live for many years. In fact, patients with alcoholic cardiomyopathy who abstain from drinking have a better prognosis than do patients with cardiomyopathy from other causes.

Physicians once believed that malnutrition was the sole mechanism by which alcohol damaged the heart. In extreme cases, alcoholics consume too many calories as drink and not enough as food, and they become malnourished. This could cause depletion of the protein in heart muscle. However, it is now recognized that in most cases, alcohol damages the heart even in the absence of malnutrition.

MODERATE USE OF ALCOHOL

A number of epidemiologic studies have suggested that the risk of heart disease is somewhat lower among people who regularly drink small amounts of alcohol, such as a glass of wine a day, than among teetotalers. Likewise, higher levels of high-density-lipoprotein (HDL) cholesterol have been reported among light drinkers than among nondrinkers. The overwhelming evidence, however, indicates that excess alcohol is harmful to the cardiovascular system. In all of the studies showing a lower than average risk among light drinkers, the highest risk was shown to be among heavy drinkers. Excess alcohol has been proved to damage the heart—and other organs, including the liver, stomach, and brain.

Alcohol Content By the Drink

Alcohol, in its pure, undiluted form, is too strong for the mouth and stomach. The type of alcohol in alcoholic drinks is ethyl alcohol.

Alcohol content is expressed in percentages by volume. Thus, the amount of liquid is not the determining factor. At a bar or party, the size of the glass in which a certain type of drink is usually served determines the amount of alcohol a person can expect to ingest. For instance, although there is a much smaller proportion of alcohol in beer than in a cocktail, beer is usually served in a mug many times the size of a cocktail glass. Below are approximations of the amounts of alcohol found in various kinds of drinks.

Beer

Most beers contain about 5 percent alcohol by volume. Malt liquors may contain up to 8 or 9 percent.

Wine

A typical table wine contains about 10 to 13 percent alcohol by volume. A wine's taste and bouquet are not indicators of alcohol content. A light, fragrant wine may contain a higher percentage of alcohol than a full-bodied wine. (Wine such as sherry or vermouth is fortified; extra alcohol is added when it is produced. It sometimes contains up to 20 percent alcohol by volume.)

Cocktails

Hard liquors including brandy, gin, vodka, and whiskey and most liqueurs contain 40 to 50 percent alcohol by volume. The proof is a measure of alcohol concentration. In the United States, proof is equal to two times the alcohol content. Thus, liquor that is 80 proof contains 40 percent alcohol by volume.

Approximate equivalents determined by the size of the conventional drink glasses:

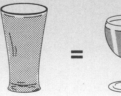

A 12-ounce mug of beer = a 4- to 5-ounce glass of wine = a 1.5-ounce shot of 80-proof liquor

The links between light drinking and cardiovascular protection should certainly not be used as an excuse for drinkers to consume additional alcohol; nor should nondrinkers start drinking in order to protect their hearts. On the other hand, for those who drink, a modest alcohol intake can be an acceptable means of stress modification. (See box, "Alcohol Content By the Drink.") A single cocktail or a glass of wine or beer at the end of a long day may be quite relaxing and beneficial. It should not be harmful unless there is a family history of alcoholism or a demonstrated sensitivity to small amounts of alcohol.

ALCOHOL ABUSE

Any use of an illicit drug can be considered abuse. The situation with alcohol, however, is more complex. Although alcohol is a drug, and a potentially harmful one, its use is legally and socially sanctioned. An estimated two-thirds of adults in the Western world use alcohol, and at least one in ten is a heavy user. Therefore, definitions of alcoholism vary.

How much alcohol is too much? The level of alcohol an individual can tolerate before showing mental and physical effects varies from person to person and may vary for the same individual depending upon the circumstances. Body size is a major determinant of how much a person can drink: Generally, the larger a person is, the more he or she can tolerate. In general, women cannot tolerate as much alcohol as men can. Until recently, it was assumed that this is because, on average, they weigh less. A preliminary study has shown, however, that women's stomachs also have less alcohol dehydrogenase, an enzyme that helps neutralize alcohol before it reaches the bloodstream. Thus, more alcohol is absorbed into a woman's bloodstream. Drinking on an empty stomach, consuming drinks in rapid succession, and drinking when fatigued can affect tolerance. In most states, the legal limit for driving is 100 mg/100 ml of alcohol in the blood. (See Figure 6.2.) But the deleterious effects of alcohol can begin with far less.

A "yes" answer to even one of the following questions should be reason to suspect alcohol abuse in an individual:

- Has alcohol ever caused lateness for or absence from work?

- Has alcohol ever caused neglect of obligations to family, friends, or job?

- Has the individual ever acted "out of character"—obnoxious, belligerent, antisocial, or even overly sociable—while drinking?

- Has the individual ever "blacked out" or been unable to remember the night before on the morning after?

Like smokers and drug abusers, alcoholics must stop denying their problem before they can start to solve it. Confronting the substance abuser is often the first step in this process. Suspicions that one—or one's friend, relative, or coworker—has a drinking problem warrant a consultation with a doctor. Local resources, including Alcoholics Anonymous chapters, are listed in the yellow pages of the telephone book.

Figure 6.2

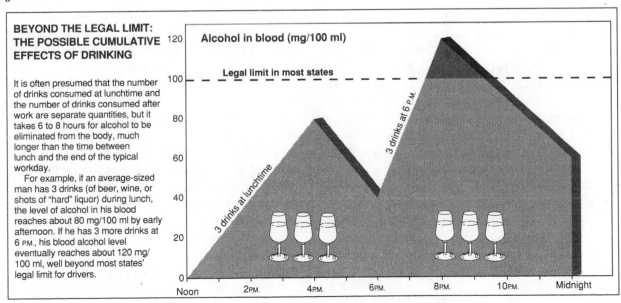

BEYOND THE LEGAL LIMIT: THE POSSIBLE CUMULATIVE EFFECTS OF DRINKING

It is often presumed that the number of drinks consumed at lunchtime and the number of drinks consumed after work are separate quantities, but it takes 6 to 8 hours for alcohol to be eliminated from the body, much longer than the time between lunch and the end of the typical workday.

For example, if an average-sized man has 3 drinks (of beer, wine, or shots of "hard" liquor) during lunch, the level of alcohol in his blood reaches about 80 mg/100 ml by early afternoon. If he has 3 more drinks at 6 P.M., his blood alcohol level eventually reaches about 120 mg/100 ml, well beyond most states' legal limit for drivers.

ILLICIT DRUGS

Like smoking and drinking, using illicit drugs can also be hazardous to the heart. The problems vary with the drug used and they range from physiologic to infectious.

COCAINE

Use of cocaine has snowballed in recent decades, along with the myth that the drug is relatively safe, especially when it is sniffed ("snorted") rather than injected or smoked as "crack." In fact, no matter how it is used, cocaine can kill. It can disturb the heart's rhythm and cause chest pain, heart attacks, and even sudden death. These effects on the heart can cause death even in the absence of any seizures, the most common of cocaine's serious noncardiac "side effects." Dabblers should beware: Even in the absence of underlying heart disease, a single use of only a small amount of the drug has been known to be fatal. Although such deaths are uncommon, they do occur.

Cocaine use is not healthful for anyone, but especially for certain groups. Although the drug has been shown to impair the function of normal hearts, it seems even more likely to cause death in people with any underlying heart disease. And when pregnant women use cocaine, they not only raise the likelihood of having a miscarriage, a premature delivery, or a low-birth-weight baby, but also of having a baby with a congenital heart abnormality, especially an atrial-septal or ventricular-septal defect.

A variety of mechanisms conspire to cause cocaine's impairment of the heart. Use of cocaine raises blood pressure, constricts blood vessels, and speeds up heart rate. It may also make blood cells called platelets more likely to clump and form the blood clots that provoke many heart attacks. In addition, cocaine's effects on the nervous system disrupt the normal rhythm of the heart, causing arrhythmias (irregular heartbeats). Recently, scientists have established that cocaine binds directly to heart muscle cells, slowing the passage of sodium ions into the cells. Cocaine also causes the release of the neurotransmitter norepinephrine (noradrenaline), a chemical messenger that stimulates the autonomic nervous system. Both changes can lead to arrhythmias.

Heart attacks in young people are rare. However, when they do occur, cocaine is frequently the cause.

Friends and even medical personnel may be slow to suspect that a heart attack is taking place because of the victim's youth; yet the percentage of cocaine-induced heart attacks that are fatal is equal to the percentage of heart attacks from other causes that are fatal. Recurrent chest pain and heart attacks have been reported among those who continue to use cocaine after surviving a cardiac complication.

INTRAVENOUS (IV) DRUGS

Using a needle to "shoot up" a drug such as heroin can lead to a deadly disease called infective endocarditis. Endocarditis is an infection of the endocardium, which includes the heart valves. Colonies of bacteria (usually streptococcus or staphylococcus), fungi, or other microbes introduced into the bloodstream via intravenous needles grow on the endocardium and can damage or destroy the heart valves. The microorganisms can also migrate through the bloodstream to other regions of the body. The clumps of microbes and their by-products can also form plugs, or emboli; if these plugs become lodged in arteries serving the lungs, heart, or brain, they can lead to pulmonary embolism, heart attack, or stroke, respectively.

Endocarditis is not confined to drug users. However, when it strikes people who do not use drugs, it tends to be confined to artificial valves or to valves that have been previously weakened by a heart condition such as rheumatic heart disease or congenital heart disease. In contrast, in most IV drug users who develop infective endocarditis, the heart valves are normal at first. It is possible that IV drug use itself makes heart valves vulnerable to infection. Particles present in the injected material may damage the valves and blood vessel linings, roughening the surface and leading to platelet clumping, thus providing likely sites for bacteria to grow.

"Street" drugs carry no verified list of ingredients. Along the way to the buyer, they pass through the hands of many distributors. Each of these dealers may "cut," or dilute, a single sample of a drug with cheaper powders such as lactose, starch, quinine, and talc. Bacteria or fungi easily find their way into the drug sample during the mixing of these substances, or when the drug is dissolved in fluid just prior to injection, or from the injection paraphernalia itself.

Early symptoms of infective endocarditis include weakness, fatigue, fever, chills, and aching joints. Without treatment, infective endocarditis is invariably fatal. However, recovery is possible when the disease is detected and treated promptly with an antibiotic that has been selected to kill the particular bacteria causing the infection. Sometimes surgery must be performed to replace the damaged valve; for example, if antibiotic treatment alone is unsuccessful, or if heart failure develops and cannot be controlled, surgery may be recommended to replace the damaged valve.

AMPHETAMINES

Like cocaine, amphetamines ("speed") raise blood pressure and heart rate. They are dangerous drugs for anyone, but particularly for people with any history of heart disease. Users of street cocaine may unknowingly consume amphetamines, as the two drugs are sometimes mixed together.

RECOGNIZING DRUG ABUSE

Warning signs of drug use include mood swings, irritability, and nervousness. Like alcoholics, drug users often miss work on Mondays, Fridays, and the day after payday. Their job performance may be erratic and marked by extra accidents and gross lapses in judgment. One may be tempted to protect drug-using friends, relatives, and coworkers. However, it is far better to confront the drug use, not cover up for it, and to urge the drug user to seek help. Many employers now offer employee assistance programs (EAPs) for workers who are having problems, including alcohol and drug abuse. For help and information, consult a doctor or check the yellow pages under "Drug Abuse Information and Treatment."

CHAPTER 7

EXERCISE

FRANS J. TH. WACKERS, M.D.

INTRODUCTION

The past two decades have seen a much-publicized fitness boom in America. From sales of aerobic dance videotapes to popular participation in marathon running, indicators abound that Americans are interested in "working out." However, there is also evidence that a significant proportion of the population, especially the young, engage in little physical activity. The increase in hours spent watching television, the epidemic rates of obesity, and the abundance of energy-saving modern conveniences all testify to the fact that many people live in a sedentary manner.

Unfortunately, exercise is often perceived by those who need it most as a painful or exhausting process. Properly performed, however, regular moderate exercise should be a life-enhancing part of health maintenance. There is no need for athletic-level effort, highly structured programs, or costly equipment to gain the benefits of increased physical activity. For those who are at high risk of cardiovascular disease, a sensible program of exercise can help reduce that risk; and for those who have had a heart attack or have other symptoms of coronary heart disease, a medically supervised program can slow or even partially reverse the loss of cardiac function.

WHY EXERCISE?

What, precisely, are the benefits of exercise? Increased protection against cardiovascular disease is a proven one, although exercise alone does not confer immunity to heart disease. Regular exercise also may work synergistically to help control a host of other independent risk factors for coronary heart disease, including obesity, stress, high blood pressure, and high levels of blood lipids, including cholesterol and triglycerides. (See Chapters 3, 4, and 12.) It is an excellent way to reduce stress, another independent risk factor for coronary heart disease. (See Chapter 8.) In addition, the initiation of an exercise program often helps stimulate or reinforce other positive life-style changes, such as better nutrition or smoking cessation. (See Chapters 5 and 6.) It promotes an enhanced self-image and sense of control.

Increased physical activity is associated with longer life, and in old age it can improve quality of life and the ability to continue enjoying work and recreation. In general, exercise provides a positive, enjoyable foundation for a healthier way of living; unlike many health-enhancing measures, it adds something pleasant to one's existence rather than taking something away.

A DEFINITION OF FITNESS

Overall physical fitness consists of several components. The most important of these for most adults is cardiovascular (aerobic) endurance, the ability of the body to take in, transport, and use oxygen efficiently to metabolize carbohydrates and fats for energy. Other components of fitness include muscular strength, flexibility, and body composition (the relative proportion of lean to fat tissue). Ideally, an exercise program will help to improve all these components, but a distinction must be made between the regular physical exertion necessary to produce cardiovascular fitness—thus helping to reduce the risk of coronary artery disease—and the level of muscle strength and endurance required for athletic competition.

It is well recognized that even moderate exercise can modify heart disease risk. An expenditure of 2,000 calories a week through exercise is generally considered sufficient. This may come from a variety of sources, including such everyday activities as housework, gardening, and walking the dog. (See Table 7.1.) Expending even a modest amount of energy is better than being sedentary. In fact, those who have been sedentary will actually derive more cardiovascular benefit from a low-level workout than those who are more fit. As their cardiovascular fitness improves, they will need to expend more energy to produce the same effect.

There are two primary modes of exercise: aerobic and anaerobic. The difference between them is important in choosing which types of activities to include in an exercise program to benefit the heart and circulatory systems.

ANAEROBIC EXERCISE

Short, intense bouts of activity, also called *isometric* exercise, do not require the muscles to burn oxygen as fuel. The familiar feelings of muscle fatigue and exhaustion result when a person crosses the "anaerobic threshold" from moderate to more intense activity, causing lactic acid to build up in the muscles in a so-called oxygen debt. Examples of isometric exercise include some types of calisthenics, as well as weight lifting and use of Nautilus machines. Isometric exercise is a good way to increase muscle strength and endurance, but it does little to improve cardiovascular fitness. Since it may cause temporary but

Table 7.1
Calories Used in Various Activities

Activity	Calories expended (per minute)
Badminton	6
Basketball	7
Bicycling, 6 mph	4
10 mph	7
12 mph	9
Bowling	4
Canoeing (2.5 mph)	4
Dancing, aerobic	9
ballroom	6
square	6
Dusting	3
Furniture polishing	6
Gardening	4
Golf, power cart	3
pulling cart	5
Horseback riding (trotting)	6
Ice skating	7
Ironing	2
Jogging, 5 mph	8
7 mph	12
Jumping rope, slow	7
medium	9
fast	11
Mopping floors	4
Roller skating	6
Rowboating (2.5 mph)	5
Rowing, machine	6
scull racing	7
Running, 8 mph	13
10 mph	17
Scrubbing floors	6
Skiing, cross-country	11
downhill, 10 mph	10
Squash and handball	10
Table tennis	6
Tennis, singles	7
doubles	6
Vacuuming	4
Walking, 2 mph	3
3 mph	5
4 mph	7

Number of calories is calculated for a 150-pound person. For a 100-pound person, reduce the calories by 0.67; for a 200-pound person, multiply by 1.33. Because individual metabolic rates vary, all numbers are approximate, but they are useful in establishing relative values of various activities.

marked rises in blood pressure, it may be ruled out for people with uncontrolled high blood pressure, or hypertension. (See Chapter 12.)

AEROBIC EXERCISE

This type of exercise improves cardiovascular health by increasing the efficiency with which the body uses oxygen for energy. (The term "aerobic" refers to the use of oxygen.) To qualify as aerobic, an activity must be of sufficient duration to require oxygen consumption. Any rhythmic activity that uses large muscle groups and can be maintained for an extended period of time will increase the body's cardiovascular endurance if performed regularly. Examples include walking, running, jogging, swimming, aerobic dancing, skating, cycling, rowing, jumping rope, and cross-country skiing.

What actually happens to the body's functioning through regular aerobic exercise? Through a process called the *training effect*, the body becomes more efficient in extracting oxygen from the blood. All the organs involved in oxygen transport—including the heart, lungs, muscles, and blood vessels—learn to work more effectively with less effort. With training, muscle fibers actually become better able to obtain oxygen from the hemoglobin in red blood cells; they extract a higher percentage of oxygen than those of an untrained person. The lungs can take in and expel a greater volume of air in a single breath. Hence, exertion produces less "huffing and puffing" than before training.

As training progresses, the heart becomes accustomed to pumping more blood in a single stroke (increased stroke volume) and is thus able to accomplish the same workload, both during exertion and at rest, with fewer beats per minute. These two effects of training explain why athletes have a slower resting pulse than untrained individuals, and why their pulse rate returns to its resting state more quickly after exertion. The resting heart rate of an athlete might be 45 to 50 beats per minute, compared to 75 to 80 beats per minute in a sedentary person. The body becomes more proficient at diverting blood to working muscles, including the heart. The heart muscle itself may enlarge somewhat in highly trained individuals, although this effect is neither harmful nor necessary to improved fitness.

Finally, exercise enables the body to burn fat more efficiently for fuel. For people trying to lose excess weight, this enhances the effect of calorie restriction and encourages the loss of fat rather than the lean body mass that is muscle. Most often, someone who has a weight problem is consuming more calories than he or she is expending; the body stores the extra calories as fat. It takes 3,500 calories to equal 1 pound of fat, so in order to lose a pound, a person must expend 3,500 more calories than he or she takes in.

Not only does exercise promote the use of fat—as opposed to muscle—for energy, but it also increases the body's demands for energy. Walking or jogging, for example, burns approximately 100 calories for every mile covered. A pace faster than a stroll adds cardiovascular benefits and increases the rate at which calories are burned, but walking at any pace will burn calories. (For the calorie expenditures of other activities, see Table 7.1.)

One reason many dieters become discouraged is that the body's metabolism usually slows down in reaction to caloric restriction; exercise can help counteract that decrease. At the same time, regular exercise helps control appetite, making it easier to stick to a moderate program of calorie restriction. Improved muscle tone contributes to a trimmer, healthier look, enhancing the effect of weight loss. Exercise simply promotes a sense of well being.

HOW MUCH EXERCISE IS ENOUGH?

The training effect of exercise depends on four variables: frequency (how often a person exercises); intensity (how strenuously or, in some cases, at what speed); duration (how long); and mode (type of exercise). Aerobic activities allowing moderate exertion over long periods are best suited to improving the vital capacity of the lungs and the efficiency of the heart. But the other factors are open to considerable variation, depending on an individual's health profile, schedule, interests, and motivation. Because these factors are interrelated, a change in one will mean an increase or decrease in the others. For example, walking a mile burns the same amount of calories as running a mile. In the running mode, the body works at a greater *intensity* but covers the ground more quickly, so the *duration* is shorter. Walking is done at a slower speed, so it takes longer to cover the same ground. A person running at 6 miles an hour will burn about 330 calories running 3 miles in 30 minutes. In order to burn approximately the same number of calories, a person walking at a lower intensity, 3 miles an hour, will either have to increase the duration to one hour or, at the same duration, to increase the frequency by dividing the walking into two half-hour sessions.

According to the American College of Sports Medicine (ACSM), the following recommendations can guide healthy adults in achieving fitness:

- *Frequency.* Exercise should be performed three to five days a week.

- *Intensity.* Intensity is expressed in terms of maximum heart rate, which is determined by subtracting one's age from 220. The maximum heart rate for a 40-year-old, for example, would be 180 (220 − 40 = 180). Exercising at this maximum, however, would soon result in exhaustion. The ACSM guidelines recommend exercising at 60 to 90 percent of maximum heart rate. Using the same example, a 40-year-old would exercise at an intensity that brings the pulse up to between 108 (180 × .60) and 162 (180 × .90) beats a minute. For nonathletes, the American Heart Association (AHA) recommends working at a target heart rate of between 60 and 75 percent of the maximum rate; older people or those in poor health may start out in the low end of the range, while better-conditioned people may start at a higher range. After six months or so, exercisers may want to work up to 75 to 85 percent of maximum heart rate. There is no need to exceed that; most people can stay in excellent condition at 75 percent. (For a fuller explanation of how to gauge the intensity of exercise, see "The Exercise Session," page 90.)

- *Duration.* Each session should last 20 to 60 minutes.

Clearly, these guidelines leave the exerciser a great deal of latitude when developing an individual plan. Is it better to exercise closer to the minimum described, or closer to the maximum? Does exceeding the maximum described above yield any additional benefits, or can it do harm?

The answers to these questions will vary, depending upon a person's initial fitness level, the potential for injury because of orthopedic or other conditions such as arthritis, and desired goals. The person who wants to improve from a good baseline level of conditioning to the status of a marathon runner will have very different requirements from the obese and completely sedentary individual who wishes to introduce some additional activity safely into his or her weekly routine. In addition, the choice of a particular activity or set of activities will reflect personal abilities, circumstances, and preferences.

In general, the greater the frequency, intensity, and duration of exercise, the more improvement can be expected in aerobic capacity. People who start an exercise program with a very low level of fitness will notice a greater initial improvement than those who start in better condition. Studies of the efficiency of exercise training tend to produce conflicting data, but they have generally shown that exercising for more than four to five days a week produces little additional cardiovascular benefit, while exercising fewer than three days a week is inadequate to achieve the training effect. The minimum level of exertion to start improving oxygen consumption is about 60 percent of maximum heart rate. This *target heart rate* changes with age and other factors.

Although it is the total amount of exercise that will improve and maintain fitness, the relationship of intensity and duration of exercise can be manipulated, as described earlier, to suit the individual exerciser. Of course, exercise must be done regularly on a long-term basis to consolidate the gains of the training period; missing a session occasionally won't set one back significantly, but some studies have shown up to 50 percent loss in fitness improvement after 4 to 12 weeks without exercise.

The question "How much is enough?" raises another question: "How much is too much?" For people at high risk for coronary heart disease (CHD) or those who already have it, this is an issue to be resolved in consultation with the physician, based on medical test results such as the exercise stress test. (See Chapter 10.) For healthy adults, there is a slight risk of injury from intense and prolonged exercise that involves jumping or pounding, such as running, jogging, and rope-jumping, or from any activity that involves overuse of certain joints, muscles, and connective tissues. Graduated, balanced workouts with appropriate warm-ups and cool-downs are the best safeguards against injury. (See Table 7.2 for sample programs.)

GETTING STARTED

Even for a healthy adult, starting an exercise program can seem a daunting task in the middle of a busy but sedentary life. The following suggestions can help such individuals to get going:

YALE UNIVERSITY SCHOOL OF MEDICINE HEART BOOK

Table 7.2
Sample Exercise Prescriptions

The following exercise programs illustrate how two very different people might approach their fitness goals. They are intended only as examples; any exercise prescription, particularly one for a person with heart disease, should be individualized under a physician's supervision. Each session should be preceded by a five-minute warm-up period (low-intensity exercise and stretching) and followed by a five-minute cool-down period. Frequency should be flexible; increase when comfortable at a certain level, and decrease or discontinue if injury or discomfort occurs.

A 35-Year-Old Individual, Healthy But Sedentary

	Week	Intensity (heart rate)	Duration (minutes)	Frequency (times/ week)
Initial Phase	1	50%	10	3
	2	60%	10	3
	3	70%	15	3
	4	70–75%	15	4
	5	75–80%	20	4
Improvement Phase	6–9	75–80%	20	4
	10–13	80%	25	4
	14–16	80%	30	4
	17–19	80%	30	4–5
	20–23	80%	30	4–5
	24–27	80%	30	4–6
Maintenance Phase	28+	80%	40–60	4–6

Note: Intensity is reflected in *target heart rate*, a percentage of the age-adjusted maximal heart rate (220 minus a person's age). Thus, for a 35-year-old, 185 beats per minute is maximal, and 60% of that figure equals 111 beats per minute.

A 60-Year-Old Individual with Stable Angina

	Week	Intensity (heart rate)	Duration (minutes)	Frequency (times/ day)	(days/ week)
Initial Phase	1	below angina threshold[1]	5–10	1	3
	2	" "	12	2	3
	3	" "	14	2	4
	4	" "	16	2	4–5
	5	" "[1]	18	1	5
Improvement Phase	6–9	" "	20	1	5
	10–13	" "	24	1	5 6
	14–16	" "	24	1	6
	17–19	" "	28	1	6
	20–23	" "	30	1	6
	24–27	" "[1]	30	1	6
Maintenance Phase	28+	" "	40+	1	6

[1]Scheduled treadmill exercise test. An exercise prescription for an individual with known heart disease is carried out under physician supervision as part of a rehabilitation program. Intensity is limited by the *angina threshold*, the heart rate at which symptoms of chest pain develop (determined during a treadmill exercise test). The goal is to reach an average heart rate just below this threshold, which varies among individuals. Intensity is readjusted periodically as threshold improves.

• *Start gradually.* One of the commonest mistakes among the would-be fitness buff is to start in a burst of enthusiasm, then give up because of exhaustion, pain, and possibly even injury. For the totally sedentary, or those with orthopedic impairments such as arthritis or severe obesity, conditioning might better begin with an upgrade in simple, everyday activities: taking the stairs instead of the elevator, for example, or parking the car farther from work and walking the rest of the way. A brisk daily walk, even one of five to ten minutes, is better than sitting still and forms the basis for progress to more prolonged and vigorous exercise. It is also unlikely to produce the kind of failure or discomfort that destroys motivation.

• *Choose enjoyable activities.* The person who hates running will never practice it regularly for a lifetime, no matter how good his or her intentions. People should take up activities that interest them and that they feel comfortable performing. A person who needs social interaction might do best in a low-impact aerobic dance class, while someone who prefers solitary pursuits might prefer a daily walk alone each dawn or dusk.

• *Anticipate obstacles, and plan around them.* For many people, "no time" is the chief excuse for not exercising. In some instances, though, a closer analysis of the daily schedule may reveal ways to include exercise, such as an early-morning run, a brisk lunch-hour walk, or an after-work swim instead of an after-work drink. Often, the extra effort to include exercise in a tight schedule pays back handsomely in stress reduction, alertness, and productivity later.

Climate may be a barrier in some areas or some seasons; for these times, indoor workouts, at home or in the setting of a health club or community fitness center, may be a valid alternative. The same logic applies to higher-crime areas where exercising outdoors alone, particularly at night, is considered unwise.

- *Encourage support from family, friends, and co-workers.* People who are trying to change their life-style need help and understanding from those around them. It may help to explain one's goals and involve others in accomplishing them—for example, by inviting a sedentary lunchtime companion to join in a noontime walk a few days each week, or planning family activities such as hiking or swimming together.

THE EXERCISE SESSION

Whether an exercise session is 20, 30, or 40 minutes long, it is essential to warm up beforehand and cool down afterward. Warming up serves several purposes. It starts channeling blood to working muscles, causes heart and respiration rates to start a gradual rise, and helps stiff muscles and joints to limber up. A good warmup may be five to ten minutes of moderately brisk walking or cycling, followed by gentle (never ballistic, or bouncing) stretches of major muscle groups. Or the warmup can simply be performing the chosen exercise at a slower pace, such as walking before running. To prevent injury, exercisers should always warm up muscles before stretching them. Stretching may be done at the end of the exercise session, immediately after the cool-down. (The cool-down lowers the heart rate, but the muscles will remain warm enough to be stretched.)

After vigorous exercise, blood tends to pool in the lower extremities unless there is an appropriate cool-down period before sitting or lying down; this cool-down might consist of slow walking, more gentle stretching, or a slow, easy five to ten minutes of the same activity pursued in the session.

How can a novice exerciser know whether he or she is working hard enough to accomplish fitness goals, but not too hard for safety? One simple method is the "talk test": A person working at a reasonable rate of aerobic exertion will still be able to talk with a companion, but will notice an increased rate of breathing and some perspiration. A more accurate

method involves determining the target heart rate for exercise training (using the 220-minus-age formula previously described) and taking the pulse to monitor whether that rate is being achieved.

People who are elderly or have coronary heart disease or other medical conditions may be instructed to start training at a lower target heart rate and work up gradually to 70 percent or more. If the pulse exceeds this rate, it is wise to slow down; if it remains below this rate, gradually increase the intensity of exercise until the target rate is achieved. (See Figure 7.1 for recommended heart rates.)

To monitor heart rate, take the pulse for 15 seconds (use the second hand of a watch, clock, or stopwatch) and multiply by 4. A pulse is found by laying the first two fingers across the inside of the wrist or *lightly* across the carotid artery, which lies on the neck to either side of the Adam's apple. There is no need to take the pulse frequently; occasional checks are adequate to determine whether target heart range has been reached.

Another key to safe and enjoyable exercise is "listening to the body." For example, heart patients may suffer a worsening of angina if they exercise shortly after eating; thus, vigorous activities should be deferred for 2 to 3 hours after eating. In the heat of exertion—especially in competitive activities such as tennis or marathon running—it is tempting to ignore cues of pain, stress, or exhaustion from the whole body or from particular joints or muscles. Avoiding injury, however, means acknowledging and responding to discomfort with a change in pace or a switch to another activity that uses different muscle groups. The expression "No pain, no gain" has been discredited by exercise physiologists, cardiologists, and other experts on fitness. In fact, one should never

Figure 7.1
Recommended Heart Rate Ranges for Cardiovascular Fitness

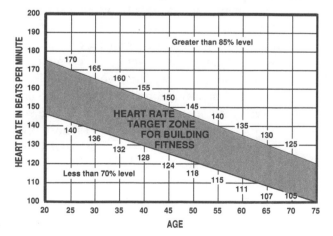

Signs of Excessive Effort

The following symptoms may indicate that an individual is exercising too hard, too long, or too often.

During or Right After Exercise
Chest pain (angina)
Light-headedness or confusion
Nausea or vomiting
Crampy pain in leg (claudication)
Pallor or bluish skin tone
Breathlessness lasting for more than ten minutes
Palpitations

Delayed
Prolonged fatigue (24 hours or more)
Insomnia
Weight gain caused by fluid retention
Persistent racing heartbeat

Source: Adapted from Steven N. Blair et al., eds., *Resource Manual for Guidelines for Exercise Testing and Prescription* (Philadelphia: Lea & Febiger, 1988), ch. 27.

work up to pain or exhaustion except as part of a diagnostic medical test. (See box, "Signs of Excessive Effort.")

In addition, exercisers should take the following special precautions:

- *Hot weather.* It is very easy for heat exhaustion and heatstroke to occur when exercising at high temperatures. Drink plenty of water before, during, and after exercise, and do not rely on thirst alone as a guide to water requirements. Wear lightweight, breathable clothing, and stop exercising at any sign of dizziness, nausea, or difficulty breathing. A number of synthetics, such as polypropylene (sold under such brand names as Thermax and Drylete), are excellent as a first layer of clothing because of their ability to wick perspiration away from the skin, keeping it dry so that it does not feel cold and clammy. Synthetics such as Gore-Tex and Thintech are good for the outer layer because they are wind- and water-resistant.

- *Cold weather.* People who ski, run, or hike in very cold temperatures should dress in warm, lightweight layers of clothing that can be removed as needed during exertion. High winds not only intensify cold, but also increase the likelihood of frostbite. Go indoors at any sign of numbness or tingling in the face or extremities.

- *High altitudes.* The thinner air at very high altitudes makes it more difficult to extract adequate oxygen from the air without an adjustment period of several days. A person who has recently arrived in a mountainous area would be wise to start even a familiar level of exercise slowly and to begin with caution any new activity such as skiing or hiking.

For other conditions that may temporarily preclude exercise, see box, "When to Defer Exercise."

THE EXERCISE PRESCRIPTION

Medical professionals often refer to an "exercise prescription" as part of an individual's health care plan. This term implies a formal, structured, and medically supervised program; but how necessary these strictures are depends on individual circumstances.

For healthy adults who simply wish to become more active, a structured exercise program such as that offered by a gym or health club is not necessary unless an individual finds it helpful for purposes of motivation and adherence. And for people under age 35 or so, with no known medical problems or risk factors for coronary heart disease, it is not necessary

When to Defer Exercise

The following are reasons to suspend a program of physical activity until a physician can be consulted:

Chest pain or progression of cardiac disease
Recurrent illness
Abnormally high blood pressure
Orthopedic problem
Severe sunburn
Severe alcoholic hangover
Dizziness or vertigo
Swelling or sudden weight gain
Dehydration
Environmental factors:
    Weather (excessive heat/humidity)
    Air pollution (smog)
Use of certain prescription drugs (ask a physician or pharmacist)

Source: Adapted from Steven N. Blair et al., eds., *Resource Manual for Guidelines for Exercise Testing and Prescription* (Philadelphia: Lea & Febiger, 1988), ch. 27.

to undergo a medical evaluation before starting an exercise program if such a program is begun gradually. Men over age 45 and women over age 50 who have been sedentary should get a physician's okay before beginning an exercise program.

Some people should begin exercising only under a physician's supervision. These include people with coronary heart disease, elderly people, and those with other medical conditions, such as asthma, arthritis, and diabetes mellitus, that may have an impact on physical activity. For them, a thorough preliminary health assessment is in order, and activity may be best followed in the form of a specified, graded regimen.

The medical assessment of physical fitness takes into account weight; age; other cardiovascular risk factors such as smoking, high blood pressure, high blood cholesterol, and a family history of heart disease; current medications (some of which can affect the output of the heart); and a history of orthopedic problems or other medical conditions. For those with coronary heart disease or a family history of premature death from heart disease, an exercise stress test, and possibly some other diagnostic procedures, may be necessary to determine a safe exercise level. (See Chapter 10.)

An exercise prescription is developed based on these factors plus the person's own interests and abilities. It may be formal or informal; weekly charts or calendars may be used to record miles walked, pace and heart rate achieved, and other variables like body weight, dietary changes, discomfort or symptoms, and mood. A good exercise prescription will allow for flexibility, variety, and incremental progress. Such a program is typically included as part of cardiac rehabilitation programs for heart attack survivors, either in the hospital or in a community-based setting. (See Chapter 28.)

Many health clubs, gymnasiums, or "cardiac fitness centers" offer clients a prescription-type exercise regimen as part of their services, but some of these can be quite expensive. Caution should be used when choosing such a facility or program. A health club or similar center should offer personnel who are trained in exercise physiology and are alert to the cautions and concerns outlined in this chapter. Facilities that concentrate on competitive or ostentatious performance, or that stress anaerobic exercises, such as yoga or weight training, to the exclusion of cardiovascular training, are to be avoided. In addition, facilities should be clean, convenient in terms of location and scheduling, and uncrowded at the times planned for attendance.

THE PAYOFF FOR HEART HEALTH

Even if physical activity did nothing for the heart, it would still be worth doing for the improvements in self-image, energy level, and mood. Adding to these rewards, though, are the very real physiological improvements in cardiovascular functioning and tangible risk reduction in the following areas:

BLOOD LIPIDS

Regular, vigorous exercise has been shown to reduce elevated levels of total and LDL ("bad") cholesterol in the bloodstream and most notably to increase levels of protective HDL ("good") cholesterol. (See Chapter 4.) Part of the increase in HDL levels seen with training may result from a concomitant decrease in body fat—another proven way to raise HDL.

BLOOD PRESSURE

Moderate exercise, especially with loss of excess weight, may lower elevated blood pressure without drugs. In fact, in about 25 percent of those with mild hypertension, these measures alone may reduce pressure to safe levels.

OBESITY

The time-honored formula for weight loss—to burn more calories than you eat—is more easily said than done, at least if diet alone is the prime weight-loss strategy. In many obese people, the basal metabolic rate is likely to go down when calories are cut back, meaning that the body is actually conserving fat in response to dieting. Exercise, on the other hand, raises the metabolic rate both during the session and, according to some researchers, for a while afterward. Thus, by exercising, it may be possible to lose weight without cutting calorie consumption; and by exercising in conjunction with calorie restriction, it may be possible to avoid the metabolic slowdown that frustrates so many habitual dieters. Supplementing calorie restriction with exercise also prevents loss of muscle along with the loss of body fat.

BLOOD CLOTTING

There is evidence that vigorous exercise reduces the stickiness of platelets, the blood components responsible for clotting. Because blood clots, or *thrombi*, are the triggers for many heart attacks and strokes in persons with atherosclerosis, this effect may further reduce the risk of such events.

DIABETES

Exercise helps make the body's use of insulin more efficient and can blunt the rises in blood sugar associated with diabetes mellitus. Better diabetic control, in turn, is linked to a lower rate of cardiovascular and other complications. The effect of exercise on obesity—often an accompaniment of diabetes—is an added benefit.

RISKS OF EXERCISE

It should be remembered that running or any other vigorous exercise does not by itself confer immunity to coronary heart disease. In fact, vigorous exercise carries a slight increased risk of sudden death, a term usually associated with fatal heart rhythm abnormalities. (See Chapter 16.) For this reason, people with a cardiovascular risk factor such as a family history of premature heart disease, high blood cholesterol, or chest pain should *not* take up exercise without medical assessment and supervision.

On the other hand, virtually everyone can enjoy the benefits of exercise if exercise programs are carefully designed to meet individual needs and if exercisers are taught to recognize warning signs that indicate they should stop and rest or possibly seek medical help. After Jim Fixx, the author who helped popularize jogging, died while running in 1984, many people became concerned about this possibility. It should be pointed out, however, that Mr. Fixx may have ignored two important factors: He was the son of a premature heart disease victim, and he was believed to have run in spite of chest pain.

WHAT RESEARCH SHOWS

The effects of exercise have been difficult to document in long-term, controlled clinical trials. This is due to the difficulty of documenting consistent and com-

parable activity levels in large groups of people. There is still no definitive survey proving that regular exercise will lower heart disease rates. However, there are numerous epidemiologic studies—that is, retrospective surveys examining the health and habits in large groups of people—that strongly suggest that the benefits of exercise include avoiding coronary heart disease and lengthening life.

In one landmark study, heart disease rates were compared in two groups of London men: bus drivers, who sat most of the day, and bus conductors, who were more active. The conductors had a significantly lower rate of heart attacks. However, this study left key questions unanswered, including whether the conductors may have been drawn to their active jobs because they were in better physical condition in the first place and whether the drivers may have been subjected to other factors, such as stress, that were not accounted for by exercise level alone. Other studies, including those of physically active men such as longshoremen, have shown an association between exertion and heart health, but again no causative link was shown; in some countries, such as Finland, physically active lumberjacks who ate that country's typical high-fat diet showed no protection against heart disease and, indeed, had a high rate of heart attacks.

The most recent, and compelling, evidence that moderate exercise can lengthen life came from a study by Ralph Paffenbarger, M.D., and colleagues at Stanford University in 1982. Among 17,000 graduates of Harvard University, aged 35 to 74, those who expended at least 2,000 calories a week in exercise (including light activities such as walking around the office) had a significantly lower death rate from heart attack than those who were sedentary. Interestingly, the death rate rose slightly at the very highest levels of exertion; moderate, rather than extremely strenuous, activity appeared to be the protective factor.

THE EXERCISE STRESS TEST

The exercise stress test, which is described in detail in Chapter 10, serves to alert the physician to the possible presence of heart function abnormalities that may be triggered or worsened by exertion. During the test, a person exercises to 85 percent of his or her maximum ability (or until symptoms of heart disease or other problems result, at which point the test is immediately stopped). Meanwhile, blood pressure, heart rhythm, and, in some cases, oxygen consumption are continuously recorded. If the results are abnormal, further testing may be recommended, based on the person's age, gender, and other risk factors. It should be noted, however, that exercise stress tests have a false positive rate (a result indicating disease when none is present) of anywhere from 15 to 40 percent; this rate is even higher in young women with no symptoms of heart disease. It may also be less reliable in trained athletes.

The stress test is especially important for determining the safe level of exercise during heart attack recovery and may be performed at intervals during cardiac rehabilitation to monitor progress.

Who needs an exercise stress test before starting a program of activity?

Definitely needed: Anyone over 40 who has symptoms or a family history of coronary heart disease, or more than two risk factors for it—including being male. (See Chapter 3.)

Possibly needed: People who are elderly or extremely sedentary, but otherwise free of cardiovascular symptoms or risk factors. The decision to perform a stress test on these individuals is made in consultation with the physician based on their overall health profile and proposed exercise goals. Also, younger people with one or two possible risk factors for heart disease may wish to consult a physician on the need for an exercise stress test, particularly if they plan to take up a new and strenuous activity.

Not needed: Young, healthy people with no cardiovascular risk factors or symptoms. The exercise stress test has been marketed by some "fitness cen-

ters" or trainers as a good tool for assessing baseline fitness and motivating improvement; however, for most nonathletes, this is a costly and inappropriate use for the test.

EXERCISE AND THE ELDERLY

It is normal for some degree of aerobic capacity to be lost along with the aging process. In many people, however, much of that loss is due to declining activity levels rather than physiological change related to age itself. A 70-year-old who exercises regularly may well be in better "shape" than a 35-year-old who is totally sedentary. Research has shown that even in old age, conditioning can improve cardiovascular endurance, muscle strength, and well-being.

In many communities, this is being acknowledged through programs aimed at offering elderly people the opportunity to exercise in a safe and pleasant manner. Older people should start at a slower pace and increase the intensity and duration of their exercise more gradually than younger people, and they should select "low-impact" aerobic activities that do not place extra stress on joints (swimming, cycling, or walking, for example). Most important, they should realize that age alone is no barrier to physical fitness, no matter how long a person has been inactive.

CHAPTER 8

STRESS, BEHAVIOR, AND HEART DISEASE

MATTHEW M. BURG, Ph.D.

INTRODUCTION

Scientists have long puzzled over the fact that many heart attacks occur in persons apparently free of risk factors such as high blood pressure, smoking, and high cholesterol. What, they ask, accounts for these heart attacks?

The answer, according to some, may lie not merely in physiology but in behavior. In the last 30 years or so, a small group of scientists has held steadfastly to the hypothesis that the way people think, feel, and act as they cope with the daily stresses of life can have a profound—and sometimes deadly—effect on their hearts. Through thousands of interviews with heart attack patients, these researchers have discerned common traits, behavioral responses, and stress reactions that appear to be associated with increased risk for heart disease. By following individuals with evidence of such patterns, they have been able to amass enough evidence to support the idea that stress and how we react to it plays an important, albeit controversial, role in the risk factor profile.

WHAT IS STRESS?

For some people, stress is the feeling of being stretched to the breaking point, like a rubber band about to snap. For others, it is the events that lead to muscle tension, tightened fists, and clenched jaws. Dr. Hans Selye, a pioneer stress researcher in the 1930s, described it as the response of the body to any of a variety of demands, such as extremes of temperature. Later researchers have defined it as the state in which individuals are faced with the need to make difficult or undesirable changes in order to adapt to events and situations in their lives. Under this definition, stress includes not only the body's response to physical and psychological demands, but the mental, emotional, and behavioral responses as well. (See box, "Signs and Symptoms of Mental Stress.") The demands may be highly significant—a death in the family, for example, or the loss of a job, or taking part in armed combat. But more often they are the ordinary hassles we all experience in the course of our daily routine—a traffic jam, a disagreement with a colleague, a deadline at work, a day that just does not go as planned. It is the way we handle these demands that has a profound impact on our health and well-being.

Not all stress is detrimental. Indeed, a certain amount of stress in life is desirable. It relieves monotony, spurs people toward worthwhile goals, and is an integral part of many pleasurable activities: the joy experienced with successful accomplishments, for example. Selye coined the word "eustress" (good stress) to refer to stress of this kind, and to distinguish it from distress, which is prejudicial to health and well-being. How can an individual tell whether the stress experienced during a difficult task is eustress

Signs and Symptoms of Mental Stress

Following is a partial list of common stress indicators. Not all of these indicators are due solely to stress; some (particularly the physical ones) may have other causes, while others may be exacerbated by stress. If you experience a number of them, however, it may be an indication that the mental stress you are under is being manifested in how you feel and the way you behave.

Physical Indicators
Facial tautness
Muscle aches, stiffness, or tension
Profuse sweating or facial flushing
Cold, clammy hands
Facial tics: rapid eye blinking or horizontal eye movement, repeatedly retracting eyelids, raising eyebrows, etc.
Tapping foot or drumming fingers
Headaches
Sleep problems
Dizziness
Gastrointestinal symptoms: nausea, stomach pains, cramps, diarrhea, constipation, indigestion, heartburn
Coughing
Fatigue
Skin disorders: rashes, hives, acne
Asthma
Back pain
Dry mouth or throat
Change in appetite (increase or decrease)
Palpitations

Emotional Indicators
Anger
Frustration
Withdrawal, lack of emotional feeling
Excessive crying, especially without obvious cause
Depression
Anxiety
Fears, phobias, panic attacks
Excessive talking or inability to express self
Irritability
Impatience
Overreaction to events
Difficulty concentrating
Forgetfulness, confusion
Feeling of time pressure

Behavioral Indicators
Rapid speaking
Rapid walking
Chain-smoking
Excessive drinking
Teeth grinding
Doing two things at once
Restlessness, pacing, inability to sit still
Nail-biting
Picking at skin on face or around nails
Hair-twisting
Eating other than when hungry
Sexual problems
Short-fuse reactions

or distress? The most apparent distinguishing characteristics is emotional: Eustress is associated with joy, exhilaration, a feeling of a job well done; distress is associated with frustration, anger, anxiety, fatigue, or a general feeling that something is wrong.

HOW STRESS WORKS

MENTAL, EMOTIONAL, AND BEHAVIORAL RESPONSES

A person faced with a particular situation assesses it to determine whether it calls for anything special—that is, he or she interprets the event. These mental responses lead the individual to take the action the situation requires. This behavioral response may be calm or, if the situation is perceived as highly demanding and upsetting, it may be associated with negative emotions such as irritation or anxiety.

For example, some people faced with a deadline experience a sense of dread and foreboding. They perceive the situation as insurmountable and become virtually paralyzed. Others are motivated by deadlines, and do their best work "against the clock." Some people can study in a crowded subway car; others find they need quiet and solitude, or concentration is impossible.

Another factor affecting how people react is their sense of having or not having control. One study found that assembly-line workers who could control the pace of work or select their work station on the line were able to work more effectively than colleagues on a "set" assembly line. The workers with some flexibility felt better at the end of the work day and had fewer stress-related problems. Other studies have found that a lack of autonomy is one of the major characteristics of a stressful job.

Yet another factor making a situation stressful is unpredictability. A loud unexpected noise makes us "jump out of our skins"; the same noise, if we know it is coming, is no more than an unpleasant sound. Similarly, it is unexpected bills and unexpected traffic jams that we find to be most taxing.

It also seems that people with "stress-buffering" resources—including a social support network, good overall health, and a clear sense of self-worth—are better able than others to deal with the stress in their lives. It appears that these resources enable a person to keep things in perspective and not become stressed as easily. They also enable a person to have a sense of being able to handle whatever comes along during the day. Last, they provide a sense of belonging and of having people around to call on in times of need.

PHYSIOLOGICAL RESPONSES

The mental, behavioral, and emotional responses described above play a key role in determining the magnitude of what is commonly called the "fight-or-flight response," an innate set of physiological changes that occur during stress and prepare the body to meet the associated demands. Humans share this response with other animals, and it has been part of our physiologic makeup since the earliest times.

The "fight-or-flight" response occurs automatically in a dangerous or challenging situation—or one that is perceived as being dangerous or challenging. Within a split second, the sympathetic nervous system "turns on" and the pituitary gland releases certain hormones that result in the pouring out of adrenaline-like substances and cortisol, which gird the body and the brain for action. In response to these hormones, many changes occur throughout the body. The heartbeat quickens, the blood pressure rises, and blood is directed to the large muscles and the brain—the areas that need it most for effective performance. Fat is mobilized from tissues in the body where it is stored and transformed into fatty acids so that it is available to fuel the muscles.

In situations of real danger, such as being caught in a fire, the physiological changes that occur with stress can be life-saving, as they ready the body for extraordinary action. When demands are physical, as they often were in earlier times, the hormones and fats released during the stress response are rapidly delivered to the muscles by the increased heart rate and blood pressure. In the muscles, they are "burned up" as the work is carried out. Thus, the sympathetic nervous system response can lead to effective mobilization of the body's resources to respond to highly challenging physical demands. While it is hard to mistake the pounding heart and sweating palms of a full-blown fight-or-flight response occurring in the face of physical threat, the response to mental challenge or to chronically stressful situations may be more subtle—and more damaging.

MENTAL STRESS AND THE DEVELOPMENT OF HEART DISEASE

Mental demands, more characteristic of modern-day life, are different from physical demands. They do not abate—there's always more to do—and hence the demands may be more continuous. Meeting mental demands requires lower, but ongoing, levels of stress hormones and fatty fuels. Yet, the physiological response to a situation is the same whether it calls for physical work or mental work. When the work to be done is mental, the hormones and fats that have been mobilized for action are not used up. The unnecessarily high heart rate and blood pressure set up a condition of increased turbulence in the bloodstream, which in turn increases the tension on the walls of the arteries; this is particularly the case in the coronary arteries, which provide the heart with its own supply of nourishment.

The increased turbulence and the circulating stress hormones may damage the lining of the arteries. When such damage occurs, platelets in the blood (which are also mobilized by the stress hormones) adhere to the injured walls in an attempt to promote a healing process. Unfortunately, the healing process results in a thickening of the arterial wall—setting the stage for a possible blockage. The thickened wall attracts other substances in the blood, most notably low-density cholesterol (LDL), which is produced by the body from mobilized fat left over from the behavioral stress response. Over time, some scientists believe, this process may also result in a speeding up of the process of atherosclerosis in the coronary arteries. It is this process of stress reactivity that many believe plays a key role in the development of atherosclerotic heart disease.

STRESS, MYOCARDIAL ISCHEMIA, AND HEART ATTACK

Whatever its cause, when the narrowing that has developed in a coronary artery grows to the point that blood flow is significantly reduced, stress can lead to a condition known as myocardial ischemia. This condition occurs when the amount of blood reaching heart tissue through the coronary arteries is not enough to support the pumping work the heart is doing. How can stress make this happen? Remember, the stress hormones cause the heart to pump harder and faster. If the blockage in the coronary arteries is severe enough, the heart may reach a point where its work cannot be supported by the amount of blood that can pass through them. Moreover, while the stress hormones cause a normal, healthy artery to dilate—that is, open wider to allow more blood to pass—they may cause an artery that is diseased by blockage to constrict or become narrower, reducing the flow of blood even further. As an example, when the blockage reaches 90 percent, the constriction caused by the stress hormones during a stress response and the blood platelets mobilized by the hormones during this response can actually cause the remaining 10 percent to be closed off, resulting in a heart attack.

When myocardial ischemia is provoked by a partially blocked coronary artery in combination with the extra demands of physical work, the effects can be felt as chest pain and other symptoms of angina pectoris. (See Chapter 11.) Sometimes, especially as a result of mental or emotional stress, the ischemia may be silent. Silent ischemia has been found in some studies to raise the risk of a significant coronary event, probably because there are no signals of pain or discomfort that cause a person to slow down or take medication. Indeed, some researchers believe that silent ischemia is one of the factors that may lead to a fatal heart attack.

PSYCHOSOCIAL FACTORS AND THE RISK OF HEART DISEASE

Today's Western society is fast-paced and challenging, and often fraught with insecurity and change. Day-to-day living is undeniably stressful, but it is not easy to measure just *how* stressful, nor to say what the effect of life stresses on any given individual's health and well-being might be. Many individuals handle day-to-day stress without major physiological responses. To delineate the effects of stress, scientists have developed a number of instruments.

One of the best-known of the self-rating scales for stress is the Social Readjustment Scale developed by Drs. Holmes and Rahe of the University of Washington in the mid-1960s. After interviewing thousands of patients, these researchers compiled a list of 43 life events that are generally perceived as stressful and ordered them according to their stressfulness. Not surprisingly, the death of a spouse heads the list, with 100 "stress points." But events that are positive (outstanding personal achievement) or that happen routinely year after year (school opening) also receive a considerable number of stress points (28 and 26 points, respectively). The critical aspect is how much life change the event requires.

Having followed their patients over a number of years, Drs. Holmes and Rahe concluded that an accumulation of 150 or more stress points in any one year is associated statistically with a significant risk of a major illness such as heart attack within the next two years. This is probably due to the amount of life change the events require and the resulting chronic activation of the fight-or-flight response. These researchers point out that while some of the stressful events are unpredictable or outside an individual's control, others can be postponed or even avoided altogether. By anticipating life changes, where possible, and by planning for them, individuals can do much to prevent too great an accumulation of stress points in a short time, and so can help keep the risk of stress-related illness down.

Many of the more stressful life events listed in the Social Readjustment Scale have a clear association with heart disease. For example, the recent death of a loved one has been connected with heart attack death. So, too, can the intense emotions that accompany a catastrophic event trigger an acute heart attack, or sudden death. In devastating earthquakes such as the one in Athens in 1981, many of those who perished died as the result of fear, not from falling debris. More recently, several fatal heart attacks occurred during the missile attacks outside Tel Aviv in February 1991.

Chronic negative emotions also can have a major impact on heart disease. Individuals who continue to be anxious and depressed as a result of a heart attack show substantially higher rates of illness (a second heart attack, restenosis of coronary arteries, or a change in the pattern of angina pain) and death than those who are able to put these feelings behind them.

In studies by Dr. Robert Karasek of Columbia University, people in different professions were asked to rate their jobs in terms of psychological demand (how taxing their work seemed, what time pressures they felt) and in terms of occupational self-esteem and autonomy. It was found that jobs that combined a high level of psychological demand with a low level of self-esteem and autonomy were associated with higher rates of heart disease; assembly-line work, in which time pressures are relentless, work is repetitive, and there is little or no autonomy, carried the greatest risk.

Women who work outside the home and also have the responsibility for children and housework are in a particularly stressful situation. They report more stress-related physical and emotional symptoms (depression, nightmares, gastrointestinal disturbance, a sense of being overwhelmed) than do either employed men or housewives. Not surprisingly, those who are lower on the socioeconomic scale and have less help at home experience more stress. They also have a greater incidence of heart disease.

Illness itself is profoundly stressful, and heart disease perhaps particularly so. This can be most evident in the year after a heart attack. After taking into account the severity of the underlying disease, researchers have found that psychological factors and stress play a key role in this circumstance. In one study, successful coping with the recuperation process was shown to be associated with a better prognosis. Cardiac patients who failed to adjust adequately to their illness while in the hospital coronary care unit, however, had higher death rates in the first six months following discharge than their better-adjusted fellow patients. In another study, male survivors of a heart attack who were socially isolated and showed high degrees of life stress (anxiety, competitiveness, sense of pressure) had a risk of death four times greater than that of men with low levels of stress and with strong social and community ties.

In the laboratory, the role of psychosocial and behavioral factors in heart disease has been explored by exposing monkeys to stresses that are designed to mirror those experienced in today's society. In a series of studies in which high-cholesterol diets were combined with social stress, it was found that the socially dominant monkeys were the ones to develop the most severe heart disease, but only when they ate a high-cholesterol diet and were housed in environments where their control or stability was threatened. The environment alone or the diet alone did not produce the same result.

What do these psychosocial factors have in common? And what is it about them that increases the risk of heart disease? The answer is not clear, but we can speculate that they all expose people to chronic, excessive psychological demand, and to chronic states of arousal that cannot be relieved, because of the absence of physical activity or escape.

THE CORONARY-PRONE STRESS RESPONSE AND TYPE A BEHAVIOR

According to many experts, there is a specific constellation of behaviors that increases the risk of heart disease in people who display these behaviors. The two California cardiologists who were the first to describe this, Drs. Meyer Friedman and Ray Rosenman, surveyed a group of fellow physicians and found that their colleagues attributed some heart attacks in their patients to competitive drive and the stresses of work, rather than to smoking, high blood pressure, or high cholesterol. They went on to study their own patients and other individuals in demanding professions, discovering that certain behaviors were more likely to exist in people with heart disease than in others. They called the combination of these behaviors the Type A behavior pattern and the absence of them Type B. The two cardiologists reported that as much as 50 percent of the population can be classified as Type A.

The Type A behavior pattern, according to Friedman and Rosenman, is characterized by a continuous, deeply ingrained struggle to overcome real and imagined obstacles imposed by events, other people, and, especially, time. (The struggle against time is so pervasive that these doctors initially gave the name "hurry sickness" to the behavior pattern they had identified.) Type A men are frequently impatient, competitive, easily irritated, quick to anger, suspicious, and hostile. They are often highly successful in their professions, but are dissatisfied with themselves. They try to do more than one thing at a time —they talk on the phone while working on the computer, or eat while driving—and are preoccupied with deadlines. They tend to speak rapidly and loudly, and often interrupt or finish others' sentences. Type A women share most of these characteristics but generally show less hostility than Type A men, perhaps because girls are taught to handle anger differently. In contrast, Type B people of both sexes are less driven and competitive, more easygoing—and usually as successful as or more successful than their Type A counterparts!

Friedman and Rosenman suggest that Type A behavior represents an effort to diminish an underlying sense of insecurity or self-doubt. Unfortunately, this behavior tends to set a self-defeating cycle in motion. Type A people "choose" more demanding situations and assess their situations as more demanding and challenging than they really are; they evaluate their response to these situations negatively, increasing the need for more aggressive striving. This aggressive striving leaves them in prolonged contact with the very situations that provoked feelings of insecurity in the first place, and the cycle is repeated.

Why are Type A persons more vulnerable to heart disease than Type B persons? It may be because they have a substantially greater sympathetic nervous system response to stressful or demanding circumstances—more stress hormones, a faster heart rate, higher blood pressure. Because Type A people tend to view a greater number of circumstances as demanding and because they place themselves in a greater number of demanding circumstances, they experience these heightened physiological responses for longer periods of time each day. Many studies have found that Type A individuals tend to maintain high levels of stress hormones throughout the daytime hours—levels that do not abate until after they have gone to sleep. Thus, the deleterious effects of stress hormones on the heart and the arteries (described previously) are greater.

How and when does Type A behavior develop? Is it inherited, or does it result from outside influences? The typical profile has been noted in children as young as 3 years, which suggests a genetic contribution. Further, studies of twins separated from birth indicate that at least some Type A characteristics are inherited. On the other hand, several theorists have suggested that Type A parents may model Type A behavior for their children, who thus imitate rather than inherit the pattern.

Dr. Karen Matthews, of the University of Pittsburgh, has noted striking parallels between the behavior of Type A adults and Type A children. Type A children, like adults, work at rapid rates (with and without deadlines), have high aspirations, and are more often impatient, frustrated, and aggressive than Type B children. As she sees it, Type A behavior may develop as the result of child-rearing practices in which parents and strangers alike urge children to achieve at higher and higher levels, but give them ambiguous standards for evaluating their performance. ("You're doing fine, but next time try harder.") This leaves the children frustrated, without a sense of belonging, and mistrustful of society. Moreover, there seems to be a snowball effect: Children react to the combination of positive evaluation ("You're doing well") and urging of improvement ("Next time, try harder") by becoming more competitive. In turn, competitive, impatient children elicit more positive evaluation and urging. The structure of the American classroom, with its reward system, its competitiveness, and its hourly bells, can be seen to encourage such behavior in children whose home environment makes them susceptible.

The Bortner Type A Rating Scale

Check the space that most clearly describes where you fall on each dimension.

1. Never late.	_ _ _ _	Casual about appointments.
2. Very competitive.	_ _ _ _	Not competitive.
3. Anticipate what others are going to say (nod, interrupt, finish for them).	_ _ _ _	Good listener. Hear others out.
4. Always rushed.	_ _ _ _	Never feel rushed, even under pressure.
5. Impatient when waiting.	_ _ _ _	Can wait patiently.
6. Go "all out."	_ _ _ _	Casual.
7. Try to do many things at once, think about what to do next.	_ _ _ _	Take things one at a time.
8. Emphatic in speech (may pound desk).	_ _ _ _	Slow, deliberate talker.
9. Want good job recognized by others.	_ _ _ _	Only care about satisfying myself, no matter what others think.
10. Fast (eating, walking, etc.).	_ _ _ _	Slow doing things.
11. Hard-driving.	_ _ _ _	Easygoing.
12. Express feelings.	_ _ _ _	"Sit" on feelings.
13. Few interests outside work.	_ _ _ _	Many interests.
14. Ambitious.	_ _ _ _	Satisfied with job.

Source: Bortner, "A Short Rate Scale as a Potential Measure of Pattern A Behavior, *Journal of Chronic Diseases,* 1969, vol.22, pp. 87–91.

MEASURING TYPE A BEHAVIOR

Type A behavior is not a personality type, but a constellation of behaviors, all contributing to a pattern. The challenge in "diagnosing" Type A is assessing the relative presence or absence of these behaviors. Two general methods have been devised for this task: structured interviews and self-report questionnaires.

The "gold standard" in Type A assessment is the structured interview method developed by Rosenman and Friedman. The interviewer asks a series of questions designed to elicit the individual's response to situations that might be met with impatience, aggression, competitiveness, and hostility. For example, subjects are asked how they react to waiting in lines, driving in slow traffic, and facing deadlines at work and problems at home. The interviewer evaluates style of response as well: displayed irritation, for example, and explosive, loud, and rapid speech. Classification of individuals is based on admission of Type A behavior ("Yes, I walk and eat fast, and I do two things at once") and on the behavior and speech patterns observed during the session; the latter two carry more weight. In a more precise format, the interview is videotaped so that the frequency and intensity of such Type A behavior indicators as head-nodding, rapid eye-blinking, hostile face set, and vehement gestures can be seen.

Self-report methods usually involve a list of items on an evaluation form that quizzes subjects about their Type A behavior. (For an example, see box, "The Bortner Type A Rating Scale.") These questionnaires have the disadvantage that responses are based on self-perceptions (subjects may be pleased to characterize themselves as ambitious and assertive, less likely to admit to being hostile or impatient). However, self-report methods are less expensive and easier to administer.

TYPE A BEHAVIOR AND THE ASSESSMENT OF RISK

Large-scale studies on Type A behavior as a risk factor for heart disease began in the early 1960s. The Western Collaborative Group Study (WCGS) fol-lowed 3,500 healthy men for more than eight years and demonstrated that (1) Type A was an independent risk factor for heart disease; (2) men characterized as Type A had roughly twice the risk of developing heart disease as their Type B counterparts; and (3) the pattern was a good predictor of a second heart attack in men who had already suffered a coronary. Similar results were found in the Framingham Heart Study.

A review of these and other studies, in 1978, supported the association of Type A behavior with an increased risk of heart disease in employed white middle-aged men. The risk appeared to be greater than that incurred by age, elevated blood pressure, elevated cholesterol, or smoking. Follow-up data from these studies as well as new data from studies conducted in Europe and the United States have given further support to these conclusions.

A number of more recent studies, however, have not found an association between Type A and recurrent heart attack or early death from heart disease. This discrepancy may stem from problems in the methods used to assess Type A in these studies. More research remains to be done, but evidence suggests some type of a causal link between the Type A behavior pattern and coronary heart disease.

The initial studies on risk-associated stress-response patterns focused on middle-aged men in white-collar jobs, but do the findings also apply to blue-collar workers? There is no clear answer. The Framingham Heart Study, which included both white- and blue-collar men, predicted a greater risk of coronary heart disease in white-collar Type A men than in their blue-collar counterparts. On the other hand, a European study of male civil servants and factory workers found that the Type A behavior pattern was a significant predictor of coronary disease in both groups.

Studies of people who have already had heart attacks indicate that Type A behavior increased the likelihood that another heart attack will occur. Dr. Lynda Powell of Yale University and Dr. Carl Thoresen of Stanford University recently demonstrated that "living a life-style of chronic struggle" is a significant predictor of recurrent heart attack, independent of the risks incurred by high cholesterol, high blood pressure, and relative weight.

The subjects of most studies on Type A behavior and heart disease risk have been men. However, some data do exist on women. In the Framingham study, Type A behavior has been shown to be a predictor of heart disease and angina in women aged 45 to 64. Among employed women, especially clerical workers, those with three or more children appear to be twice as likely to develop heart disease as those who have no children. Overall, heart disease was found to be four times more prevalent in Type A working women than in Type B working women. The women in Thoresen's study who were at the greatest risk of a second heart attack were extremely anxious, accommodating, tolerant, and unlikely to express their anger. In contrast, the men most at risk scored high on hostility and anger.

With children, the question is whether the Type A behavior pattern continues over time—that is, whether it will persist into adulthood and put these children at risk for heart disease in their adult years. A study at the University of Stockholm showed that Type A–related behavior—including aggressiveness, hyperactivity, overachievement, and high ambition—measured in 13-year-olds remained the same at age 27. From other studies we know that Type A attributes assessed during college predict heart disease later in life. We also know that coronary artery disease is a gradually progressive disease that begins in childhood. While this evidence is compelling, a definitive study is needed to clarify the true role of Type A behavior through the life span.

MODIFYING THE RISK OF STRESS

Like the risks of smoking, high blood cholesterol, and high blood pressure, the risks associated with stress and behavior can be modified. A number of activities and learned responses can have a beneficial effect on stress. For example, regular aerobic exercise can reduce the level of stress-related hormones circulating in the blood. (See Chapter 7.) Even the moderate exertion of a brisk walk at the end of the day can be beneficial, because it may help to "burn off" the excess hormones produced by hours of stress.

For some, individual counseling and psychotherapy are helpful; many experts consider that the changes brought about by this approach are the most profound and long-lasting. Group therapy has also proved useful, especially with people who have been bereaved, and with those who have had traumatic experiences. Building, or rebuilding, a network of supportive interpersonal relationships can help moderate the effects of life stress and provide protection from its consequences. There is growing evidence that "loners" and people without strong attachments to others are especially vulnerable to stress. Caring for a pet provides a "buffer" against stress for some individuals.

RELAXATION TECHNIQUES

Simple relaxation techniques can easily be learned. (For an example, see box, "The Relaxation Response.") If practiced regularly, they reduce the degree and duration of sympathetic nervous system arousal produced by stress. Yoga, transcendental meditation, and t'ai chi have similar effects.

There are also more formal programs that teach relaxation techniques. In Progressive Muscle Relax-

The Relaxation Response

According to Dr. Herbert Benson of Harvard University, the relaxation response is an innate mechanism that can be used to counteract the effects of the innate "fight-or-flight" response. One technique for eliciting the response is as follows:

1. Sit quietly in a comfortable position. It is important that there be no undue muscular strain in the body.

2. Close your eyes.

3. Beginning at your feet and progressing up to your face, relax all your muscles and keep them relaxed.

4. Breathe through your nose, naturally and evenly, becoming aware of your breathing. As you breathe out, say a short phrase or single word, such as "ONE," silently to yourself. The repetition of the word or phrase helps break the train of distracting thoughts.

5. Continue for 10 to 20 minutes. (You may open your eyes to check the time, but do not use an alarm.) At the end of that time, sit quietly for several more minutes, at first with your eyes closed and then with them open.

6. Do not worry about how well you are performing the technique, but adopt a passive attitude. If distracting thoughts occur, disregard them and redirect your attention to the repetition of the word or phrase.

ation, therapists teach a series of muscle tension and relaxation exercises, lasting five to ten seconds for each muscle group. Patients are instructed to note the difference between sensations associated with tension and those associated with relaxation. Deep breathing is added for further relaxation. With training and continued practice, subjects can recognize the initial sensations associated with sympathetic activation and achieve a relaxed state that reduces physiological arousal but does not prevent them from functioning effectively.

BEHAVIOR MODIFICATION TECHNIQUES

Among stress reduction treatments, the best-documented are the behavior modification techniques. In most of these methods, patients receive training in deep muscle relaxation and practice relaxation responses during imagined stressful situations, such as being behind a slow driver or having to wait for change at a cash register. Special focus is placed on helping people recognize their arousal cues. Patients are also taught to examine their mental and emotional responses and to restructure them in a nonstressful way. These interventions are not aimed at changing the value people place on achievement, but at changing the style in which they strive toward their goals. In healthy individuals, changes have been documented in psychological symptoms and, in some cases, in cholesterol and blood pressure levels.

Patients with coronary heart disease respond well and benefit from treatment aimed at stress reduction, according to several investigations. In one long-term study conducted by Dr. Nancy Fraser-Smith at McGill University in Montreal, patients who received stress management services were found to experience fewer complications or cardiac events than patients who did not receive these services. In another large-scale study, the Recurrent Coronary Prevention Program in San Francisco, post-heart-attack patients who exhibited Type A behavior were assigned either to a group that received behavioral modification training plus cardiac counseling (regarding such risk factors as diet or exercise) or to a group that received cardiac counseling alone. Those in the behavior modification group learned how to recognize their exaggerated physiological, mental, and behavioral reactions to stressful situations. They were taught how to relax physically and mentally, as an alternative response. Lectures, demonstrations, role-playing, and behavioral drills helped them develop new, non–Type A coping skills. After the first year, people in this group showed a lessening of their Type A behavior; four and a half years later, they were found to have approximately half the number of heart attack recurrences as the group that received only cardiac counseling.

Most experts believe that behavior modification programs are worthwhile for at-risk individuals. In general, they say, it depends on the person: his or her history, condition, preferences, and, especially, willingness to participate. Among the techniques most widely used are the following.

Biofeedback

In biofeedback training, people are provided with continuous information that tells them how their bodies are responding, and then they are taught to control certain stress-related physiologic responses. Stressful challenges are presented and the body's response is measured and "fed back." The feedback may be audio, using beeping sounds that denote a rise in blood pressure, or visual, using graphs on a monitor showing heart rate. For example, to reduce blood pressure, a "constant cuff" obtains beat-by-beat measurements of relative pressure and emits a tone when pressure rises. The patient is instructed to "keep the sounds off." To help patients reduce cardiac arrhythmias, or abnormal heart rates, biofeedback trains them to alternately accelerate and decelerate the rate, by noting the difference on a pulse monitor. Having learned how to manipulate the rate, patients are then able to maintain it within a fixed range. Biofeedback is known to be moderately effective—as effective as relaxation training. Because equipment is required, however, it is more expensive to administer.

Anxiety Management Training

Anxiety management training is a brief, three-stage cognitive-behavioral program to provide subjects with stress management skills that can be easily applied to tension-producing situations. The program includes practice in imagery, in increasing awareness of physical sensations, and in deep relaxation techniques. A special offshoot of the therapy, which emphasizes the modulation of responses when the stressors have to do with time urgency, has been designed for cardiac rehabilitation programs. Anxiety management training has shown some promising results in controlling high blood pressure.

*Anger Management Training/
Stress Inoculation Therapy*

Anger management training, or stress inoculation therapy as it is sometimes called, is an effort to modify anger and hostility by teaching effective coping skills. As in anxiety management training, there are three phases to the treatment. In the first, the therapist helps the individual observe and focus on his or her individual perceptions of a situation as anger-arousing and to record responses to such situations in a diary. Individuals are taught to discriminate between what is a positive display of anger and what is not. In the second phase they learn to use coping strategies—relaxation procedures, meditation, and humor, for example—to help replace angry thoughts with thoughts that are more adaptive. Assertiveness training is employed to teach nonaggressive communications in which patients learn to express negative sentiments without antagonizing others.

The third phase involves role-playing; the person is presented with provocative situations that he or she is likely to encounter in real life. Under supervision of the therapist, the patient learns to manage them with the newly acquired coping skills. Stress inoculation training, often used in cardiac rehabilitation, has been found especially effective in reducing high blood pressure.

All programs mentioned above are safe, as long as they are properly administered. It is important for persons seeking a behavior modification program to make certain it is run by a qualified health professional, preferably in a medical setting.

WHEN SHOULD TREATMENT BE SOUGHT, AND BY WHOM?

People can rely on common sense and the examples of the signs and symptoms of stress listed in the earlier part of this chapter to answer these questions. In general, however, the services of a psychologist trained in stress management and stress reduction techniques may be beneficial to people who:

- Work in a demanding job and find that they experience more than five of the signs and symptoms of stress on a regular basis.

- Are experiencing one or more major life events such as the death of a loved one, a new home, or a divorce.

- Recognize themselves in the description of attributes associated with the Type A behavior pattern.

- Have heart disease (heart attack, angina pectoris). This is particularly helpful for people who also have characteristics of Type A, or are finding that the adjustment to life with heart disease leaves them feeling chronically anxious, worried or depressed.

SUMMARY

Stress in itself is not necessarily a negative condition; in fact, it can have positive effects, giving individuals an added "edge" to do their best in challenging situations. But it can be detrimental if it is not handled properly.

A physiologic holdover from ancient times, the fight-or-flight response to a stressful situation helps the body mobilize for physical defense. When it occurs in response to mental stress, however, the hormones and fatty fuels it unleashes can be excessive and thereby set the stage for coronary heart disease or exacerbate existing myocardial ischemia. Among other things, these changes can raise the heart rate and increase the blood pressure by constricting the blood vessels, both of which can result in angina pectoris or other manifestations of myocardial ischemia.

Whether responses to stress are inherited traits or learned behavior is not yet clear; however, research has clearly shown that there are certain types of behavior that raise the risk of heart disease. This constellation of traits—which includes anger and hostility, extreme competitiveness, and preoccupation with time pressures—is sometimes referred to as Type A behavior. Fortunately, it can be modified with counseling and behavior modification training. Other useful antidotes to stress include aerobic exercise, relaxation exercises, and meditation, or just plain reading a book or taking a walk.

Although much has been learned in 30 years of scientific investigation, the exact roles of stress and behavior in heart disease need greater examination. They are, perhaps, the most difficult risk factors to study, yet it is only through research that we will find the clues to effective prevention and treatment.

PART III

STEPS IN MAKING A DIAGNOSIS

CHAPTER 9

HEART DISEASE SYMPTOMS

LAWRENCE S. COHEN, M.D.

INTRODUCTION

Each year about 500,000 people die from heart attacks. An additional 500,000 undergo coronary artery bypass surgery or balloon angioplasty for advanced heart disease. Early recognition and treatment of heart disease is vital to prevent some of these events. In cases of heart attack, it could save thousands of lives each year; in other types of heart disease, early intervention is likely to be more effective than treatment begun after the disease has advanced.

There are basically seven classic symptoms of heart disease which, when recognized by simple observation and combined with an individual's age and family history of heart disease, can lead to an accurate and early diagnosis. (See Table 9.1.) Not all people with heart disease will experience symptoms, and in some cases symptoms that are suggestive of heart disease will be due to another cause. However, the presence of any of the symptoms discussed in this

Table 9.1
The Classic Symptoms of Heart Disease

Symptom	Most common cause	What to do
Dyspnea	Altered heart function	See a physician
Chest pain	Coronary artery disease	Call a physician or go to an emergency room
Palpitations	Extra beats	Abstain from coffee, cigarettes, and get adequate rest. (If dizziness or chest pain accompany palpitations, consult a physician.)
Syncope	Heart rhythm disturbance	See a physician
Edema	Cardiac dysfunction and/or abnormalities of veins in lower extremities	See a physician
Cyanosis	Pulmonary insufficiency	See a physician
Fatigue	Lack of sleep	Get adequate rest

chapter should serve as a possible early warning to seek advice from a physician.

DYSPNEA (SHORTNESS OF BREATH)

Dyspnea, a medical term for shortness of breath, may be the earliest and most common symptom of heart disease. Everyone experiences shortness of breath occasionally, so it is important to discern when it is appropriate and when it is not. It is normal for an individual to feel short of breath after heavy exertion such as running or walking up a flight of stairs, or after sexual intercourse. It is *abnormal* to experience shortness of breath after routine walking, walking a few steps, or while at rest. Thus, when dyspnea is inappropriate to the activity, it may be considered a symptom of heart disease or, in some cases, of another illness, such as asthma.

A change in symptoms is another sign that medical attention should be sought. Dyspnea should be of particular concern if it begins suddenly. The abrupt onset of dyspnea is often due to heart failure, whereas chronic shortness of breath is more likely to be a symptom of coronary artery disease or valvular heart disease or of another condition, such as chronic lung disease or emphysema.

Dyspnea, however, may not always be easy to recognize, because it is a subjective symptom; some individuals can experience inappropriate shortness of breath, yet be unaware of it or deny it, while others may appear to be breathing normally, yet feel short of breath.

There are three basic types of dyspnea that are generally investigated when a physician is making a diagnosis: cardiac, pulmonary, and functional (psychological).

Cardiac dyspnea generally occurs when the heart's pumping action has become weakened or something obstructs the free flow of blood through the heart into the blood vessels. Poor pumping quality can be due to weakened heart muscle caused by coronary artery disease; narrowing of a valve between the heart's pumping chambers can also prevent blood from flowing from chamber to chamber. If too little blood is pumped forward with each beat there is a buildup of pressure in the lungs.

Diminished pumping quality creates shortness of breath because blood and fluids begin to back up. Pressure increases in the heart and ultimately in the lungs via the pulmonary veins. This added pressure in the pulmonary veins results in a leaking of fluid from the bloodstream into the air sacs in the lungs. As the amount of fluid increases in the air sacs, breathing becomes more difficult. In addition, fluid may also back up into the lower legs, causing swelling.

With or without fluid accumulation in the air sacs, the buildup of pressure in the pulmonary veins also can cause the lung tissue to lose its suppleness and create the sensation of labored breathing.

Pulmonary dyspnea, or shortness of breath as a result of lung disease, is usually due to the narrowing or stiffening of the airways, which makes it physically difficult to get air in and out of the lungs. People with asthma or emphysema often experience pulmonary dyspnea; this may occur when engaging in movements that prevent the lungs from expanding properly, even such simple ones as bending over or getting dressed.

Distinguishing between cardiac dyspnea and pulmonary dyspnea is not always simple, but people with pulmonary dyspnea, whose lungs have lost their suppleness over a long period of time, tend to breathe more slowly and deeply, especially in moving air out of the lungs, whereas those with cardiac dyspnea tend to move air in and out of the lungs in short, shallow breaths.

Functional (or psychological) dyspnea is usually brought on by feelings of anxiety. In this case, breathing tends to be shallow and rapid, causing hyperventilation. This type of dyspnea may be even more dramatic than shortness of breath caused by mild heart failure. The most severe example is the shortness of breath that ensues after a panic attack. The dyspnea usually will go away with exercise or if the person takes slow, deep, controlled breaths or, if the dyspnea is extreme, holds the breath. Psychological dyspnea is often characterized by a sensation of difficulty in getting air in.

Even though this is a psychological rather than a cardiac condition it should not be ignored. When panic disorder is diagnosed, it can be successfully treated by a variety of means, including anti-anxiety drugs or talk therapy, or both.

Other major causes of shortness of breath include pneumothorax, pulmonary embolism, and paroxysmal nocturnal dyspnea.

Pneumothorax, or a collapsed lung, is a relatively uncommon condition that occurs when air escapes through a leak in one of the air sacs in the lung and builds up in the chest cavity. Its onset is sudden, it may not be accompanied by any other sign of heart or lung disease, and it is not necessarily a sign of illness. It may occur spontaneously or as a result of injury. It is sometimes seen after heavy exertion in otherwise healthy athletes.

Pulmonary embolism, or a blood clot in the lungs, is a problem in people who are bedridden or recuperating from major surgery. It occurs more frequently after pelvic or hip surgery, because patients tend to be immobilized for a long period of time; lack of exercise limits the return of blood flow from the legs. Pulmonary embolism also may occur, usually within 48 hours, in people who have experienced a bone fracture.

Travelers should note that sitting for long periods of time in a car or an airplane can increase the risk of pulmonary embolism. Stopping the car periodically to move around and stretch or getting up and walking down the aisle at least once an hour on a cross-country flight lowers the risk by promoting blood flow to and from the legs. Pulmonary emboli (more than one clot) may also be found in persons with phlebitis or inflammation of the deep veins in the legs. A clot forms in the veins and is thrown off into the circulation system, ultimately getting trapped in an artery in the lung.

Paroxysmal nocturnal dyspnea is characterized by waking up short of breath after about two hours of sleep. It results from a transfer of fluid that accumulates in the legs during the day and is reabsorbed into the bloodstream at night. The result is an added workload on the heart and the buildup of pressure in the lungs.

CHEST PAIN

Pain in the chest is the second most common symptom of heart disease and may be due to angina, a heart attack, dissection of the aorta, or an inflammation of the lining of the heart called pericarditis, all of which are described below. (See box, "Possible Causes of Chest Pain.") But not all chest pain is due to heart problems. Pain in the chest may originate from a variety of other structures in the chest cavity, including the aorta, the pulmonary arteries, the pleura (the lining of the lungs), the esophagus, or even the stomach. Other superficial causes of chest pain may be a pulled muscle in the chest wall, strained cartilage, irritated joints, or pinched nerves in the thoracic spine.

Chest pain may also occur when organs below the chest cavity become irritated or diseased, such as a

---

Possible Causes of Chest Pain

1. Coronary heart disease
2. Esophagitis
3. Gallbladder disease
4. Peptic ulcer
5. Hiatus hernia
6. Musculoskeletal pain
7. Cervical spine disease
8. Dissecting aneurysm
9. Pulmonary embolus and other lung disorders
10. Mitral valve prolapse
11. Pericarditis
12. Anxiety states

---

gallbladder that is blocked by stones, an ulcerated stomach, or an inflamed pancreas. Heartburn caused by stomach acid refluxing into the esophagus is also commonly confused with chest pain.

Although chest pain may have many different causes, people who experience it should always let their physician decide whether it is related to heart disease. Any steady, squeezing pain in the center of the chest that lasts for more than two minutes may be a symptom of heart disease and should not be ignored. Some people who have died from heart attacks might have been saved had they not delayed seeking treatment because they misinterpreted the pain or believed it would go away.

When a physician evaluates chest pain in a patient, he or she considers the quality of the pain, its duration, the precipitating factors, where it appears to be emanating from, and where it goes.

Angina pectoris, or chest pain from the heart, which was first described by the British physician William Heberden more than 200 years ago, occurs because the heart muscle is not receiving enough oxygen to function properly. The heart, like any muscle, requires a steady and adequate supply of oxygen to expand and contract.

The heart muscle receives its primary oxygen supply from the coronary arteries. When these arteries become narrowed, usually because of cholesterol plaque formation, the blood supply, and thus the amount of oxygen, reaching the heart may be insufficient. When the heart muscle's demand for oxygen becomes greater than the supply, which generally occurs during exertion or moments of great anxiety, pain fibers in the muscle are stimulated and angina occurs. Most people describe the quality of angina as a pressure in the chest or as if the heart were being squeezed in a vise.

Common activities that increase the demand for oxygen and cause angina include jogging, carrying a suitcase while running to catch a plane, walking briskly up the stairs, and emotional engagements (such as a family argument or a dispute at work) that cause the heart to beat faster and the blood pressure to elevate. Oxygen demand also may exceed the supply after a big meal, when blood and oxygen are diverted from the heart to the stomach and intestinal tract. An easy way to remember the major causes of angina is to think of the so-called three E's: exercise, emotion, and eating.

The pain during angina may be confined to the center of the chest or may also radiate from the center of the chest to the shoulders and down the inside of the left arm. At times it can radiate to the jaw and be confused with a toothache. It generally lasts for two to three minutes and usually subsides when the person stops the activity and rests. When arteries are severely narrowed, angina may occur at rest or after only minimal activity.

Depending on the degree of the narrowing in the coronary arteries, the onset of angina after exertion may be rapid or delayed. The greater the narrowing, the more rapid the onset of angina and the longer it may persist.

A heart attack occurs when one of the arteries supplying blood to the heart muscle becomes completely blocked by a combination of the long-standing cholesterol plaque and a blood clot at the site of the narrowing. In most cases, the plaque has broken through the smooth lining of the artery and attracts sticky substances in the blood, called platelets and fibrin, which accumulate and form a clot.

The pain of a heart attack often radiates to the same areas as in angina, but it will be of longer duration than angina and it does not go away with rest. Although some heart attacks can be "silent" (occurring without pain), the nature of the pain is most often severe and may be accompanied by nausea, clamminess, sweating, and the feeling of great anxiety or dread. A heart attack may occur during heavy exertion, but it happens more frequently at rest. The most common time of day for a heart attack to occur is from 6:00 A.M. to noon.

Sometimes a panic attack can mimic a heart attack. This tends to occur primarily in younger people who have an anxiety disorder. Panic attacks also are more likely to be experienced by women than by men. But whether the chest pain is of cardiac or psychological origin, any of the above symptoms in a person over 40 years of age warrants a phone call for medical care.

Dissection of the aorta is another cause of chest pain. This occurs when the major artery leading away from the heart undergoes a disruption in the inner layers of its lining. Blood enters between the layers, then is pushed along the length of the artery in a pulsing fashion that creates severe pain. Dissection most frequently occurs at the site of a ballooning out or weakening of the aorta and is called an aortic aneurysm. It is most often seen in elderly people with a history of high blood pressure, but it can occur at younger ages with rare medical conditions such as the Marfan syndrome, in which people characteristically are very tall, with long arms and legs. For example, there have been rare but unfortunate cases in which basketball or volleyball players have died suddenly from the Marfan syndrome.

The pain from a dissecting aneurysm may radiate from the front of the chest to the back, or outward from between the shoulder blades. Fainting may occur when blood flow to the brain is blocked, and stroke may occur when the carotid artery is blocked. The condition should always be treated as a medical emergency. It is fatal in more than 50 percent of untreated patients. Fortunately, this is rather rare.

Pericarditis can cause chest pain when the thin, smooth double membrane of the heart becomes inflamed. Both the heart and lungs are covered by this type of cellophane-like membrane. The pain is caused by friction as the two inflamed layers rub against each other with the normal movement of the heart. Pericarditis is usually the result of an infection with a virus, most commonly the Coxsackie virus Type B.

In the early stages, pericarditis may be difficult to distinguish from a heart attack. The diagnosis may be confirmed if a "rub" is heard with a stethoscope. This occurs as the two membrane layers rub together. Although it is less common, pericarditis may be caused by a chest injury, such as hitting the steering wheel of car in a traffic accident. A malignant tumor also can cause pericarditis when it invades the chest cavity. This is rare but may occur with lung or breast cancer, or with a lymphoma in the elderly. Tuberculosis, which is being seen more frequently in underprivileged populations and in people with the human immunodeficiency virus (HIV), also may cause pericarditis.

Functional, or so-called psychological, chest pain is more difficult to diagnose because in some cases it may actually have a physical basis. This condition is being studied in a group of middle-aged women who experience chest pain but who are found after diagnostic tests to have normal coronary arteries. The new evidence suggests that a hormonal imbalance may contribute to the pain. Some doctors are calling this condition microvascular angina. Replacement estrogen therapy may be extremely therapeutic.

PALPITATIONS

Ordinarily, people are unaware of their heartbeat, and for good reason: The heart of an average person beats about 500,000 times per week.

Palpitation is the awareness of one's heartbeat and is often quite disturbing when it occurs. Physicians say it is one of the symptoms most likely to bring a patient to the office for an evaluation of heart disease.

Palpitations are different from the expected pounding one feels after exercise or heavy exertion. People who experience palpitations often describe the sensation as a fluttering—like a bird beating its wings in the chest—or a thumping, flip-flopping, skipped heartbeat, or a pounding in the chest or neck region.

The most common form of palpitation is not due to heart disease, but may simply be a heightened awareness of the heartbeat because of anxiety or tension. Palpitation is often experienced during a panic attack along with symptoms of tingling and shortness of breath caused by hyperventilation.

Palpitations also may be sensed in the presence of premature ventricular or atrial beats. The heart normally beats in a steady rhythm, like a drummer in a marching band. On occasion, an extra beat will occur prematurely and the regularity of the heart rhythm will be disturbed. This premature beat, as it is called, will be followed by a heavy beat, as if the heart were trying to catch up. This will be felt as an extra beat. Even though palpitations are most often not due to heart disease, they should always be brought to the attention of a physician if they happen repeatedly.

Palpitations not related to heart disease may be brought on by exercise, eating, emotions, smoking, drinking alcohol or caffeine-containing beverages, or taking certain prescription drugs.

Irregular or very rapid heartbeats, known as arrhythmias, may occur in people without heart disease but may also be indicative of cardiac problems. Ex-

tremely rapid heartbeats that occur without exertion are often due to conditions called *supraventricular tachycardia* or *paroxysmal atrial tachycardia*, indicating that the rapid heartbeat is originating in the upper, or atrial, chambers of the heart. Usually the individual feels well except for the palpitations, which are generally short-lived. Nevertheless, anyone who experiences a series of rapid heartbeats without exertion, especially when the condition persists more than a few minutes, should have a medical evaluation.

Most serious is a condition called *ventricular tachycardia*, which generally occurs in people with well-established heart disease. Here the arrhythmias originate in the ventricular, or lower, pumping chambers of the heart during ventricular tachycardia, the individual will often feel quite weak and short of breath because the amount of blood the heart is able to pump out is greatly reduced.

Frustrating to both patients and doctors is that palpitations often subside before they can be evaluated by examination. It is important for individuals to remember when they occur and how they feel. A Holter monitor examination or transtelephonic monitoring can often help diagnose otherwise elusive symptoms.

SYNCOPE (FAINTING SPELLS)

Syncope simply means fainting or the sudden loss of consciousness. Fainting usually results after the brain has been deprived of oxygen and blood for about ten seconds. Syncope can be caused by any number of conditions that result in the deprivation of oxygen and blood from the brain. (See box, "Causes of Faint-

Causes of Fainting

1. Low blood pressure
2. Carotid artery narrowing (stenosis)
3. Slow heart rate
4. After coughing (cough syncope)
5. During urination (micturition syncope)
6. Cardiac arrythmias
7. Hypoglycemia (low blood sugar)
8. Aortic valve narrowing (stenosis)
9. Epilepsy

ing.") The general causes of fainting include cardiac problems, diseases of the brain, and a variety of abnormalities of the arteries and veins that secondarily cause inadequate blood flow to the brain. Most commonly, it is caused by an abnormal reaction of the vagus nerve, which can temporarily cause a slow heart rate and a decrease in blood to the brain. This phenomenon, known as a vasovagal response or vasovagal syncope, can be caused by fright (as sometimes happens when donating blood), pain, or trauma.

Syncope is considered a potentially serious symptom, although most of the time it has a benign cause. For example, Victorian ladies who swooned when overwhelmed by a great emotional event did not have a serious underlying disease.

The most common cardiac cause of syncope is an irregular heartbeat or arrhythmia, especially a type of arrhythmia called heart block. This condition is characterized by an extremely slow heartbeat that results in an inadequate blood and oxygen supply being pumped to the brain. Very rapid heartbeats (usually more than 150 beats per minute) also can cause the heart to pump inefficiently, sending an insufficient amount of blood to the brain.

Syncope also may be due to an obstruction in the blood vessels in the neck that carry blood and oxygen to the brain. A very narrowed valve leading out of the heart may prevent adequate blood from reaching the brain; this also can cause syncope. Or a heart attack may result in fainting when the heart muscle becomes severely weakened and stops pumping temporarily. This is not, however, a common symptom of heart attack.

When fainting occurs frequently, it may be due to a narrowing of the carotid arteries, which serve as conduits for blood and oxygen to the brain. Less common, and generally less serious, is fainting that occurs with a condition resulting from an overactive carotid sinus reflex. This occurs when a person turns his or her head and activates the reflex, which temporarily slows the heart rate and decreases blood pressure.

Some people can experience syncope after standing still, especially with the knees locked for long periods of time, as do soldiers standing at attention, or people at a cocktail party in a hot room, or singers standing in a church choir. Blood pools in the legs, leading to an inadequate blood flow to the heart and then to the brain. In younger people, this is probably only a temporary condition that can be relieved by changing posture, moving the legs around, or sitting down.

Fainting can also be caused by an abnormal metabolic condition, such as occurs when a diabetic patient takes too much insulin. If an individual's blood sugar levels fall too low, the blood may not be able to carry enough oxygen to nourish the brain.

Micturition (urination) syncope is a form of fainting that typically occurs in the middle of the night in elderly men with prostate problems. This happens when blood flow is temporarily diverted from the brain as the individual stands from a reclining position or when he must bear down in order to urinate. This is not common, but should be considered before a lot of tests to look for more serious problems are scheduled.

Other noncardiac causes of syncope include hyperventilation, hysteria, and epilepsy.

EDEMA

Edema is a swelling or puffiness of tissue around the ankles, legs, eyes, chest wall, or abdominal wall. The swelling is due to retention of water or lymph fluid in the cells of the tissue. Technically, edema is classified as a sign, rather than a symptom, because it is physically observable. For example, a sign of a broken arm is severe swelling, while the symptom is pain.

Edema is a common sign of heart disease. The site of edema serves as a signal for several different problems with the heart. If the muscle of the right side of the heart is weakened and the pumping quality is diminished, edema may be noted in the abdomen or legs as pressure builds behind the right heart.

Swelling that occurs in the ankles in the evening after standing during the day may indicate that an individual is retaining salt and water, which may be the result of right-sided heart failure. (If the left side of the heart is weakened, pressure will build in the pulmonary veins, then the lungs, and also lead to dyspnea, but not edema.) This may also be the result of gravity in people who are sedentary; the lack of exercise results in blood being retained in the lower legs and not returning to the heart. Individuals with varicose veins and other abnormalities in the veins of the lower extremities may develop ankle edema as well.

A second major cause of edema is kidney disease, sometimes called nephrotic syndrome. This means the kidney is not getting rid of salt and water adequately and allows fluid to build up in the body.

Edema may also be caused by liver disease. Albumin, which is made by the liver, is a vital protein in the blood that keeps fluid from escaping from the blood vessels into the surrounding tissues. Liver diseases, such as cirrhosis caused by alcoholism, affect the production of albumin and cause edema.

At times, edema may result from an allergic reaction to substances such as foods, insect venom, or drugs such as the ACE inhibitors, which are used to treat heart failure or high blood pressure. This syndrome is sometimes called angioneurotic edema. It may be characterized by local hives or swelling at the site of a bite or sting, or by a generalized systemic reaction that includes swelling around the eyes and swelling of the tissues of the throat, leading to asphyxiation. Fortunately, this symptom is rare.

Edema also may result secondarily from interference with the lymphatic system. This occurs sometimes in women who have undergone surgery for breast cancer that included removal of the lymph nodes in the axillas or armpits. Similarly, cancer that has spread to the lymphatic system may lead to swelling of the arms or legs.

Edema is nearly always considered abnormal and a potential sign of disease. However, there is probably no cause for concern when edema occurs on a hot day when an individual has consumed a generous amount of water and salty foods. It also is not uncommon for the ankles and feet to swell somewhat during late pregnancy and in travelers who have been sitting for a long period of time.

CYANOSIS

Cyanosis is the bluish discoloration of the skin and mucous membranes. It is caused by too little oxygen-carrying hemoglobin in the blood that flows through the capillaries. The discoloration usually is most apparent in the fingernail beds and around the lips. Like edema, cyanosis is more a sign of heart disease than it is a symptom. Most people are familiar with cyanosis from historical accounts of the so-called royal blue bloods of England. A common and familiar type of cyanosis is that which occurs when an individual has been outside in the cold for too long.

There are two primary types of cyanosis: central cyanosis and peripheral cyanosis. The first type, from which the term "blue blood" originated, is due to an inherited form of heart disease. In central cyanosis, there is an abnormal mixing of venous blood with arterial blood. Venous blood is normally bluish in color because it is carrying little oxygen, having given

up its oxygen to the tissues. Arterial blood is red because it has become enriched with the oxygen inhaled through the lungs.

Central cyanosis generally occurs when the venous and arterial blood are mixed together in the heart, either because of a congenital opening between the left and right sides of the heart or because of a genetically defective heart in which there is a common mixing chamber. It may also be a result of advanced lung disease, such as emphysema, which prevents arterial blood from absorbing enough oxygen.

Peripheral cyanosis is the type commonly caused by exposure to cold temperatures. This occurs when the body attempts to conserve heat for vital organ functions by constricting the capillaries of the skin and slowing the blood flow. The body tissues respond by removing excessive amounts of oxygen from the capillary blood. Peripheral cyanosis can occur in anyone following exposure to the cold, but may also occur in people with diseased arteries.

The two types of cyanosis are generally easily differentiated by their observable signs. People with peripheral cyanosis display the bluish discoloration only on skin surfaces, primarily the fingers, cheeks, nose, and outer areas of the lips. The color returns when the areas are warmed. Those with central cyanosis also display discoloration around the conjunctiva of the eyes and inside the oral cavity, including the tongue.

In addition to the congenital defects that characteristically cause central cyanosis, it can also be the result of severe heart disease and cardiogenic shock—shock caused by the heart's failure to pump adequately.

FATIGUE

While fatigue is a common complaint of patients with heart disease, it is also a very elusive and subjective symptom—a common symptom of many physical diseases as well as depression. Basically, cardiac-related fatigue will be of recent onset. The individual will begin the day with a relatively normal energy level, then become increasingly tired through the day to the point of exhaustion. This is because the heart muscle has become weakened and lost its ability to pump enough blood and oxygen for the body to function normally.

Fatigue associated with the diminished pumping ability of the heart is often described by individuals as weakness or heaviness of the legs. Such individuals also tend to eat poorly and may develop malnutrition. This type of fatigue may occur with or without shortness of breath.

Heart disease patients also may experience fatigue because of their medications. Fatigue may be noted in about 10 percent of people on blood-pressure-lowering drugs.

Other physical causes of fatigue include anemia and most major chronic diseases, including hypothyroidism, diabetes mellitus, and lung disease.

People who feel tired when they awaken and remain tired throughout the day with little variability are more likely to have a psychological disorder than heart disease. Fatigue is a major and common symptom of undiagnosed depression. It may also occur temporarily in people who are under a lot of stress or who simply have not been getting enough sleep.

Finally, there is some good news for healthy elderly individuals who experience fatigue because they chronically wake up too early in the morning. New research on sleep/wake cycles is showing that early-morning awakening, which generally means waking up at around 4:00 A.M. and being unable to return to sleep, is a common finding in the elderly. Because these people may find it impossible to go back to sleep, they often will feel fatigued in the early evening and be ready for bed by 7:00 P.M. Researchers have discovered that aging can set the normal biological clock back by several hours. Experiments in resetting the biological clock with timed exposures to light and dark are now proving successful in reducing fatigue. When heart disease and psychological problems have been eliminated as a cause of fatigue in older individuals, a referral to a sleep center may be of benefit.

CHAPTER 10

DIAGNOSIS

BARRY L. ZARET, M.D.

INTRODUCTION

Over the past thirty years, the ability to diagnose heart disease has improved dramatically, largely because of the evolution of new, increasingly sophisticated cardiac-testing techniques that include electrocardiography, exercise stress testing, radio-isotope studies, echocardiography, and cardiac catheterization.

Despite these technological advances, the initial diagnosis of heart disease is still supported by two low-technology, low-cost cornerstones: the medical history and physical examination. When carefully performed and properly interpreted, the history and the physical will yield an accurate diagnosis in many, if not the majority of cases. Signs and symptoms such as chest pain, shortness of breath, and an abnormal pulse, coupled with detailed cardiopulmonary examination and a careful history that may reveal major risk factors, have proved over and over their value in establishing a diagnosis.

After an initial presumptive diagnosis is made based on the findings of the history and physical, cardiac testing can be used to establish the diagnosis and determine the functional capability of the patient, the severity of the disease, and the category of risk into which the individual falls. With varying levels of detail and precision, diagnostic tests can establish or confirm the presence of blockages in the coronary arteries, the degree of blockages, damage to the heart muscle, enlargement of the heart chambers, congenital heart defects, abnormalities of the heart valves, and electrical disturbances that interfere with the rhythm of the heartbeat.

Thus, a major value of cardiac testing is its ability to increase the precision of the diagnosis, enabling today's physician to prescribe the treatment with the greatest likelihood of success for each individual patient. In many situations, judiciously ordered tests may also be used to uncover a cardiac abnormality even when there are no signs or symptoms.

The choice of tests and the order in which they are used is guided by the findings of the history and physical and by the physician's clinical judgment. For example, if a patient's symptoms are similar to those of congestive heart failure, the physician will recognize that heart failure is associated with poor heart muscle function and that a radioisotope study is an excellent method of evaluating the degree of heart muscle damage. If the patient has a heart murmur, the physician will suspect a lesion of a heart valve; in this case, echocardiography is warranted because it allows the physician to see the valve actually functioning.

In general, the diagnosis of heart disease progresses in a stepwise fashion from the simplest, least invasive, least expensive, and least risky method. As more information about a patient's condition is accumulated, appropriate decisions can be made regarding the use of more sophisticated and more invasive diagnostic procedures. The following sections describe each of these tests in detail and generally in the order in which they might be ordered—though not all of them would be used in any one patient. Many patients with heart disease may require only one, or at most two, tests to make an accurate diagnosis. (The role of these diagnostic procedures is also discussed in individual chapters on specific types of heart disease.)

THE GENERAL EXAM

THE ELECTROCARDIOGRAM

The electrocardiogram (ECG) is one of the simplest and most routine tests used by cardiologists. It is often the first test used to follow up the medical history and physical exam. Millions of ECGs are now performed each year in doctors' offices and in hospitals because the test is noninvasive, does not entail any risk to the patient, and yields valuable information about a wide variety of heart conditions. (See box, "Electrocardiogram.")

The primary purpose of the ECG is to yield information about heart rhythms and electrical configu-

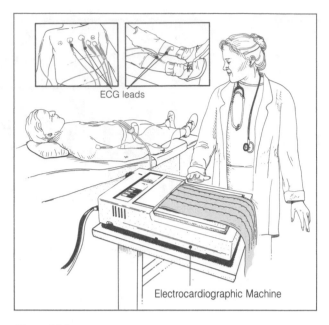

ECG leads

Electrocardiographic Machine

Figure 10.1
An electrocardiogram (ECG) records the heart's electrical activity through electrodes, or leads, attached to the chest or ankles. The impulses are transmitted to a machine with special needles that move over a continuous strip of paper, recording the results.

Electrocardiogram

Description
Electrode leads are attached to the patient's arms, legs, and chest, and, while the patient lies still, they measure and record the electrical activity of the heart, which is printed out in the form of a series of waves representing each heartbeat.

Major Uses
Provides initial evaluation of patient with suspected heart disease
Can usually detect the presence of heart attack, old or current
Detects and defines disturbances in heart rhythm
Detects wall thickening (hypertrophy)

Advantages
Totally noninvasive and safe
Can be obtained quickly and easily
Relatively low cost

Disadvantages
Often nonspecific
May not always be sufficiently precise for detailed diagnosis

Availability
Readily available in all health care facilities and virtually all cardiologists' and internists' offices

rations that may provide clues to a heart problem or heart attack. Irregular heartbeats, or arrhythmias, are a major factor leading to sudden death, which accounts for about 60 percent of heart attack deaths in this country. (See Chapter 11.)

Normally, the heartbeat originates from a specialized group of cells in the right atrium. These cells are technically called the sinoatrial node, but are more commonly referred to as the heart's natural "pacemaker." The electrical signal, which makes the heart muscle contract and pump blood, travels from the pacemaker through the left and right atria to the atrioventricular (AV) node. The AV node then directs the signal through fibers in the ventricles.

Damage to the heart muscle in the area of the pacemaker, the AV node, or anywhere along the electrical signal's pathway can lead to an abnormal rhythm. An ECG also can reveal evidence of muscle damage from a previous heart attack, enlargement (hypertrophy) of the heart, and a variety of conduction disturbances. The particular findings will determine the type of interim treatment that may be needed and indicate which, if any, additional tests should be ordered next.

The electrical activity of the heart is monitored through a series of electrical leads placed on each limb and across the chest. (See Figure 10.1.) These leads act as sensors for the electrical pathway in the heart muscle. The results are printed out on a strip of paper in the form of continuous wavy lines, representing outputs from combinations of 12 leads. (See

Figure 10.2.) The configuration of these waves may provide important information concerning the nature of the individual's cardiac problem.

Each wave on the printout of the ECG is broken into segments designated by the letters P, Q, R, S, and T. Each segment represents a different stage of the contraction and relaxation of the heart muscle, corresponding to the emptying and filling of blood in the atria and ventricles. The beginning of the heartbeat, in which stage the right atrium contracts, is designated by the P wave. The QRS segments of the wave represent the contraction of the ventricles. The T wave represents the repolarization of the electrical current and the end of one heartbeat (relaxation phase of the heart cycle). Studies have shown that a flattening or depression of the normal configuration of the ST segment is an important indicator of permanent or temporary damage to the heart muscle caused by lack of oxygen.

Two examples of results of an ECG illustrate the rational ordering of tests. The presence of ST segment depression on an ECG in a patient with symptoms of coronary artery disease may indicate the need for an exercise stress test to learn more about the extent of ischemic disease and whether it is due to blockages in the coronary arteries. The finding of increased voltage on the ECG might indicate excessive heart-wall thickening (known as hypertrophy) and indicate the need for an echocardiogram to measure heart-wall thickness and function.

No special preparation is necessary for an electrocardiogram. The patient will be asked to remove clothing above the waist. While he or she lies down, a gel-like paste will be applied to areas of the upper arms, chest, and legs so that cloth patches attached to the ECG leads can be affixed. The test generally lasts about five minutes.

Signal-Averaged Electrocardiogram

A still investigational form of electrocardiographic testing is the signal-averaged electrocardiogram (SAECG), or late potential study. This test picks up small currents that are present in the electrical pathway long after normal muscle activation. These currents, called late electrical potentials, are generally found in areas of injury. For this test, a regular electrocardiogram is taken, but for a longer period of time (perhaps up to 30 minutes). A computer is used to superimpose the resulting signals on top of each other and create an averaged ECG which is then analyzed to detect late potentials. The presence of these late potentials indicates a propensity for developing heart rhythm disturbances. (See Chapter 16.) This test is one way of evaluating individuals suspected of having certain types of rhythm abnormalities.

CHEST X-RAY

A second routine test often used initially after the medical history and physical examination is the chest X-ray. Approximately 750,000 chest X-rays are performed by cardiologists each year. The small amount of radiation involved in the exposure from a single X-ray is minimal and should not be of concern to the patient. There are no other risks involved in X-rays; they are painless, fast, and relatively inexpensive.

Figure 10.3
Chest X-ray in a patient with Marfan syndrome and an aortic aneurysm. There is a large outpouching of the aorta noted in the upper right-hand corner. This is an aneurysm characteristic of this disorder.

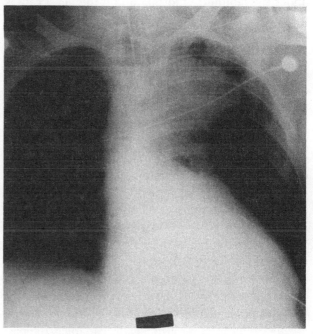

Figure 10.2
This is a normal electrocardiogram (ECG) with the P wave representing contractions of the atria, the QRS segment representing contractions of the ventricles, and the T wave representing the return of the electrical impulses to zero.

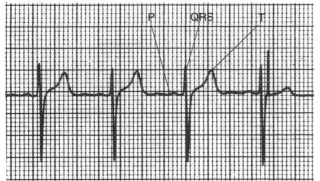

The main advantages of the chest X-ray are in differentiating primary lung disease from heart disease and in providing a clear view of anatomical abnormalities such as heart enlargement or congenital defects.

Generally, the chest X-ray is used to define enlargement of the heart or pulmonary vessels; detect the presence of calcium deposits, which may indicate muscle scarring or blockages in the arteries; show any dilation of the aorta (expansion may be due to Marfan's syndrome or aortic aneurysm); and indicate the presence of fluid in the lungs when congestive heart failure is suspected. (See Figure 10.3.)

HOLTER MONITORING

In some cases, a physician may want to know what happens to an individual's heart rate over a longer period of time than can be measured with an electrocardiogram in a single office visit. The Holter monitor provides a means of recording an ECG continuously on a small cassette tape, usually for 24 hours, while the patient goes through normal daily activities. Potentially serious arrhythmias are the primary indication for using a Holter monitor, although it is increasingly used in the diagnosis of silent ischemia. (See box, "Holter Monitor.")

A patient undergoing a Holter monitor test will be asked to wear a small cassette recorder on a shoulder strap or belt. (See Figure 10.4.) The continuous ECG reading is produced via several electrical leads from the recorder that are attached to the patient's chest under the clothing. Information on the heart rate is recorded on a cassette tape, which later will be played back through a computer, analyzed, and printed out in the same manner as a standard ECG.

The data will indicate at which point or points during the recording period the patient experienced abnormal heart rhythms. Some devices allow the patient to insert markers into the recording to indicate the time of day any symptoms were felt. The patient is often asked to keep a diary to note the type of activity in which he or she was engaged when the arrhythmia occurred.

If rhythm disturbances are serious enough to warrant treatment with an antiarrhythmic drug, the Holter monitor may be used for a longer period of time to determine whether the medication is effective. This information is crucial because the effectiveness of a particular drug and the effective dose may vary widely among patients. (See Chapter 16.)

The Holter monitor also has the capability of dem-

Holter Monitor

Description
Uses a portable recording device, worn by patient under clothing and attached to the chest via electrode leads and patches, to record an electrocardiogram continuously over an extended period, usually 24 hours.

Major Uses
Documents and classifies arrhythmias
Assesses results of antiarrhythmia medications, cardioversion, or ablation
Diagnoses "silent" ischemia

Advantages
Produces "hard-copy" graph of abnormalities
Noninvasive
Very reliable
Allows assessment during patient's typical daily activities

Disadvantages
No identification or warning of serious arrhythmia as it occurs
May often require more than 24 hours to detect an event

Availability
Almost all hospitals, as well as many cardiologists' offices

onstrating the presence of myocardial ischemia via ST segment depression. For this reason, Holter monitoring has become a potentially important new tool for detecting "silent ischemia" during routine activities of everyday life.

There are a variety of Holter monitors in use. Some record continuously, while others begin recording only when the patient senses a rhythm disturbance and activates the device. Some newer models are programmed to sense abnormalities and begin recording automatically.

Although all of the various Holter monitors are effective, none is free from error, which most commonly is the false appearance of tachycardia. Usually recording errors are due to a loose electrode or to the patient's inadvertently scratching an electrode. But errors also may occur when batteries are low or when a previously used tape has not been completely erased. While false readings may result in an inaccurate diagnosis, this outcome is uncommon.

Holter monitoring involves no risk or discomfort. There is no special preparation for the test, although men may need to have small areas of the chest shaved. Patients can carry on their normal daily activities, although they must avoid showering.

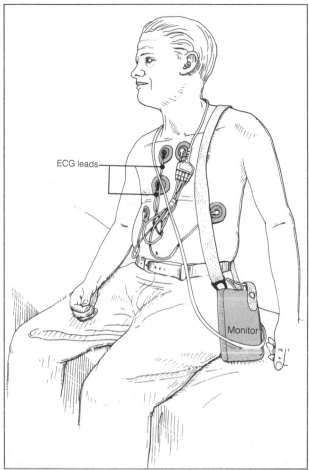

Figure 10.4
For an ambulatory electrocardiogram (ECG), also called Holter monitoring, a person wears a shoulder harness holding a portable tape recorder connected to electrodes attached to the chest. It is worn, usually for a 24-hour period of time, under clothing, and the person is monitored while going about his or her normal activities.

ECHOCARDIOGRAPHY

Echocardiography is one of the most important non-invasive techniques used in the diagnosis of heart disease today. Approximately 970,000 echocardiograms are performed each year.

Echocardiograms are obtained by reflecting high-frequency sound waves off various structures of the heart, then translating the reflected waves into one- and two-dimensional images. New experimental techniques are also producing finely detailed three-dimensional images of the heart's anatomy. (See box, "Echocardiography.")

The advantages of echocardiography over other diagnostic techniques are many. It is painless, risk-free, and ideal for diagnosing problems in children and pregnant women for whom X-rays would be inappropriate, and it requires no preparation of the patient. Echocardiography is most commonly used for diagnosing conditions that require knowledge of the anatomy of the heart, such as valve disease, ventricular enlargement, and congenital heart abnormalities. It is widely employed in the diagnosis of pericardial effusion (fluid around the heart) and is the best technique for diagnosing idiopathic hypertrophic subaortic stenosis, a relatively common condition in which a portion of heart muscle has become excessively thickened.

Echocardiography also is the preferred method for identifying intracardiac masses such as tumors and blood clots. It can be used to monitor the effectiveness of treatment for high blood pressure by taking periodic measurements of the size of the left ventricle and the thickness of its wall. Recent studies have shown that left ventricular enlargement diminishes with effective hypertension treatment.

Echocardiography

Description
Patient sits or lies down while technician holds a transducer—a small device that both emits and records sound waves—against the chest in order to produce different views of the heart in motion.

Major Uses
Measures heart size, function, and thickness of muscle
When combined with the Doppler technique, measures blood flow through heart chambers, as well as flow through and pressure gradients across valves to determine the degree of narrowing, regurgitation, or calcification
When combined with stress test, evaluates wall motion of ventricles and other physical characteristics of the heart under stress
Identifies tumors or clots within heart
Detects congenital abnormalities

Advantages
No pain or risk
Noninvasive
Reduces need for cardiac catheterization
Very reliable

Disadvantages
Cannot measure ejection fraction as precisely as MUGA
Good images cannot be obtained in 5% to 15% of patients, especially those who have broad chests or are obese

Availability
Most medium-sized hospitals and all large medical centers, many cardiologists' offices

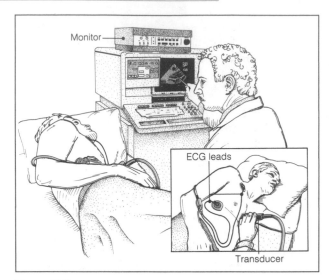

Figure 10.5
An echocardiogram uses sound waves, emitted and received by a microphone-like device called a transducer, to examine the heart. The results are translated into a picture on a television screen.

When combined with the Doppler technique, which records changes in frequency of sound waves, echocardiography can be used to measure blood flow through heart valves and calculate pressure differences across valves. Doppler echocardiograms are the best way to determine the degree of narrowing, calcification, or leakage of a valve. The technique also provides measurements of blood flow within the heart's chambers to assess their function while pumping and resting (systolic and diastolic function), and blood flow in the major blood vessels and peripheral vessels in the arms and legs.

Echocardiography techniques also are being applied to exercise testing so that the motion of the walls of the ventricles and other physical characteristics of the heart under stress can be studied. A stress echocardiogram is done immediately following an exercise stress test or after the injection of the drug dobutamine, which produces a stress on the heart similar to exercise. Failure of a part of the heart to contract well often indicates that under conditions of stress, part of the heart does not receive enough blood and is supplied by a narrowed coronary artery.

The recent development of transesophageal echocardiography, a procedure in which the sonar device is attached to a relatively long, narrow tube and inserted into the esophagus, permits physicians to monitor heart function during surgery more closely. This is more complicated and slightly riskier than routine echocardiography.

No special preparation is necessary for this test. It can be performed in a hospital outpatient department or at a patient's bedside and is available in some cardiologists' offices. (See Figure 10.5.) A colorless gel is applied to the patient's chest and a transducer—a small device that both emits and records sound waves—is held against the chest in various locations to produce different views of the heart. The test takes from 10 to 30 minutes, depending on the number of views and whether the Doppler technique is used.

EXERCISE STRESS TESTING

The exercise stress test, sometimes referred to as a treadmill test, is essentially an electrocardiogram taken while an individual walks on a treadmill or pedals a stationary bicycle. (See Figure 10.6.) It is used to determine the functional capability of the heart, or in other words, its level of fitness. (See box, "Stress Test.")

As the name "exercise stress test" implies, the patient is exercised in order to create a greater level of work, or stress, for the heart. Exercise testing can reproduce symptoms, such as chest pain (angina pectoris), that a patient may encounter during physical exertion in the course of everyday activities. It allows a physician to determine the amount of exertion under which the patient experiences chest pain, while monitoring specific functions of the heart—primarily the heart rate and blood pressure.

A stress test is usually sustained until pain is provoked, significant changes in the electrocardiogram

Figure 10.6
An exercise electrocardiogram (ECG) is usually performed using a treadmill or stationary bicycle. The test measures the capacity of the heart at work.

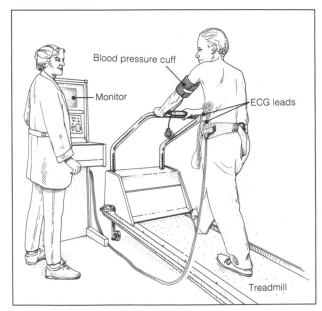

Stress Test (Exercise Stress Test)

Description
Individual walks on treadmill or pedals exercise bicycle at increasingly higher levels of exertion while heart rate and rhythm, blood pressure, and, sometimes, oxygen consumption are monitored.

Major Uses
Evaluates chest pain

Establishes severity of coronary disease

Screens people at high risk of coronary disease

Checks effectiveness of antianginal drugs

Screens older adults (especially males) before they begin strenuous exercise or activity programs

Advantages
Very high safety rate

Identifies cardiac problems that do not show up at rest or with moderate activity

Reliable results

Noninvasive

Simulates stress to heart in everyday activity

Not difficult to perform or repeat

Less expensive than isotope (thallium) stress tests

Disadvantages
Generally cannot be used on patients with abnormal resting ECG

Relatively high false positive rate (15%—40%), especially in young women who have no symptoms of coronary disease

Relatively high false negative rate (15%—30%), especially in men

Can only be used with individuals capable of strenuous exercise on a treadmill or exercise bicycle

Availability
Readily available at hospitals, many cardiologists' offices, and exercise training facilities

---

(ECG) occur, or a target heart rate is achieved. These changes or symptoms will not usually occur during a traditional, resting ECG. The ECG component of the stress test allows for the detection of an abnormality even if pain is not provoked. Electrocardiogram abnormalities are thus a fundamental part of the diagnostic capabilities of the exercise test.

The exercise stress test may reveal the presence of myocardial ischemia (inadequate blood flow to the heart), left ventricular dysfunction (decreased pumping ability), or ventricular ectopic activity (heart rhythm abnormalities originating in the ventricle). It also provides information on the relationships among these findings.

The most common indication for an exercise stress test is the evaluation of chest pain, which may or may not be angina pectoris. Angina occurs when the heart's demand for blood and oxygen exceeds its supply, a condition known as myocardial ischemia. Blockages in the coronary arteries are the main cause of ischemia, but angina usually will not occur at rest unless the blockages are extremely severe. The rate at which the heart's demand for blood and oxygen exceeds the supply during an exercise test generally reveals the severity of the disease. If angina occurs rapidly with little exertion, the blockages are likely to be extensive and the chance of a future heart attack significant.

The stress test is often used to determine the level of heart function and prognosis in a patient with established ischemic heart disease, particularly after he or she has had a heart attack and has been stabilized. It is also a source of clues about the cause of angina that is not easily controlled with medication, and a way of measuring heart function following balloon angioplasty or coronary artery bypass surgery. In nonacute settings, it is widely used to monitor the progress over time of treatments such as angioplasty, bypass surgery, medication, and life-style changes.

Less frequently, exercise testing may be part of a physical examination for healthy, middle-aged individuals who do not have symptoms of heart disease. In this case, it is used to establish cardiac fitness for certain occupations (such as piloting commercial aircraft), or when such individuals have been sedentary and want to start a program of vigorous exercise, such as jogging.

For reasons not completely understood, stress tests are less accurate in young women without symptoms than in men without symptoms. Because the rate of false positives (an indication that heart disease is present when it is not) is higher in these asymptomatic women, stress tests are generally not recommended unless heart disease is strongly suspected.

In the past few years, exercise stress testing has become an important tool for diagnosing a condition known as "silent" ischemia, which means ischemia without chest pain. During that time, cardiologists have come to realize that the majority of ischemic episodes are silent—as many as 75 percent, according to some studies.

Silent ischemia is often detected in unsuspecting individuals when exercise stress testing is performed as part of a routine physical. However, there is currently much debate over whether the general public should be screened for ischemia via exercise stress testing. Because stress testing is relatively expensive, widespread screening for low-risk populations is not likely to be recommended in the near future. Still, individuals who have a family history of heart disease, or major risk factors, might consult their doctors about exercise stress testing, even if they have no symptoms.

The goal of the stress test is to reproduce symptoms or the appropriate physical state within the first 6 to 15 minutes of physical exertion. This goal is achieved by periodically increasing the speed and incline of the treadmill or the resistance of the pedals on an ergometer (stationary bicycle). A briefer test may not provide enough exertion to reproduce symptoms, while a longer, less rigorous one may tire a patient before symptoms can occur.

The heart's specific level of function is graded using a scale of metabolic equivalents (METs), which represent the workload on the heart during the exercise test. One MET is the amount of energy expended while standing at rest. The patient's score will be determined by the number of METs required to provoke symptoms.

More than a million stress tests are performed each year, with a very low risk of complications. The chance of a nonfatal heart attack occurring during an exercise test is about 1 in 100,000. The risk of complications is presumably highest in patients with severe heart disease.

There is no special preparation for a stress test. Individuals scheduled for this test may be advised to have only a light breakfast or lunch at least two hours before the test, in order to minimize any possibility of nausea that might be brought on by heavy exercise. They are also advised to wear rubber-soled shoes and loose, comfortable clothing, such as shorts or sweatpants and a T-shirt. In order to be sure that the ECG electrodes stay in place, men may need to have small areas of the chest shaved. For the same reason, both men and women are advised not to use body lotion.

The stress test begins and ends with a regular (resting) ECG (see earlier discussion of the electrocardiogram), and blood pressure is taken periodically. The entire test takes about 30 to 40 minutes, with the treadmill or ergometer portion lasting no more than 15 minutes.

NUCLEAR CARDIOLOGY

The use of radioactive substances to learn about the function of the heart was first suggested as early as 1927. Scientists at that time discovered that they could inject a radioisotope into the blood via a vein in one arm and, using a simple radiation detector, track its arrival in the other arm a short time later.

Today, nuclear cardiology has become a sophisticated, essentially noninvasive method of evaluating heart disease. Nuclear studies may be ordered early in the diagnostic process, before heart disease has been clearly established, or used to evaluate heart function following a heart attack or other major cardiac event.

The results of nuclear studies will determine whether further testing is necessary and, if so, what type. If the results indicate that ischemia is present and is due to blockages in the coronary arteries, angiography, a type of cardiac catheterization (discussed later in this chapter), will be seriously considered.

Although the term "nuclear" sometimes frightens patients, these procedures pose no danger. The radioisotopes used in most studies contain only a minute amount of radiation, remain in the body for a short period of time (usually four to six hours), and are well tolerated by patients. The procedures entail an extremely low risk for adults. Fetuses, however, have a lower tolerance of radiation, so such tests are inappropriate for pregnant women and nursing mothers.

Although nuclear technology has evolved only in the past 30 years, the basic principle is the same as envisioned in 1927: A small amount of a short-lived radioisotope is injected into the bloodstream; then a radiation-detecting device is used to follow its progress and specific uptake through the circulatory system.

In nuclear cardiology procedures, a scintillation camera (see Figure 10.7), also called a gamma camera, is used to detect the radiation (gamma rays) emitted by the isotope; a computer then collects and processes the data, quantifying the information and displaying it as still pictures of the heart. Three-dimensional images, or tomographs, can be obtained by taking multiple pictures from a variety of angles in a single plane. The computer processes this information and develops a three-dimensional reconstruction.

MAJOR USES

Nuclear cardiology has two primary functions: assessing the performance of the heart, and studying its viability and metabolism and the flow of blood into the heart muscle. Such testing is probably the most precise means currently available to detect the pres-

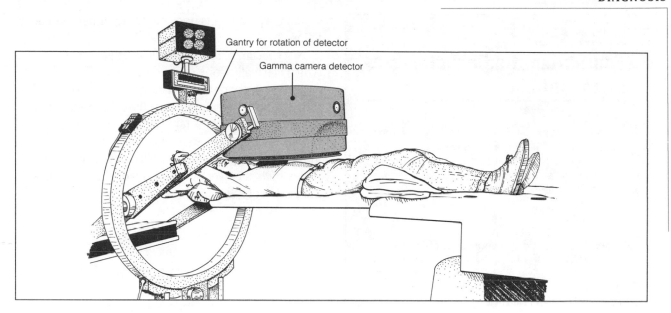

Gantry for rotation of detector

Gamma camera detector

Figure 10.7
A thallium scan begins with an intravenous injection of the isotope thallium. This accumulates in the normal heart muscle and is visible on a picture made with a gamma camera. In this illustration, the camera is capable of rotating around the patient so that three-dimensional tomography (SPECT) can also be obtained.

ence of ischemic damage to the myocardium (heart muscle) and to demonstrate how well the heart's ventricles are functioning. Because of the accuracy and relative ease of testing, nuclear studies are increasingly used in major hospitals to measure this ventricular function immediately following treatment of a heart attack with a thrombolytic (clot-dissolving) drug.

The two major functions of nuclear testing are accomplished by using two general types of radioisotopes. For measuring the heart's performance, the isotope used most often is technetium-99m. This isotope stays in the bloodstream as the blood circulates through the heart, allowing the technician to see the volume of blood being pumped from the ventricles and the flow of the blood through the valves. To study the heart muscle itself, the most commonly used isotope is thallium-201, which is taken up by heart muscle from the bloodstream. The resulting pictures show a contrast between areas of the heart muscle that are functioning normally and receive an adequate blood supply and those that are damaged and thus do not receive an adequate supply. Studies using thallium-201 are known as perfusion imaging and are currently the most widely used tests in nuclear cardiology.

EQUILIBRIUM RADIONUCLIDE ANGIOCARDIOGRAM (MUGA SCAN)

The test most commonly used to assess heart function or performance is the equilibrium radionuclide an-

giogram, more commonly known as the MUGA (mul tigated graft acquisition) test or MUGA scan. For this test, the patient is injected with the technetium isotope, which remains in the blood for several hours. Gamma rays are detected and ECG information accumulated over the course of several hundred heartbeats. This information is analyzed by a computer, which summarizes it and generates a moving picture of the beating heart. (See box, "MUGA Scan.")

The MUGA test reveals information about the functioning of the left ventricle, the heart's main pump. The information of greatest interest is the ejection fraction, which is the amount of blood squeezed from the left ventricle with each heartbeat. Within limits, the greater the ejection fraction, the greater the likelihood that the patient has a normal heart. A low ejection fraction will indicate a weakened ventricle, which may be due to blockages in the arteries that supply the heart muscle, to valve defects, or to a primary problem with the heart muscle itself. The ejection fraction of the right ventricle can also be measured. Damage to the right ventricle may indicate the presence of chronic lung disease, usually acquired pulmonary hypertension.

Other uses of performance testing include the diagnosis of congenital heart disease and the assessment of surgery to repair a congenital defect. It is also beneficial in the diagnosis of valvular heart disease, either at rest or combined with an exercise test. Within this context, a normal ejection fraction may indicate the presence of a primary valve disease that is amenable to surgical replacement. However, poor

MUGA Scan (Equilibrium Radionuclide Angiocardiogram)

Description
After receiving a small injection of a radioisotope, the individual lies on a table while a scintillation camera records images (linked to the electrocardiogram) of various parts of the heart in motion.

Major Uses
Evaluates cardiac function

Measures the ejection fraction (how much blood is pumped from the left ventricle with each heartbeat)

Shows how different regions of the heart are contracting

Advantages
Relatively noninvasive

Gives the most accurate measurement of heart function, namely ejection fraction

Produces reliable results that can be repeated without difficulty

Disadvantages
Requires the injection of a small amount of radioisotope

May not be possible to obtain the most accurate information if there is a very irregular heart rhythm

Availability
Readily available at hospitals, noninvasive laboratories, and in a limited number of doctors' offices

ejection fraction in the presence of a valve problem is more likely to indicate primary disease of the heart muscle, or valve disease that has progressed beyond the point of surgical repair.

More recently, cardiologists have learned that the MUGA scan is quite useful for monitoring the diastolic function of the heart, or how the left ventricle fills with blood between heartbeats. A substantial number of elderly patients with coronary artery disease or congestive heart failure can have a normal ejection fraction and normal squeezing, or pumping, of the ventricle, but have poor diastolic function (abnormal filling of the ventricle because of increased stiffness). This monitoring ability has important implications for the treatment of people with congestive heart failure because of poor filling, a condition managed quite differently from routine heart failure, in which the problem is poor pumping rather than poor filling.

No special preparation is needed for this test, which is usually done on an outpatient basis in a hospital or independent laboratory. Discomfort, if any, is momentary, during the injection of the isotope. The patient then lies on a table while scanning pictures are taken, a process that can last from 10 to 15 minutes, depending on the information sought. The only risk, which is extremely low, is from the exposure to the radioisotope.

VEST SCAN

One of the newest applications of radioisotopes in heart performance studies is ambulatory monitoring using a miniaturized radionuclide detector, called a VEST, that is worn by the patient. The technique may be used to monitor patients with unstable coronary syndromes or to monitor heart function prior to hospital discharge in people who have undergone thrombolysis for a heart attack. The test procedure is the same as for the MUGA scan, except that the patient wears the miniaturized equipment for about four to six hours and can move around freely during that time.

PERFUSION (BLOOD FLOW) IMAGING

In perfusion imaging, a radioisotope is injected into the bloodstream and absorbed by the heart muscle as it passes through the heart's chambers. The basic principle is that healthy heart muscle cells will absorb the isotope almost immediately; those that are transiently ischemic (not receiving an adequate blood supply) will take longer to absorb it, and those that have been permanently scarred by a heart attack will not absorb the isotope at all. Thus, by comparing two or even three sets of pictures taken over time, the cardiologist can make an accurate assessment of heart muscle damage.

Test results that are normal indicate an extremely low risk of a coronary event in the following year, while positive results will identify a majority of patients who are at high risk. Absorption by the lungs of a lot of the isotope is an indication of poor heart function during exercise and is a poor prognostic sign.

THALLIUM STRESS TEST (THALLIUM SCAN)

Perfusion imaging is used in combination with an exercise stress test or, for patients who cannot tolerate exercise, with a drug that produces the same effect. For patients who have heart disease or are strongly suspected of having it, the thallium stress test more accurately defines the extent of existing damage and much more sensitively predicts future heart attacks than standard ECG exercise testing or chest pain alone. The number of cases of heart disease detected with thallium scans is about 20 percent greater than it would be with exercise testing alone. (See box, "Thallium Stress Test.")

The thallium stress test begins in the same way as a regular stress test, with a resting ECG, regular blood pressure monitoring, and exercising with gradually increased speed or resistance on the treadmill or bicycle ergometer. An intravenous infusion of sugar water is started in advance. When the individual has exercised to peak exertion, a very small amount of thallium is administered through the intravenous line, and then he or she continues to exercise for one minute more. After that point, exercise is stopped and the patient lies on a special table under a scanning camera. By this time the thallium has traveled throughout the body and is concentrated in the heart, where it is picked up by the camera in a series of pictures. This process takes approximately 20 to 45 minutes.

When a patient is too sick to tolerate, or is physically unsuited for, a treadmill or a stationary bicycle, dipyridamole (Persantine) or adenosine may be injected prior to the thallium.

Both drugs increase blood flow, thus producing the same cardiac effect without having the patient undergo physical exertion. Studies have shown that this technique is just as effective as exercise testing.

After the initial set of pictures, the individual will be asked to remain relatively quiet for two to three hours, during which time limited beverages, but not food, will be allowed. This period is followed by a second set of pictures, representing the heart in its resting state. In some cases, a third set of pictures is taken 24 hours later.

Thallium Stress Test (or Dipyridamole Thallium)

Description
After standard exercise stress test (see previous description), patient is injected with thallium radioisotope, then lies on a table while a gamma-detection camera is used to track uptake of the thallium in heart muscle; photos are repeated in 2–3 hours. Patients who cannot exercise are given the drug dipyridamole or adenosine to simulate effects of exercise.

Major Uses
Diagnosis of coronary disease
Determines extent of diagnosed coronary disease
Assesses effectiveness of angioplasty
Evaluates patients with abnormal ECG

Advantages
Measures the percentage of heart muscle not receiving adequate oxygen
Can identify problems with heart's blood supply during exercise in patients who have no ECG changes or symptoms
Low false positive and false negative rate
Identifies more cases of previously undetected heart disease than standard stress test
Dipyridamole or adenosine test can be done on patients who cannot exercise

Disadvantages
Time-consuming
Expensive
Requires IV injection of the radioisotope thallium

Availability
Most hospitals and many hospital outpatient facilities

OTHER ISOTOPE AND IMAGING TECHNIQUES

SINGLE PHOTON EMISSION COMPUTED TOMOGRAPHY

Thallium scans are usually done with a gamma detection camera. At many medical centers, a detection technique called single photon emission computed tomography, or SPECT, may be used to obtain three-dimensional thallium images of the heart. Although SPECT is slightly more expensive than standard nuclear imaging techniques, it may be superior in detecting individual lesions in the coronary arteries, in pinpointing the location of damaged and ischemic heart muscle, and in assessing the effects of treatment for ischemic heart disease. From the patient's point of view, the procedure itself is the same as that using the more traditional camera, only in this case, the camera rotates around the patient. In this way, it accumulates enough information to create three-dimensional images.

Relatively new nuclear imaging agents that may potentially replace thallium in standard techniques as well as SPECT are technetium-labeled isonitrile and teboroxime. Both agents are able to create much sharper images than thallium, and each has other unique advantages as well.

New monoclonal antibodies (cellular substances produced in laboratories through cloning techniques) that can target specific areas of the heart muscle have recently been developed. These antibodies are "tagged" with a radioisotope and tracked and imaged with highly advanced imaging techniques as they collect in the heart muscle. Still experimental, but with potential for clinical application in the near future, antibodies can define areas of the heart muscle that have been irreversibly damaged by a heart attack and cannot recover, even if blood flow is restored. This has important implications for treatment.

POSITRON EMISSION TOMOGRAPHY

A major research tool in the area of cardiac nuclear imaging is three-dimensional positron emission tomography (PET), which measures the metabolic activity of the heart, or, in other words, how the heart uses fuel, as well as blood flow (perfusion). Positron emission tomography is potentially important because it produces a very accurate definition of areas of the heart muscle that remain viable following myocardial infarction. But because PET is quite expensive and requires highly specialized equipment, it is not used routinely in the diagnosis of heart disease. In the near future, however, this important new technology may become more available clinically.

COMPUTED TOMOGRAPHY

Although computed tomography, commonly called CT scan, is often used in diagnosing stroke, its use in heart disease is generally reserved for diagnosing diseases of the aorta. The technique, from the patient's point of view, is similar to other scans, but the scanning camera is rotated 360 degrees around the patient, who lies on a special table. New tomography techniques are being studied experimentally at this time and may be used clinically in the future.

MAGNETIC RESONANCE IMAGING

Pictures of the heart in exquisite anatomic detail are possible with magnetic resonance imaging, or MRI. For now, expense and limited availability restrict the use of this sophisticated technique more to research, at least as far as heart disease is concerned. Further, it requires the patient to lie still in a small space for an extended period, making it impractical for patients who are acutely ill and difficult for people who are claustrophobic. In the future, however, MRI may become useful in a hospital setting for diagnosing various types of cardiac disease.

CARDIAC CATHETERIZATION

Cardiac catheterization is the process of inserting a thin, hollow tube into a blood vessel in the leg (or, rarely, the arm), then passing it into or around the

Figure 10.8
Cardiac catheterization performed from the leg near the groin. A small incision is made in the leg near the groin, and the catheter is inserted through a sheath into a blood vessel and carefully threaded up the aorta and into and around the heart.

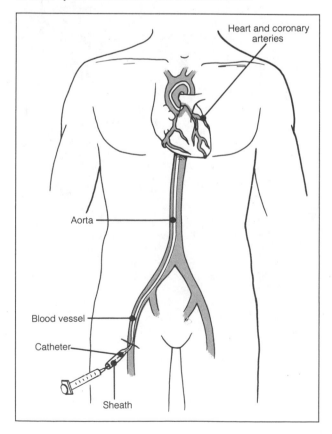

heart in order to obtain information about cardiovascular anatomy and function. (See Figure 10.8.) First attempted experimentally on humans in 1929, cardiac catheterization evolved into wide clinical use in the 1940s. It is most commonly employed for evaluating disease of the coronary arteries, as well as valvular, congenital, and primary myocardial diseases. More than 900,000 cardiac catheterization procedures are performed in hospitals each year, making it one of the most widely used advanced diagnostic tests.

Catheterization of the coronary arteries, called coronary arteriography, is considered the "gold standard" against which all other methods of diagnosing coronary artery disease are compared. The findings from coronary artery catheterization are almost always compared with the findings from nuclear studies and exercise stress tests. In this manner, the important correlation is made between the anatomic site of the problem and its clinical and physiologic consequences.

Cardiac catheterization has three main uses, the first two being routine with all catheter procedures:

- The measurement of heart function by taking pressure readings around valves and within ventricles, arteries, and veins, using special catheters.

- The visualization of the ventricles, coronary arteries, and other vessels following injection of radiopaque contrast dye, which is used to produce X-ray movies called cineoangiograms or, simply, angiograms. The procedure itself is known as angiography.

- The biopsy of heart muscle via the insertion of biopsy instruments into the catheter. Microscopic examination of the biopsied tissue helps assess the possibilities of transplant rejection and diagnose heart muscle diseases and inflammatory heart diseases such as myocarditis. Biopsy is performed only if there are specific indications of disease.

Angiography is particularly useful for diagnosing congenital abnormalities, for examining overall patterns of contraction of the ventricles, and for identifying blood vessels anywhere in the body—but especially the coronary arteries—that are narrowed or obstructed. (See box, "Cardiac Catheterization and Coronary Angiography.")

Various methods of injecting the dye can provide

Cardiac Catheterization and Coronary Angiography

Description
A small tube (catheter) is advanced into and around the heart through an artery or vein in the groin or arm in order to measure pressures within the heart and produce angiograms (moving X-rays) of the coronary arteries, left ventricle, and, where appropriate, other cardiac structures.

Major Uses
Evaluates individuals with chest pain or other cardiac disease
Defines function of the heart
Defines narrowing or leaking of the heart valves
Helps identify candidates for bypass surgery and angioplasty

Advantages
Provides precise anatomic information
Reliable

Disadvantages
Invasive procedure
Very small, but significant, risk of artery blockage at the site of catheter introduction, embolism, or heart attack

Availability
Readily available at mid-size hospitals and major medical centers and in a few free-standing (but usually hospital-affiliated) laboratories

---

different types of information. Dye can be injected and allowed to circulate through the vessels to produce a larger view of vascular and coronary anatomy, or it can be injected selectively at individual sites. For example, a simple way to demonstrate whether a valve is functioning is to inject dye from the tip of the catheter at a point just beyond the opening of the valve. If blood is being pumped through the valve normally, the dye will be pushed away by the force of the blood flow, revealing a characteristic pattern of dye removal. On the other hand, if there is valvular regurgitation—the backward flow of blood through a valve—the dye released in this area will move backward.

Coronary arteriography provides an anatomic map of the coronary arteries and a relatively clear picture of the location of blockages, their shape, and their degree of narrowing. From this information, a physician can also assess the volume of blood that is flowing through the coronary arteries and the degree of ischemia in the heart muscle.

During angiography, the physician may also catheterize the left ventricle and inject dye to determine the overall ventricular function, or make measurements of left ventricular pressure and directly view the contraction of the ventricle. Comparing information from the left ventricle (generally systolic and diastolic volume and the ejection fraction) will help identify areas of the heart muscle that may benefit from bypassing a blocked coronary artery.

Cardiac catheterization is usually performed as an inpatient procedure requiring a one-night hospital stay. In specific instances, the test may also be performed on an outpatient basis—the patient has the test in the morning and goes home in the early evening. In either case, the patient will be asked not to eat for at least six hours prior to the procedure and will be given a sedative for relaxation. The area where the catheter will be inserted, usually the groin, may be shaved. The procedure itself takes place in a catheterization laboratory, commonly referred to as a cath lab, where the patient will lie on a padded table under a fluoroscope (moving X-ray camera). The patient receives an injection of local anesthesia at the site of the incision, and an intravenous infusion (IV line) may be started.

To perform cardiac catheterization, the doctor inserts the catheter through a large-diameter needle and hollow sheath into an artery (to examine the left side of the heart) or a vein (to examine the right side of the heart). Using the fluoroscope for guidance, the doctor threads the catheter through the vein or artery into the heart, during which time the patient may feel some pressure, but no pain.

Once the catheter is in place, pressure readings (described above) may be taken in several locations and dye may be injected through the catheter. During the release of the dye, the patient may feel some nausea, hot flashes, and the need to urinate. These sensations generally pass quickly. At various times during the procedure, the patient may be asked to cough, pant, or breathe deeply. The procedure usually lasts one to two hours. Afterward, the patient is usually wheeled back to his or her room. The leg through which the procedure was performed is immobilized to ensure that there is no bleeding. This is usually done by placing a sandbag on the insertion site for 8 to 12 hours (or less for patients who are having an outpatient catheterization). If the procedure was performed through an incision in the arm stitches will be required and a splint may be used to immobilize the arm for 24 hours.

The patient may have solid food immediately if desired. He or she will be offered pain medication once the anesthesia wears off and will generally be discharged from the hospital the following morning.

RISK

In general, cardiac catheterization is considered to be a very safe procedure with little risk of complications. Nevertheless, an invasive procedure such as this has more potential for complications than the noninvasive procedures described earlier in this chapter. For this reason, most catheterization procedures are performed in a hospital or an outpatient center attached to a hospital so that rapid access to emergency services will be available should a serious complication such as a ruptured artery or embolism occur. In fact, the American College of Cardiology and the American Heart Association generally recommend against having cardiac catheterization done in an outpatient clinic that is not connected with a hospital. The primary factors that influence the risk are the level of experience of the team performing the procedure and the patient's general health and severity of heart disease. The risks of cardiac catheterization are divided into two types: those that can arise in the artery in which the catheter is inserted due to complications, and those that can occur in the arteries under study.

When local complications occur, they consist mainly of damage or bruising of the artery at the site where the catheter is inserted. The second group of complications are more serious and include the formation of blood clots, heart attack because of blocked blood flow to the heart by the catheter, sudden arrhythmias, stroke, and allergic reactions to the dye.

Discomfort may be unavoidable in some patients. About 10 percent develop nausea and vomiting immediately after the injection of contrast material, and a smaller percentage have allergic reactions to the dye, including headache, sneezing, chills, fever, hives, itching, or shock.

SUMMARY

Different types of cardiac testing can provide a large amount of information. In many cases, only one type of test may be necessary; in others, combining the results of two or more tests may yield greater precision in the diagnosis.

It is important to understand that a patient who undergoes a large battery of tests is not necessarily receiving superior medical care, nor that care is substandard when relatively few tests have been ordered. The number and type of tests used will vary from patient to patient, depending on the type and severity of disease.

It is appropriate, however, for the patient as a consumer to ask the physician at any stage of the diagnosis why a particular test is being performed and what information the test is expected to yield. Cardiac testing should always flow in a rational order from the findings of the history and physical and from the results of each test used in the course of the diagnosis. This rational order of testing will minimize unnecessary costs and risks to the patient.

PART IV

MAJOR CARDIOVASCULAR DISORDERS

CHAPTER 11

HEART ATTACKS AND CORONARY ARTERY DISEASE

LAWRENCE DECKELBAUM, M.D.

INTRODUCTION

Coronary artery disease has probably affected human beings throughout history, but it is only in the last century or so that it has emerged as a leading cause of death. The first description of the symptoms of coronary artery disease was written in 1768 by William Heberden, an English physician. Dr. Heberden coined the term "angina pectoris"—from the Latin, *angere*, which means to strangle or distress, and *pectoris*, "of the chest"—and his classic description still holds true today:

There is a disorder of the breast, marked with strong and peculiar symptoms considerable for the kind of danger belonging to it, and not extremely rare, of which I do not recollect any mention among medical authors. The seat of it, and sense of strangling and anxiety, with which it is attended, may make it not improperly be called Angina pectoris.

Those, who are afflicted with it, are seized while they are walking and more particularly when they walk soon after eating, with a painful and most disagreeable sensation in the breast, which seems as if it would take their life away, if it were to increase or to continue; the moment they stand still, all this uneasiness vanishes.

Although the relationship between angina pectoris and diseased coronary arteries was established just a few years later, it was not until the early 20th century that the medical profession gave widespread recognition to coronary artery disease as a major cause of death. Such recognition may have been slow in coming because the disease was not widely prevalent until around the middle of the 19th century. With the advent of improved sanitation, immunization, and other advances in public health, the death toll from infectious diseases—previously the leading cause of death—dropped. In industrialized nations, these advances in public health coincided with life-style changes, such as adoption of a diet high in meat and other fatty foods, an increase in cigarette smoking, and a more sedentary life-style. It was at this time that the death rate from heart attacks began to soar. (See Chapter 3.)

According to statistics compiled by the Centers for Disease Control, almost one in two Americans dies of cardiovascular disease. The total annual toll is more than 975,000; of these, about 500,000 die of heart attacks. The large majority of heart attacks results from coronary artery disease, a condition that afflicts about 5 million Americans.

Of course, mortality statistics are only part of the story—coronary artery disease also affects life-style, productivity, and the economy. According to 1991 figures compiled by the American Heart Association and the National Center for Health Statistics, about 6 million Americans have a history of a heart attack, angina, or both. Although the likelihood of a heart attack increases with age, a large number of Americans—mostly men—are struck down during their most productive years. About 45 percent of heart attacks occur before the age of 65, with 5 percent before age 40. The American Heart Association puts the total annual cost of cardiovascular disease at $94.5 billion, a figure that includes both direct medical costs and estimated lost productivity resulting from disability.

Fortunately, the number of deaths from coronary artery disease—while still unacceptably high—has been steadily declining since the late 1950s. In 1950, the age-adjusted death rate from heart attacks was 226 per 100,000 Americans. By 1986, this had dropped by nearly half to 129 per 100,000. For example, the five-year survival rate of patients with angina improved from 75 percent in the years 1950 to 1970, to 87 percent during 1970 to 1975. Much of this improvement is undoubtedly the result of improved medical care. But altered life-style factors such as smoking cessation and a reduction in fat consumption are also believed to lower the risk of premature death from a heart attack.

ANATOMY OF THE HEART

The normal human heart has two major coronary arteries, so named because, together with their branches, they surround the heart like a crown (or *corona*). From its branch off the aorta, the left main coronary artery quickly divides into two vessels: the left anterior descending artery and the circumflex artery. Another vessel, the right coronary artery, comes off the aorta and supplies blood to the right and bottom parts of the heart. The three vessels supply all the oxygenated blood necessary to keep the heart's muscle and electrical conduction system functioning and viable. (See Chapter 1.)

Although the body's entire volume of blood passes through the heart's chambers approximately every 60 seconds, only about 5 percent of the total amount of oxygenated blood is available for the heart's own energy needs. The coronary arteries (which are 3 to 5 millimeters or ⅛ to ⅕ of an inch in diameter) are the sole conduits for this supply. Because heart muscle (myocardium) extracts oxygen from arterial blood with maximum efficiency, any increase in the heart's workload requires an increase in the blood supply. When there is an imbalance between the available supply of blood (oxygen) and demand for blood (oxygen), the heart muscle becomes oxygen-deprived, a condition known as myocardial ischemia. Without adequate blood flow to the heart muscle, the heart itself is unable to function properly.

OXYGEN DEPRIVATION (ISCHEMIA)

For the majority of people suffering from coronary artery disease, the supply of oxygenated blood is reduced due to a progressive narrowing of the open channels (the interior lumens) of the coronary arteries. This is due to atherosclerosis, a disease in which scattered lesions, known as atherosclerotic, plaques or atheromas, appear on the inner wall of the coronary artery. See Figure 11.1, a series of illustrations showing how an artery becomes blocked. (The word *atheroma* comes from the Greek for porridge, because atheromas contain a porridgelike mixture of cholesterol, fat, and fibrous or scarlike tissue.)

The first signs of atherosclerosis can appear at an early age. A significant proportion of males in their teens and early 20s may already have fatty streaks and other evidence of the disease on the walls of their coronary arteries—as was first demonstrated by autopsies conducted on young American soldiers killed during the Korean War. The buildup of atherosclerotic plaque is a gradual process, however, and it may take upward of 20 years or more from the first appearance of fatty streaks before the coronary arteries are blocked enough to produce symptoms such as angina or shortness of breath. Symptoms usually do not occur until the coronary artery has been narrowed by about 50 to 70 percent. Even with significantly clogged coronary arteries causing ischemia, however, many people do not experience symptoms. This is referred to as silent ischemia.

The exact causes of buildup of atherosclerotic

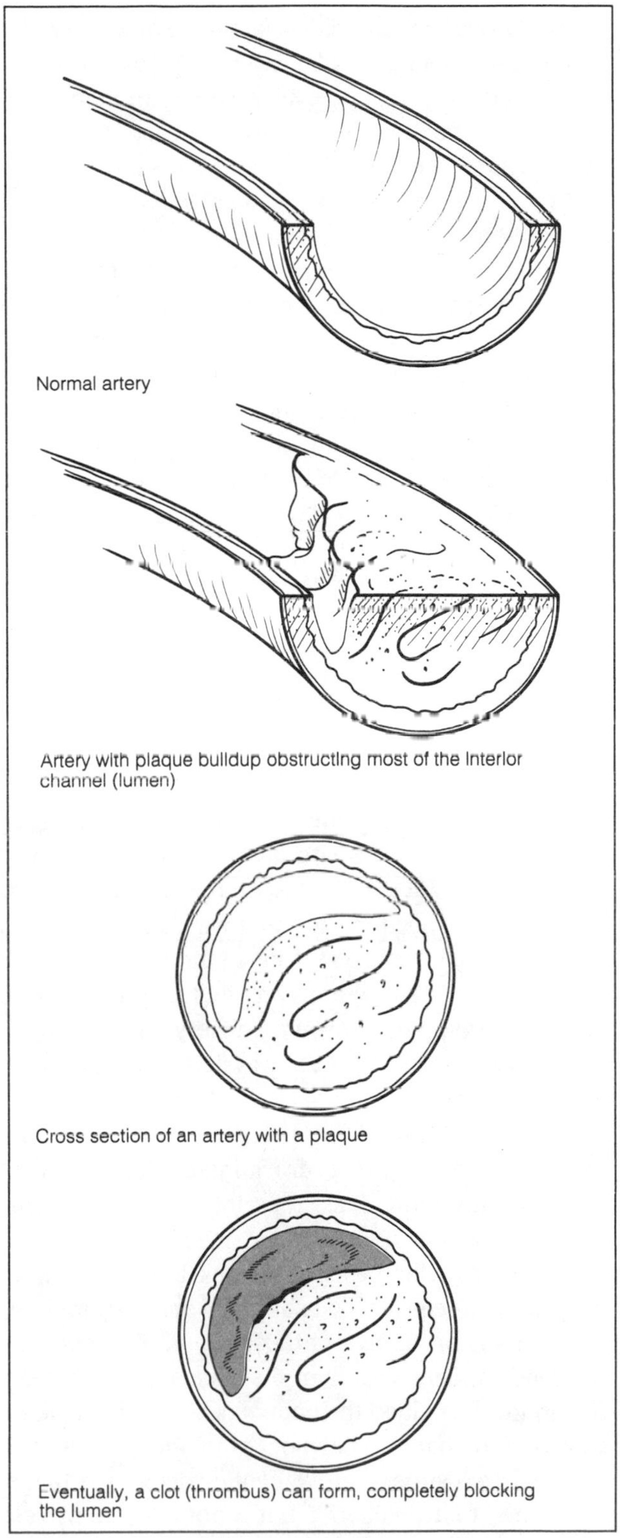

Normal artery

Artery with plaque buildup obstructing most of the interior channel (lumen)

Cross section of an artery with a plaque

Eventually, a clot (thrombus) can form, completely blocking the lumen

Figure 11.1
How a normal artery may become blocked by fatty plaque.

plaque are not understood, nor is it possible to pinpoint how they begin or what their course will be. However, evidence based on a number of long-term studies (such as the Framingham Heart Study, which has examined the health of several thousand men and women in the Boston suburb of Framingham from 1948 to the present day) has enabled us to identify which *risk factors* increase the likelihood that someone will develop atherosclerosis. These risk factors include some that are controllable, such as smoking, hypertension, and elevated blood cholesterol, as well as age, gender, family history, and other factors that are beyond our control. (See Chapter 3.)

In addition to atherosclerotic plaque buildup, spasms of the muscles that encircle the coronary arteries can also interrupt the coronary blood supply. In 85 percent of people who have coronary artery spasms, atherosclerosis is also present. In about 10 to 15 percent of people with typical anginal chest pains, spasms may be the sole cause of the oxygen deprivation (ischemia) and resulting pain.

Some people who experience angina may have normal coronary arteries. The angina some of these people experience may be caused by a constriction or narrowing of the aortic valve. In others—who may have no evidence of coronary artery spasm, heart valve disease, or left ventricular heart muscle abnormality—there is no clear reason for the angina. These people generally have an excellent overall prognosis.

An inability to deliver adequate oxygen during rest or periods of increased demand can result in ischemia manifested by angina and other symptoms. Factors affecting the heart muscles' demand for blood include blood pressure, heart rate, and the size of the left ventricle.

A sizable percentage of people suffer from chronically high blood pressure. In addition, blood pressure temporarily rises during exercise or periods of stress. (See Chapter 12.) The heart rate is increased by exertion, fever, stress, and an overactive thyroid. Enlargement of the main pumping chamber—the left ventricle—is commonly the result of hypertension or certain heart valve disorders. All of these conditions result in increased work for the heart and the need for more oxygen. If this cannot be supplied, symptoms may occur.

SYMPTOMS

The primary symptom of coronary artery disease is chest pain or *angina*, which is not itself a disease but a set of symptoms closely corresponding to Heberden's original description. A person suffering from angina may clutch a fist to the chest while describing

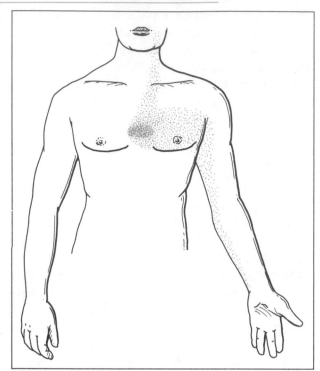

Figure 11.2
The shaded areas show locations for angina. It occurs most frequently or classically in the center of the chest (most heavily shaded area), but it may also radiate to the whole chest, neck, jaw, and down the arms, particularly on the left side. Angina can also occur in these places without occurring in the center of the chest.

a feeling of discomfort or pain, often using such words as "pressure" or "heaviness." This pain is usually located in the center of the chest but may radiate to or occur only in the neck, shoulder, arm, or lower jaw, particularly on the left side. (See Figure 11.2.) Brief sharp stabbing or sticking pains confined to a small area of the chest are rarely caused by angina.

For most people, these symptoms almost always occur during or after physical activity and/or emotional stress and are more likely to occur following a meal or in cold weather. People who have what is known as stable angina can often predict with reasonable accuracy the amount of activity that precipitates an attack—sometimes to the point of knowing how many stairs they can climb before pain begins. Typical activities that might bring on angina include walking up several flights of stairs, climbing a hill, or other sudden vigorous activities, such as running for a bus or playing tennis. A change in anginal pattern, such as increased frequency of angina or the new onset of angina at rest, is referred to as crescendo or unstable angina.

Angina may be more likely to occur following a meal, because blood pools in the stomach and the intestinal tract during digestion, increasing the work of the heart. During cold weather, angina may also be more frequent because vessels may go into spasm, increasing the work of the heart while simultaneously decreasing the blood supply to the heart. In general, anginal symptoms usually fade and disappear when the person ceases the particular activity that provoked them.

Ischemia may occasionally occur without symptoms of angina or other discomfort, so-called "silent ischemia." Some patients may experience only silent episodes of ischemia, whereas others have episodes with and without angina. The potential danger of silent ischemia is that someone may not be aware of the reduced blood flow to the heart muscle and might, therefore, be less likely to cease the activity precipitating it. The diagnosis, significance, and treatment of silent ischemia are areas of active research.

DIAGNOSIS

Angina is a clinical diagnosis; however, diagnosing coronary artery disease purely on the basis of symptoms may be difficult. The discomfort of angina is not always experienced in the same way, and a patient's symptoms may be vague. Chest pain can also occur in a variety of other conditions that may exist alone or may accompany coronary artery disease. It is, therefore, important for the physician to distinguish between anginal pains and chest pain from other sources. (See Table 11.1.) Anginal pain usually begins gradually and lasts for several minutes, generally fading when the individual stops the activity that precipitated the attack or takes a medication such as nitroglycerin, which widens (dilates) the coronary arteries and increases blood supply to the heart muscle.

Angina is probably not the cause of the chest discomfort if it lasts less than 5 seconds or more than 20 minutes (provided the patient is not having a heart attack), if the pain is sharp or "stabbing," if it is precipitated by a sudden movement or deep breath, if it is confined to a small area, if it is not relieved by rest or cessation of physical activity (again, provided the patient is not having a heart attack), or if the chest wall is tender to the touch.

The sources of chest pain that mimic angina include esophageal or stomach disorders (for example, reflux of stomach acid into the esophagus, resulting in "heartburn"), pain due to obstruction of the bile duct, inflammation of the cartilage of the chest wall, and arthritis of the bones in the neck.

Table 11.1
Identifying Causes of Chest Pain

Causes	Type of chest pain and other symptoms	Causes	Type of chest pain and other symptoms
Blood clot in the lung (pulmonary embolism)	Chest pain accompanied by breathlessness, faintness, cough bringing up bloody phlegm, blueness (cyanosis) around the mouth.	Lack of oxygen in the heart (angina)	Dull, heavy, constricting pain in the center of the chest that can spread to throat and upper jaw, back, and arms (mainly left arm). Pain appears when person is active and disappears when activity stops and person rests. Can be accompanied by difficult breathing, sweating, nausea, and dizziness.
Broken rib	Pain in or near the chest area that increases with pressure or movement; area around fracture may be swollen and bruised.		
Collapsed lung (pneumothorax)	Usually sudden sharp chest pain on one side of the body, accompanied by breathlessness; may be discomfort rather than pain, may include pain at the bottom of the neck and tightness across chest.	Nerve infection (shingles) in the chest area	Intense, knifelike pain in one area of the chest that precedes, by several days or less, a rash (groups of blisters on the skin—much like chicken pox—above the affected nerve); pain continues through and after rash appearance.
Heart attack	Crushing pain in the center of the chest, accompanied by difficult breathing, sweating, nausea, or a feeling of faintness.		
Heartburn and hiatus hernia	Painful burning sensation in the chest that becomes worse when person bends forward or lies down; person may also experience belching and regurgitation of acidic fluid.	Pneumonia	Respiratory illness, including cough and fever, precedes other symptoms, including chest pain, shortness of breath, chills, sweating, bloody or yellow phlegm, or delirium.
Infection of the airways in the lungs (acute bronchitis)	Pain in the upper chest that worsens when coughing; deep cough that brings up grayish or yellowish phlegm from the lungs.	Pulled muscle in the chest area	Pain, stiffness, or tenderness in the chest area as a result of overstretching a muscle (for instance, while working out); area may become swollen as a result of internal bleeding.

Disorders of the heart can also result in anginalike symptoms. These include an elevated pressure in the lungs (*pulmonary hypertension*) or a blood clot in an artery supplying the lungs (*pulmonary embolism*), resulting in lack of oxygen delivery to the lung tissue. Inflammation or infection of the tough outer sac that covers the heart (*acute pericarditis*) can produce persistent chest pain, which usually comes on suddenly and is aggravated by coughing or movement.

Further complicating the difficulty of making a diagnosis of coronary artery disease on the basis of symptoms alone is the existence of *silent ischemia*. Some people—who may or may not also occasionally experience anginal discomfort—can show all the clinical signs of an attack of angina and yet may not feel any discomfort at the time. This syndrome appears to be more common in persons with diabetes.

The presence of chest discomfort in someone who

has several risk factors for heart disease strongly suggests to the physician that the patient has coronary artery disease. However, accurate diagnosis of coronary artery disease in these people (and those with chest pain who do not fit the risk profile) may require some of the following tests.

ELECTROCARDIOGRAPHY

The electrocardiogram (ECG), a graphic record of the electric currents generated by the heart, is an essential tool for the diagnosis of coronary artery disease. An ECG taken while a person is resting (a resting, or baseline, ECG) will not show evidence of lack of oxygen in the heart muscle—unless the patient is having an attack of angina at the time—but it can demonstrate the presence of a previous heart attack or other changes suggesting that the heart muscle may not be receiving an adequate blood supply.

The baseline ECG can provide a considerably more useful diagnosis if the patient experiences angina during testing. The test can then not only show that inadequate oxygen is reaching the heart muscle, but also give an idea of which artery is blocked and the extent of heart muscle that may be at risk.

The exercise ECG—popularly known as an exercise stress or tolerance test—is another useful tool for diagnosis. While being monitored, the patient engages in physical activity of progressive intensity, usually on a treadmill, stationary bicycle, or stair-climbing device. Exercise is usually continued until the heart rate reaches 85 percent of a calculated so-called maximum level—about 220 minus the person's age (for a 60-year-old person, about 160 beats per minute), or until symptoms of fatigue or chest pain or significant ECG changes are noted.

If coronary arteries are healthy, they dilate or open up to supply the extra blood and oxygen necessary to sustain the extra heart muscle workload. If this occurs, the electrocardiogram shows few changes. If the arteries are narrowed or go into spasm, however, portions of the heart muscle do not get enough blood and ECG changes will occur.

If changes occur at low work levels after only a few minutes and/or at a heart rate of only about 100 beats per minute, this suggests that coronary heart disease may be fairly severe. It is also useful to monitor a patient's blood pressure and heart rate during the test, because a drop in blood pressure during exercise also implies that the extent of coronary artery disease may be severe. The exercise ECG can correctly identify about 65 to 75 percent of people with coronary artery disease.

Holter monitoring, or the ambulatory ECG, which is worn for 24 to 48 hours, may be a useful tool in diagnosing some cases of angina. ECG changes may be recorded during episodes of angina. Like other tests in cardiology, it may not be necessary in all cases.

RADIOISOTOPE SCANS

Thallium-201 is an isotope that is used for diagnosing coronary artery disease. This radioactive substance is injected and passes through the bloodstream into the heart muscle cells. The distribution of thallium is recorded with a gamma camera, and areas of heart muscle that are not getting sufficient oxygen show up as "cold spots" in which the blood flow did not deliver thallium or the heart muscle cells did not take it up. Combined with the exercise ECG, an exercise thallium test helps to correctly identify about 90 percent of people with coronary obstructions. This test also helps to locate the specific sites of lesions. Recently, new radioisotope agents have become available that may replace thallium-201 in the future. (See Chapter 10.)

Another diagnostic tool, multigated acquisition scan (MUGA), which uses the radioisotope technetium, can also provide information on the size and contraction pattern of the left ventricle. Contraction abnormalities that are induced by exercise can indicate coronary artery disease. Ischemic or infarcted (dead, due to a heart attack) regions of the heart usually contract abnormally.

People who are unable to tolerate an exercise test because of orthopedic problems or impaired leg circulation (see Chapter 17) can be effectively tested using thallium combined with a potent drug, dipyridamole (Persantine). Dipyridamole causes the coronary arteries to dilate (as they should to satisfy the increased demand for oxygenated blood created by exertion) and thus increases the blood flow. If there are blockages in an artery, the increase of flow does not occur and a "cold spot" is imaged. This test compares favorably with exercise thallium imaging.

ECHOCARDIOGRAPHY

Portions of the heart can be seen using an ultrasound method called echocardiography. The echocardiogram is a useful diagnostic tool for determining impaired function and increased thickness of the walls of the left ventricle as well as for helping to rule out other cardiac problems such as valve disease. (See Chapter 14.) As with the MUGA, abnormalities in ventricular contraction (wall motion abnormalities) can be documented by the echocardiogram during exercise or pharmacologic stimulation. A diagnosis of angina and/or coronary heart disease can usually be made without the use of this test, however.

CORONARY ANGIOGRAPHY

X-ray imaging of the coronary arteries can be performed in a cardiac catheterization laboratory. Here, with the patient under mild sedation, an opening is made to a blood vessel in the groin or arm, and a thin tube is threaded up through the vessel to the heart. A dye that shows up on X-ray is injected into the coronary vessels to outline their lumen, and into the left ventricle to assess its contraction. This sequence of events is captured on motion-picture X-rays (angiograms).

Coronary angiography provides the "gold standard" diagnosis of the extent and location of disease in the coronary arteries. Angiography also gives a clear indication of whether the left ventricle is functioning well. A stenotic or narrowed vessel can be identified by an indentation or narrowing in the column or channel of dye in the vessel due to the obstructing plaque or clot. The severity of the stenosis can be quantified by the percent of the narrowing of the dye channel. An occluded vessel can be identified because it contains little or no blood and hence shows little or no dye beyond the blockage.

People are sometimes fearful of this procedure because it does carry a small risk of mortality (0.1 percent) or adverse reactions such as heart attack or stroke (less than 3 percent), but the potential life-saving benefits of an accurate diagnosis may outweigh by far the modest risk. Obviously, however, all people with angina do not need catheterization. The cardiologist will usually consider whether the diagnostic benefits exceed the potential risks given any of the following situations:

- A patient who is under medical treatment combined with life-style changes continues to suffer from incapacitating angina. Such people can usually be relieved of their pain by coronary bypass surgery or angioplasty, and coronary angiography is necessary to determine whether their arteries are suitable for either procedure.

- An electrocardiogram and other tests suggest that a patient risks damage to a considerable portion of the heart muscle (for example, the patient who has marked electrocardiogram [ECG] changes after only a few minutes of a stress test). Certain severe anatomic subsets of coronary artery disease (as shown using coronary angiography) are better treated with coronary bypass surgery.

- Coronary angiography may sometimes be suggested to evaluate the coronary anatomy and hence better advise a patient about his or her prognosis or treatment options.

DETERMINING TREATMENT

The choice of treatment depends on both the need to relieve symptoms and the need to identify those at increased risk of death. For example, in a large study of patients with chronic stable angina who were undergoing treatment in Veterans Administration facilities, it was shown that 35 percent of those who had obstructions of the left main coronary artery died within four years with medical treatment alone. This compared with a four-year death rate of 27 percent for patients who had obstructions of three vessels, a 12 percent death rate for patients who had obstructions of two vessels, and a 2 percent death rate for patients with obstructions of one vessel. (Fortunately, obstructions of the left main coronary artery are not too common.)

It is useful in deciding treatment to determine the specific type of angina that is present. People with coronary artery disease may be affected by what seems to be either stable exertional angina or vasospastic (for example, Prinzmetal's) angina. (See box, "Complications of Angina.")

Complications of Angina

The medical problems that can arise from coronary artery disease are:

- *Heart rhythm disorders (arrhythmias),* which are disturbances in the heart's electrical activity. In people with coronary artery disease, the arrhythmias are likely to have been caused by damage to certain areas of the heart muscle through lack of oxygen (ischemia) or heart attack (infarction). Electrical instability is probably the major cause of sudden death in people with coronary artery disease. When heart rhythm disorders are the major clinical manifestations of coronary artery disease, therapy focuses primarily on preventing arrhythmias using medical, electrical, or in refractory cases, surgical therapy. (See Chapter 16.)

- *Unstable angina or angina which becomes progressively more severe regardless of treatment.* A person with this kind of angina may find that the frequency and severity of chest pain increases, and attacks may occur during rest or may be provoked by less effort than usual. This type of angina may also occur in people who previously have not had angina; the attacks increase in frequency and severity and may occur during rest or be precipitated by less and less physical activity each time. This angina is not well controlled by medication.

- *Angina that cannot be controlled.* This unstable angina often serves as a forewarning of impending heart attack. People who suffer from unstable angina should be hospitalized— preferably in a coronary intensive care unit— and treated with bed rest and medication. Aspirin and the drug heparin, a blood thinner administered intravenously, have been shown to reduce the incidence of heart attacks in people with unstable angina. Coronary angiography (chest X-ray of dye-filled blood vessels) should be considered to determine the extent and location of any narrowing of the coronary arteries and to help decide whether angioplasty or bypass surgery should be performed.

- *Heart attack.*
- *Sudden death.*

Stable exertional angina is caused by an imbalance between the coronary blood supply and demand resulting from a fixed or stable obstruction of one or more of the coronary arteries. Oxygen deprivation usually occurs at about the same point during exertion, and people can generally predict the factors that provoke an attack. Pain can usually be alleviated with medication and/or by stopping the activity that pre-

cipitated the attack. In addition, medication generally helps to reduce the frequency of the attacks or, often, eliminates them by decreasing the heart's blood (oxygen) requirements or by increasing blood (oxygen) supply.

People with vasospastic angina, which is caused by arterial spasms, may often have a fixed blood vessel narrowing, but of a kind or degree in which constriction of the blood vessel also plays an important role in the onset of oxygen deprivation. Angina is less predictable in these people. They may experience days when there is little or no chest pain regardless of the amount of physical activity or days when angina is sparked by even slight exertion. In fact, angina frequently occurs even when the person is resting or asleep. Vasospastic angina usually responds to medications that alleviate or prevent vessel spasms.

DRUG THERAPY

A variety of medications are used to treat angina. (See Chapter 23.) These medications work either by reducing the oxygen demand of the heart, by helping increase the supply of blood, or by doing both. Often, two or more medications will be prescribed together because they can complement each other's actions and may reduce the necessary dose of any one drug, thus minimizing side effects.

The oldest and most frequently used coronary artery medications are the *nitrates*. Nitrates dilate veins, causing blood to pool in the veins and thus reducing the amount of blood returning to the heart. This has the effect of decreasing the size of the left ventricle, reducing the work of the heart (lowering heart muscle demand for oxygen), and lowering the blood pressure. Nitrates may also increase the supply of oxygenated blood by causing the coronary arteries to open more fully, thus improving blood flow. Nitrates also relieve coronary artery spasm. They do not, however, appear to decrease the strength of the heart's contraction. Nitrates are available in the form of nitroglycerin tablets, long-acting tablets, topical ointments, and time-release medicated patches that attach to the skin.

During an attack of angina, nitroglycerin tablets are taken under the tongue (sublingually), where the medication is quickly absorbed into the bloodstream. The medication begins to work within five minutes, and its beneficial effects last from 10 to 30 minutes.

Because of its rapid effect and short duration of action, sublingual nitroglycerin is generally used for relief of individual angina episodes rather than for sustained treatment.

Isosorbide dinitrate is a long-acting nitrate. It takes 3 to 15 minutes to take effect, and its benefits last from one to two hours when it is taken sublingually. The benefits of oral forms of isosorbide dinitrate last from four to six hours, depending on the size of the dose; there is also a longer-acting sustained-release form.

Transdermal nitroglycerin disks are patches worn on the skin; the nitroglycerin is absorbed into the bloodstream to provide continuous delivery of medication for up to 24 hours. However, it is generally recommended that the patch be removed during some part of each day to prevent the buildup of tolerance to the drug's effects.

BETA BLOCKERS

Beta blockers were first introduced in the early 1970s and have become one of the most useful types of drugs to treat coronary artery disease (and effort-induced angina in particular). Beta blockers work by blocking or inhibiting certain receptors in the heart.

During exercise or emotional stress, adrenalinelike products are released and normally stimulate these receptors (beta-adrenergic receptors) to transmit messages to the heart to speed up and pump harder. By blocking these beta receptors and reducing the heart's workload (lowering heart rate and strength of contraction), beta blockers effectively reduce the demand of the heart muscle for oxygen during physical activity or excitement. This helps prevent oxygen deprivation to areas of the heart muscle. Beta blockers also help to lower blood pressure, which further reduces the work of the heart.

The drugs may be used alone or in combination with others that relieve angina; the effects of beta blockers are particularly complemented by nitrate therapy. Beta blockers currently on the market include propranolol (Inderal), nadolol (Corgard), timolol (Blocadren), pindolol (Visken), betaxolol (Kerlone), metoprolol (Lopressor), atenolol (Tenormin), acebutolol (Sectral), and penbutolol (Levatol).

CALCIUM CHANNEL BLOCKERS

Calcium plays an important role in the contraction of the smooth muscle cells of both the heart and the arteries. Calcium blockers or antagonists work by blocking the channels through which calcium would normally enter these cells. By helping to block smooth muscle contraction which causes arteries to narrow, the medication helps keep the vessels dilated, thereby improving blood flow.

The calcium antagonists commonly used in the United States are nifedipine (Procardia), nicardipine (Cardene), verapamil (Calan, Isoptin), and diltiazem (Cardizem). Although their clinical effects and chemical structures are different, they all work by reducing the ability of calcium to enter heart muscle and vascular smooth muscle cells. As a result, they are effective in treating coronary artery spasm and increasing blood flow by dilating the arteries. The heart's workload is also decreased because the drugs lower blood pressure and decrease the strength of the heart's contractions.

Calcium channel blockers may often be prescribed as an addition to a regimen consisting of a beta blocker and a nitrate, particularly for people whose anginal discomfort has persisted despite the use of the latter medications. Verapamil and diltiazem have also been used to treat heart rhythm disorders. Caution in the use of these drugs is necessary in people with any significant degree of heart block (abnormality of the heart's normal rhythm electrical conductive system) or poor left ventricle function.

COMBINATION DRUG TREATMENT

Effective treatment for people with severe angina often involves using a combination of drugs, most often a nitrate, a beta blocker, and a calcium channel blocker. For people with less severe angina, there are several options. Broadly speaking, beta blockers are often the treatment of choice for angina that is usually brought on by an increase in heart work or oxygen demand. For people with angina in which vessel spasms are likely to play a significant role, calcium channel blockers may be the drugs of choice. Nitrates are generally used in conjunction with either drug.

Aspirin therapy is also being frequently recommended for people with coronary artery disease. Aspirin has an antiplatelet effect that reduces the risk of clot formation in a coronary artery. Platelets are a type of blood cell. They are instrumental in clot formation that can occur at the site of a plaque and further decrease blood flow through a coronary artery, often resulting in a heart attack. Aspirin has been shown to be beneficial after a heart attack and for reducing the risk of a heart attack in people who suffer from unstable angina and possibly also in people who suffer from stable angina.

ANGIOPLASTY AND SURGERY

Two options for interventional or surgical treatment of angina are currently available and widely used: balloon angioplasty (also called percutaneous transluminal coronary angioplasty or PTCA) and coronary artery bypass surgery.

Angioplasty involves inserting a thin tube (catheter) with a deflated balloon on its tip through an incision into a blood vessel in the groin or the arm and threading it through the major arteries until it reaches the coronary arteries. The catheter is then positioned so that the balloon rests within the blockage, at which point the physician inflates the balloon, thereby flattening and cracking the plaque or other obstruction against the vessel wall and also stretching the vessel open with the pressure. When the balloon is deflated and removed, the blocked vessel remains less obstructed.

This procedure was first performed in humans in 1977. More than 200,000 Americans now undergo it each year, with an overall initial success rate approaching 90 percent, according to the National Heart, Lung, and Blood Institute's registry figures for 1985 and 1986. Approximately 30 percent of patients undergoing angioplasty experience a recurrence of artery narrowing (restenosis) within six months, although they may benefit from repeat angioplasty. The mortality rate is around 1 percent, with a 4 percent chance of complications that might require emergency coronary artery bypass surgery.

Care in selection of patients is important to the success of angioplasty. Ideally, the patient should have only one or two vessels obstructed (although multivessel angioplasty is increasingly being used), and the obstructions should be in sections of the artery that can be reached easily by the catheter. Improvements in technique, along with new developments in the field, make angioplasty an increasingly effective method of treating coronary artery disease. However, angioplasty is not initially successful in some cases. Studies are under way to compare angioplasty to medical therapy in patients with predominantly single vessel disease and to surgery in patients with multiple vessel disease. (See Chapter 24 for further details.)

Coronary artery bypass surgery is one of the most common and successful major surgeries performed today. Although this operation was first performed as recently as 1967, about 320,000 bypass procedures are now done in the United States each year. The principal behind the coronary bypass operation is to provide new conduits to bypass obstructed or narrowed sections of the coronary arteries. These new conduits can be fashioned from lengths of a vein removed from the leg (the saphenous vein) or from an artery of the chest wall (the internal mammary artery). This procedure takes place in an operating room, with the patient deeply anesthetized. His or her heart is stopped, and blood is circulated through the body by a pump outside of the body (a heart-lung machine).

Coronary artery bypass surgery has a relatively low mortality rate (1 to 2 percent in people with good heart muscle function), although there is also a 5 to 10 percent risk of a heart attack during or immediately after the operation. Coronary artery bypass surgery provides complete relief from anginal pain in about 70 percent of people and partial relief in another 20 percent. The clearest indication for bypass surgery, therefore, is for patients who continue to have incapacitating angina despite being on a good medical program.

There is evidence that coronary artery bypass surgery improves the longevity of certain people—notably, those with blockages of the left main coronary artery branch and those with disease in all three coronary arteries and impaired function of the left ventricle. There is little proof that surgery improves the survival rate of people with narrowing in one or two arteries alone, but a major study showed that quality of life (symptoms) improved in patients in all categories. Because of improvements in operative technique, coronary artery bypass surgery is now an option for elderly people, as well as for people suffering from other diseases—such as diabetes mellitus—in conjunction with coronary artery disease. It is, however, an expensive operation with a significant recovery period. (See Chapter 25 for a more detailed discussion.)

LIFE-STYLE MODIFICATION

Life-style changes are an important part of any treatment regimen for angina. Some changes may be useful in reducing the frequency of attacks by identifying and modifying the activities and situations that precipitate these attacks. Changes may be relatively minor, such as avoiding exertion after a heavy meal or using a golf cart instead of walking. Emotional upset should be avoided as much as possible, and air conditioning may be considered a necessity for patients with coronary artery disease who live in hot, humid climates.

Long-term changes that reduce known cardiovascular risk factors are also helpful, because they can help not only to prevent further damage to the arteries but also, in some instances, actually to reverse the damage.

For smokers, smoking cessation is the first and most efficacious life-style modification that can be undertaken. Studies have shown that if a person quits smoking altogether, the risk of a heart attack returns within 3 to 5 years to a level similar to that of nonsmokers in the same age group. (See Chapter 6.)

Changes in diet are also a vital part of reducing the continued development and progression of atherosclerosis. Reducing the total calories and the intake of saturated fats and dietary cholesterol while increasing the intake of starches and high-fiber food may significantly lower blood cholesterol levels. (See Chapter 5.)

Regular aerobic exercise has many possible beneficial effects: controlling weight, lowering blood cholesterol, improving cardiovascular tone, reducing stress, and providing a general feeling of well-being. The conditioning effect of exercise also increases a person's ability to perform a greater amount of work with the use of less oxygen. (See Chapter 7.)

Exercise need not be strenuous, but it is important that it be energetic enough to gradually raise the heart rate and that it be performed *regularly* (a minimum of three to five days a week). Brisk walking for 30 to 45 minutes is inexpensive, requires no skill, and puts little burden on knees, back, or hips. Exercises that produce a sudden strain—such as lifting heavy weights—should be avoided or conducted under a physician's guidance. They have relatively little cardiovascular benefit, and the sudden increase of blood pressure that such activities produce may precipitate an attack of angina.

Reducing stress can be a valuable adjunct to any life-style modification. While stress has been only tenuously linked to high blood pressure and coronary artery disease, reduction of stress can benefit the body as a whole. It is important to realize that stress does not arise just from having a lot to do; rather, it comes from feelings of being overwhelmed and unable to cope, from feelings of hostility and from an inability to relax or enjoy leisure time. Regularly setting aside time to pursue an enjoyable activity (such as listening to music), meditation, and in some cases, psychological counseling, can all help reduce stress. (See Chapter 8.)

HEART ATTACK

A heart attack, known medically as *acute myocardial infarction* or an acute MI, is a major and all too common medical emergency. Each year, there are about 1.5 million heart attacks in the United States, leading to more than 500,000 deaths. Most of these deaths—more than 300,000—are sudden, occurring before the patient even reaches the hospital.

The vast majority of heart attacks are a direct result of coronary artery disease. A blood clot or muscular spasm in a narrowed coronary vessel may suddenly block it completely, triggering an infarction in the area of the heart muscle that is normally nourished by that artery. (The *myocardium* is the muscular wall of the heart. *Infarction* is a term to describe the death of some of this vital tissue because it has been deprived of blood and oxygen.)

A myocardial infarction can be dangerous because irreparable heart damage may develop within a short time after the muscle is deprived of oxygen. An infarction that affects as little as 10 percent of the myocardium can cause death if it involves a critical area such as the papillary muscle (the muscle supporting the heart valve) or if it precipitates an irregular rhythm or perforation of the heart wall. Still, heart attack patients often survive much larger infarctions, affecting up to 30–40 percent of the myocardium, if a less critical area is involved.

The severity of the heart attack depends on several factors, including:

- *The site of the coronary artery that is blocked.* Blockages of the left main and the left anterior descending arteries are usually more life-threatening than blockage of the right coronary artery.

- *Cardiac arrhythmias.* Blockage of a coronary artery can cause a serious heartbeat irregularity (arrhythmia) that may result in sudden death. For example, blockage may cause a malfunction of the heart's electrical impulse system, leading to an inefficiently rapid beat (tachycardia) or an ineffective fluttering of heart muscle (ventricular fibrillation). Ventricular fibrillation is fatal unless blood flow is restored with cardiopulmonary resuscitation and the normal heartbeat restored with drugs or electric shock therapy (defibrillation). Serious arrhythmias may also arise later, after the acute phase of a heart attack, if certain areas of the ventricular wall have been damaged. (See Chapter 16.)

- *Collateral circulation.* When a key coronary vessel slowly becomes blocked over a period of months or years, the heart muscle's demand for oxygen prompts other vessels and their branches to widen and even extend into the oxygen-deprived area to provide an alternative blood source. In effect, a gradual natural coronary bypass takes place. This is referred to as "collateral" coronary blood flow, which can be a saving grace if the original vessel becomes totally occluded. Collaterals are credited with saving many older heart attack patients. The sudden, fatal heart attacks that sometimes strike younger men or women may be more serious because the blockage occurs in a vessel serving an area for which collaterals have yet to develop.

WARNING SIGNS AND SYMPTOMS

Heart attacks vary in severity and in symptoms. The one clear rule is that whenever heart attack is suspected, the person must be taken to a hospital as quickly as possible. About 60 percent of all heart attack deaths occur within the first hour. Yet, according to the American Heart Association, at least half of people suffering a heart attack delay seeking help for two or more hours.

The initial pain of a heart attack is often intense— a *crushing* feeling or pressure in the middle of the chest. But in other cases it is much less severe; the pain may be no more than an unusual dull, aching sensation that persists. Or there may be a strong squeezing sensation inside the center of the chest. Some people experience burning feelings, while in some cases, they simply feel bloated. Sometimes, there is virtually no pain. (These are referred to as silent heart attacks.)

When pain occurs, it most often is focused beneath the sternum (breastbone). Or it may spread out, encompassing all of the chest, the shoulders and arms (the left arm more often than the right), and even the neck and the jaws. For some people, this chest pain seems very much like, albeit more severe than, the angina pectoris that they had previously experienced. In unusual instances, there is little or no pain, although there may be other symptoms. If an anginal

episode lasts for more than 10 or 15 minutes and it is not relieved by up to three nitroglycerin tablets (given every few minutes), it is a sign that a heart attack may be occurring.

Cold sweats are common just before or during a heart attack. The person may be dizzy or weak or may feel faint; loss of consciousness can also occur. The pulse may be rapid and shallow or irregular. Nausea, vomiting, and other gastrointestinal symptoms are common. A person having a heart attack also may be short of breath. He or she may be weak, pale, and extremely anxious. (For information on how to help victims of a heart attack and other cardiac emergencies, see box "What You Can Do" and Chapter 27.)

Prompt emergency care not only saves many lives but it also helps minimize the damage of a heart attack. Many ambulances and other emergency vehicles are now equipped with life-saving equipment. In fact, many are actually mobile coronary care units, and the emergency medical teams are trained in administering life-saving treatment even before the patient reaches the emergency room. In most communities, emergency medical service (EMS) workers, ambulance drivers, firemen, and others are now trained to stabilize heart attack patients before and while transporting them to the emergency room. (See Chapter 27.)

Even in the face of marked symptoms of a heart attack, there is a natural tendency to wait and see if the pain or discomfort in the chest is from heartburn or some other harmless ailment. But, if it is a heart attack, irreversible damage may occur within hours if not minutes. Perhaps more important, some of the most potent new drugs that can prevent death of heart muscle work only if they are given within the first four to six hours of the heart attack. Thereafter, they may be less beneficial.

Preferably, treatment should be sought at a hospital with a 24-hour-a-day emergency room that is continuously staffed by doctors. If the choice presents itself, one should go to a hospital with an intensive care unit (ICU) or, preferably, one with a specialized ICU called a coronary care unit (CCU).

IN THE EMERGENCY DEPARTMENT

When you accompany a person with a suspected heart attack to the emergency department, ask immediately for a doctor or a nurse and clearly an-

What You Can Do

These are the American Heart Association's instructions for use with a possible heart attack victim:

Know the warning signals of a heart attack

- Uncomfortable pressure, fullness, squeezing or pain in the center of the chest lasting two minutes or longer.

- Pain spreading to the shoulders, neck, or arms.

- Severe pain, lightheadedness, fainting, sweating, nausea, or shortness of breath.

- Not all these warning signs occur in every heart attack. If some start to occur, however, don't wait. Get help immediately. Delay can be deadly.

Know what to do in an emergency

- Find out which area hospitals have 24-hour emergency cardiac care.

- Determine (in advance) the hospital or medical facility nearest home and office, and tell family and friends to call this facility in an emergency.

- Keep a list of emergency rescue service numbers next to the telephone and in a pocket, wallet, or purse.

- If any chest discomfort lasts 15 minutes or more, call the emergency rescue service.

- If getting to the hospital is faster by car, do not wait for an ambulance.

Be a heart saver

- If someone is experiencing the signs of a heart attack—and the warning signs last two minutes or longer—act immediately.

- Expect a "denial." It's normal for someone with chest discomfort to deny the possibility of something as serious as a heart attack. But don't take "no" for an answer. Insist on taking prompt action.

- Call the emergency service, or

- Get to the nearest hospital emergency room that offers 24-hour emergency cardiac care.

nounce that a heart attack patient has arrived. After an examination, the nurses and doctors can determine whether it really is a heart attack or some other perhaps less serious problem.

Emergency department nurses and physicians often can diagnose a typical heart attack by looking at the patient. (They may see several heart attack victims each day.) Even so, looks can be deceptive, and a diagnosis must be confirmed by talking to and examining the patient and by taking an electrocardiogram (ECG) and administering a series of blood tests.

The heart may be beating too rapidly (tachycardia) or too slowly (bradycardia). The blood pressure, too, may be elevated, or more commonly it may be on the low end of normal. The ECG typically shows irregularities, particularly changes in the Q waves, ST segments, and/or T waves. (See Figure 11.1.) Doctors often can deduce from the ECG which coronary vessel is afflicted.

A blood specimen should be drawn quickly and then tested for the presence of enzymes that are secreted by heart muscle cells that may have been injured, a strong indication of muscle damage or death (infarction). Treatment starts immediately, particularly if the patient's heart has stopped or he or she is unconscious.

A defibrillator will be deployed at once if the heart is fibrillating. A jolt of electricity is passed through the heart, between paddle-shaped electrodes held against the chest. This electric shock often interrupts arrhythmias and restores the heart to normal (sinus) rhythm. If the heart has stopped, doctors will compress the chest, up and down, trying to maintain the heart's pumping action. (See Chapter 27.)

Over the past decade, the most recent innovation in the treatment of heart attack patients has been the use of clot-dissolving or thrombolytic agents, a technique called reperfusion therapy. Most heart attacks result from the formation of a blood clot within a coronary artery that is narrowed by atherosclerosis or spasm, and it is possible to restore blood flow to the heart by dissolving this clot (thrombus).

Because the lack of blood and oxygen causes progressive death of myocardial cells, it is important to administer the thrombolytic agent as soon as possible. In more than two-thirds of cases, if the thrombolytic agent is administered within 6 hours of the onset of the heart attack, the blood clots can be dissolved and the blood flow restored, thereby salvaging heart muscle. Studies have clearly shown that early administration of thrombolytic agents results in better survival and better heart function following myocardial infarction.

The earliest thrombolytic agents were streptokinase (Kabikinase, Streptase) and urokinase (Abbokinase). More recently, t-PA (tissue plasminogen activator) and anistreplase (Eminase) have been introduced for clinical use in the United States. TPA (alteplase or Activase) is a genetically engineered agent that contains a natural human substance that activates an enzyme that dissolves the blood clot. Although the agent is most effective when given early, in selected patients, the myocardium can be salvaged when the thrombolytic agent is given later. These drugs have revolutionized the care of heart attack patients and have reduced the death rates by about 20 percent.

In addition to thrombolytic agents, aspirin and heparin may also be administered. The drug heparin is given intravenously and interferes with normal blood clotting. These drugs can prevent a clot in the artery from growing larger or from reforming after it has been dissolved by the thrombolytic agent.

Additional drugs are often administered early in the course of a heart attack. Morphine may be injected or infused through an intravenous line to relieve pain. This old, powerful narcotic agent is extremely effective and is still the standard for pain relief. Oxygen may be given through a face mask or nasal prongs to improve the oxygen content of the blood still flowing to the heart. Intravenous beta blockers and nitroglycerin may also be administered in an attempt to limit the size of the heart attack. Sometimes drugs used to treat or prevent irregular heart rhythms will also be given. (See Chapter 23 for more information on cardiovascular drugs.)

The aim of all of these therapies is to restore blood flow, restore a regular heartbeat, and then give the damaged heart time to recover. For some people, however, these medical treatment methods are not effective and the blocked artery may fail to open. In some cases, further treatment, such as angioplasty or coronary bypass surgery, may be necessary.

An angiogram, an X-ray showing dye-filled blood vessels, can indicate where the blockage is located, and balloon angioplasty may be used to open the obstruction. In some patients who have extensive blockage—sometimes in two or more vessels—an emergency coronary artery bypass operation may be performed. Coronary artery bypass surgery can be performed on an emergency basis, is relatively safe, and, in most cases, is quite effective.

A variety of other procedures may be deployed in the CCU to assist heart attack victims, especially those who show signs of heart failure. In one, a balloonlike device (an intra-aortic balloon catheter) is inserted inside the aorta, the body's largest artery which rises from the heart. The balloon can be inflated rhythmically from outside the body. This forces blood into the aorta and forward through the circulatory system, thereby assisting the weakened heart. In essence, the balloon is an auxiliary pump that temporarily carries some of the load when the heart is weakened by a heart attack.

HOW CORONARY CARE UNITS HELP

Much of the recent improvement in heart attack treatment comes from specific new developments—better ways to detect heart damage and improved drugs or other treatments. Still, a major factor in decreased heart attack mortality is the development of total, integrated care, with an emphasis on monitoring heart function, that is provided through coronary care units (CCUs). These are areas in the hospital reserved for heart patients and are staffed by specially trained doctors, nurses, and technicians. CCU workers can follow a patient's status in minute detail, using sophisticated computerized electrocardiograms (ECGs) and other monitoring methods. The patient is attached on an ongoing basis to an ECG monitor that sounds an alarm when an irregular heartbeat develops. Defibrillators and other life-saving equipment are on hand and can be used within minutes if a problem suddenly arises.

When the patient's heart and other vital organs are again functioning in a stable way, usually within a few days, he or she may be moved out of the CCU into an ordinary hospital room. The hospital stay for a heart attack can vary from one to three weeks, depending upon the severity and extent of heart damage and the occurrence of any complications. The heart begins to heal during the first several weeks after a heart attack by forming scar tissue to replace the damaged or dead heart cells. Although scar tissue strengthens the injured part of the heart muscle, it cannot contract like normal heart muscle. Therefore, the remaining heart muscle must compensate by working or contracting harder to pump blood. In addition to scar formation, collateral blood vessels (see above) may develop to bring more blood to the surrounding damaged but living heart cells in the border regions of the myocardial infarction.

The presence and extent of the heart attack can be definitively diagnosed by serial electrocardiograms,

YALE UNIVERSITY SCHOOL OF MEDICINE HEART BOOK

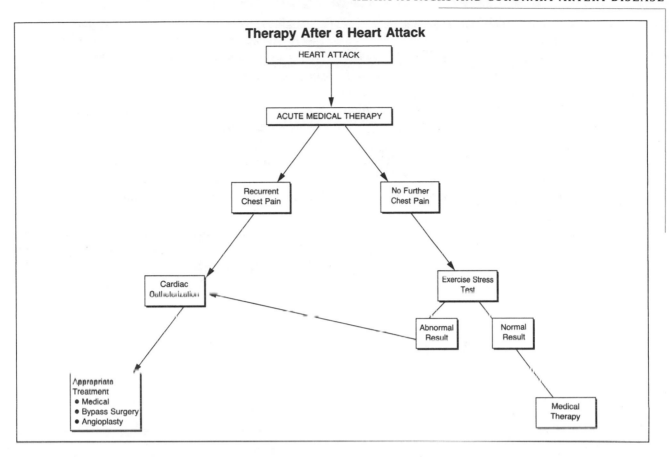

Therapy After a Heart Attack

blood tests (that measure enzymes released from dying heart cells), and possibly by an echocardiogram or radionuclide scan to image how the various regions of the heart muscle (for example, left ventricle) are pumping. A severe or large heart attack can be complicated by: rupture of the heart wall; low blood pressure; fluid buildup (congestion) in the lungs due to inability of the heart to pump adequate amounts of blood; blood clots in the heart or legs; irregular heart rhythms such as tachycardia or fibrillation; and recurrent chest pain, either due to an inflamed heart sac (pericarditis) or recurrent angina.

In this era of thrombolytic therapy in which it is frequently possible to successfully reopen a previously occluded artery, it is important to evaluate patients for their risk for another heart attack. (See box, "Therapy After a Heart Attack.") A successfully opened stenotic artery can reocclude with new clots in up to one-fourth of patients within days or months following the initial heart attack. Therefore, patients frequently have an exercise stress test prior to hospital discharge to ascertain if they are at high risk for another heart attack. Recurrent angina or a positive stress test usually leads to catheterization and evaluation for coronary artery angioplasty or bypass surgery.

The total recovery from a heart attack usually takes two to three months. During this time, the patient should try initially to reduce the strain on the heart by resting, and then to improve heart function by gradually increasing activities and starting routine exercise. The exact activity prescription for a heart attack patient depends on the size and complications of the heart attack, the level of activity before the heart attack, and how the heart responds to increased activity.

Heart attack patients are often maintained on treatment with aspirin and beta blockers, which have been shown to decrease the risk of subsequent heart attacks, as well as treatment with other antianginal drugs as needed. The goal of rehabilitation is to gradually increase one's activities to the point of resuming a reasonable life-style. (See Chapter 28.)

Initial avoidance of extreme stress or exercise and extremes of hot and cold temperatures is important to minimize the risk of putting too much stress on the heart or of precipitating angina. A physician can usually guide the resumption of activities based on the severity of the heart attack and data from an exercise stress test. Most activities of daily living, including sexual activity, can usually be resumed within three to six weeks after a heart attack. It will also be important in the rehabilitation period to decrease cardiac risk factors (see Chapter 3).

Feelings of anxiety, anger, and depression are not uncommon during the acute and chronic phases of a heart attack. It is important, however, to realize that most patients recover well from this life-threatening event.

THE PAYOFF: SALVAGED LIVES

The death rate from acute heart attack has dropped significantly over the last two or three decades. In part, this is because there are about 25 percent fewer heart attacks. There has also been a similar 25 percent reduction in fatalities from heart attacks. A significant part of this reduction in deaths is due to newer treatments, careful observation and management of patients in CCUs, and improvement in other facets of heart attack care.

Heart attack survivors require shorter hospitalizations than before. They also tend to be healthier —less disabled—after their heart attacks because of improved treatment methods. Skillful coronary care limits the damage and disability. Most heart attack patients now can regain normal or near-normal lifestyles, and some actually enjoy better health than before their heart attacks.

CHAPTER 12

HIGH BLOOD PRESSURE

MARVIN MOSER, M.D.

INTRODUCTION

High blood pressure, or hypertension as the disease is known medically, is our most common chronic illness. Estimates of exactly how many Americans have high blood pressure vary—the American Heart Association and the National Heart, Lung, and Blood Institute put the figure at about 55–60 million, but some of the individuals included in this estimate may only have had transient elevation of pressure; a more accurate estimate is probably 35–40 million. In either calculation, the number of people affected and the amount of the nation's health budget that goes toward treating high blood pressure or its complications are huge.

Because high blood pressure is the leading cause of strokes and a major risk factor for heart attacks, one of the most important aspects of preventive cardiology should be to identify as many people who have the disease as possible and to take steps to lower the blood pressure before it causes damage to the blood vessels, heart, kidneys, eyes, and other organs. Fortunately, the last 30 to 35 years have seen remarkable advances in the treatment of high blood pressure, with major payoffs. The death toll from strokes is down by more than 54 percent and heart attack mortality has dropped by more than 45 percent

since 1973–74. At that time, the National High Blood Pressure Education Program directed at both physicians and the general public raised consciousness about the dangers of untreated high blood pressure and the importance of early effective treatment. We are now reaping the benefits of this and other major programs.

Even so, it's still too early to declare victory over high blood pressure. Despite massive public education programs, misconceptions about the disease abound. Many people still harbor misconceptions about what constitutes an elevated blood pressure (see box, "Common Facts and Myths"), and there probably still are many people whose high blood pressure has not been diagnosed—especially in minority populations. There also are several millions of others whose hypertension has been diagnosed but who are not being adequately treated to normal blood pressure levels.

WHAT IS HIGH BLOOD PRESSURE OR HYPERTENSION?

To understand why lowering high blood pressure is so important in preventing heart and blood vessel

Common Facts and Myths

Myth: Tense, uptight people are the most likely to develop high blood pressure.

Fact: Many people have the mistaken notion that the term "hypertension" refers to a person's emotional or psychological state. In fact, hypertension refers to the excessive ("hyper") pressure ("tension") exerted against the artery walls, and has nothing to do with psychological stress or tension. Stress or tension may produce a temporary rise in blood pressure, but many calm people have hypertension, and, conversely, many tense, jittery people have normal blood pressure.

Myth: Older people need a higher blood pressure to ensure a steady supply of blood to the brain.

Fact: Normal blood pressure, even in the very elderly, produces adequate blood to the brain. In fact, numerous studies show that older people with normal blood pressure have a lower death rate than those with hypertension.

Myth: Side effects from drugs that lower high blood pressure are worse than the disease.

Fact: Doctors today have dozens of antihypertensive medications that they can use to structure a treatment program. If one medication causes side effects, chances are that alternatives exist that are equally effective and that can be easily tolerated. There is also no evidence to support claims that antihypertensive drugs themselves cause damage to the brain, heart, or kidneys or increase mortality. In fact, scores of studies show just the opposite; when medications are used to reduce high blood pressure, the death rate and incidence of complications fall.

Myth: High blood pressure is mostly a disease of aging.

Fact: People of all ages develop high blood pressure. While it is true that blood pressure tends to rise with age, hypertension is most often diagnosed in early adulthood or middle age.

Myth: The damage caused by high blood pressure cannot be reversed.

Fact: Many people have the mistaken idea that it does little good to treat high blood pressure once it has damaged the heart, kidneys, or blood vessels. This assumption is not true. Treatment of even advanced high blood pressure can reverse varying degrees of damage. For example, recent studies show that treatment can help reverse enlargement of the heart's main pumping chamber (a condition called left ventricular hypertrophy) and thereby help prevent heart failure.

diseases, it is important to know something about the basic physiology involved. As noted in Chapter 1, the blood circulates through some 60,000 miles of blood vessels. (See color atlas, #4.) With each heartbeat, 2 or 3 ounces of freshly oxygenated blood are forced out of the heart's main pumping chamber, the left ventricle, into the aorta, the body's largest artery.

The circulatory system can be likened to a tree. The aorta is comparable to the main tree trunk. It branches into smaller arteries (like the thick branches that come off the main trunk), which in turn divide into even smaller vessels (like smaller branches and twigs) called arterioles, which carry blood to the capillaries (like the leaves). Capillaries are the microscopic vessels that supply blood, with its load of oxygen and other nutrients, to each cell in the body. After the oxygen is used up, the blood returns to the heart via a branching system of veins.

A certain amount of force is needed to keep blood moving through this intricate system of blood vessels. The amount of force that is exerted on the artery walls as blood flows through them is what we refer to as *blood pressure*. The "head" of pressure comes from the heart, but it is the smallest arteries, the arterioles, that actually determine how much pressure is registered in the blood vessels. To raise blood pressure, the arterioles narrow or *constrict*; to lower it, they open up or *dilate*.

Exactly how much pressure is needed varies according to the body's activities. For example, the heart does not need to beat as fast or as hard to keep blood circulating when you are resting as it does when you are exercising. During exercise, however, more blood is needed to carry oxygen to the muscles, so blood pressure rises to meet increased demand. The heart pumps faster and pushes out more blood with each beat. In other situations, such as when someone stands up suddenly after lying down, the body must make an almost instantaneous adjustment in blood pressure in order to ensure a steady supply of blood to the brain. Blood vessels in the abdomen and legs constrict and the heart speeds up. Sometimes there may be a slight delay in this adjustment, and as a result, you may feel dizzy for a few seconds. This is more common in older people whose blood vessel reflexes might be impaired. A longer delay can bring on a fainting spell, which is the body's way of increasing the flow of blood to the brain (when someone lies down, blood flow to the brain increases).

Similarly, some people feel light-headed, or even faint, after standing for long periods, during which time blood may collect or "pool" in the legs, thereby reducing the amount that is available to carry oxygen to the brain. Good examples of this bodily response are the numerous instances of healthy soldiers who fainted after standing at attention for long periods of time in hot weather. Other reflexes may be triggered and result in a sudden loss of blood to the brain and an episode of light-headedness or fainting. These episodes are not serious but can be frightening. An example of this response is fainting after only a small amount of blood is drawn for a blood test. A nerve reflex slows the heart and causes blood vessels to dilate or open up. Less blood gets to the brain and fainting occurs. As we all know, if the affected individual rests quietly for just a few minutes, all is well.

Blood pressure is regulated by an intricate system of hormonal controls and nerve sensors, and it may vary considerably during the course of a day. Typically, blood pressure is low when you are resting or asleep, and higher when you are moving about or under stress. For example, when you are frightened or angry, the adrenal glands pump out epinephrine and norepinephrine, stress hormones that are commonly referred to as adrenaline. These hormones, which are responsible for the body's fight-or-flight response, signal the heart to beat faster and harder, resulting in increased blood pressure and flow to the muscles. It is apparent that pressures are typically lowest between 1:00 and 4:00 or 5:00 A.M., rise rapidly during "arousal" from sleep between 6:00 and 8:00 A.M., remain at approximately the same levels during the afternoon and evening, and decrease from about 11:00 to 12:00 at night.

WHAT CONSTITUTES HIGH BLOOD PRESSURE?

Blood does not flow in a steady stream; instead, it moves through the circulatory system in spurts that correlate with the heart's beats. The heart beats about 60 to 70 times a minute at rest and may speed up to 120 to 140 or higher during vigorous exercise. It is not contracting or squeezing all the time, however; after each contraction, the heart muscle rests and gets ready for the next beat. Blood pressure rises and falls with each beat. Thus, blood pressure is expressed in two numbers, such as 120 over 80, or 120/80. The higher number, which is called *systolic* pressure, represents the maximum force that is exerted on the walls of the blood vessels during a heartbeat. The lower number, which is referred to as the *diastolic*

pressure, is the amount of force exerted when the heart is resting momentarily between beats.

Blood pressure is usually measured with a device called a sphygmomanometer (pronounced sfig-moe-man-*om*-e-ter), which consists of an inflatable rubber cuff, an air pump, and a column of mercury or a dial or digital readout reflecting pressure in an air column. Readings are expressed in millimeters of mercury or mm Hg. (See Figure 12.1.) The cuff is wrapped around the upper arm, and the inflatable cuff is tightened until blood flow through the large artery in the arm is halted. As air is pumped into the cuff, it pushes up a column of mercury or air, in the case of the simpler machines.

The person measuring the blood pressure places a stethoscope over the artery just below the cuff and listens for a cessation of the sound of blood coursing through the artery. He or she then begins to release air from the cuff, allowing blood to flow through the artery again. As air is released, the column of mercury or air begins to fall, and the person listens for the first thumping sound that signals a return of blood flow into the vessel over which the stethoscope has been placed. The height of the column of mercury or the air pressure on the dial at this sound indicates the systolic (or higher) pressure. More air is released

Figure 12.1
Blood pressure is measured using a device called a sphygmomanometer, which consists of an inflatable cuff that goes around the arm. The blood pressure reading is obtained from the height of a column of mercury which is connected to the cuff.

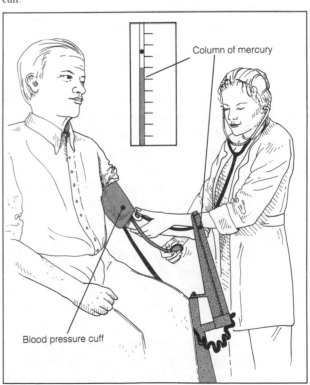

Column of mercury

Blood pressure cuff

Monitoring Your Own Blood Pressure

Most people with hypertension do not need to measure their blood pressures at home. Some, however, find home monitoring reassuring. It is important to remember that an occasional high reading does not necessarily mean that your blood pressure is "out of control."

In some instances, home monitoring may provide useful information for your doctor, especially if you are starting a new drug regimen or experiencing symptoms, such as dizziness. If you do monitor your blood pressure at home, you should take your machine with you periodically when you visit your doctor so that he or she can check whether it is correctly calibrated.

Before starting home monitoring, ask your doctor or nurse to show you the proper way to use your machine. Most people find the electronic machines that do not have a separate stethoscope easier to use than the nonautomated ones. But they may not be quite as accurate. Whichever model you use, follow the instructions from the manufacturer and your doctor. Special points to remember include:

- Avoid caffeine (coffee, tea, colas, etc.) for at least 30 minutes before measuring your blood pressure. The same goes for cigarettes or nicotine gum. Both caffeine and nicotine raise blood pressure and can give a falsely high reading.

- If you are experiencing dizziness or feelings of faintness, try taking your blood pressure immediately after standing up to see if it differs from pressure taken while sitting.

from the cuff, and pressure continues to fall. The height of the mercury or the level of air pressure when the thumping sound of blood ceases, indicating the pause between heartbeats, is the diastolic pressure.

People with high blood pressure can learn to monitor their own pressure (See box, "Monitoring Your Own Blood Pressure"), although for most it is not necessary.

As noted earlier, blood pressure varies considerably during the course of an average day. It also varies according to age—a baby's blood pressure may normally be 70/50, whereas the average blood pressure in an adult is about 120/80. Until recent years, there was no clear agreement among physicians as to what constituted high blood pressure, but now it is generally agreed that blood pressure readings that

are *consistently* above 140/90 warrant a diagnosis of hypertension, and the higher the readings, the more serious the disease. (See Table 12.1.) A reading of about 140/90 does not necessarily indicate that the condition requires immediate therapy, but it does suggest follow up and some treatment.

STEPS IN ESTABLISHING A DIAGNOSIS OF HIGH BLOOD PRESSURE

A diagnosis of high blood pressure should not be based on a single reading, except when it is extremely high—for example, above 170–180/105–110. Other-

Table 12.1
Recommendations for Management of Various Blood Pressure Levels

Range (mm Hg)	Diagnosis	Recommended activity
Diastolic		
below 85	Normal blood pressure	Recheck within 2 years.
85–89	High normal blood pressure	Recheck within 1 year.
90–104	Mild hypertension	Confirm within 2 months.
105–114	Moderate hypertension	Therapy should be undertaken.
above 115	Severe hypertension	Begin therapy with medication.
Isolated systolic hypertension, when diastolic blood pressure is below 90 (mostly seen in older individuals)		
below 140	Normal blood pressure	Recheck within 2 years.
140–159	Borderline isolated systolic hypertension	Confirm within 2 months.
160–199	Isolated systolic hypertension	Confirm within 2 months. Therapy should be instituted if pressure remains elevated.
above 200	Isolated systolic hypertension	Begin therapy with medication.

wise several measurements taken over a period of time are generally needed to confirm a diagnosis. This is why single readings obtained at health fairs or other blood pressure screening events are often misleading. In addition, the electronic machines used for self-measurement at airports or in pharmacies are often poorly calibrated or improperly used and may give false readings (usually on the high side). Although hypertension screening has its place, people should understand that readings obtained are only an indication to follow up more carefully, and do not justify a definite diagnosis of high blood pressure or hypertension. Unfortunately, many people are unduly frightened, on the basis of just one blood pressure recording, into thinking they have hypertension.

The circumstances under which blood pressure is measured must also be taken into consideration. For example, a blood pressure reading taken when a person is under severe stress may be misleadingly high. Similarly, a high reading may be obtained if blood pressure is measured soon after a person has had a couple of cups of coffee or smoked a few cigarettes. Thus, if possible, a person should avoid smoking and/or drinking coffee, cola, or other sources of caffeine for about one to two hours before having blood pressure measured.

In a physician's office or clinic, blood pressure is usually measured after the doctor has asked questions about the patient's health history. This also gives the patient a few minutes to relax, although some people remain anxious. (See box, "White-Coat Hypertension.") Two readings may be taken—the first with the person seated, and the second while standing. The reading while standing may be especially useful in older persons whose pressures may fall when they stand up. And it can help to guide treatment decisions, since some blood-pressure-lowering drugs may cause a greater decrease in standing than in sitting blood pressures. Blood pressure may be measured several times during the visit, especially if the first reading was on the high side. The results of all the readings are then usually averaged.

In an adult, blood pressure recordings need only be repeated every one to two years if pressures are below 140/90. If the average falls in the mild to moderate range of high blood pressure, about 140/90 to 160/100, an appointment for additional measurements will be made to confirm the diagnosis. However, very high diastolic blood pressure readings (more than 110 to 115 mm Hg) during the course of an office visit justify starting treatment. If an elevated blood pressure is present in individuals below 60 years of age, both the systolic and diastolic levels are usually high—for example, above 140 systolic and 90 diastolic. In older people, however, there is a form of hypertension called isolated systolic hypertension. The systolic, or upper, reading may be high, for example, 150–180, but the diastolic, or lower, reading is below 90. (See Table 12.1.) This type of hypertension also results in an increased risk of stroke, heart attack, or heart failure.

In addition to measuring blood pressure, the doctor will also look for signs of organ damage, if the readings are high. Specifically, the examination will include:

- *Inspection of the eyes.* The eyes are the only place in the body where blood vessels can be looked at directly. By shining a bright light into the eye and inspecting its interior with an ophthalmoscope (a special magnifying device), the doctor can inspect the blood vessels for thickening or narrowing, changes that are characteristic of high blood pressure. He or she will also look for tiny hemorrhages inside the eye, another possible sign of damage from high blood pressure.

- *Examination of the heart.* This includes a careful examination using a stethoscope to listen for any unusual sounds or beats and palpation of

White-Coat Hypertension

Some people have elevated blood pressure readings in a doctor's office, but their blood pressures will be normal or near-normal when measured at home or at work. This is referred to as *white-coat hypertension*. Some doctors believe that it is not necessary to treat this type of high blood pressure on the theory that if the pressure is normal most of the time and elevated due to the stress of being in a doctor's office, this elevation is of little importance.

While it is true that some patients are nervous in a doctor's office and therefore may experience a rise in blood pressure, we believe that white-coat hypertension should not be ignored. If blood pressure rises in a doctor's office, chances are it goes up at other times, too. We are all under some kind of stress daily. Research indicates that these spikes in blood pressure are significant, and that appropriate treatment to avoid them should be instituted. In a follow-up study of patients with labile (unstable) or high normal blood pressure, it was found that enlargement of the heart may occur over time. In general, treatment guidelines are the same as for sustained high blood pressure.

the heart impulse to judge heart size. An electrocardiogram will measure the heart's electrical activity and help to determine if the heart is enlarged.

- *A check of blood flow in the arteries.* Pulses will be felt at various parts of the body, including the wrists, neck, and ankles. The doctor may use a stethoscope to listen to blood flowing through the carotid artery, the large blood vessel in the neck that carries blood to the brain. A humming noise (called a bruit) may indicate a narrowing of this artery. Similarly, the doctor will probably listen for bruits in the abdominal arteries that carry blood to the kidneys. If a specific kind of bruit or murmur is found it may indicate that the high blood pressure has resulted from a narrowing of one of the arteries of the kidneys.

- *Examination of the kidneys.* By pressing on the abdomen, a doctor may be able to tell if the kidneys are enlarged, which may indicate a specific type of hypertension. This type of high blood pressure is rare.

- *A check for an enlarged thyroid.* A swelling in the neck (a goiter) may be a sign of an overactive or underactive thyroid, conditions that can elevate blood pressure.

In addition to the physical examination, the doctor will likely order a urinalysis to check for possible kidney damage or a bladder infection, and blood tests, especially to measure blood sugar (glucose) and cholesterol levels and to estimate kidney function. Any abnormality in either the physical examination or lab studies that indicates possible damage to the heart, kidneys, eyes, or blood vessels (the major "target"

Tests That Are Often Overused

In the majority of patients, hypertension and possible target-organ damage can be diagnosed on the basis of a routine patient history and a physical examination that includes an electrocardiogram, a few blood tests, and a urinalysis. Additional testing may be warranted in special cases, but often, expensive tests and procedures fail to provide additional information that is of value in determining effective treatment. As a general rule, a test is not needed unless it is likely to produce information that alters therapy or helps determine prognosis. Some of the most overused tests in the management of high blood pressure include the following.

ECHOCARDIOGRAM

In this test, high-frequency sound waves are "bounced off" the heart to create an image of its structures. Many doctors recommend echocardiograms, which cost from $250 to as much as $450, for hypertensive patients to determine whether they have an enlarged heart or thickened heart muscle, a common consequence of long-term high blood pressure. It may be of academic interest to know whether a patient has an enlarged heart. In our experience, however, the knowledge is unlikely to alter the approach to treatment, especially in dealing with mild to moderate high blood pressure without evidence of heart failure.

24-HOUR BLOOD-PRESSURE MONITORING

This test, which costs $200 to $300, requires that a patient wear a portable device that measures

and records blood pressure every 15 or 30 minutes over a 24-hour period. The theory is that such monitoring may provide useful additional information about fluctuations in a patient's blood pressure as he or she goes about normal activities. There is no scientific evidence, however, that such a test is better than periodic blood pressure measurements in a doctor's office or pressures taken at various intervals at home. The National High Blood Pressure Program concurs that such testing is not indicated for the vast majority of patients with high blood pressure.

EXERCISE TOLERANCE OR STRESS TEST

This examination entails taking a continuous electrocardiogram and periodic blood pressure measurements while exercising, typically on a treadmill or stationary cycle. Many doctors urge an exercise test for patients with high blood pressure, presumably to detect possible coronary artery disease. An exercise test may be justified for patients who plan to embark on a rigid exercise conditioning program, especially if they have other cardiovascular risk factors such as a family history of early heart attacks or elevated blood cholesterol, or if they smoke. But for most patients with mild to moderate high blood pressure, an exercise test is not needed to establish a diagnosis or to institute effective treatment. A typical exercise tolerance test costs $200 to $300, an expense that cannot be justified for most patients with high blood pressure in the absence of other evidence of heart disease.

organs of high blood pressure) may warrant additional testing. (See box, "Tests That Are Often Overused.") In most cases, however, a diagnosis of high blood pressure and its severity can be established accurately by repeated measurements with a sphygmomanometer and a few simple tests.

WHAT CAUSES HIGH BLOOD PRESSURE?

In the majority of cases—over 90 percent—no specific cause for the elevated blood pressure can be identified. In this case, the elevated blood pressure is referred to as *primary* or *essential hypertension.* Some researchers believe that this type of high blood pressure may be due to hormonal factors relating to the handling of salt by the kidneys and/or to the elaboration of certain substances that cause constriction of blood vessels. These are probably genetically determined, but certain environmental factors, such as a high-salt, low-potassium diet and *chronic* stress, may play some role.

In up to 10 percent of patients, high blood pressure may be a consequence of another disorder, or a side effect of medication. This type of hypertension is referred to as *secondary hypertension. It is important to remember that these cases are relatively uncommon.* However, some of the more common causes of secondary hypertension include the following.

KIDNEY DISORDERS

About 4 percent of all cases of high blood pressure can be traced to some type of kidney (renal) disorder. The kidneys work in several ways to help regulate blood pressure. For example, they are instrumental in regulating the body's fluid volume and its balance of sodium (salt) and water. If the kidneys conserve too much sodium, the body's fluid volume increases. In turn, this increased fluid volume puts an increased burden on the heart to maintain an adequate flow of blood to tissues and causes blood pressure to rise. The kidneys also produce renin, an enzyme that plays a key role in regulating blood pressure. (See the discussion below of renovascular hypertension.)

About 2 to 3 percent of all cases of high blood pressure are the result of recurrent kidney infection or a bout of nephritis (a kidney infection caused by

strep bacteria). But almost any *chronic* kidney disorder can result in elevated blood pressure. An example is damage to the kidney's blood vessels caused by diabetes.

As a rule, doctors will probably suggest specific tests of kidney function in cases of high blood pressure that do not respond to conventional antihypertensive (blood-pressure-lowering) therapy, especially if a urinalysis shows protein in the urine—an indication of impaired kidney function. It should be noted, however, that long-standing, poorly controlled hypertension by itself can *cause* kidney damage. In fact, about 25 percent of patients who require kidney dialysis have renal failure that is due to hypertension. This is especially true in the African-American population.

RENOVASCULAR HYPERTENSION

The renal arteries, which carry blood to the two kidneys, branch off from the abdominal aorta. A narrowing in one or both of the renal arteries results in reduced blood flow to the kidneys. This prompts the kidneys to attempt to raise blood pressure in order to improve their own blood supply. To do this, the kidneys increase their secretion of renin, an enzyme that, through a series of biochemical changes in the kidneys and lungs, gives rise to a substance called *angiotensin II.* This is a powerful *vasoconstrictor,* a medical term used to describe substances that cause blood vessels to narrow, or constrict. This constriction results in increased blood pressure. This substance also increases the secretion of a hormone, aldosterone, which leads to a retention of salt and water—further increasing blood pressure.

Renovascular hypertension is rare (accounting for 1 to 2 percent of all cases of hypertension), but it is relatively more common in elderly persons who may have widespread hardening of the arteries. It tends to occur more frequently in smokers. It sometimes occurs in children, as a result of infection or an inflammatory condition. In fact, renovascular hypertension is one of the more common causes of high blood pressure in young children, and should be suspected in any youngster under the age of 10 to 12 with elevated blood pressure. Less commonly, renovascular hypertension may be due to an inflammatory disorder that affects the muscles that encircle the arteries and control their diameter. This type of renovascular hypertension occurs more frequently in young women, although it is occasionally seen in men. It also tends to develop more frequently in smokers than in nonsmokers.

Renovascular hypertension can be diagnosed by studies in which a contrast dye is injected into a vein or artery to visualize the kidneys' blood vessels on X-ray film. Widening or opening up the narrowed renal artery will often cure this type of high blood pressure. The widening may be accomplished by angioplasty, a procedure in which a catheter with a balloon tip is inserted into the renal artery. The balloon is inflated at the site of narrowing to stretch the artery and increase blood flow. In some cases, surgery may be necessary to put in a bypass graft or bridge around the narrowed segment of the artery. The cure rate is high in carefully selected cases.

ADRENAL TUMORS

The two adrenal glands, which rest atop each kidney, secrete a number of hormones, including aldosterone. This hormone is instrumental in maintaining the body's fluid and electrolyte or mineral balance by regulating potassium secretion and prompting the kidneys to conserve sodium. In rare instances (fewer than 0.5 percent of all cases of hypertension), an adrenal tumor develops and production of aldosterone is increased. The elevated aldosterone results in the body's excreting too much potassium and conserving too much sodium. The extra sodium increases the body's fluid volume, leading to high blood pressure. These tumors are benign except in extremely rare instances.

This type of hypertension is rare, but should be suspected if a person develops high blood pressure and experiences other symptoms, such as muscle weakness, thirst, and excessive urination. Younger women are more susceptible to this disease than other people. But one should also keep in mind that excessive thirst and urination may be symptoms of other illnesses, such as diabetes. A diagnosis can be established by blood and urine studies and a computed tomography (CT) scan of the adrenal glands. CT scan is an examination that uses a computer to create a cross-sectional view of internal organs from multiple X-rays. Removal of the adrenal tumor usually cures the high blood pressure. If, however, excessive aldosterone secretion is due to overactive adrenal glands instead of a specific tumor, medication can be prescribed to block the hormone's action.

PHEOCHROMOCYTOMA

This is another very rare type of secondary hypertension that is related to a different type of a tumor of the adrenal gland called a pheochromocytoma. This type of tumor, which is benign in about 90 percent of all cases, produces different types of hormones, specifically adrenaline-like substances. As noted earlier, these hormones are instrumental in the body's fight-or-flight response. They serve to get us ready for emergencies or help us to exercise vigorously. Adrenaline increases the heart rate, elevates blood pressure, and helps increase blood flow to leg muscles. In addition to elevated blood pressure, the hormone elaborated by a pheochromocytoma may cause palpitations, tremors, clammy skin, jittery feelings, and facial and body sweating even in a cool room. The symptoms, including high blood pressure, may come and go.

The tumor usually develops on the adrenal glands, but in fewer than 10 percent of even these rare cases, it arises elsewhere in the body, usually along the aorta or spine, in the chest, or in the bladder. There are, however, only a few of these tumors reported yearly worldwide. If a pheochromocytoma is suspected, the patient may be asked to collect his or her urine over a 24-hour period; this is then analyzed for excessive amounts of adrenaline. X-ray studies or a CT scan may be ordered to locate the tumor(s), which can then be removed surgically. This removal usually cures the high blood pressure unless it has been present for some time, in which case antihypertensive medication may still be needed to keep blood pressure within normal limits.

DRUGS

Some drugs that are used for other conditions can raise blood pressure. Examples include birth control pills, the use of which may result in a *small* rise of 5 to 10 mm Hg in many women and a greater increase in about 1 in 30 to 50 women. The use of cortisone or other steroid medications and of certain nonprescription drugs, including some cold remedies, diet pills, arthritis medications such as the nonsteroidal anti-inflammatory agents Indocin, Naprosyn, etc., and nasal decongestants, may also increase blood pressure. Glycyrrhizic acid, an ingredient in natural licorice candy, can also raise blood pressure if consumed in large quantities. In almost all of these cases, blood pressure usually returns to normal when the causative substance is stopped. In some instances, the use of one of these medications may unmask a previously undiagnosed case of hypertension.

HYPERTENSION IN PREGNANCY

There is a type of hypertension that may develop in the last three months of pregnancy as part of toxemia of pregnancy. (See Chapter 19.) Since blood pressure levels in pregnancy are usually on the low side of normal (90–110/70–75), any increase to levels of above 135–140/85–90 should be considered as elevated, and some treatment should be instituted.

WHO DEVELOPS HIGH BLOOD PRESSURE?

High blood pressure develops in all social and economic groups, and affects both men and women. It generally begins in adulthood between the ages of 35 and 50, although it also occurs to a lesser extent among children and younger adults. Hypertension is rather uncommon in preadolescent children, but blood pressure should be checked at age 2 to 3 and again at age 13 to pick up the rare cases. The younger the age, the more probable that a secondary cause of hypertension will be found. Some people are more susceptible to hypertension than others, including:

- *African-Americans.* Not only are blacks twice as likely as whites to develop hypertension, but their disease is also more severe.

- *People with a family history of the disease.* Babies born to parents who have hypertension tend to have higher-than-average or more variable blood pressures throughout infancy and childhood, and are more likely to develop hypertension at a relatively early age. This tendency strongly suggests that there is a genetic basis for at least some cases of high blood pressure. It does not mean, however, that if both parents have hypertension the offspring will always develop high blood pressure.

- *People with diabetes.*

- *People who are overweight.*

Epidemiological, or population, studies suggest a number of other factors that may increase the risk of having high blood pressure. These include consuming large amounts of salt (sodium) and alcohol (more than the equivalent of 3 to 4 ounces of alcohol daily), smoking cigarettes, and following a diet low in po-

tassium. The exact mechanisms by which these factors raise blood pressure have not been clearly identified; some people appear to be more susceptible to them than others. For example, a high-salt diet may raise blood pressure only in people who have a genetic tendency to conserve sodium. Similarly, many people who consume excessive amounts of alcohol have normal blood pressures.

LONG-TERM EFFECTS

Hypertension is often referred to as the silent killer because it usually does not produce definite symptoms until it reaches an advanced stage. The first indication of high blood pressure may be an event such as a stroke or heart attack. Untreated high blood pressure is the major cause of strokes; it is also one of the major risk factors for a heart attack. Even before one of these events occurs, however, and even though a person may feel well, hypertension, if untreated, is taking its toll on vital organs throughout the body. Fortunately, as noted earlier, the consequences of hypertension can be largely prevented by lowering high blood pressure into the normal range and keeping it there.

ARTERIES

High blood pressure speeds up the process of hardening of the arteries in both large blood vessels such as the aorta and its major branches and the smaller arteries. The increased pressure on the inner walls of blood vessels makes them more vulnerable to a buildup of fatty deposits, a process called atherosclerosis. This blood-vessel damage may not produce symptoms until it reaches an advanced stage, and then symptoms or findings will depend upon the site of the atherosclerosis. For example, *angina*, the chest pains that are a sign that the heart muscle is not getting enough blood, is caused by severely narrowed and clogged coronary arteries. Narrowed arteries in the lower legs can make it painful and difficult to walk, a condition called *intermittent claudication.* (See Chapter 17.)

Clots, or *thrombi* as they are known medically, are more likely to form in arteries that have been narrowed by deposits of fatty material. A clot in a coronary artery (a *coronary thrombosis*) can result in a heart attack; one in the carotid artery or a blood vessel in the brain (a *cerebral thrombosis*) can cause a stroke.

High blood pressure that persists untreated for many years also increases the likelihood of an aneurysm, the ballooning out of a weakened segment of an artery (similar to a blister that forms over a weakened spot of a balloon). In time, these aneurysms may rupture, often with life-threatening consequences. For example, a ruptured aneurysm in the brain can cause a cerebral hemorrhage and a stroke. A ruptured aneurysm of the aorta can lead to fatal internal hemorrhaging if it is not repaired immediately.

High blood pressure also damages the small arteries, but in a different manner. The muscles that form the lining of these vessels become thickened, constricting the vessels and obstructing blood flow through them. If this happens to the arterioles in the kidney, it can lead to progressive renal damage. Similarly, a thickening and hemorrhaging of the tiny arteries in the eyes can result in a loss of vision.

HEART

The heart is one of the major target organs of long-term hypertension. Hypertension forces the heart to work harder in order to sustain an adequate blood flow to the tissues, resulting in an enlarged heart. The heart is composed mostly of muscle tissue, and any muscle that is strained will become larger (witness what happens to the biceps muscles of weight lifters). In the early stages, the enlarged heart muscle has the added strength needed to pump blood against the increased pressure in the arteries. In time, however, the enlarged heart may become stiff and weak, and unable to pump efficiently. This can lead to heart failure, a condition in which the heart is unable to pump enough blood to meet the body's needs. Just a few decades ago, heart failure usually progressed rapidly, with increasing disability and eventual death. Today, however, it can generally be controlled with medications, enabling most patients to lead normal lives for many years. And most important, recent studies show that with effective treatment of high blood pressure, much of the heart enlargement actually can be reversed. In the 1940s and early 1950s, the most common cause of heart failure was hypertension. Today this complication is extremely rare—high blood pressure is being effectively treated, and heart enlargement and heart failure are actually being prevented.

BRAIN

The circulatory system is designed to ensure a steady supply of blood and oxygen to the brain. When the body senses a decrease in blood flow to the brain, it takes immediate action to remedy the situation by raising blood pressure and by diverting blood from other organs and sending it to the head. The heart speeds up and vessels in the abdomen and legs contract, allowing more blood to get to the brain. If the carotid artery and other blood vessels that supply blood to the brain become clogged with fatty deposits, vital blood flow to the brain may be diminished. In such a situation, the risk of a stroke increases. For example, a stroke may occur if a portion of a vessel is blocked by a clot. Blood flow to a portion of the brain ceases and the tissue supplied by the clotted vessel is damaged. More seriously, a stroke may be caused by a cerebral hemorrhage. A stroke may occur when an artery that is weakened by long-term hypertension or atherosclerosis develops an aneurysm and ruptures.

Often, the blockage is temporary, causing only a brief interruption of blood flow. This is called a *transient ischemic attack* (TIA) or *ministroke*. (See box in Chapter 18, "Common Warning Signs of Stroke and Transient Ischemic Attack.") Although the episode usually passes within minutes, it warrants medical attention, because TIAs may be precursors of full-blown strokes. In addition, repeated TIAs may result in some loss of mental function, known as *TIA dementia*. If portions of the brain are repeatedly subjected to periods of lack of oxygen, brain tissue may be permanently injured. (See Chapter 18.)

KIDNEYS

Each kidney contains a million or more tiny filtering units called nephrons. Each day, more than 400 gallons of blood flow through the kidneys, where waste products are filtered out and excreted in the urine and nutrients and other useful substances are returned to the bloodstream. Sustained high blood pressure forces the kidneys to work even harder. The increased blood pressure may eventually damage some of the tiny blood vessels within the kidney and reduce the amount of blood available to the filtering units. In time their ability to filter the blood efficiently is reduced. Protein may be excreted in the urine rather than returned to the bloodstream because of damage to the delicate excreting mechanism, and waste products that are normally eliminated from the body may build up in the blood. This accumulation can lead to a condition called *uremia,* and eventually to kidney failure, requiring periodic dialysis to cleanse the blood.

Like the other organs that may be damaged by high blood pressure, the kidneys can be spared if effective antihypertensive treatment is started early and normal blood pressure maintained. Unfortunately, some patients still avoid drug treatment of their high blood pressure because of erroneous reports that diuretics or other antihypertensive drugs will cause rather than prevent kidney damage. There is no scientific evidence to back these reports; indeed, numerous well-controlled studies show just the opposite—that treatment with diuretics and other medications markedly lower the risk of kidney failure caused by high blood pressure if blood pressure is maintained at normal levels.

EYES

As noted earlier, the eyes contain tiny blood vessels that are vulnerable to damage from high blood pressure. After many years of poorly controlled hypertension, the retina or the screen in back of the eye may be damaged because of a decrease in blood supply; hemorrhages and/or fatty deposits may occur. This condition is referred to as *retinopathy.* This situation is more common in people with poorly controlled diabetes; the risk is increased if the patient also has high blood pressure.

At one time, poorly controlled high blood pressure was a major cause of diminished vision and blindness. This is no longer true, thanks to effective antihypertensive drug therapy.

TREATMENT OF HIGH BLOOD PRESSURE

The development of a variety of effective medications to control high blood pressure is one of major accomplishments of medical science since the 1950s. Before then, treatment was limited to strict restriction of sodium, radical surgical procedures, and drugs such as phenobarbital that were not particularly effective. All too often, patients developed malignant or accelerated hypertension, a complication marked

by rapidly rising blood pressure, usually culminating in a stroke, heart or kidney failure, or some other catastrophic event. In fact, this is what led to a crippling stroke in President Woodrow Wilson in 1917 and what killed President Franklin Roosevelt in 1945. In the late 1940s, it was not uncommon to find that every third or fourth bed in a hospital was occupied by a patient with some kind of complication of hypertension. A decade later, the first effective antihypertensive drugs were introduced, and today, dozens of medications that lower blood pressure are available. As a result, malignant hypertension is now so rare that it is considered a medical oddity. Even at a major center like the Yale–New Haven Hospital, it is unusual to find more than just a few patients in the entire facility who are there because of high blood pressure. This change is exciting.

Many misconceptions persist about when and how high blood pressure should be treated. Most doctors agree that even mild hypertension (repeated readings over 140/90) should be treated. (Treatment may not

Illustrative Case

The following case illustrates the reason why we feel strongly that readings above 140/90 should not be ignored.

About four years ago, a 48-year-old man came in complaining of a slight early-morning headache in the back of his head, and some shortness of breath. He was not a person who had neglected himself. He was relatively thin, did not smoke, and exercised regularly. He noted that his blood pressure had been elevated at pressures of about 145/90 to 160/95–100 for the past five years; he had been told by his doctor to reduce stress and salt intake, to exercise, and not to worry. His pressure had remained within this range, but he had developed symptoms and had come because he did not feel well (he had felt fine for three to four years). On examination, his blood pressure was 160/100. The electrocardiogram showed evidence of some heart enlargement, and he had some narrowing of the blood vessels in his eyes. In other words, he had begun to show changes indicating damage from his untreated high blood pressure. We started him on medication and his pressure returned to normal; his heart size also normalized. However, not everyone with untreated elevated blood pressure and target-organ damage does well. We know that we can still help at this point, but the outcome is usually better if treatment is started early, before damage occurs.

merely imply the use of drugs, as discussed below.) Some dissenters, however, advocate waiting until blood pressure reaches a higher level (blood pressures above 145–160/95–105) before initiating treatment. (See box, "Illustrative Case.")

Numerous studies showing decreased mortality and target-organ damage document the benefits of treating mild high blood pressure. These studies, carried out in the United States, Europe, and Australia, have involved over 40,000 men and women between about 40 and 80 years of age. They have demonstrated not only that lowering blood pressure will prevent progression to more severe hypertension, but that effective therapy also prevents heart attacks, heart enlargement, heart failure, strokes and stroke death, and progression of kidney damage. In other words, the occurrence of cardiovascular disease can be markedly decreased in both sexes and, importantly, in both young and elderly individuals by modern treatment of high blood pressure. Before initiating drug therapy, however, most doctors put patients on a trial of three to six months of non-pharmacologic life-style modifications, unless pressures are very high (greater than 160–180/100–110). These nondrug treatments include the following.

REDUCING SODIUM INTAKE

Early in the century, doctors first recognized that sodium restriction lowered high blood pressure. (Ordinary table salt is made up of sodium and chloride, and sodium is a major ingredient in many flavorings and preservatives.) Before the development of effective antihypertensive medications, a strict low-salt diet such as the rice and fruit diet developed by Dr. Walter Kempner at Duke University Medical Center was one of the most effective treatments for high blood pressure. The problem, of course, was that most patients had difficulty sticking to such a restrictive diet. In the days when we had nothing else to offer, some patients did stay on this diet for long periods of time. Today's low-salt diet allows many more foods and flavorings and does not have to be nearly as rigid. Care must be taken in selecting from a large variety of processed foods—our major source of sodium—if sodium is to be restricted. (See Table 12.2.) If it proves ineffective, other methods of treatment are available.

In reducing sodium intake—as in all aspects of life-style modification—common sense and moderation should prevail. Contrary to popular belief, scientific data do not confirm that salt is a major cause of high blood pressure or that eliminating it from your diet will always prevent high blood pressure. Sodium is probably a contributing factor only among people who are salt-sensitive, i.e., whose blood pressure goes up or down as they eat more or less sodium. Only about a third of hypertensive Americans may fall into this category. For reasons that are not completely understood, African-Americans tend to be more sodium-sensitive than Caucasians. Since many of the ethnic dishes favored by African-Americans are high in salt, this may be one reason that high blood pressure is more prevalent and severe in this segment of the population.

The typical American diet provides about 10 to 15 grams of salt (about 3–4 teaspoonfuls) a day, which is far more than we need. For most people, this extra sodium is not a hazard. The exceptions are the hypertensive patients who may be salt-sensitive. The American Heart Association believes that there is enough justification to urge all people to reduce their salt intake. The latest federal dietary guidelines also urge reducing salt intake. Still, many health experts feel that these guidelines are too broad, and that they should be applied mostly to those who are likely to be salt-sensitive, especially those with a strong family history of high blood pressure.

So, what should you do if you have a strong family history of hypertension in both parents and you hope to prevent hypertension, or you have a higher blood pressure than normal and you would like to lower it without any drugs?

Try to reduce your salt intake to about 1–1½ teaspoonfuls (about 4–6 grams) a day. You can do this by:

- Not using salt on food at the table.
- Avoiding obviously salty foods—processed meats, peanuts, pretzels, ketchup, and so forth.
- Using less salt in cooking and using other spices or condiments, such as salt-free herb mixtures.

If you are salt-sensitive, this degree of sodium restriction will probably work in many cases; if not, other measures can be used to lower blood pressure.

Some individuals are able to restrict salt to a great degree (to about 2 grams or less per day) without being miserable. It is possible that this degree of restriction may be more helpful in either preventing or treating high blood pressure—but there is no guarantee, and it does represent a sacrifice and a major change in life-style.

Table 12.2
Common High-Salt Foods

Food	Amount	Sodium (mg)	Calories	Food	Amount	Sodium (mg)	Calories
Bacon (Canadian broiled/fried)	1 slice	442	65	Peas (canned)	1 cup	493	150
Biscuits	1 oz	185	104	Peanuts (roasted and salted)	1 oz	138	170
Broth (canned beef or chicken)	1 cup	782	16	Pickle (dill medium)	1	928	5
Bologna (beef)	1 slice	230	72	Pickle relish (sweet)	1 tbsp	107	21
Bouillon				Pizza (cheese, regular crust)	¼ of a 12-inch pie	673	326
beef	1 cup	1,358	19	Potato chips (Lay's)	1 oz	260	150
chicken	1 cup	1,484	21	Pretzel twists (hard)	10	1,010	235
Catsup (Heinz Ketchup)	1 tbsp	156	16	Salmon (canned pink)	⅔ cup	387	141
				Saltines	4 oz	123	48
Cheese (cheddar)	1 oz	176	114	Sardines (canned in oil)	4 oz	735	175
Coffee cake (made with self-rising flour)	1 medium piece	310	232	Sauerkraut (canned)	⅔ cup	666	21
				Sausage (pork)	1 link	1,020	265
Corned beef	1 slice	294	46	Soups (commercially prepared)			
Corn chips	1 oz	210	153	chunky chicken, canned, ready to serve	1 cup	887	178
"Fast foods"							
Big Mac	1	963	541	chicken noodle, canned, made with water	1 cup	1,107	75
Vanilla shake	1	250	324				
Frankfurter (beef)	1	461	145	chicken noodle, dry	1 cup	1,284	53
Ham (regular, 11% fat)	1 slice	373	52	Soy sauce (La Choy)	1 tbsp	975	8
				Spinach (canned)	7¾ oz	519	42
Lima beans (canned)	8½ oz	536	41	Tomato juice (canned or bottled)	1 cup	878	45
Milk							
1% fat	1 cup	123	102	Tuna (canned light in water)	6½ oz	523	184
chocolate, 1% fat	1 cup	152	158				
Olives (green)	3	385	15	Worcestershire sauce	1 tbsp	147	12
Pancakes	1 oz	412	164				

MAINTAINING A MODERATE ALCOHOL INTAKE

As noted earlier, there is some evidence that a moderate intake of alcohol may actually help lower the risk of cardiovascular disease. There is also evidence that an intake of more than 3 ounces of alcohol a day may increase the risk of developing high blood pressure or cardiovascular disease. The Joint National Committee on Detection, Evaluation, and Treatment of High Blood Pressure recommends that people should drink "no more than 1 ounce of ethanol a day." This amount is contained in 2 ounces of 100-proof whiskey, about 8 ounces of wine, or about 24 ounces of beer.

All bets are off, however, if there is a strong family history of alcoholism or a sensitivity to small amounts of alcohol. In these cases, a person should not drink any alcohol regardless of the recommendations.

The good news is that alcohol in moderation is acceptable in most people. But drinking more than a few drinks a day might be harmful, not only to the brain and liver, but also to the cardiovascular system. In a number of cases blood pressure has become easy to control once patients have reduced their excessive intakes of alcohol.

LOSING EXCESS WEIGHT

It has long been known that people who are obese (20 percent or more above desirable weight) have an increased incidence of high blood pressure. They also are more likely to have high blood cholesterol and to develop diabetes. In many of these overweight and/ or diabetic patients, losing excess weight will normalize blood pressure and may also control the diabetes. *This is probably the most important thing other than stopping smoking that someone can do to reduce his or her risk of heart disease and possibly to reduce blood pressure.*

A common-sense diet that reduces the intake of total calories and fats (especially animal and other saturated fats) and emphasizes complex carbohydrates (starches) as the major diet component (55 to 60 percent of calories consumed) may help control many of the risk factors that predispose to early cardiovascular disease. Crash diets should be avoided. Although they may produce a fast weight loss, in more than 90 percent of cases, the pounds are quickly regained once the diet is stopped. Instead, strive for gradual weight loss—1 or 2 pounds a week—and undertake a moderate increase in physical activity. Such a program is more likely to achieve long-term weight control than a crash diet. (See Chapter 5.) There are no miracle diets. If the first ten miracle diets really worked, they would still be in use. Instead we have a new miracle diet—seven-day, four-week, Beverly Hills, Scarsdale, California, and on and on—every few months, just long enough for the book author or the diet center to get rich and walk away. *Consumers beware when it comes to the quick fix in the world of diets.*

INCREASING PHYSICAL ACTIVITY

Moderate exercise, combined with weight reduction and a low-salt diet, is an important component in any nondrug treatment program for high blood pressure. Some studies have shown that increased exercise can produce a modest lowering of blood pressure. It also helps burn up some calories and control excess weight, and it adds to the sense of well-being. A recent well-controlled 4-month study reported, however, that blood pressure was no more reduced in those who completed a regimen of vigorous aerobic exercise than it was in the control group.

Exercise need not be a regimented or rigorous cardiovascular conditioning program—activities such as taking a brisk walk, playing tennis regularly, cycling, and swimming all provide excellent means of relaxation and provide almost all of the benefits in terms of reducing cardiovascular risk that are derived from vigorous exercise. (See Chapter 7.) Nor is it necessary to set aside a time to exercise every day unless you want to—studies show that 15 to 30 minutes of moderate exercise three times a week provide the desired results. The exercise should be convenient and enjoyable; otherwise, you're likely to give up after

an initial burst of enthusiasm. Remember, too, that many day-to-day activities—walking up two or three flights of stairs, working around the house or yard—are excellent forms of exercise. A long-term study of nearly 17,000 Harvard alumni found that those who burned an extra 2,000 calories a week in moderate activities such as recreational sports, or walking or climbing up several flights of stairs a day, had a lower death rate than their more sedentary counterparts. (Again, see Chapter 7.)

A moderate exercise program plus a low-salt diet may lower blood pressure by anywhere from 1 to 10 mm Hg systolic and 1 to 8 mm Hg diastolic. If you start with a pressure of 145/95 and are one of the lucky responders, your pressure may decrease to below 140/90 and you will not have to take medication. Unfortunately, and contrary to what some popular media tell us, nondrug treatment methods will be effective in only 20 to 25 percent of cases of high blood pressure. Moreover, some nondrug treatments are highly questionable. (See box, "Alternative Nondrug Treatments of Questionable Value.") So although we all would like to be in control of our own destiny and not depend on medications, the majority of individuals with hypertension will have to take some medication to bring their blood pressures down to normal levels.

ANTIHYPERTENSIVE DRUGS

Unfortunately, many misconceptions persist regarding antihypertensive drugs; some of these are based on exaggerated reports of negative side effects. Pressure from industry to make newer drugs seem better also results in dissemination of the "dangerous" side effects of the older drugs. Reports may be misleading or based on inconclusive or incomplete data.

The public and doctors alike should not be pressured by pharmaceutical companies to change treatment practices. The bottom line is, if you are feeling well and your blood pressure is well controlled, do not let yourself or your doctor be persuaded to change medication unless there is a very good reason.

As already noted, many well-controlled studies have demonstrated that drug therapy for mild, moderate, or severe high blood pressure results in lowered death rates and fewer complications such as heart attacks and strokes.

Many patients have been lead to believe that anti-

Alternative Nondrug Treatments of Questionable Value

A number of so-called natural therapies have been advocated in the treatment of high blood pressure. Patients with high blood pressure are understandably swayed by glowing reports of supposedly effective treatments that do not require drugs, dietary restrictions, and other facets of traditional blood-pressure-lowering therapy. The major problem is that little scientific evidence demonstrates that these treatments have a sustained or reliable effect in lowering high blood pressure. Some may be beneficial adjuncts to medical treatment, but they are not acceptable alternatives or substitutes. The most common alternative therapies are the following.

BIOFEEDBACK TRAINING

Biofeedback is a process in which a person learns to control certain bodily functions that normally are involuntary. During biofeedback training, special equipment is used to show the patient how he or she can alter physical responses. The patient is hooked up to sensors, typically electrodes that are attached to the scalp or hand-held devices that measure heart rate and temperature changes. These changes are transformed into electronic impulses and presented on a video screen. By observing the screen, the patient can learn to alter some physiologic responses.

When used to treat hypertension, the sensors monitor changes in blood pressure. The patient watches the monitor and observes what seems to lower it, and then consciously tries to control blood pressure by concentrating on whatever it is that produces the reduction. The objective is eventually to control blood pressure without having to use the biofeedback equipment. A person may be able to produce a transient reduction in blood pressure using biofeedback techniques. Some studies have suggested that regular biofeedback sessions can produce more sustained reductions, but these results have not been replicated in long-term controlled scientific experiments. Biofeedback requires a great deal of discipline and dedication— beyond what can be expected of a typical patient. Thus, any short-term reduction in blood pressure is unlikely to be sustained once he or she resumes normal activities. Biofeedback, therefore, has little use as a definitive treatment of hypertension, other than in a small number of people.

HYPNOSIS

During hypnosis, a person enters a trancelike state in which his or her entire concentration is focused on a specific object or subject. It is akin to being totally absorbed in a daydream and oblivious to what is going on around you. During hypnosis, breathing and pulse rates slow down, and blood pressure may drop. There is also a reduced sensation in the peripheral nervous system. (This results in reduced sensitivity to pain, explaining why a person under hypnosis can perform such painful tasks as walking on nails or hot coals.) Like biofeedback, hypnosis may produce a temporary reduction in blood pressure, but there is no evidence of long-term benefits.

MEDITATION, YOGA, AND OTHER RELAXATION TECHNIQUES

These techniques are useful in overcoming tension or stress. Typically, the person is taught to relax by sitting quietly with eyes closed and taking slow, deep breaths while concentrating on a calming image or word. After a few minutes of such activities, there may be a modest lowering in blood pressure. Practiced regularly, these techniques can help a person achieve a more relaxed outlook and enhanced sense of well-being. They may even enable a person to reduce his or her dosage of medication. But they are not considered a definitive alternative therapy for high blood pressure.

FAD DIETS

Every few years, a new diet comes on the scene that promises to lower blood pressure (and cure a variety of other ailments) without resorting to drugs. Usually, these diets allow a limited number of low-salt, low-fat foods (for example, rice, grapefruit, oatmeal, and other such foods). Such a regimen may result in a loss of weight and a lowering of blood pressure. But it is also a boring, nutritionally unbalanced regimen that is difficult if not impossible to maintain. Before long, the person resumes his or her former eating habits, and weight as well as blood pressure go back up. These diets are not to be recommended as preferred therapy for high blood pressure.

hypertensive drugs always produce some side effects —ranging from lethargy and mental depression to impotence—that can make life miserable. While all drugs, even simple aspirin, may cause side effects in some people, the fact is that fewer than 5 to 10 percent of people experience annoying reactions to blood-pressure-lowering drugs. There are now so many drugs to choose from that if one produces side effects or is not effective, a satisfactory alternative almost always can be found. Patients should nevertheless be aware of the possible side effects of a particular drug so that they can report them to the doctor. (See box, "Questions You Should Ask Your Doctor About Your Therapy.")

In arriving at the most appropriate antihypertensive regimen for an individual patient, a physician considers many factors, including the patient's age and race and the presence of other disorders such as diabetes, kidney failure, or heart disease. Cost may also be a consideration, since some of the newer drugs are much more expensive than older medications that may be just as effective. Even so, it may be necessary to try a number of drugs before arriving at the best regimen that controls blood pressure with minimum side effects. The major classes of antihypertensive drugs are outlined below; specific medications and their cost and side effects are described in more detail in Chapter 23.

DIURETICS

Diuretics, commonly referred to as water pills, lower blood pressure by increasing the kidney's excretion of sodium, which in turn reduces the volume of blood. Their long-term effect is to dilate blood vessels, which reduces pressure in the blood vessel walls. These are among the older antihypertensive agents, having been introduced for use in the United States in 1957. They are still widely used, either alone or in conjunction with other antihypertensive drugs. There are several types of diuretics, which are classified according to their site of action in the kidney. The thiazide diuretics, which work in the tubules (the structures that transport urine in the kidneys), are the most commonly used.

The loop diuretics, more potent than the thiazides, are so named because their site of action is in the loop of Henle, the area near where waste is filtered from the blood. They are usually prescribed when a thiazide diuretic proves insufficient or for patients with heart failure or compromised kidney function.

A third type, the potassium-sparing diuretics, works in the area where potassium is excreted. They prevent the excessive loss of potassium that sometimes occurs with the thiazides. Since they have a less potent antihypertensive effect, they are often given in conjunction with a thiazide or loop diuretic.

Diuretics are highly effective, generally well-tolerated, and less expensive than most other antihypertensive medications. (See Chapter 23 for details.)

BETA BLOCKERS

These drugs, which were first introduced in the United States in the 1960s to treat angina, lower blood pressure by working through the autonomic (auto-

---

Questions You Should Ask Your Doctor About Your Therapy

If you are diagnosed as having high blood pressure, you undoubtedly will have many questions, especially if you are given medications. Don't hesitate to question your doctor, and if you experience side effects, let him or her know about them. It may be a good idea to take notes or ask your doctor for printed material. (An excellent booklet entitled *High Blood Pressure and What You Can Do About It* is available free of charge from the National High Blood Pressure Information Center, 120/80 NIH, Bethesda, MD 20892.) If the cost of your medication is a problem, ask your doctor if there is a generic equivalent or other medication that is less expensive but equally effective. Other questions you should ask regarding antihypertensive medications include:

- How often should I take my medication? Should I take it with food or on an empty stomach?

- What medications, including over-the-counter remedies, should I avoid?

- Are there foods or drinks (including alcohol) that I should avoid?

- What should I do if I forget to take my medication as scheduled?

- What are the possible side effects? Which ones are likely to pass with time? Which are signs to call you?

- How often should I have a medical checkup and pressure reading?

Source: Adapted from the National High Blood Pressure Education Program, National Institutes of Health, 1989.

---

matic) nervous system. Specifically, they block responses from the beta nerve receptors. This serves to slow down the heart rate and to reduce the amount of blood that the heart pumps every minute. Blood pressure is lowered. Beta blockers also block the effects of some of the hormones that regulate blood pressure.

Beta blockers may be prescribed as the initial drug to lower blood pressure, or they may be given along with a diuretic or other antihypertensive drug. In general, beta blockers are more effective in younger patients with rapid heartbeats. Since they relieve angina, they may be the drug of choice for patients who have this problem along with high blood pressure. For reasons that are not fully understood (it may be related to different levels of a hormone from the kidney), African-Americans do not seem to respond as well as Caucasians to beta blockers, although there are exceptions. Since beta blockers may constrict peripheral blood vessels, they generally are not recommended for patients with circulatory problems in their hands or legs. They also are contraindicated for patients with asthma or heart failure because their use tends to cause a narrowing of the bronchial tubes in the lungs (especially at higher doses), in addition to reducing the strength of the heart's pumping action.

Most patients, however, tolerate beta blockers well, especially if they are administered in low doses along with a diuretic or other antihypertensive drug. In some patients, however, they may cause sexual impotence. Other possible side effects include depression, vivid dreams, and feelings of lethargy. (See Chapter 23.)

CALCIUM-CHANNEL BLOCKERS

These are relatively new drugs that work by blocking the passage of calcium into the muscle cells that control the size of blood vessels. All muscles need calcium in order to constrict; when the muscles of the arteries are prevented from constricting, blood vessels open up (dilate), allowing blood to flow more easily through them. Blood pressure is reduced.

Calcium-channel blockers are effective as initial treatment in about 30 to 40 percent of patients. They also may be added to a diuretic or other antihypertensive medication. They are generally well tolerated, but they are more costly than diuretics and beta blockers. Thus, many doctors still recommend that these older drugs be used first. (See Chapter 23.)

ANGIOTENSIN CONVERTING ENZYME (ACE) INHIBITORS

These are also relatively new drugs. They work by preventing the formation of angiotensin II, a substance derived from the action of renin, an enzyme produced by the kidneys, and angiotensin I, a naturally occurring body chemical. Angiotensin II is a powerful vasoconstrictor that raises blood pressure by causing the arterioles to narrow. Angiotensin II also stimulates the release of aldosterone, the hormone that promotes the retention of sodium and fluid.

ACE inhibitors do not appear to be as effective as diuretics or calcium blockers in lowering blood pres-

sure in African-Americans. However, they may be among the first-choice drugs for hypertensive patients with kidney disease, diabetes, or heart failure. They are more effective when combined with small doses of a diuretic. They may be an appropriate alternative for patients who suffer impotence from beta blockers, diuretics, or other medications. Their high cost may be a drawback for many patients. (See Chapter 23.)

ALPHA-BLOCKING DRUGS

Like beta blockers, these agents work through the autonomic nervous system, but they block a different type of nerve receptor, the alpha receptors that promote constriction of the arterioles. Blocking constriction promotes dilation of vessels and lowers blood pressure. Alpha blockers inhibit the effects of norepinephrine, one of the adrenal hormones that raise blood pressure as part of the fight-or-flight response. Thus, alpha blockers may be a first-choice drug in treating patients with pheochromocytoma, the tumor that produces excessive amounts of adrenaline-like products.

Alpha blockers are usually prescribed along with other antihypertensive drugs, such as a beta blocker and/or a diuretic. One of their major side effects is orthostatic hypotension, a drop in blood pressure when a person abruptly stands up; this can result in fainting, especially in the elderly. Thus, care is needed to avoid sudden movements when taking this medication, especially when first starting the drug. In general, alpha blockers are not as effective for initial therapy as some of the other blood-pressure-lowering medications. Several medications are now available that combine the effects of blocking both the beta and alpha receptors. (See Chapter 23.)

VASODILATORS

As their name indicates, these drugs lower blood pressure by dilating, or opening up, arteries, thereby facilitating blood flow through them. Vasodilators are usually prescribed along with other drugs such as a beta blocker and a diuretic. Some produce a very rapid reduction in blood pressure, especially when administered by injection. Thus they may be useful in treating a hypertensive crisis. For chronic use, several office visits may be needed to fine-tune the dosage. Side effects may be annoying, and blood-pressure-lowering effects may be less when these drugs are used as initial treatment. One drug in this category, minoxidil, has gained considerable media attention because of one of its side effects, promotion of hair growth. It has been formulated into a topical preparation that is now marketed as a remedy for baldness. (See Chapter 23.)

PERIPHERAL ADRENERGIC ANTAGONISTS

These drugs, which are among the older antihypertensive agents, lower blood pressure by inhibiting the release of norepinephrine or by blocking its activities. Reserpine, the oldest drug in this category, is derived from rauwolfia plants and has been used in India and other Asian countries for many years as a sedative. This effect remains a major drawback to the continuing use of the drug to treat high blood pressure. Some patients complain that it dulls mental acuity and makes them feel lethargic. This can be at least partly overcome by giving it in small doses with other antihypertensive drugs, such as a diuretic. In any event, medications in this class should not be prescribed for patients who have suffered episodes of mental depression. This is the least expensive of all the antihypertensive medications and, in combination with a diuretic, is effective in lowering blood pressure.

CENTRALLY ACTING DRUGS

Drugs in this category reduce nerve impulses from the brain to the sympathetic nervous system. They lower blood pressure by opening up (dilating) peripheral arteries; they may also cause the heart to beat more slowly.

Centrally acting drugs are not widely used in the initial treatment of high blood pressure; instead, they are given along with a diuretic or other antihypertensive drugs when these drugs alone do not produce an adequate reduction in blood pressure. They may cause a number of side effects, including muscle weakness, fatigue, drowsiness, depression, dry mouth, and constipation. One drug in this category, clonidine, has an added use in some people, namely, minimizing withdrawal symptoms during smoking cessation or in an alcohol detoxification program. (See Chapter 23 for specific details about antihypertensive drugs.)

SUMMARY

There is little doubt that the next few years will see the development of newer and more effective blood-pressure-lowering drugs. In the meantime, however, we can continue to utilize the available treatments with the expectation that the majority of hypertensive patients can have their pressures normalized. We can also expect that as more people are treated there will be a further reduction in cardiovascular disease rates.

CHAPTER 13

HEART VALVE DISEASE

JEFFREY R. BENDER, M.D.

INTRODUCTION

The human heart is an efficient muscular pump that has four chambers—two atria and two ventricles—each closed off by a one-way valve. In the course of a day, the heart contracts and expands on average 100,000 times, pumping approximately 2,000 gallons of blood. By opening and closing in a synchronized manner, the four valves keep the blood flowing in a forward direction.

Blood from the veins enters the heart via the right atrium. It has a high content of carbon dioxide (a result of body metabolism), but is relatively depleted of oxygen, which has been absorbed by the body's tissues. After filling, the right atrium contracts, sending the blood through the tricuspid valve, which opens into the right ventricle. Blood is pumped through the pulmonary valve into the lungs. From the lungs, where it has been enriched in oxygen and depleted of carbon dioxide, the blood returns to the left atrium. It is then pumped through the mitral valve into the left ventricle. Finally, it is pumped out through the aortic valve into the aorta and the rest of the circulatory system.

HOW VALVES WORK

To control the flow of blood, all valves have thin flaps of muscle tissue, called leaflets or cusps, that open to let the blood through and close to prevent it from flowing backward. The mitral and tricuspid valves are shaped somewhat like parachutes. When open, their leaflets—three in the tricuspid and two in the mitral valve—form a ring resembling the wide end of a funnel. The leaflets are connected by chords—strings of strong fibrous tissue referred to as *chordae tendineae*—to muscle bundles in the chamber walls. Contraction of these muscles pulls the chords, and the leaflets snap shut, closing off the heart chamber. Valves act like gates that open when pressure behind them builds up, and close after blood has passed through and pressure is reduced.

The aortic and pulmonary valves have no chords but consist of petal-like flaps of tissue—two in the pulmonary and three in the aortic valve—at the exit from the chamber, which are flung open by the flow of blood and fall back together to close off the ventricle once the blood has been ejected.

The mitral and aortic valves are the most common

167

sites of heart valve disease, because of their location on the left side of the heart. The left chambers have a greater workload, because they pump blood to the entire body, whereas the right chambers push blood only to the lungs. Any abnormality in the valves of the left atrium and ventricle is more likely to produce symptoms and be quickly noticed by both patients and physicians.

Two major problems may arise in the functioning of the valves: They may fail either to open fully or to close properly. The narrowing of a valve, called stenosis, occurs when the leaflets become rigid, thickened, or fused together, reducing the opening through which the blood passes from one chamber to another. As its flow is obstructed, the blood accumulates in the chamber, causing the heart to work harder in order to push it through. (See Figure 13.1.)

When the valve fails to close properly—a condition referred to as insufficiency and also called incompetence or regurgitation—a portion of the ejected blood flows backward. For example, if the aortic valve is unable to close properly, some of the blood that is pumped forward from the left ventricle to the aorta leaks back into the ventricle. In severe cases, as much as 90 percent of the entire pumped volume may flow back. To compensate for the leak, the heart must enlarge in order to pump out an extra volume of blood with each beat, which significantly increases its workload.

Figure 13.1
Diagram of the heart showing aortic and mitral valve stenosis, in which the valves are narrowed and unable to open fully. This results in an inadequate amount of blood flowing into the aorta (aortic stenosis) or left ventricle (mitral stenosis).

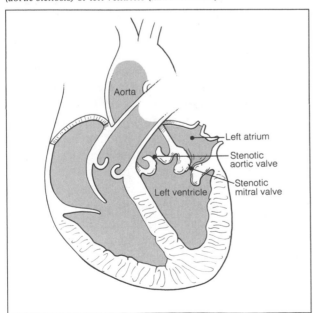

In some cases, stenosis and insufficiency may occur together. This happens when the leaflets become shrunken and stiff and the valve is fixed in a half-open position.

Valvular stenosis and insufficiency can gradually wear out the heart. At first, heart muscle dilates and thickens. This enables it to compensate for the extra work and allows the heart to supply an adequate amount of blood to the body. Eventually, however, the enlarged heart may grow weaker and become unable to pump blood as efficiently as before.

(Specific valve disorders are discussed at the end of the chapter.)

COMPLICATIONS AND SEQUELAE OF HEART VALVE DISEASE

The major complication of heart valve disease is congestive heart failure, a condition that occurs when the heart is unable to pump out an adequate volume of blood. Blood backs up, engorges the veins in the lungs and other parts of the body, and causes a congestion of fluid in body tissues. Fluid may collect in the lungs, obstructing the passage of air and oxygen exchange and interfering with breathing. During the day, when the person spends a great deal of time in the upright position, it may also build up fluid in the legs. Therefore, breathlessness, which is characteristic of congestive heart failure, is a major symptom of heart valve disease, along with swelling of the ankles. Other symptoms may include fatigue, fainting, palpitations, and chest pain. (See Chapter 14.)

Heart valve disease can also lead to heart muscle disease and disruption of the heartbeat—complications often associated with congestive heart failure. Another serious complication is formation of blood clots, which may become detached and travel through the bloodstream (at which point they are known as emboli). If one of these gets stuck in a small blood vessel, the organ affected may not get enough blood. A clot in the brain may cause a stroke. An embolus to the leg may result in pain, discoloration, or, in extreme instances, gangrene. Clots may form because the surface of a damaged valve is roughened; this interferes with the smooth and steady flow of blood, creating areas where it stagnates or swirls in place. Sticky substances in the blood congregate and a clot forms.

Many diseases of the valves take 20 to 30 years to develop, and by the time a patient becomes aware of

Table 13.1
Typical Prophylactic Antibiotic Schedule

Dental Procedures and Surgery of the Upper Respiratory Tract

Category of patient	Medication	Category of patient	Medication
Patients at risk (includes those with prosthetic heart valves and other high risk patients)	3 grams oral amoxicillin 1 hour prior to procedure and then 1.5 grams 6 hours after initial dose	Patients considered to be at a high risk who are allergic to amoxicillin, ampicillin, and penicillin	1 gram of vancomycin given by IV over 60 minutes, begun 60 minutes before procedure; no repeat dose necessary
Patient allergic to amoxicillin/penicillin	800 milligrams erythromycin 2 hours prior to procedure and then 400 milligrams, then ½ the dose 6 hours after initial dose or 300 milligrams clindamycin 1 hour before procedure and 150 milligrams six hours after initial dose		

Gastrointestinal and Genitourinary Tract Procedures

Category of patient	Medication	Category of patient	Medication
Patients unable to take oral medication (pills)	2 grams ampicillin by injection or IV 30 minutes before procedure and then 1 gram 6 hours after initial dose or Initial ampicillin followed by 1.5 grams of amoxicillin orally (suspension) 6 hours later or 300 milligrams of clindamycin IV 30 minutes before procedure and 150 milligrams 6 hours after initial dose	Most patients	2 grams of ampicillin given by injection plus 1.5 milligrams per kilogram (not to exceed 80 milligrams) gentamicin 30 minutes before procedure, followed by 1.5 grams of oral amoxicillin 6 or 8 hours after initial dose
Patients considered to be at a high risk who are not candidates for the standard regimen	2 grams of ampicillin plus 1.5 milligrams per kilogram (not to exceed 80 milligrams) gentamicin given by IV or injection 30 minutes before procedure followed by 1.5 grams of amoxicillin orally 6 or 8 hours after the initial dose	Patients allergic to amoxicillin, ampicillin, or penicillin	1 gram of vancomycin given by IV over 60 minutes plus 1.5 milligrams per kilogram (not to exceed 80 milligrams) gentamicin, given by injection or IV, 60 minutes before procedure; may be repeated once 8 hours after initial dose
		Alternate regimen for low-risk patients	3 grams of amoxicillin orally 1 hour before procedure and 1.5 grams 6 hours after initial dose

Note: In patients with compromised renal function, it may be necessary to modify or omit the second dose of antibiotics. Intramuscular injections may be contraindicated in patients receiving anticoagulants.

Source: Adapted from *Prevention of Bacterial Endocarditis,* by the Committee on Rheumatic Fever, Endocarditis and Kawasaki Disease. *JAMA* 1990; 264:2919–2922. Also excerpted in *J. Am. Dent. Assoc.* 1991.

the symptoms, the condition has often progressed to an advanced stage. Many damaged valves, however, may not cause any trouble at all, and people with one or more abnormal valves can go through a normal life. Often a routine physical examination will detect a murmur, suggesting that one of the heart valves is roughened or diseased. The murmur results from blood moving through a narrowed valve or blood swirling back and forth through a valve that remains partially open. People with slightly damaged valves may require no treatment, but may receive advice on prophylactic measures, such as taking antibiotics before dental and surgical procedures to reduce the risk of a valve infection called endocarditis. (See Table 13.1.)

Although the decrease in rheumatic fever, an important cause of valve problems, has led to a drastic reduction in the incidence of some forms of valve disorders in the United States, heart valve disease remains a relatively common form of cardiac disease. However, advances in diagnostic and surgical procedures, as well as a greater general awareness of cardiovascular disorders, have greatly improved survival rates in the past 20 to 25 years. A murmur that indicates a possible heart valve problem may not be of any significance or cause for concern. A patient who has been told he or she has such a murmur may simply have to be followed more carefully than someone without the problem.

CAUSES OF HEART VALVE DISEASE

RHEUMATIC FEVER

In the past, heart valve disease in the United States was usually caused by rheumatic fever, an inflammatory condition that often starts with a strep throat (a streptococcal bacterial infection). Fortunately, it is an uncommon disease today.

It can affect any tissues in the body, including the joints, the brain, and the skin, but, most important, it can scar the heart muscle, and particularly the heart valves. Damage is caused not by the bacteria themselves, but by an autoimmune response—a process in which the body, while fighting the bacterial infection, mistakenly begins to damage its own tissues. Rheumatic fever usually affects children 5 to 15 years old, but its consequences, referred to as rheumatic heart disease, can smolder throughout a lifetime.

No laboratory test offers a definitive diagnosis of rheumatic fever, but the condition can be recognized by a series of characteristic signs, including mild fatigue, fever, and pain and swelling of the joints, which may emerge several weeks after all symptoms of a streptococcal infection have disappeared. Except for acute cases, symptoms of heart trouble generally appear much later in life, some 20 years after the initial infection. If a streptococcal sore throat is treated promptly, rheumatic fever and heart disease usually can be prevented. It is therefore important to diagnose the condition early and use the appropriate antibiotic. A course of penicillin or another antibiotic for seven days will usually control most cases of streptococcal infection. There exist, however, rare cases when antibiotics suppress the infection but rheumatic fever and rheumatic heart disease develop. Some patients who develop heart valve disease many years later are not even aware of having had rheumatic fever.

Antibiotic treatment has dramatically reduced the incidence of rheumatic heart disease and associated deaths in industrialized countries. Although rheumatic heart disease still affects some 2 million Americans and continues to be an important cause of valve problems, many of these cases represent instances of residual disease from an era when antibiotics were not commonly used. *Non*rheumatic causes of heart valve disease today are by far more common in the United States.

INFECTIVE ENDOCARDITIS (BACTERIAL ENDOCARDITIS)

Another inflammatory condition that can lead to heart valve disease is infective endocarditis—an infection of the endocardium, the lining that covers the inner walls of the heart's chambers and the valves. It occurs when bacteria, fungi, or other microorganisms multiply on the valves' inner lining and form small, warty nodules or cauliflower-like polyps. Since the condition is most often caused by two types of bacteria, streptococci and staphylococci, it is frequently referred to as bacterial endocarditis. Fatigue, a low-grade fever, weakness, and joint aches may indicate that this disease is present. In persons with heart valve disease, of course, these symptoms do not always indicate endocarditis and may just be the flu, for example. However, a heart infection should be considered.

Endocarditis is twice as common in men as in women, and it seldom occurs in people whose valves are completely normal and healthy. In fact, it is relatively uncommon even in people with heart valve disease. It often results from an untreated infection elsewhere in the body, and usually affects the valves that have a congenital abnormality or that have already been damaged by rheumatic fever or another form of disease. It is also seen in people who have artificial valves. Another group at risk are drug abusers who use contaminated hypodermic needles.

Colonies of microorganisms that grow on the endocardium can cause holes in the valve, distort its shape, and completely disrupt its function. Clusters of infectious organisms may stimulate the formation of emboli, which travel through the circulation and end up blocking small blood vessels. The infection may take an acute form and lead to heart failure and death if left untreated, or it may linger undetected for much longer before producing disturbing symptoms. To prevent the occurrence of endocarditis in patients who have damaged or artificial valves, the American Heart Association recommends that antibiotics be taken before dental treatment, surgery involving the respiratory tract, gastrointestinal or genitourinary surgery, invasive diagnostic procedures, or any other procedure that may stimulate the release of bacteria into the bloodstream.

MYXOMATOUS DEGENERATION

In the elderly, one of the most common causes of heart valve disease is a process called myxomatous degeneration, which usually affects the mitral valve that connects the left atrium and ventricle. This dysfunction stems from a series of metabolic changes in the course of which the valve's tissue loses its elasticity, becomes weak and flabby, and becomes covered by a buildup of starch deposits. The chords that control the opening and closing of the valve may break off. It is not known what triggers myxomatous degeneration. Many elderly people with this condition are unaware of it and have no symptoms or other adverse effects.

CALCIFIC DEGENERATION

Another common cause of heart valve disease in the elderly is calcific degeneration, a process in which calcium deposits build up on the valve. This type of tissue degeneration usually causes aortic stenosis, a narrowing of the aortic valve. It may also affect part of the mitral valve, causing it to become leaky or regurgitate. In many elderly persons, aortic stenosis may not manifest any symptoms.

CONGENITAL ANOMALIES

Heart valve disease may also result from congenital abnormalities, problems that are present from birth. The most common congenital defect is a misshapen aortic valve, which has two leaflets instead of three and is therefore referred to as bicuspid. The defect does not usually produce any symptoms, although such a valve is more prone to develop an infection. The defect may be corrected by surgery, which is usually not performed unless there are symptoms or repeated valve infections. Most of the time this is not a serious problem. Congenital malformation may also be present in the mitral valve, which results in mitral stenosis.

OTHER CAUSES

Finally, heart valve disease may be a result of other heart disease, particularly coronary artery disease or a heart attack. These conditions can cause injury to one of the papillary muscles that support the valves, so that it doesn't close properly. Heart attacks, for example, often disrupt the closing of the mitral valve, leading to mitral regurgitation.

DIAGNOSIS

Valve disorders can usually be diagnosed by listening to the heart with a stethoscope. While no sound is heard when blood flows through a normal valve, its passage through a diseased valve creates a whooshing noise, referred to as a murmur. The heart sounds normally consist of regular double throbs—one heard upon the simultaneous closing of the mitral and tricuspid valves, and the second heard immediately afterward, when the aortic and pulmonary valves close almost at the same time. Heartbeats sound like lub-dub, lub-dub. When a valve is damaged and fails to close or open completely, blood will create a swirling current as it is squeezed through a narrow opening or regurgitated in the wrong direction, and a murmur is produced. In the case of stenosis, the sound may be a rough, short, low-pitched murmur; with a valve insufficiency, the sound may be higher-pitched, softer, and longer.

Murmurs are present in a great number of healthy people and do not necessarily indicate disease. Physicians can usually tell when murmurs or any deviations from the normal heart sounds signal a cause for concern. An electrocardiogram (ECG) and chest

X-ray are two diagnostic techniques that can provide important information about heart size and activity. They may, for example, reveal that the heart is enlarged, which is often a sign of heart valve or other cardiac disease. However, while both these methods are useful for detecting valve disorders, they are not especially helpful in making a specific diagnosis. Listening with a stethoscope is actually more helpful.

A major diagnostic tool in assessing valve disorders is echocardiography, a noninvasive and painless procedure that has revolutionized the evaluation of heart diseases. In echocardiography, high-frequency sound waves (like sonar waves) are bounced off the heart's tissues, allowing physicians to visualize the shape and motion of the valves, the size of the valve's opening, and the thickness of chamber walls. One variety of this procedure, called Doppler echocardiography, makes it possible to measure the speed and flow of blood and is particularly helpful in assessing to what extent a valve is stenotic or leaky. While these procedures are more definitive, they are expensive and often not necessary for making a diagnosis.

Once a valve disorder has been detected, if less invasive procedures have failed to provide sufficient information about it, or if surgery is being considered, diagnosis is usually established on the basis of cardiac catheterization. Fortunately, this procedure is rarely necessary for making a diagnosis, but it is often indicated prior to surgery. A thin plastic tube called a catheter is inserted into the patient's artery and guided to the heart. When the catheter is in place, a chemical dye is injected through the tube. The dye shows up on the X-ray, allowing physicians to visualize the inside of the heart, to see whether all the blood is flowing in the proper direction or if there is any backflow, and to assess the function of the chamber muscle and the performance of natural or prosthetic valves. In addition, it displays any blockage of coronary arteries, which can accompany a valve disorder and can be corrected at the same time as valve surgery is performed. (For more information, see Chapter 10.)

TYPES OF HEART VALVE DISEASE

MITRAL VALVE PROLAPSE

This disease is also known as click-murmur syndrome, floppy-valve syndrome, balloon mitral valve, and Barlow's syndrome. It is a deformity of the mitral valve that may prevent its leaflets from closing properly. One or both leaflets may be bulging, or the entire valve may be out of its normal position. Depending on the degree of the deformity, the prolapse can lead to mitral regurgitation.

Mitral valve prolapse is the most common type of valvular disorder, and perhaps the best known to the general public. Although a larger number of cases than in the past are now being diagnosed by physicians, most of these are mild, and the increase probably reflects a heightened awareness of the disorder rather than an actual increase in the incidence rate of new cases. The prevalence (total number of cases) is unknown, but the syndrome is believed to affect, to some extent, 5 to 10 percent of the population in the United States. Women are affected by mitral valve prolapse much more often than men. One possible explanation is that in women the mitral valve tends to be larger in relation to the left ventricle than in men, and may therefore tend to fit less well.

The disorder is believed to be primarily hereditary, as approximately half of family members of people with mitral valve prolapse also have been found to be affected. It is often associated with myxomatous degeneration, and it may be a part of genetic diseases involving other organs of the body. The disorder tends to be more easily detected in adolescents and young adults. It is usually recognized by characteristic clicks and murmurs that can be heard with a stethoscope.

In the vast majority of patients, mitral valve prolapse is very mild and produces no symptoms at all. Unfortunately, many individuals with a mitral-click syndrome or mitral prolapse have become anxious or overly concerned as a result of excessive emphasis by their doctors on this murmur or their disease. Symptoms that do appear are often vague and cannot always be attributed to the valve defect. They may include palpitations, breathlessness, chest pain, and fatigue. While for many years the disorder was thought to be associated with nervousness, weakness, anxiety, and various other forms of malaise, most experts today discount this connection for lack of firmly established evidence. There may be some association between mitral valve prolapse and an overactive sympathetic or automatic nervous system.

Generally, when there are no symptoms or when symptoms are mild, no treatment is required. In a very small number of patients, however, mitral valve prolapse can result in mitral insufficiency. Extra beats or episodes of tachycardia may also become frequent enough to cause symptoms. In some cases of mitral insufficiency, patients may be advised to refrain from strenuous activities such as competitive sports. Unusual or rapid rhythms may be relieved by the use of beta blockers, which help to slow down the heart rate.

People with mitral valve prolapse are also at an increased risk of developing infective endocarditis. This is particularly true of patients in whom the prolapse causes mitral insufficiency; these people should consult their physicians regarding possible preventive antibiotic treatment.

MITRAL STENOSIS

While in infants mitral stenosis can, in rare cases, be caused by congenital abnormalities, in adults it usually develops as a result of rheumatic fever suffered in childhood. With the decrease in the incidence of rheumatic fever, the incidence of this type of valvular disorder has dropped sharply in recent years.

Symptoms of mitral stenosis are slow to develop and usually do not appear until 10 to 20 years after an episode of rheumatic fever. The disorder is usually diagnosed when patients are in their 30s or 40s. Once symptoms appear, they tend to progress.

Since the mitral valve is located between the left atrium or upper heart chamber and the left ventricle, the major pumping chamber, its stenosis or narrowing results in an increase in the pressure in the left atrium. This pressure is transmitted back through veins to the lungs, causing congestion of the air passageways. The buildup of pressure, fluid, or both in the lungs is one manifestation of congestive heart failure and results in dyspnea (shortness of breath), the major symptom of mitral valve stenosis. It should be understood that heart failure may be serious but does not imply that the heart is unable to function. Many patients whose failure has been controlled are able to live long, productive lives. Mitral stenosis can be aggravated by atrial fibrillation, a condition in which the atrium weakens and moves in fine, quivery movements instead of a pumping action. The result is that blood is not pumped efficiently into the lower heart chambers.

Patients with mitral stenosis who develop heart failure are treated with diuretics. If they develop atrial fibrillation they may be given digitalis, quinidine, or a similar drug, as well as blood-thinning medications (anticoagulants) to prevent clots. In severe cases, the valve may have to be widened in an operation called mitral valvotomy. It can also be widen by a balloon catheter during cardiac catheterization, a procedure called valvuloplasty. This valve can also be replaced if repair is not feasible.

MITRAL REGURGITATION

Mitral regurgitation is most often caused by rheumatic heart disease, a type of degeneration of the valve, dysfunction of the muscles that control the closing of the valve, or rupture of the valve's chords. A heart attack may result in mitral insufficiency if a portion of the heart that supports the position of the valve is disrupted. Prolapse of the mitral valve may also be associated with insufficiency. In rare cases, insufficiency is a result of a congenital defect or disorder.

As in the case of stenosis, mitral regurgitation may be present without symptoms for many years. If a great deal of leakage occurs between the atrium and ventricle and this persists over long periods, in time pressure will build up in the lungs and breathlessness will result. In acute cases, such as those following a heart attack or damage caused by infective endocarditis, symptoms may be sudden and severe. Patients may go into heart failure, and urgent therapy becomes necessary.

There are no medications that will help to heal the valves; therapy is directed toward relief of shortness of breath and various other changes that may occur. These include diuretics, digitalis, and quinidine. Severe cases are more likely to be treated by surgical valve replacement rather than repair. Some patients with mitral regurgitation are at a high risk of endocarditis and should receive prophylactic (preventive) antibiotic treatment before any procedure, from dental work to major surgery, that may involve possible blood infections. There are many older people who function without difficulty despite having had rheumatic fever and mitral insufficiency in childhood.

AORTIC STENOSIS

There are three major causes of aortic stenosis: calcific degeneration or deposits of calcium on the valve (primarily affects the elderly), congenital abnormality (uncommon), and rheumatic fever. Even in the case of a congenital defect, symptoms are most likely to appear only in adulthood. Whether the cause is rheumatic, degenerative, or congenital, the leaflets of the valve are usually covered with calcium deposits, which can completely distort their shape. While the condition may produce no symptoms for many years, it may cause chest pain, fainting, and shortness of breath during exercise if narrowing of the valve becomes severe. The disorder is recognized by a characteristic murmur; it can become quite loud and is usually easily recognized when listening with a stethoscope.

Stenosis of the aortic valve obstructs the flow of blood from the left ventricle, causing it to enlarge or thicken and eventually weaken over time. Under normal conditions, even in the presence of aortic stenosis, the ventricle can maintain the output of blood to the body at a regular level by pumping harder, but at times of physical exertion it may not be able to maintain an output of blood sufficient to supply blood to the brain. Fainting may result. Patients with aortic stenosis should refrain from strenuous activity. Moderate exercise is usually well tolerated. Surgical repair of severe aortic stenosis has been successfully performed in thousands of people. The presence of a narrowed aortic valve may result in less blood getting into the coronary arteries which supply blood to heart muscle. Angina may result even after moderate exercise. This may be a sign that the valve should be repaired.

AORTIC REGURGITATION

In its acute form, aortic regurgitation usually occurs as a result of an infection that leaves holes in the valve's leaflets, but this condition is uncommon. The chronic form, which is more common, is usually a consequence of the widening of the aorta in the region where it connects to the valve, or from valve disease, rheumatic fever, etc. In most cases, it is not known what causes the widening of the aortic ring, which prevents the valve from properly closing off the left ventricle. Sometimes the aorta may be widened due to a genetic disorder, such as Marfan syndrome, a congenital disease of connective tissue. In the past, aortic insufficiency was frequently caused by syphilis, but since the advent of penicillin for treating syphilis, this is no longer the case.

Aortic regurgitation, like other valve abnormalities, often produces no symptoms for many years. Breathlessness, sometimes accompanied by chest pain and ankle swelling, may be noticed after many years if the condition is severe. The constant swirling or regurgitation of blood results in a dilation or enlargement of the left ventricle. Eventually, the burden becomes too great and the blood backs up. If symptoms are severe, valve replacement may become necessary. The acute form of the disorder may lead to heart failure and requires emergency surgery and valve replacement.

TRICUSPID STENOSIS AND REGURGITATION

These disorders account for less than 5 percent of valvular disease. They seldom occur as a single symptom; they usually accompany other types of valve problems or cardiac abnormalities. Abnormalities of the tricuspid valve are generally caused by rheumatic fever or metabolic abnormalities affecting the heart. Among the major symptoms they produce are swelling of the legs and fatigue.

PULMONARY STENOSIS AND REGURGITATION

These disorders—particularly pulmonary stenosis—are also rare and are primarily due to congenital defects. Children born with a severely narrowed pulmonary valve may require immediate surgical intervention for survival.

TREATMENT

DRUGS

None of the drugs prescribed for valve disorders are curative; rather, their major functions are to reduce the severity of symptoms, possibly reduce the workload of the heart, and prevent complications. Digitalis medications are most often used in patients with heart valve disease. They increase the heart's efficiency in pumping blood and may help relieve the symptoms of heart failure. Digitalis-like medications also help in managing some arrhythmias (abnormalities of the heartbeat) that may occur as a result of valve disorders. Other classes of drug that may be prescribed for the symptoms resulting from heart-valve disorders include:

- *Vasodilators.* These drugs dilate blood vessels and are used to treat congestive heart failure associated with heart valve disease (usually valvular insufficiency). They help to reduce the pressure against which the heart must pump. These drugs include the ACE inhibitors, nitroglycerin, and prazosin (Minipress), among others.

- *Diuretics.* These remove salts and water from the body. They reduce the workload on the heart (which may be overburdened by the presence of a valve disorder) by decreasing the volume of blood that needs to be pumped. Diuretics include furosemide (Lasix) and hydrochlorothiazide combinations (Hydrodiuril), among others.

- *Anticoagulants.* These include medications such as warfarin (Coumadin), which help to prevent formation of blood clots that may block blood vessels.

- *Antiarrhythmics.* Drugs such as quinidine and procainamide help control arrhythmias, or irregular heartbeats, which are fairly common in heart valve disease.

(For more information about these medications, see Chapter 23.)

BALLOON VALVULOPLASTY

This relatively new technique is increasingly used as an alternative to surgical repair of valvular stenosis. A deflated balloon attached to the end of a catheter is introduced through an artery into the heart to the center of the valve opening and then inflated. The method, which is used primarily to correct the narrowing of the mitral and occasionally the aortic valves, can alleviate symptoms and partially clear the obstruction. While somewhat less effective than surgery, it is a much simpler, safer, and less expensive procedure, although it is not yet clear whether it can provide a permanent solution to valve stenosis. Balloon valvuloplasty is more successful in repairing the mitral valve than in repairing aortic stenosis. In elderly patients who might not tolerate surgery or where a long convalescence should be avoided, the procedure may be helpful in relieving symptoms.

SURGICAL REPAIR

Surgical treatment is reserved for severe cases of heart valve disease when symptoms suggest progression of the disease. Thus, in the case of stenosis, it is usually performed if the opening of the mitral valve is less than a quarter of its normal size or the opening in an aortic valve is a third of normal. During the operation, the surgeon can stretch and open the valve's leaflets; this may not completely correct the obstruction but can reduce the symptoms.

In case of a tear, the surgeon may repair the leaky valve by suturing and tightening the leaflets or chords. When leaflets of the mitral valve fail to close, it may be possible to pull the base of the valve to-

gether or make the whole valve smaller, to facilitate the closure. In the majority of cases, however, a severely stenotic valve, particularly if it is also leaky or insufficient, has to be replaced.

VALVE REPLACEMENT SURGERY

This type of surgery is usually recommended when the damage to the valve is severe enough to be potentially life-threatening. There may, for example, be a risk that the valve disorder could cause sudden death, as in the case of severe aortic stenosis. The mitral and aortic valves, which are the gates controlling blood flow into and out of the heart's two main pumping chambers, are the ones that most often need to be replaced.

There are two types of prosthetic valves that can be used to replace the original valves: mechanical and biologic. Mechanical valves are made of synthetic materials: metal alloys, carbon, and various plastics. They come in two major designs. One, called a caged-ball valve, consists of a small cage containing a ball that pops up when blood is ejected and then drops down to seal the chamber. The other, referred to as tilting-disk valve, consists of a round disk pivoting inside a ring, which can tilt to a horizontal or vertical position to let the blood through or prevent its flow.

Mechanical valves are more durable than biologic ones and can last for 20 years or more without having to be replaced. They do, however, tend to promote abnormal clot formation, so patients must take anticoagulant drugs as a preventive measure. Thus, mechanical valves cannot be implanted in patients who have bleeding problems, ulcers, or other conditions precluding a long-term use of anti-blood-clotting medications. Biologic valves may also be preferred in elderly patients, when the issue of durability is less crucial.

Biologic valves can be composed of animal or human valve tissue. Because of the scarcity of human valves available for transplantation, pig valves, specially processed and sutured into a synthetic cloth, are most often used. They are well tolerated by the human body and are much less likely to require blood-thinning therapy, but they tend to be less durable; after 10 years, some 60 percent need to be replaced.

(For more information on surgical repair and replacement, see Chapter 25.)

CHAPTER 14

HEART FAILURE

ROBERT SOUFER, M.D.

The heart's primary function is to pump blood to all parts of the body, bringing nutrients and oxygen to the tissues and removing waste products. When the body is at rest, it needs a certain amount of blood to achieve this function. During exercise or times when greater demands are placed on the body, more blood is required. To meet these variable demands, the heartbeat increases or decreases, and blood vessels dilate to deliver more blood or constrict during times when less blood is required.

When a person is diagnosed with heart failure, it does not mean the heart has stopped working, but rather that it is not working as efficiently as it should. In other words, the term "failure" indicates the heart is not pumping effectively enough to meet the body's needs for oxygen-rich blood, either during exercise or at rest. The term *congestive* heart failure (CHF) is often synonymous with heart failure but also refers to the state in which decreased heart function is accompanied by a buildup of body fluid in the lungs and elsewhere. Heart failure may be reversible, and people may live for many years after the diagnosis is made. (See box, "Classifications of Heart Failure.")

Heart failure may occur suddenly, or it may develop gradually. When heart function deteriorates over years, one or more conditions may exist. (See box, "Effects of Heart Failure.") The strength of muscle contractions may be reduced, and the ability of the heart chambers to fill with blood may be limited by mechanical problems, resulting in less blood to pump out to tissues in the body. Conversely, the pumping chambers may enlarge and fill with too much blood when the heart muscle is not strong enough to pump out all the blood it receives. In addition, as the architecture of the heart changes as it enlarges, regurgitation of the mitral valve may develop, making the heart failure even worse.

WHO DEVELOPS HEART FAILURE?

There are an estimated 2 million people in the United States with heart failure. The incidence of chronic congestive heart failure—the number of new cases developing in the given population each year—has increased in recent years. This is possibly a result of the overall decline in deaths from coronary (ischemic) heart disease, an improvement attributed to medical advances and the fact that people are living longer.

The most common cause of congestive failure is coronary artery disease—narrowing of the arteries supplying blood to the heart muscle. Although coronary disease often starts at an early age, congestive failure occurs most often in the elderly. Among people more than 70 years old, about 8 out of 1,000 are diagnosed with congestive heart failure each year. The majority of these patients are women, probably because men are more likely to die from coronary artery disease before it progresses to heart failure.

Heart failure is also associated with untreated hypertension, alcohol abuse, and drug abuse (primarily cocaine and amphetamines) at any age. Hyperthyroidism and various abnormalities of the heart valves (particularly aortic and mitral) are among the

Classifications of Heart Failure

The New York Heart Association developed a system that has been used for many years to provide a standardized set of criteria for the classification of heart failure based on the severity of the condition. This is evaluated by symptoms and ability to function.

- Class I: no undue symptoms associated with ordinary activity and no limitation of physical activity
- Class II: slight limitation of physical activity; patient comfortable at rest
- Class III: marked limitation of physical activity; patient comfortable at rest
- Class IV: inability to carry on any physical activity without discomfort; symptoms of cardiac insufficiency or chest pain possible even at rest

Effects of Heart Failure

- Strength of muscle contractions is reduced.
- Ability of the heart chambers to fill with blood is limited, so there is less blood to pump out to tissues in the body.
- The pumping heart chambers fill with too much blood; the heart muscle is not strong enough to pump out all the blood it receives.

other disorders that can cause heart failure. In addition, viral infection or inflammation of the heart (myocarditis) or primary heart muscle disease (cardiomyopathy), and in rare instances, extreme vitamin deficiencies, can result in heart failure. (See Chapters 13 and 15.)

SIGNS AND SYMPTOMS

Depending on the underlying causes, heart failure can be either acute (intense but not long-lasting) or chronic (protracted over a long time). When heart failure occurs, the forward flow of blood is slowed down, the quantity of blood pumped is less than adequate, and the pressure rises in the chambers of the heart, causing blood that is returning to the heart to back up in the lungs or veins. Excessive fatigue may be an early symptom. (See box, "Symptoms of Heart Failure.") Some excess fluid may be forced out of the blood vessels into the body's tissues. It then settles in the feet, ankles, and legs, and sometimes also in the abdomen and liver.

Dyspnea, or shortness of breath, resulting from increased pressure, fluid, or both in the lungs, is a common symptom of congestive heart failure. Although breathlessness is most likely to be noticed during exercise (known as dyspnea on exertion, or DOE), it can also be a problem at rest, particularly when the patient is lying down (when it is known as orthopnea). Individuals with orthopnea find that the condition feels worse when they are in a reclining position because the backflow of fluid and buildup in pressure from the heart interferes directly with the free flow of oxygen in the lungs.

Normally, oxygen is easily exchanged through the thin spongy tissue of the lungs. (See Figure 14.1.) If this tissue becomes waterlogged, as it does in heart failure, less oxygen can be transferred to the blood. If there is not enough oxygen, certain reflexes stimulate faster breathing. People with lung congestion as a result of heart failure usually have to prop themselves up with extra pillows in order to sleep. The number of pillows used may indicate to a physician the extent of the heart failure. When an individual wakes at night because of shortness of breath from

Symptoms of Heart Failure

- Shortness of breath (dyspnea)
- Shortness of breath when lying down (orthopnea)
- Shortness of breath while sleeping (paroxysmal or intermittent nocturnal dyspnea)
- Buildup of fluid in the lungs (pulmonary edema), frequently causing a person to cough up blood-tinged sputum
- Buildup of excess fluid (edema) in other parts of the body, causing weight gain, swelling of the ankles, legs, and back, and in extreme cases fluid accumulation in the abdomen (ascites)
- Fatigue, weakness, and an inability to exert oneself physically or mentally
- Blueness of the skin (cyanosis)

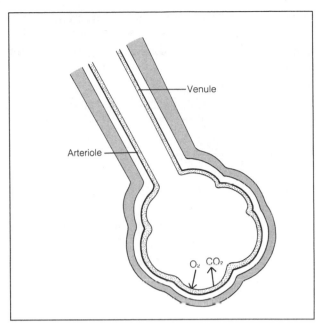

Figure 14.1
This diagram of an alveolus (air sac) shows the exchange of carbon dioxide (CO_2) and oxygen in the lung.

When a marked excess of fluid accumulates in the lungs, it is known as pulmonary (lung) edema. This condition is often, but not always, acute and is frequently associated with coughing up blood-tinged, pinkish-colored sputum.

Inefficient circulation may also manifest itself as fatigue, weakness, and an inability to exert oneself physically or mentally because less blood and oxygen reach the brain. Older people in particular may suffer from confusion and impaired thinking ability.

LEFT SIDE OR RIGHT SIDE?

The particular symptoms that an individual experiences are determined by which side of the heart is involved in the heart failure. (See box, "Symptoms of Left-Side and Right-Side Heart Failure.") For example, the left atrium (upper chamber) receives oxygen-

fluid settling in the lungs, the condition is known as paroxysmal (intermittent) nocturnal dyspnea. A person suffering from this typically will wake up short of breath about two to three hours after going to sleep. Standing or sitting often relieves symptoms.

One of recent history's most noted patients with heart failure was President Franklin Delano Roosevelt. He had severe hypertension that led to an enlarged heart and eventually to heart failure. For months, he was unable to lie flat in bed, so he slept in a chair. He was told that he had bronchitis, allergies, and the flu. Finally, the right diagnosis was made and treatment started. However, this was before the development of effective drugs to lower blood pressure and to treat advanced heart failure. At the time of President Roosevelt's death of a massive stroke on April 12, 1945, his blood pressure ranged between 180/110 and 230/130.

The infiltration of the body with fluid can cause more than breathing problems and sleepless nights. Patients may weigh more, because of the excess water retention, and they may have edema (swelling) of the skin and soft tissues, usually in the feet, ankles, or legs, and sometimes in the lower back. This swelling is characterized by a gradual filling out after the area is depressed with a finger. (See Figure 14.2.) In extreme cases, fluid will accumulate in the abdomen. This is called ascites and is caused when swelling of the gastrointestinal tract forces fluid through the capillaries into the abdominal cavity. Ascites usually occurs only in severe chronic heart failure.

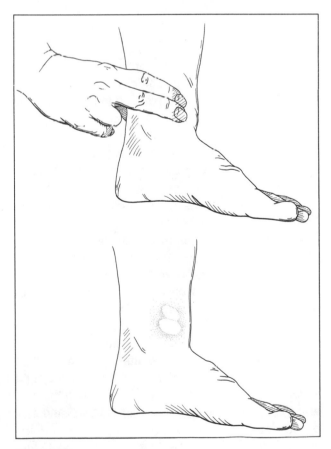

Figure 14.2
Edema is swelling of the extremities caused by excess fluid buildup. A sign of edema in the ankles is an indentation that remains momentarily when a finger is pressed into the skin and then removed.

Symptoms of Left-Side and Right-Side Heart Failure

Symptoms of left-side heart failure

- Fatigue
- Shortness of breath (dyspnea)
- Shortness of breath when lying down (othopnea)
- Paroxysmal (intermittent) nocturnal dyspnea
- Accumulation of fluid in the lungs (pulmonary edema), frequently causing a person to cough up blood-tinged sputum

Symptoms of right-side heart failure

- Swelling (edema)
  Dependent edema (edema that travels by gravity to the lowest portions of the body)
  Enlargement or swelling of the liver (hepatomegaly)
  Buildup of fluid in the abdominal cavity (ascites)
  Edema of the skin and soft tissues, causing swelling of the feet, ankles, and legs
- Excessive urination at night caused by fluid redistribution while a person is sleeping lying down (nocturia)

pendent (edema that travels by gravity to the lowest portions of the body), edema that results in enlargement or swelling of the liver (called hepatomegaly), ascites, and edema of the skin or soft tissues (only in some cases).

Because congestive heart failure causes the body to fill with excess fluids, the kidneys may not be able to dispose of the extra sodium (a component of salt) and water, a condition known as kidney failure. (Again, the term "failure" implies that the kidneys have failed and will not recover. However, as in the case of heart failure, the kidney changes may be temporary, and proper treatment may correct much of the problem.) Sodium that would normally be eliminated through the urine remains in the body, causing it to retain even more water, thereby aggravating the problem of excess fluid associated with congestive heart failure.

DIAGNOSIS

A stethoscope can be used to detect rales, crackling noises that are caused by the movement of excess fluid in the lungs. This can help locate where fluid has accumulated. By listening to breathing sounds or thumping the chest, a physician can usually tell when fluid from the lungs has leaked (pleural effusion) into the chest cavity. The fluid will also appear as a cloudy area on X-rays. The stethoscope can also detect the sounds of the heart chambers filling and emptying and the heart valves opening and closing throughout the cardiac cycle. Abnormal variations in these sounds can aid the physician in diagnosing and monitoring heart failure, because the condition is associated with one or two abnormal sounds in addition to the two sounds usually heard with the healthy heart. Another symptom, blueness of the skin (called cyanosis) accompanied by coolness and moisture, most often in the fingers and toes, indicates low levels of oxygen in the blood (called hypoxia). Edema is detected by pressing the finger against the ankle or skin and noting how long it takes the depression to refill. Liver enlargement is felt by examining the abdomen. The neck vein may also be distended. (See box, "Signs of Heart Failure During an Examination.")

A number of sophisticated diagnostic techniques may also be employed to diagnose and monitor heart failure and heart function. The two main noninvasive

ated blood from the lungs and passes it on to the left ventricle (lower chamber), which pumps it to the rest of the body. When the left side isn't pumping efficiently, blood backs up in the vessels of the lungs, and sometimes fluid is forced out of the lung vessels and into the breathing spaces themselves. This pulmonary congestion causes shortness of breath. The other major symptoms of left-sided heart failure are fatigue, dyspnea (orthopnea, paroxysmal nocturnal dyspnea), and the sputum production (sometimes bloody) that comes from pulmonary congestion.

Right-sided failure occurs when there is resistance to the flow of blood from the right heart structures (right atrium, right ventricle, pulmonary or lung artery) into the lungs or when the tricuspid valve, which separates the right atrium from the right ventricle, fails to work properly. This results in a backup of fluid and pressure in the veins that empty into the right side of the heart. Pressure then builds up in the liver and the veins in the legs. The liver enlarges and may become painful; swelling of the ankles or legs occurs.

The major symptoms of right-sided heart failure are edema and nocturia (excessive urination at night caused by fluid redistribution while a person is lying down). The different types of edema possible are de-

---

Signs of Heart Failure During an Examination

In the heart

- Heart enlargement
- Increased heart rate (tachycardia)

In the lungs

- Crackling noises (rales) heard through a stethoscope indicating a buildup of fluid in the lungs
- Leakage of fluid from the lungs (pleural effusion) into the chest cavity

In other areas

- Swelling (edema) of the skin and soft tissues, usually noted in the feet and ankles
- Edema of the lower back (sacral edema)
- Buildup of fluid of the abdominal cavity (ascites)
- Increased size of liver (hepatomegaly)
- Ascites

---

techniques for this purpose are the echocardiogram and the radionuclide angiocardiogram. (See Chapter 10.) Both tests can quantify the level of heart dysfunction and distinguish between generalized as opposed to regional dysfunction.

In cardiac catheterization, a thin tube is introduced through a vein or artery into the heart. The procedure determines whether there are blockages in the blood vessels and measures pressures in various chambers of the heart. (See Chapter 10.)

The electrocardiogram (ECG) provides a graphic record of the heart's electrical impulses; it can detect increased wall thickness (called hypertrophy), heart enlargement, or various rhythm changes in heart failure. The ECG may also be used to monitor the effects of drug treatments on the heart. Chest X-rays can also detect an enlarged heart.

CAUSES

An array of different problems can cause congestive heart failure. (See box, "Causes of Congestive Heart Failure.") Among them is coronary (ischemic) heart disease resulting from insufficient blood flow to the myocardium, or heart muscle. This is usually caused by atherosclerosis, the buildup of fatty substances or plaque on the walls of the arteries that carry blood to the heart muscle. The heart's ability to perform decreases because ischemia results in the delivery of less oxygen and fewer nutrients to the heart muscle.

A heart attack may also cause congestive failure. During a heart attack, the heart muscle is deprived of oxygen, resulting in tissue death and scarring. The development of heart failure depends on the extent and location of scarring. (See Chapter 15.)

Long-standing high blood pressure is another common cause of heart failure. Because there is greater resistance against which the heart must pump, the heart muscle works harder. This results in an enlargement of the heart muscle, especially of the left ventricle, the heart's main pumping chamber. Eventually, this enlarged muscle tissue weakens, setting the stage for heart failure, especially if the pumping ability of the enlarged chamber greatly decreases.

Arrhythmias (irregular heartbeats) can lead to heart failure, but they usually have to be severe and prolonged, with a rapid rate of more than 140 beats per minute, and must often occur in the presence of an already weakened heart. They change the pattern of filling and pumping of blood from the heart. This condition may also lower output of blood to the point of heart failure. (See Chapter 16.)

Diseased heart valves are another cause of heart failure, which results when a narrowed or leaking valve fails to direct blood flow properly through the heart. The problem may be congenital (inborn) or due to an infection such as endocarditis or rheumatic fever. This increases the heart's workload, thereby in-

---

Causes of Congestive Heart Failure (CHF)

- Coronary (ischemic) heart disease resulting from insufficient blood flow to the heart muscle (myocardium)
- A heart attack, resulting in acute damage and then scarring of heart muscle tissue
- Chronic high blood pressure
- Major cardiac arrhythmia
- Diseased heart valve(s)
- Diseased heart muscle
- Congenital heart disease

creasing risk of developing heart failure. (See Chapter 13.)

Cardiomyopathy, a disease of the heart muscle itself, can also lead to heart failure. Causes of cardiomyopathy include infection, alcohol abuse, and cocaine abuse. When heart failure seems to have no known causes, it is known as idiopathic heart failure. (See Chapter 15.)

HOW THE BODY TRIES TO PROTECT ITSELF

When one system of the body is not functioning optimally, other systems may attempt to take over to make up for the problem. In the case of heart failure, several types of compensation are possible.

First, the heart chambers may enlarge, and the heart may beat more forcefully to pump out more blood for the body's needs. In time, the overworked heart muscle enlarges (much as skeletal muscles grow larger during weight muscle training), creating increased muscle fibers with which the heart can pump more forcefully.

Second, the heart may be stimulated to pump more often, thereby increasing its output.

Third, a compensation mechanism called the renin-angiotensin system may be initiated. When the lack of blood volume coming from the heart (cardiac output) results in a decrease in the amount passing through the kidneys, the kidneys respond by stimulating the system to secrete hormones that prompt the kidneys to retain salt and water, and thereby increase blood volume. This is an attempt to compensate for the decrease in output of the heart. This leads to a rise in blood pressure as the body attempts to circulate the extra fluid volume and also ensures that adequate oxygen reaches the brain, kidneys, and other vital organs.

These compensation mechanisms keep the failing heart functioning almost normally in the early stages of heart failure. As the disease progresses, however, compensation mechanisms cannot maintain proper circulation. It may take years for a heart to go through the stages of enlarging, working harder, and finally breaking down. In many cases, as when a person has hypertension, heart failure is preventable if blood pressure is treated adequately.

TREATMENT

Whenever possible, the best treatment of congestive heart failure is one of prevention. This includes diagnosing and treating high blood pressure and attempting to prevent atherosclerosis. Other important preventive steps include not smoking, using alcohol in moderation if at all, and abstaining from cocaine and other illicit drugs. A prudent diet, regular exercise, and weight control are also important.

When a patient is diagnosed as having heart failure, the first treatment is often restriction of dietary sodium. Drugs may be prescribed as well. Diuretics, available since the 1950s, are often used to help the kidneys get rid of excess water and sodium, thereby reducing blood volume and the heart's workload. (See Chapter 23.)

Digitalis, a drug that has been used since the 18th century, is still a component of modern therapy. It is prescribed to strengthen the heart's pumping action. Patients taking both diuretics and digitalis may need to supplement their levels of potassium.

Newer drugs for the treatment of heart failure include vasodilators, which cause the peripheral arteries to dilate, or open up. This reduces the work of the heart by making it easier for blood to flow. Among the newest vasodilators used for heart failure are the angiotensin-converting enzyme (ACE) inhibitors, which may be used, along with diuretics, in patients with mild-to-moderate or severe congestive failure. ACE inhibitors, which include captopril (Capoten) and enalapril (Vasotec), block the production of a substance called angiotensin II, a potent constrictor of blood vessels. If blood vessels are dilated, the amount of work needed for the heart to pump blood forward is decreased.

Other drugs used in the treatment of heart failure include calcium-channel blockers, which dilate blood vessels; beta blockers, which slow the heart (used only in unusual circumstances); and medications that affect various heartbeat irregularities. Most cases, however, respond to diuretics and digitalis, especially when ACE inhibitors are added.

Sometimes, surgery proves effective. When heart failure is due to valvular disease, surgical implantation of an artificial heart valve or valve repair may alleviate the problem. Surgery may also be helpful in correcting congenital heart defects that can lead to heart failure. Coronary artery bypass graft surgery and catheterization using a balloon to flatten fatty deposits (called angioplasty) are among the therapeutic techniques used to prevent and treat heart failure caused by occluded, or blocked, arteries.

Heart transplants are a last resort in treating severe heart failure caused by diseased heart muscle. Although the success rate of heart transplants has significantly improved, the cost of the operation and the shortage of donor organs makes it impractical except as a last resort.

PROGNOSIS

The outlook for most people with heart failure is dependent upon the cause of the heart failure and the overall degree of cardiac dysfunction. An estimated 50 percent survive more than five years after diagnosis. That figure, however, is an average of all patients with varying levels of severity of the disease. The prognosis for a specific person with heart failure depends to a large degree on effects of the disease, such as the level of blood output of the left ventricle, or his or her ability to exercise, as well as other factors, including age, overall health, and other medical conditions. The sooner heart failure is diagnosed and action is taken to control the problem, the better.

In many cases, heart failure can be effectively treated to prevent or slow the progression of the disease and to alleviate its symptoms. Therapy can achieve several goals: It can improve the performance of the left ventricle, prevent further deterioration of heart function, improve a patient's ability to exercise, and improve quality of life.

In addition, it is possible that in selected instances, early, effective treatment may increase a person's likelihood of improved survival.

CHAPTER 15

HEART MUSCLE DISEASE

FORRESTER A. LEE, M.D.

Compared with other cardiovascular diseases, heart muscle disease (cardiomyopathy) is relatively rare. In its most common form, the disease accounts for only 50,000 new cases in the United States each year, while the annual number of stroke cases, for example, reaches 500,000. Unlike many other cardiovascular disorders that tend to affect the elderly, cardiomyopathy commonly occurs in the young and can have a tragically brief course.

Cardiomyopathy (*cardio* meaning heart, *myopathy* meaning muscle disease) refers to a group of disorders that directly damage the muscle of the heart walls. In these disorders, all chambers of the heart are affected. The heart's function as a pump is disrupted, leading to an inadequate blood flow to organs and tissues of the body. Depending on the nature of the injury or abnormality in the heart muscle and the resulting structural changes in the heart chambers, one of three types of nonischemic (not caused by heart attack) heart muscle disease may be present: *dilated congestive, hypertrophic,* or *restrictive.* (See Table 15.1.)

Massive or multiple heart attacks may also lead to severe heart damage as a result of a disruption of blood supply to heart muscle. The damage can result in functional impairment and structural abnormalities similar to those found in the other types of cardiomyopathy. This type of heart disease, resulting from coronary artery disease, is called *ischemic car-*diomyopathy. When used alone, however, the term "cardiomyopathy" refers to heart muscle disease that is not caused by heart attacks.

DILATED CONGESTIVE CARDIOMYOPATHY

This is the most common type of heart muscle disease. It is generally called either dilated or congestive cardiomyopathy. This type of disease damages the fibers of the heart muscle, weakening the walls of the heart's chambers. Usually, all chambers are affected, and depending on the severity of the injury, they lose some of their capacity to contract forcefully and pump blood through the circulatory system. To compensate for the muscle injury, the heart chambers enlarge or dilate. The dilation is often more pronounced in the left ventricle, the heart's main pumping chamber. (See Figure 15.1.)

Dilated cardiomyopathy causes heart failure—an inability of the heart to provide an adequate supply of blood to the body's organs and tissues—which, if left untreated, is always associated with excess fluid retention, congestion in the lungs and liver, and swelling of the legs. Fluid retention occurs during heart failure because many organs fail to receive suf-

Table 15.1

Types of Heart Muscle Disease (Cardiomyopathy)

Type	Therapy
Dilated congestive: Cavity of the heart is enlarged and stretched. Cause is usually unknown.	When underlying cause is unknown, treatment focuses on relieving symptoms and improving function. Drugs used include digitalis and digoxin (Lanoxin and others), diuretics such as furosemide (Lasix and others), steroids to relieve inflammation, and ACE inhibitors such as captopril (Capoten). When symptoms cannot be relieved, heart transplant may be considered.
Hypertrophic: Muscle mass increases, causing chest pain, palpitations, and possibly fainting during physical activity. May be genetically acquired.	Limit stressful physical activity, and use medication, including beta blockers or a calcium channel blocker such as verapamil (Calan, Isopton, Verelan). If medication does not relieve symptoms, undergo surgical removal of excess muscle tissue that obstructs blood flow in the heart chambers. If surgery does not help, heart transplant may be considered.
Restrictive: Abnormal cells, proteins, or scar tissue infiltrate the heart, causing the chambers to become thick and bulky. Most common cause in the United States is a disease (amyloidosis) that is associated with cancers of the blood.	Treated with medications that alleviate symptoms (see dilated congestive section above). No cure exists.

Type	Therapy
Ischemic (related to coronary artery disease):	Treated with medications that relieve symptoms of heart failure and coronary artery disease (see above). Angioplasty and coronary artery bypass grafting may help increase blood flow to the heart, enhancing heart muscle function. When neither drug therapy nor surgery helps, heart transplant may be considered.

ficient blood flow. The kidneys respond to this lack of blood supply by retaining more than the usual amount of salt and water. With time, excess fluid retention leads to congestion in the lungs and other organs. At the end of the day, much of the retained fluid gravitates to the lower portions of the body and causes swelling in the legs. (See Chapter 14 for more information on heart failure and its symptoms.)

THE COURSE OF DILATED CARDIOMYOPATHY

When the chambers dilate, the muscle fibers in the heart walls stretch, enabling them to contract more forcefully. (This is characteristic of all muscles.) Growth of muscle tissue, which can to some extent rebuild damaged areas of the heart wall, also helps to keep up normal function. If the injury to the heart muscle is relatively mild, new muscle growth and the process of fiber stretching, which occurs roughly in proportion to the muscle damage, can partially restore cardiac function. If, however, injury is severe, the heart's function deteriorates. When damage to the heart is chronic or recurrent, as may occur with a prolonged exposure to excessive amounts of alcohol or infection, chamber dilation may be slow and progressive. Eventually, the enlarged, thin-walled ventricles become flabby and cannot generate sufficient pressure to pump blood effectively throughout the body.

Dilated cardiomyopathy typically leads to a steady deterioration in heart function, although the course

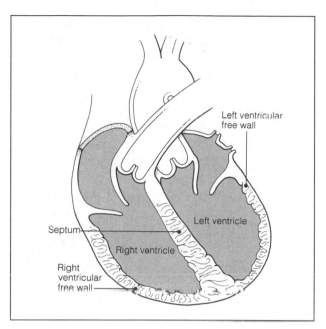

Figure 15.1
In dilated cardiomyopathy, the cavity of the heart is enlarged and stretched.

of the decline varies greatly and is difficult to predict for any given patient. Most patients go through periods of relatively stable heart function that may last several months or even years. However, the majority eventually succumb to complications of the disease. Most commonly, they die of progressive heart failure that is not amenable to treatment, although some die suddenly and unexpectedly.

Most instances of sudden death are believed to result from ventricular fibrillation—an abnormally fast and irregular heart rhythm with ineffective contractions that causes death within minutes. Patients with dilated cardiomyopathy are at risk of sudden death because the underlying disease process disrupts the normal electrical pathways of the heart, possibly causing rhythm disturbances.

Less often, sudden death may result from an embolus—a blood clot that dislodges from one of the heart chambers, travels to another vital organ, such as the brain or lungs, and obstructs the blood supply. Poor circulation and stagnation of blood in the dilated heart chambers provide favorable conditions for blood clot formation.

SYMPTOMS AND CAUSES OF DILATED CARDIOMYOPATHY

The main symptoms of dilated cardiomyopathy are those of congestive heart failure—breathlessness or fatigue during physical activity and swelling of the lower legs. Some patients, especially those who lead a sedentary life, may experience few symptoms and be unaware that the heart is failing. With advanced disease, symptoms may occur with minimal activity or even in the absence of physical exertion.

In more than 80 percent of cases, the cause of dilated cardiomyopathy is unknown. Major causes of the disease are inflammation of the heart muscle (myocarditis), excessive alcohol use, poor nutrition, and, rarely, complications arising shortly before or after childbirth (peripartum) and genetic disorders. (See box, "Causes of Dilated Congestive Cardiomyopathy.")

HEART MUSCLE INFLAMMATION (MYOCARDITIS)

Most cases of dilated cardiomyopathy probably result from inflammation of the heart muscle (myocarditis), but not all cases of heart muscle inflammation lead to dilated cardiomyopathy. In fact, myocarditis is often categorized as heart muscle disease in its own right. In Western Europe and the United States, myocarditis occurs most often as a complication of a viral disease, but it is a rather rare complication. Viral infections are believed to cause indirect damage to the heart. The invading virus provokes proteins that normally are confined within heart muscle cells to become exposed to the bloodstream. This sets off an inflammatory process as the body mistakenly assumes these newly exposed proteins belong to foreign cells and attacks them in the same way it fights viruses and bacteria. The unfortunate result is inflammation and injury to the body's own tissues—in the case of myocarditis, the tissues of the heart.

Many organisms can infect and injure the heart muscle. Coxsackie Type B, a virus among those that

---

Causes of Dilated Congestive Cardiomyopathy

In many cases, the cause cannot be identified. When causes are known, they include:

- Inflammation of the heart muscle (myocarditis), either infectious or noninfectious
- Excessive alcohol consumption
- Nutritional deficiencies
- Complications arising shortly before or after childbirth (peripartum)
- Genetic disorders

usually infect the gastrointestinal tract, is believed to be the most common offending agent. Many other viruses, such as those of polio, rubella, and influenza, have been associated with myocarditis. It is not clear why the same viruses cause myocarditis in some patients and different diseases—gastroenteritis, pneumonia, or hepatitis, for example—in others.

Myocarditis can occur as a rare complication of bacterial infections, including diphtheria, tuberculosis, typhoid fever, and tetanus. Other infectious organisms, such as rickettsiae and parasites, may also cause inflammation in the heart muscle. In Central and South America, myocarditis is often due to Chagas disease, an infectious illness that is transmitted by insects.

Noninfectious causes of myocarditis are numerous, but all of them are rare. They include systemic lupus erythematosus, a disease in which the body attacks its own organs and tissues; adverse or toxic drug reactions; and radiation-induced heart injury as a complication of cancer radiotherapy.

Often myocarditis, particularly in its mild form, produces no symptoms at all. However, it is frequently accompanied by an inflammation of the heart's outer membrane—the pericardium. Inflammation of the heart lining is called pericarditis and, unlike myocarditis, can cause severe pain that typically gets worse when the person takes a deep breath or changes position.

Myocarditis may start as a flulike illness that lingers longer than the usual several days. If significant muscle damage and weakening of the heart's chambers occur, symptoms of heart failure may develop. A month or two later, the symptoms of flu—weakness and malaise—merge with symptoms of heart failure—fatigue during physical activity and shortness of breath. If the illness is persistent and progressive, symptoms eventually become disabling enough for the person to consult a physician. By this time, however, the infecting organisms usually cannot be detected or cultured from the heart or other places in the body. By the time the patient seeks medical help, all traces of the infecting organism or disease process that may have triggered the condition may be undetectable.

In some cases, the injury to the heart muscle is mild but persists or recurs intermittently over many years. Symptoms of heart failure sometimes appear 20 to 30 years after the initial viral illness. Patients usually do not recall having had a viral infection and often mistakenly interpret the symptoms as a sign of age until progressive heart disease produces more obvious signs of congestion and heart failure.

Myocarditis is usually diagnosed after it has reached an advanced stage and produces heart failure. Physical examination and a chest X-ray usually reveal signs of lung congestion and heart enlargement. An electrocardiogram may show changes of heart damage, and an echocardiogram demonstrates the characteristic abnormalities of severe myocarditis—enlargement of all heart chambers and poor contraction of the heart muscle. In acute myocarditis, a heart biopsy, in which a small sample of muscle tissue is removed from the heart chamber for laboratory examination, may be performed to document the presence of an ongoing inflammatory process. In cases of infectious myocarditis, however, it is usually impossible to grow the infecting organism from samples of the heart tissue.

Mild cases of myocarditis with no signs of heart failure are usually not diagnosed and consequently remain untreated. When treatment is given, it is aimed at eliminating the underlying cause. When the cause is unknown, steroids (cortisone) are sometimes prescribed to reduce inflammation. (This approach to therapy has not yet been shown to be beneficial but is currently under study.) Medications are also prescribed to relieve the symptoms of heart failure. (See Chapters 14 and 23.) During the acute phase of myocarditis, patients are advised to rest and gradually return to a more active life-style once evidence disappears of ongoing inflammation and heart injury. (See box, "Guidelines for Cardiomyopathy Patients.")

Many cases of myocarditis cause minimal heart damage. Heart function fully recovers in these mild cases. Occasionally, severe cases of myocarditis also clear up spontaneously and leave little permanent damage. More typically, however, severe inflammation produces chronic, progressive, and irreversible heart damage.

Left untreated, myocarditis may lead to a severe form of pulmonary edema, or lung congestion, in which fluid leaks from the blood into the tissues and air spaces of the lung. The onset of this can be quite rapid, often waking the patient from sleep. Such patients are severely disabled and require emergency treatment. It must be emphasized, however, that myocarditis is rare and that viral infections rarely result in heart muscle damage.

ALCOHOL

In Western countries, excessive alcohol consumption is a major cause of cardiomyopathy. Alcohol can damage the heart directly by exerting a toxic effect on heart muscle cells. Severe heart damage may also

YALE UNIVERSITY SCHOOL OF MEDICINE HEART BOOK

Guidelines for Cardiomyopathy Patients

- To detect cardiomyopathy in its early stages, watch out for its early symptoms. Shortness of breath may constitute the first warning and therefore should never be disregarded as simply a sign of aging.

- Because hypertrophic cardiomyopathy can be passed on as a genetic trait, children of people with this condition should be evaluated by a cardiologist.

- When possible, eliminate all factors causing or contributing to heart muscle disease, such as excessive alcohol consumption.

- Keep salt intake to a minimum to decrease the tendency toward lung congestion and possibly reduce the need for diuretics.

- Losing weight is an effective way to decrease the workload of an impaired heart, but it may not eliminate all symptoms.

- Quitting tobacco use is essential, since smoking constricts blood vessels and increases the work of the heart.

- Any disorder that can impair heart function, such as high blood pressure, should be treated and controlled.

- While rest is recommended during the acute inflammatory stage of myocarditis, it is essential that patients lead as normal a life as possible after that. Adopt a life-style as vigorous as possible within the capacity of the heart muscle—that is, its ability to provide an adequate blood supply to meet the demands of the body. In other words, do not go beyond the body's limits. Avoid sudden stresses, like lifting heavy objects or exercising with free weights. Instead, opt for types of exercise —such as walking, bicycling, swimming—that are ideal for patients with cardiovascular disease. *Caution:* People with hypertrophic cardiomyopathy should consult a physician before choosing an exercise regimen.

- Inquire about heart transplant if symptoms are not well controlled with medications. Modern scientific advances have made heart transplantation a feasible alternative for some patients with severe cardiomyopathy.

result from nutritional deficiencies that occur when alcohol is the person's main source of caloric intake. In some drinkers, alcohol primarily attacks the liver, causing cirrhosis, and in others, mainly the heart, but severe damage usually does not occur in both organs at the same time.

Alcoholic cardiomyopathy can develop after five to ten years of excessive alcohol use. Examples of excessive amounts are two-thirds of a pint of whiskey or gin, one quart of wine, or two quarts of beer daily, although individual susceptibility to and tolerance of alcohol varies greatly. Most patients with this type of cardiomyopathy are males, possibly because there are more heavy drinkers among men than women.

NUTRITIONAL ABNORMALITIES

Cardiomyopathy can also be caused by severe nutritional deficiency (which can also be related to alcohol use). The heart muscle, like any other muscle, can be damaged by chronic deficiency in certain vitamins, particularly vitamin B-1, or in minerals. In some developing countries, nutritional-deficiency-related cardiomyopathy is more common than coronary artery disease, the predominant form of heart disease in the United States.

PERIPARTUM CARDIOMYOPATHY

For an unknown reason, cardiomyopathy sometimes develops in connection with pregnancy and is referred to as peripartum (*peri* meaning around or at the time of, *partum* meaning labor or childbirth) cardiomyopathy. During the last month of pregnancy or within several months following delivery, the woman develops heart muscle inflammation that appears to be unrelated to any infection or other known causes. The condition may result in severe and irreversible heart failure, although many patients recover completely. Women who survive the illness are at a high risk of developing this type of heart muscle disease in subsequent pregnancies. Peripartum cardiomyopathy occurs with particularly high frequency in African-American women in the United States and is a common cause of heart failure among women of childbearing age in some African countries.

GENETIC DISORDERS

Dilated cardiomyopathy is known to develop in patients with some genetic disorders that affect the muscles or nerves of the back, arms, and legs. (Such diseases include progressive muscular dystrophy, myotonic muscular dystrophy, and Friedreich's ataxia.) There are also cases when dilated cardiomyopathy is not associated with muscle disorders but appears to be genetic in origin because several members of the same family are affected. However, because no abnormal gene has been identified, it is uncertain whether clustering of this condition within some families results from genetic or environmental factors.

DIAGNOSIS OF DILATED CARDIOMYOPATHY

In most cases, dilated cardiomyopathy is preceded by heart muscle inflammation that produces flulike symptoms such as fever, chills, and muscle aches. These symptoms are so common and vague that the cardiomyopathy is usually not diagnosed until heart muscle injury has caused impaired heart function and produced symptoms of heart failure.

Diagnosis is based on assessing the size and function of the heart chambers. A chest X-ray typically reveals the main features of dilated cardiomyopathy: an enlarged heart and fluid congestion in the lungs. An electrocardiogram may show evidence of heart damage. Characteristic abnormalities can also be detected using echocardiography or radionuclide angiography, often called the MUGA scan (equilibrium radionuclide angiocardiogram).

If diagnosis remains in doubt, heart catheterization, sometimes accompanied by a heart biopsy, may be performed. Catheterization allows a physician to measure pressures in the heart chambers and to see the heart's structures when a contrast dye is injected into its chambers and vessels through the catheter— a thin plastic tube that is inserted in an artery or vein and threaded through it to the heart. During the procedure, X-ray images of the heart are recorded on film or videotape. In biopsy, a small sample of tissue is removed from the heart wall and examined under a light or electron microscope. The combined findings of catheterization and heart biopsy usually make it possible to distinguish dilated cardiomyopathy from other forms of heart disease.

Tests may also be used to rule out recognized causes of dilated cardiomyopathy. In most cases no cause can be established. However, blood tests, for example, may sometimes show that the patient has had a recent viral infection known to be associated with cardiomyopathy.

TREATMENT

When the cause of dilated cardiomyopathy is known, therapy is aimed at treating the underlying disorder, such as a curable infection or nutritional deficiency. For example, in the case of heart muscle disease caused by alcohol consumption, treatment entails total abstinence. Alcoholic cardiomyopathy is one of the few for which there exists a specific treatment, and patients with this type of heart muscle disease have a good prognosis if they follow the prescribed treatment.

Because in most cases the cause of dilated cardiomyopathy is unknown, treatment focuses on relieving the symptoms and improving the function of the injured heart chambers. Patients receive medications that enhance the contraction capacity of the heart muscle. The few drugs that produce this effect work indirectly, by increasing the level of calcium inside the heart cells. (Calcium initiates heart muscle contractions.) Digitalis and its derivatives such as digoxin (Lanoxin and others), the oldest and best-known of such drugs, are usually administered orally but may, in some circumstances, be given by an intravenous injection. More potent cardiac stimulants such as dobutamine (Dobutrex), dopamine (Intropin), and amrinone (Inocor), can be given only intravenously and are therefore primarily reserved for use in the hospital in more serious situations. Oral forms of such medications are currently being developed.

Diuretics are prescribed to relieve lung congestion and remove excess body fluid. Commonly referred to as "water pills," they facilitate the kidney's excretion of excess salt and fluid into the urine. While these drugs, which reduce congestion and swelling, are an essential part of heart failure therapy, patients can help the physician decrease the dosages of diuretics by limiting the amount of salt in their diet.

Function of the impaired heart can be significantly improved by altering the conditions under which it must work. Because the body responds to heart failure by constricting blood flow to all but the most vital organs, drugs that dilate blood vessels (vasodilators) reduce the work of the heart by decreasing resistance to bloodflow. Angiotensin-converting enzyme (ACE) inhibitors, a class of vasodilators, are particularly effective in heart failure treatment.

In the presence of an active inflammation in the heart (usually confirmed by heart biopsy), anti-inflammatory drugs such as steroids (cortisone) may be prescribed. Although these medications have been extensively studied, it has not been proved whether they benefit patients with newly diagnosed dilated cardiomyopathy.

In the early, acute stages of cardiomyopathy, when signs of heart inflammation and ongoing muscle injury are present, patients are told to rest. With recovery from acute illness, they are advised to engage in regular physical activity to the extent that their heart function permits.

In extreme cases, when cardiomyopathy has progressed to the point when medical treatment can no longer relieve the symptoms, a heart transplant may be considered. Transplants increase life expectancy in persons with advanced heart failure who might otherwise be expected to live less than six months. Currently, 80 to 90 percent of heart transplant recipients survive at least one year, and more than 75 percent survive five years. The scarcity of donor organs and the high level of sophisticated care required for a successful transplant make this option available only to a small number of patients—approximately 2,000 per year in the United States.

PROGNOSIS

By the time patients with dilated cardiomyopathy develop heart failure symptoms, the disease has usually reached an advanced stage and prognosis is poor. About 50 percent of patients achieve the average survival rate five years after initial diagnosis, and 25 percent survive ten or more years after diagnosis. These statistics have not changed significantly in several decades, although current forms of therapy for heart failure offer promise that this bleak prognosis may improve.

HYPERTROPHIC CARDIOMYOPATHY

This rare disease is the second most common type of cardiomyopathy. Hypertrophic cardiomyopathy is also known as idiopathic hypertrophic subaortic stenosis (IHSS) or asymmetric septal hypertrophy (ASH). The disease is characterized by a disorderly growth of heart muscle fibers causing the heart chambers to become thick-walled and bulky. All the chambers are affected, but the thickening is generally most striking in the walls of the left ventricle. Most commonly, one of the walls, the septum, which separates the right and left ventricles, is asymmetrically enlarged. The distorted left ventricle contracts, but the supply of blood to the brain and other vital organs may be inadequate because blood is trapped within the heart during contractions. Mitral valve function is often disrupted by the structural abnormalities in the left ventricle with backward leakage of blood. (See Figure 15.2.)

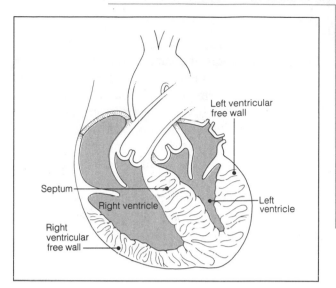

Figure 15.2
In hypertrophic cardiomyopathy, the muscle mass of the left and occasionally the right ventricle is enlarged, causing the heart chambers to stiffen. The septum between the ventricles often becomes disproportionately thickened; this is noticeable when it is compared to the freestanding portion of the left ventricular wall.

Fainting during physical exertion is often the first and most dramatic symptom of hypertrophic cardiomyopathy. During periods of exertion, as the body stimulates the heart to beat more forcefully, blood has a greater tendency to become trapped within the vigorously contracting chambers. As a result, the person may faint or, in extreme cases, die. Unexplained death during athletic activity always leads physicians to suspect undiagnosed hypertrophic cardiomyopathy. Several world-class athletes have suffered this type of sudden death in the past few years.

COMPLICATIONS OF HYPERTROPHIC CARDIOMYOPATHY

The walls of the hypertrophied heart are not always adequately nourished by blood vessels. This leads to muscle injury and scarring—a common complication of hypertrophic cardiomyopathy. In advanced stages of the disease, the thickened, deformed, and scarred walls of the heart prevent the chambers from contracting effectively and filling up completely, leading to severe loss of heart function.

Sudden death—the most unpredictable and devastating complication of this type of cardiomyopathy—is most commonly caused by ventricular fibrillation, abnormally fast and disorganized contractions of the left ventricle that interfere with effective pumping. The hypertrophied heart is prone to fibrillation because the disorderly overgrowth of muscle creates abnormal sites and pathways for the heart's electrical activity.

CAUSES OF HYPERTROPHIC CARDIOMYOPATHY

Hypertrophic cardiomyopathy is usually congenital. In half of the cases, the patient has inherited an abnormal gene from one parent. The pattern of genetic transmission is termed "autosomal dominant." This means that a copy of the gene from only one parent is needed for the disease to develop in the child. However, some siblings in the family may carry the gene but have hardly any trace of hypertrophic cardiomyopathy while others may die at a young age.

In the rest of the cases, neither parent carries a gene for hypertrophic cardiomyopathy, and the child is believed to develop the disease because of a spontaneous gene mutation.

SYMPTOMS OF HYPERTROPHIC CARDIOMYOPATHY

People with hypertrophic cardiomyopathy may experience a variety of symptoms during the course of the disease. Some have absolutely no symptoms for years and are only diagnosed after having an electrocardiogram for another reason, or when they come for an examination because a family member is known to carry the disease. Sometimes the disorder is detected for the first time at autopsy after the patient's death.

Although predisposition for developing hypertrophic cardiomyopathy is present from birth, the abnormal heart muscle proliferation may actually begin during the adolescent growth spurt. In such cases, symptoms may develop rather abruptly during teenage years.

Fainting upon exertion and chest pain similar to the angina of coronary artery disease may be early symptoms of hypertrophic cardiomyopathy. Some patients experience palpitations because of abnormal heart rhythms. Eventually, symptoms of congestive heart failure may become prominent.

DIAGNOSIS OF HYPERTROPHIC CARDIOMYOPATHY

The most important diagnostic tool in assessing hypertrophic cardiomyopathy is echocardiography. It provides images and reveals blood flow patterns that allow physicians to identify the distinctive abnormalities in the heart walls and valves. Other characteristic features of the disease are often recorded on chest X-rays, on electrocardiograms, and during cardiac catheterization.

TREATMENT

When hypertrophic cardiomyopathy is severe, patients are advised to limit stressful physical activity, particularly strenuous competitive sports. They may also be given drugs to relieve symptoms. Traditionally, drugs called beta blockers have been used to prevent a rapid heartbeat and decrease the excessive force of contractions. Antiarrhythmic drugs are often prescribed to treat abnormal heart rhythms. In the past decade, calcium channel blockers, particularly verapamil (Calan), have been shown to be especially effective for relief of symptoms. Like beta blockers, calcium antagonists reduce the force of the heart's contractions, but they also increase the flexibility of the bulky heart chambers. These combined effects increase the efficiency of pumping and reduce congestion.

Surgery may be performed in people with hypertrophic cardiomyopathy whose symptoms are not relieved by medications. The surgeon may remove the excess muscle tissue that obstructs the blood flow in the heart chamber.

PROGNOSIS

The course of hypertrophic cardiomyopathy varies. The condition may remain stable over decades or may progress slowly. Approximately 4 percent of people with the disease die annually, most of them from sudden death, which may occur at any stage of the disease. The younger the age at which the disease appears, the higher the risk of sudden death.

SPECIAL RISKS OF HYPERTROPHIC CARDIOMYOPATHY FOR YOUNG ATHLETES

People who regularly participate in strenuous physical exercise, such as professional athletes or those who train for marathons, may experience changes in the function and structure of their hearts. These adaptations, which include a slower than normal heartbeat and an overall enlarged heart, enable the heart to deliver more oxygen to the tissues in the limbs in order to sustain and enhance athletic performance.

Heart muscle thickness may increase in an athlete's heart. Generally, this is nothing to worry about, but athletes—especially teenagers—should be monitored to ensure that hypertrophic cardiomyopathy is not an underlying cause of heart enlargement.

A good deal of publicity was given to this disease when Hank Gathers, the college basketball star, died suddenly in 1990 while playing in a conference championship game for Loyola Marymount in Los Angeles. Gathers was known to have an enlarged heart and was taking medication at the time of his death. Most often, though, a young athlete with this condition is not aware of it.

Although these incidents seem to make headlines frequently, they are relatively rare. According to the *American Journal of Diseases of Children*, each year there are 1 or 2 cases per 200,000 athletes 30 years old and younger. Of those few cases, hypertrophic cardiomyopathy is involved about 60 percent of the time. Even so, anyone who begins participating in a new sport should undergo a complete medical history and physical examination—including orthopedic, neurologic, and cardiovascular assessment. If hypertrophic cardiomyopathy is diagnosed, the athlete should avoid strenuous sports.

HYPERTROPHIC CARDIOMYOPATHY CAUSED BY DRUG THERAPY

A number of drugs can have toxic effects on the heart. Perhaps most damaging are the chemotherapy drugs doxorubicin (Adriamycin and Rubex) and daunorubicin (Cerubidine). Although they are effective in the treatment of leukemia and other cancers, large doses can be toxic to heart muscle. Changes in the radionuclide angiocardiogram (See Chapter 10) may help detect this type of reaction.

Drugs used to treat emotional and psychiatric problems can also alter heart function. Phenothiazine drugs such as chlorpromazine (Thorazine) and thioridazine (Mellaril) and tricyclic antidepressant drugs such as imipramine (Tofranil) and amitryptyline (Endep and Elavil) may cause electrocardiographic abnormalities and heart rhythm disorders.

If possible, these drugs should be avoided by anyone with a history of heart disease. In any case, people taking these drugs, especially large or continuous doses of them, should undergo heart examinations, including electrocardiograms, to detect toxic effects. If these are detected, the drugs will most often be discontinued, and alternate treatment will be instituted.

RESTRICTIVE CARDIOMYOPATHY

Restrictive cardiomyopathy is extremely rare. In this type of heart muscle disease, abnormal cells, proteins,

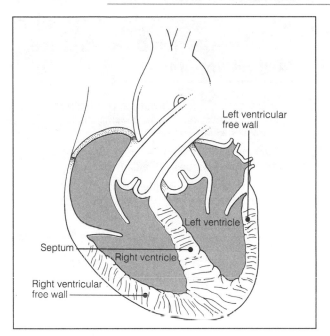

Figure 15.3
In restrictive cardiomyopathy, abnormal cells, proteins, or scar tissue infiltrate the heart, causing the chambers to become thick and bulky.

or scar tissue infiltrate the muscle and structures of the heart, causing the chambers to become stiff and bulky. The heart may initially contract normally, but the rigid chambers restrict the return of blood to the heart. As a consequence, high pressures are needed to fill the heart chambers, forcing the blood back into various tissues and organs—the lungs, abdomen, arms, and legs. Eventually, heart muscle is damaged and contractions impaired. (See Figure 15.3.)

CAUSES OF RESTRICTIVE CARDIOMYOPATHY

The most common cause of restrictive cardiomyopathy in the United States is amyloidosis, a disease that is sometimes associated with cancers of the blood. In amyloid heart disease, abnormal proteins are deposited around the heart cells, making the chambers thick, inflexible, and waxy in appearance. Other rare diseases can also fill the heart's walls with abnormal cells or excessive scarlike tissue. For example, sarcoidosis (a disease characterized by the growth of numerous tumors called granulomas throughout the body), hemochromatosis (a metabolic disorder characterized by a buildup of iron in the body), endomyocardial fibrosis (an abnormality of heart muscle tissue), and some cancers that metastasize into the heart walls are all possible causes. (See box, "Possible Causes of Restrictive Cardiomyopathy.")

Possible Causes of Restrictive Cardiomyopathy

- *Amyloidosis:* The heart muscle is infiltrated by amyloid, a fibrous protein, causing the heart chambers to stiffen.

- *Sarcoidosis:* An inflammatory disease that affects many tissues, especially the lungs.

- *Hemochromatosis:* Iron deposits form in the tissues, impairing heart function (and also resulting in liver disease and diabetes).

- *Endomyocardial fibrosis:* A progressive disease characterized by fibrous lesions on the inner walls of one or both ventricles. A frequent cause of heart failure in Africa.

SYMPTOMS OF RESTRICTIVE CARDIOMYOPATHY

The major symptoms of restrictive cardiomyopathy stem from the stiffening of the chambers, which impedes blood return to the heart. Congestion occurs in the lungs but is typically most severe in the organs of the abdomen (the liver, stomach, and intestines) as well as the legs. Patients tend to tire easily and complain of swelling, nausea, bloating, and poor appetite. Symptoms of advanced restrictive cardiomyopathy typically include significant weight loss, muscle wasting, and abdominal swelling. Patients with this condition are commonly misdiagnosed initially as having cirrhosis or cancer.

DIAGNOSIS AND TREATMENT OF RESTRICTIVE CARDIOMYOPATHY

It is occasionally possible for a physician to suspect the diagnosis based on a patient's symptoms of heart disease and the presence of an underlying disease. Imaging techniques that show details of the heart walls and function help a physician detect the restrictive movements of the heart chambers. Such techniques include echocardiography, computerized tomography (CT) scanning, and magnetic resonance imaging (MRI). Definitive diagnosis can be made by biopsy of the heart muscle.

Accurate diagnosis is important, since restrictive cardiomyopathy shares many clinical features and symptoms with a more treatable form of heart disease, constrictive pericarditis. Pericarditis is an inflammation and thickening of the membrane surrounding the heart—the pericardium. Severe or chronic pericarditis may lead to pericardial constriction, which disrupts the filling of the heart in the same manner as do the stiff chambers of restrictive cardiomyopathy. Constrictive pericarditis can often be treated effectively with surgery. In contrast, most forms of restrictive cardiomyopathy cannot be cured, and treatment is focused on alleviating symptoms.

CARDIOMYOPATHY FROM LACK OF OXYGEN (ISCHEMIA)

Severe heart injury caused by a major heart attack or multiple smaller heart attacks may result in heart enlargement and thinning of the chamber walls—abnormalities resembling those observed in dilated cardiomyopathy. This type of heart disease, called ischemic cardiomyopathy, typically develops in patients with severe coronary artery disease, often complicated by other conditions such as diabetes and hypertension.

Heart failure symptoms in ischemic cardiomyopathy are similar to those found in dilated cardiomyopathy. However, ischemic disease is more likely to be accompanied by symptoms of coronary artery disease, such as angina (chest pain). Diagnosis is typically based on a history of heart attacks and studies that demonstrate poor function in major portions of the left ventricle. The diagnosis can be confirmed by coronary angiography, which reveals areas of narrowing and blockage in the coronary blood vessels.

Patients with ischemic cardiomyopathy are treated with medications that relieve heart failure symptoms and improve blood flow through the diseased coronary arteries (nitroglycerine, some types of calcium channel blockers, and ACE inhibitors). When symptoms of heart failure and coronary artery disease cannot be controlled with medications, coronary angioplasty or surgery may be considered. Angioplasty and coronary artery bypass grafting may help increase blood flow to the heart, which in turn enhances heart muscle function.

When heart failure symptoms are advanced and cannot be improved by drug therapy or surgery, patients may be referred for a heart transplant. Patients with ischemic cardiomyopathy now account for approximately half of all heart transplant recipients.

CHAPTER 16

HEART RHYTHM DISORDERS

CRAIG A. McPHERSON, M.D., AND LYNDA E. ROSENFELD, M.D.

INTRODUCTION

Heart rhythm disorders, called arrhythmias, pose one of the paradoxes of medicine. Almost anyone's heart will occasionally produce an extra beat or two, and the distressing symptoms that may accompany the extra beats, such as palpitations or dizziness, do not necessarily signal a serious health problem. Yet an undetected arrhythmia also may set off a chain of events leading to sudden death from cardiac arrest. In the United States, more than 300,000 deaths result each year from sudden cardiac arrest. When confronted with a patient who has an arrhythmia, a physician's task is to assess the risks and need for treatment, offer a course of treatment that will prevent adverse consequences, and relieve any discomfort. Because treatment with medication may have ill effects, a decision as to whether to treat at all or how to treat requires careful weighing of the disorder and the person in whom it occurs.

Abnormal heart rhythms fall into two general classes: excessively slow heart rates, known as bradyarrhythmias or bradycardias, and overly rapid heart rates, known as tachyarrhythmias or tachycardias. (See box, "Types of Arrhythmias.")

Extra or "skipped" heartbeats most often occur in hearts that are otherwise normal. Coronary artery disease, heart valve disease, heart muscle disease, and other cardiac disorders also may underlie more serious arrhythmias, but the immediate cause for an abnormal heart rhythm is a malfunction in the heart's electrical system. Without its electrical conduction system, the heart would be a mass of muscle incapable of coordinated pumping. The layout and timing of the heart's circuitry provide an exquisite solution. (See Figure 16.1.) This circuitry, however, can also break down.

THE ELECTRICAL SYSTEM OF THE HEART

The sinus node (SN), located at the top of the right atrium near the point where blood returns from the upper body, is the heart's pacemaker. Specialized cells in the sinus node send out electrical impulses that normally range between 60 and 100 per minute. As these impulses spread, they stimulate the muscle tissue of the left and right atria, causing contractions. The electrical impulses travel to the atrioventricular node (AV node), which is located in the septum (a wall of fibrous tissue that separates the two ventricles, the heart's major pumping chambers, from each other).

Electrical current moves faster than blood, so the atrioventricular node acts as a stop sign to delay the

Types of Arrhythmias

Slow heart rhythms

- Sinus bradycardia: heart rate slower than 60 beats per minute

- Sick sinus syndrome: failure of the sinus node to generate or conduct impulses properly

- Heart block: malfunction of the electrical conducting system between the atria and the ventricles

Rapid heart rhythms

- Supraventricular tachycardias: abnormally rapid rhythms that arise in the atria or the atrioventricular node

- Atrial flutter: a "circus current," triggered by an extra or early beat, that travels in regular cycles around the atrium, pushing the atrial rate up to 250 to 350 beats per minute

- Atrial fibrillation: a chaos of uncoordinated beats, with the atrial rate at more than 350 beats per minute, that causes the atria to quiver

- Paroxysmal supraventricular tachycardia (PSVT): a supraventricular tachycardia that causes a sudden increase in the heart rate, to between 140 and 250 beats per minute

- Wolff-Parkinson-White syndrome: presence of abnormal conduction pathways that bypass the normal atrioventricular node; tends to result in recurrent tachycardias

- Premature ventricular contractions (PVCs): early or extra beats that commonly occur in normal hearts, but can cause problems in unhealthy hearts; usually safe but can cause ventricles to lapse into fatal ventricular fibrillation or ventricular tachycardia

- Ventricular tachycardias: abnormally rapid rhythms that arise in the ventricles; potentially more serious than supraventricular tachycardias

- Ventricular fibrillation: ventricles quivering and ceasing to pump blood effectively; death possible within three to four minutes if patient is not treated

impulses long enough for the blood pumped by the atria to fill the ventricles. Then the signal enters a "superhighway" of conducting fibers, the His-Purkinje system, that branch left and right to direct the impulse first to the bottom and then up the sides of

Figure 16.1
This rendering of the heart's electrical conduction system shows electrical impulses traveling from the sinus node through electrical pathways to the atria, causing them to contract. The impulses travel to the atrioventricular (AV) node and then to the Bundle of His, the right and left bundles, and through the Purkinje fibers to the bottom and sides of the ventricles. The result is a smooth contraction from atria to ventricles that then forces blood up and out through the valves leading to the major arteries. (See Atlas 3B for four-color rendition.)

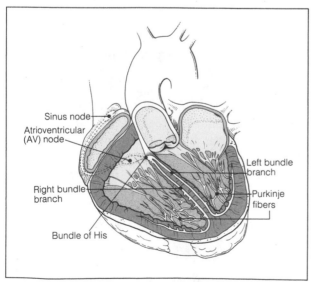

the ventricles. The result is a smooth surge of muscular contraction in the ventricles that squeezes the blood up from the floors of the chambers. The blood is then forced through valves that lead to the major arteries. Thus, it begins its journey to the lungs or to the rest of the body.

In order to adjust its pumping rate to meet the range of physical demands encountered in daily life, the heart must be able to receive brain, hormonal, and reflex signals. Physical exertion or emotional arousal can stimulate the sympathetic nerves, a part of the involuntary (autonomic) nervous system that also tends to constrict blood vessels. Its effects can almost triple the heart rate and nearly double the heart's pumping strength. Conversely, stimulation of the other division of the autonomic nervous system, the parasympathetic, or vagal, nerves, which often occurs during sleep, slows the heart rate. However, vagal stimulation can also occur during the course of daily life. In fact, the heart rate may slow enough to cause fainting. For example, some people experience this sudden, intense parasympathetic stimulation at the sight of blood.

People are usually unaware of this ongoing adjustment of heart rate that takes place as they move from quiescence to activity, from waking to sleeping. Yogis and others trained in meditation, however, are able voluntarily to slow their own heartbeats. In contrast, a person suffering an anxiety attack may feel his or her heart racing. The increase in heart rate during panic, to as fast as 170 beats per minute, is caused not only by strong stimulation of the sympathetic nerves, but also by a flood of adrenaline (epinephrine), secreted by the adrenal gland, that reaches the heart through the circulatory system.

Normal heart rates vary with each individual and factors such as cardiovascular conditioning, so casual comparisons of pulse rates can be misleading. For instance, a highly fit athlete at rest will have a slower pulse (45 to 60 beats per minute) than a sedentary individual (65 to 80 beats per minute). If both the sedentary person and the athlete run up a flight of stairs, both heart rates will increase, but the athlete's will not increase as much as and will return to normal sooner than that of the sedentary person, primarily because his or her muscles use oxygen much more efficiently.

Abnormal heart rates and rhythms also have variable causes and consequences in different people. The degree of symptoms alone does not necessarily indicate the seriousness of the underlying disorder. As a consequence, anyone experiencing any of the symptoms outlined should consult a physician.

SYMPTOMS OF ARRHYTHMIAS

Symptoms arise from both slow or fast arrhythmias, but they may be different from person to person. The classic symptoms of arrhythmias include palpitations, dizziness, fainting, chest pain, and shortness of breath. Of course, some of these may not occur, even with serious arrhythmias. People may experience palpitations as missed beats, "skips," "thumps," "butterflies," "fluttering," or "racing"; the palpitations may come in single or multiple beats and may be felt anywhere from the stomach to the head. People often become more aware of palpitations before going to sleep at night, particularly when they lie on the left side of the body. At this time they are free from distractions, and the bed may act like a drum, amplifying heartbeats.

Palpitations may not be especially bothersome, but light-headedness or fainting (syncope) caused by irregular, rapid, or slow rhythms is harder to ignore. These symptoms usually do not occur unless the heart rate becomes very slow (less than 35 to 45 beats per minute) or extremely rapid (more than 150 beats per minute). In other words, the heart rate rhythm disturbance usually must entail more than just a few

extra beats. The individual passes out because the erratically beating heart fails to pump enough blood to the brain.

A fainting spell caused by heart rhythm abnormalities usually begins with light-headedness rather than the spinning (vertigo) associated with dizziness. The first sensation may be of falling. If the individual recovers before actually passing out, the symptom is known as presyncope. Fainting without warning, however, may occur and may cause injury. If the person is driving a car or operating heavy machinery, fainting obviously can lead to an accident. Any sudden blackout, in the absence of a history of other causes, may indicate an arrhythmic disorder.

The chest pain and shortness of breath that may accompany an arrhythmia usually occur because a rapid heartbeat has put a strain on the heart muscle, which becomes starved for oxygen. The symptoms may be similar to those of angina—pain or pressure originating from the heart but felt anywhere from the stomach to the jaw, including the back, and sometimes associated with nausea or sweating. These symptoms are not common in younger persons who may experience irregular or rapid heartbeats. They are more frequently noticed in older persons with underlying heart disease. Some patients may feel discomfort simply because of the rapid thumping of the heart against the chest.

SLOW HEART RHYTHMS (BRADYCARDIAS)

SINUS BRADYCARDIA

Doctors define sinus bradycardia as a heart rhythm slower than 60 beats per minute that originates from the normal pacemaker. Almost anyone, however, can go about normal activities with this heart rate. During deep sleep or in young, well-conditioned people, the normal heart rate may actually be as slow as 30 to 40 beats per minute. The heart of a trained athlete can pump more than the usual volume of blood with each beat, making more rapid rates unnecessary.

A slow heart rhythm becomes abnormal when it diminishes the heart's output of blood to the rest of the body enough to cause symptoms ranging from fatigue and shortness of breath to fainting spells. Exercise and increased activity often bring on these symptoms when the heart rate fails to increase to meet the body's needs.

Failure of the sinus node to generate or conduct impulses properly (a condition often referred to as sick sinus syndrome) may underlie some slow heart rhythms. Age or disease may damage the sinus node, excess fibrous or scar tissue may accumulate and interfere with its function, or the autonomic nervous system may fail to regulate its activity properly. A number of antiarrhythmic, antihypertensive, and other drugs can also have adverse effects on sinus node function. (See Chapter 23.) Physicians have recently recognized that children and adolescents who had heart disease at birth (congenital heart disease) that has been surgically corrected may develop sinus node dysfunction in their teens or adulthood. This is a result of scarring from either instrinsic disease or the surgical procedure. (See Chapter 25.)

HEART BLOCK

Slow heart rhythms may also result from the improper transmission of electrical impulses through the atrioventricular node or any of the heart's specialized conduction pathways, despite their normal generation by the sinus node. Doctors often call the condition "heart block," which should not be confused with blockage in the coronary arteries. (See Chapter 11.)

The level of impairment is expressed in degrees. First-degree heart block denotes slow conduction time in the atrioventricular node. Heart rate and rhythm are normal.

Second-degree heart block is diagnosed when some impulses from the atria intermittently fail to reach and activate the ventricles, resulting in a varying number of "dropped beats." Included in this category is a condition known as the Wenckebach phenomenon. This occurs when there is a progressive delay in each ventricular response, resulting in a periodic omission of a single ventricular contraction.

Third-degree heart block, also called complete atrioventricular block, occurs when no impulses from the atria reach the ventricles. If ventricular action is to continue, the heart must rely on an independent junctional or ventricular pacemaker. Sometimes there is a lag before this independent pacemaker takes over. During this time, there is no ventricular contraction, and the person may faint. This is called an Adams-Stokes attack. Usually, though, the ventricular pacemaker eventually establishes a slow rhythm (20 to 45 beats per minute) that is unrelated to the atrial impulses.

The most common causes of heart block are inflammation and scarring of the conducting tissue, which often result from coronary artery disease or hypertension and the "wear and tear" associated with the aging process. These other parts of the conduction system can also be adversely affected by drugs that interfere with proper sinus node operation. Heart block can occur at any age, although it most often develops in later years. Some children may be born with the condition because of an immune response transmitted from their mothers, a defect in the conducting tissue, or small tumors that disrupt the electrical pathways. These cases are rare.

Symptoms of heart block are similar to those of sinus node disease. They vary depending on the severity and location of the block. Patients with complete block are at greatest risk for fainting or congestive heart failure.

RAPID HEART RHYTHMS (TACHYCARDIAS)

Abnormally fast heart rates are classified into two types: supraventricular (meaning "above the ventricle") tachycardias—those that arise in the atria or the atrioventricular node—and ventricular tachycardias. In both instances, an extra or early beat may trigger the rapid rhythms. Although the sinus node develops as the specialized site of impulse production, all cardiac muscle cells retain the capacity to become pacemaker cells. Normally, the pacemaking activity of the sinus node suppresses impulse production by other cells, but if conductance to some part of the heart muscle is blocked, or if the heart is overstimulated, islands of cells may express their latent impulse-production ability, resulting in extra beats. In other words, impulses are fired from one or more locations in addition to the normal pacemaker, the sinus node.

Extra or early beats arising in the atria are called premature atrial contractions (PACs), atrial premature beats, atrial ectopic beats, or atrial extrasystoles. Such extra beats often occur in normal hearts and are usually harmless. They can, however, cause palpitations, as well as trigger supraventricular tachycardias. Many of these episodes are not serious and can easily be treated.

ATRIAL FLUTTER AND FIBRILLATION

Among the most common supraventricular tachycardias are atrial flutter and fibrillation. They can occur together and may arise in a heart that is otherwise normal and healthy. Flutter results when an extra or early beat triggers a "circus circular current" that travels in regular cycles around the atrium, pushing the atrial rate up to 250 to 350 beats per minute. The atrioventricular node between the atria and ventricles will often block one of every two beats, keeping the ventricular rate at about 125 to 175 beats per minute. This is the pulse rate that will be felt, even though the atria are beating more rapidly. At this pace, the ventricles will usually continue to pump blood relatively effectively for many hours or even days. A patient with underlying heart disease, however, may experience chest pain, faintness, or even heart failure as a result of the continuing increased stress on the heart muscle. In some individuals, the ventricular rate may also be slower if there is increased block of impulses in the AV node, or faster if there is little or no block.

If the cardiac impulse fails to follow a regular circuit and divides along multiple pathways, a chaos of uncoordinated beats results, producing atrial fibrillation. Fibrillation commonly occurs when the atrium is enlarged (usually because of heart disease). In addition, it can occur in the absence of any apparent heart disease. The atrial rate shoots up to more than 350 beats per minute and the atria fail to pump blood effectively, quivering like "a can of worms" or "a bowl of jelly," as it has been variously described. The ventricular beat also becomes haphazard, producing a rapid irregular pulse. Although atrial fibrillation may cause the heart to lose 20 to 30 percent of its pumping effectiveness, the volume of blood pumped by the ventricles usually remains within the margin of safety, again because the atrioventricular node blocks out many of the chaotic beats. The ventricle may contract at a rate of only 125 to 175 beats per minute.

Sleep deprivation, excessive caffeine, street drugs such as amphetamine and cocaine, and excessive alcohol consumption increase the heart's susceptibility to developing atrial flutter or fibrillation. So can heart valve disease, overactivity of the thyroid gland, lung disease, and inflammation of the membranous sac that covers the heart (a condition known as pericarditis). Atrial flutter or fibrillation may go unrecognized by the patient, but they may cause palpitations or light-headedness. Such symptoms are generally not life-threatening, and many people live long and well despite atrial flutter or fibrillation if the rate is controlled.

Though usually harmless, atrial flutter and fibrillation can pose serious risks. In a diseased heart, such arrhythmias can diminish cardiac function and lead to heart failure. Episodes of atrial fibrillation that persist more than several days also carry an additional risk of stroke, because stagnating blood in the atria may clot, producing clumps of clotted blood, which if discharged from the heart (emboli) may be carried to the brain and produce a stroke.

PAROXYSMAL SUPRAVENTRICULAR TACHYCARDIAS (PSVTs)

In this type of rapid heart rhythm, patients experience heart rates in the range of 140 to 250 beats per minute. These episodes often occur first in youth, but may also emerge later in life. While they may be distressing, such attacks are seldom life-threatening. They typically occur in patients who have been born with an extra circuit or pathway between the atria and the ventricles. Such extra circuits occur most commonly within the atrioventricular node, but in an average of 1 or 2 out of 1,000 births, so-called accessory pathways or bypass tracts (sometimes more than one is present) form separate conduction routes. These routes may link the atria and the ventricles at locations quite distant from the atrioventricular node.

Paroxysmal supraventricular tachycardias may be triggered by an ectopic (literally, "out-of-place") beat, originating in either the atria or the ventricles. If this tachycardia is started by a premature atrial contraction, because the extra atrial beat comes prematurely in the heart's rhythm cycle, the atrioventricular node or the extra circuit may be blocked. The impulse takes the available route and the ventricles contract. But now the previously blocked path has regained its ability to conduct, and the impulse that has just activated the ventricles is passed back to the atria. Impulses begin to travel around the circuit loop formed by the bypass tract and the atrioventricular node, and a rapid heart rate ensues. The resulting heart rate determines the time required for the impulse to travel around the circuit.

When evidence of a different conduction pathway between the atria and ventricle shows up on the ECG of a patient who experiences symptoms of this type of arrhythmia or atrial fibrillation, the condition is often referred to as *Wolff-Parkinson-White syndrome*, or WPW. (It is named for the three physicians who first described its most common form.) It should be emphasized that Wolff-Parkinson-White syndrome and related conditions may pose no serious threat if properly treated. Wolff-Parkinson-White syndrome may also be associated with recurrent tachycardias despite medical therapy. In unusual situations, a more serious form of abnormal heartbeat may occur in people with Wolff-Parkinson-White syndrome. This occurs as ventricular fibrillation where the main pumping chamber beats irregularly at more than 200 beats per minute, and it may result in death.

Like those of other supraventricular tachycardias, the symptoms of this syndrome may not emerge until later in life as the normal conduction system and bypass tract undergo changes. Triggering beats also become more common with age, and may result in more frequent episodes of tachycardia.

VENTRICULAR ARRHYTHMIAS

In contrast to supraventricular arrhythmias, ventricular arrhythmias are potentially more serious and are more often, but not always, associated with structural heart disease. Premature ventricular contractions (PVCs) are the most common form. Like premature atrial contractions, premature ventricular contractions are early or extra beats that commonly occur and are innocuous in normal hearts, but can cause problems in unhealthy hearts. In rare circumstances, premature ventricular contractions can cause the ventricles to lapse into ventricular fibrillation; the heart quivers and ceases to pump blood effectively, and death can occur within 3 to 4 minutes.

Prevention of these potentially dangerous contractions is crucial, because few victims of sudden cardiac arrest survive without immediate first aid. In cities such as Seattle, Washington, vigorous promotion of citizen training in cardiopulmonary resuscitation (CPR) has improved survival rates for victims of ventricular fibrillation. Even so, only 20 to 30 percent of such patients recover and continue to lead normal lives.

Long-term prevention of ventricular fibrillation remains difficult. Unlike atrial arrhythmias that have no symptoms, ventricular arrhythmias or premature ventricular contractions that cause no discomfort can indicate an increased risk of life-threatening ventricular tachycardia or fibrillation, especially in patients with heart disease or a family history of sudden death, although most of the time, these individual contractions are not serious. A physician may need to perform certain tests to aid in the assessment of the risk of these extra beats.

DIAGNOSIS

The techniques used to diagnose and monitor cardiac arrhythmias have become increasingly sophisticated.

The most basic tool is the electrocardiogram (ECG). Adhesive electrodes applied to the chest and limbs connect to a machine that can detect the pattern of minute electric currents in the cardiac muscle and print it out on a strip chart. Electrocardiograms performed to evaluate arrhythmias are most useful if done while symptoms are occurring, which may not be possible if symptoms are brief, infrequent, or absent. Because activity often provokes arrhythmias, an exercise test with electrocardiographic monitoring may prove helpful. (See Figures 16.2, 16.3, 16.4, 16.5, and 16.6 for ECGs showing different heart rhythm disorders.)

The use of computers to enhance and process the electrocardiogram signal (signal-averaged ECG) has improved the test as a means of predicting the risk of potentially dangerous ventricular arrhythmias. Transtelephonic electrocardiograms enable the patient to record his or her own electrocardiographic signal during symptoms and to send the recording to a doctor by telephone. Electrocardiograms using electrodes that are swallowed or inserted through the mouth into the esophagus are called transesophageal ECGs. This technique may be useful in more difficult cases to diagnose atrial arrhythmias, because the esophagus lies directly behind the atria.

Holter monitors are portable electrocardiogram recorders that patients wear for extended periods, usually 24 to 48 hours. Recorded on tape, the test results are then analyzed by computer. Holter monitors enable a physician to obtain a record of the patient's heartbeat during ordinary activities and may be especially useful for detecting the more serious types of premature ventricular contractions that may be associated with an increased risk of ventricular fibrillation.

Electrophysiology studies form the leading edge of arrhythmia diagnosis and treatment. These studies are not necessary in the vast majority of patients with arrhythmias, but in special cases, they can be extremely useful. Guided by an X-ray picture, physicians thread electrodes via a catheter (a thin, flexible tube) through veins in the arm, neck, shoulder, or groin into the heart, where they can be used to make detailed recordings of the heart's electrical activity. The electrodes can also be used to mimic patterns of extra beats that normally occur in everyday experience to see if they provoke arrhythmias and to assess the effectiveness of therapy.

Electrophysiology studies are usually recommended for survivors of sudden cardiac arrest in order to determine the best means of preventing a recurrence. Other likely candidates include patients

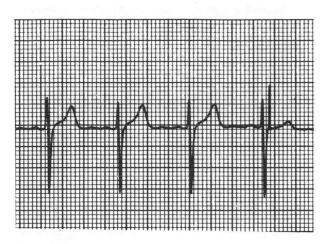

Figure 16.2
ECG Showing Normal Heart Rhythm

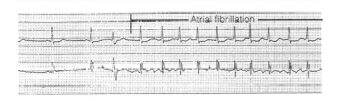

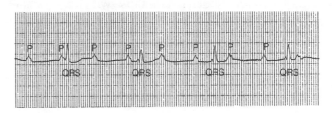

Figure 16.5
Heart Block

This electrocardiogram shows "complete heart block." The P waves, representing electrical activity of the natural pacemaker and upper heart chambers (atria), occur at a rate of 94 beats per minute. The QRS complexes, representing contraction of the lower pumping chambers (ventricles), occur at a rate of 44 beats per minute. None of the signals from the upper chambers are getting through to the lower chambers because of a "block" of the electrical circuits connecting them. The lower chambers are beating at a slow rate, which, fortunately, they are capable of generating on their own when no signals come from above. This backup or reserve rhythm is slow and not coordinated with the upper chambers, so pumping of blood becomes inefficient and reduced. There is no reserve pumping capability when needed, such as with physical exertion. This causes the symptoms of fatigue and exhaustion. Implantation of an artificial pacemaker usually restores a normally coordinated heart rhythm.

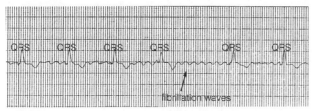

Figure 16.3
ECGs Showing Atrial Fibrillation

In the top panel, the first two beats are normal, the third is a premature atrial contraction, and the fourth marks the beginning of atrial fibrillation during which the heart rate averages 130 beats per minute and the pattern of the beats is irregular. The lower panel shows sustained atrial fibrillation.

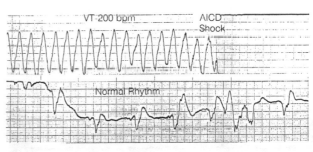

Figure 16.6
Electrical Conversion of Ventricular Tachycardia

This electrocardiogram demonstrates an attack of ventricular tachycardia, a dangerously rapid heart rhythm that can lead to fainting or, in some instances, death. In this case, the patient did not respond to rhythm-regulating medication, and an automatic defibrillator was surgically implanted. The defibrillator detects the abnormal rhythm and delivers an electric shock that terminates the irregularity and restores normal rhythms.

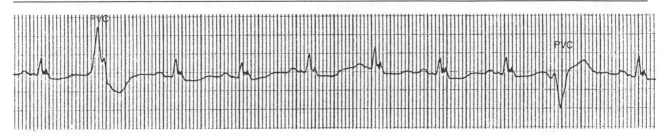

Figure 16.4
Premature Ventricular Contractions

This electrocardiogram shows a regular rhythm that is punctuated on two occasions (indicated by arrows) by premature ventricular contractions (PVCs). Because these beats arise in the bottom pumping chambers and activate the heart in abnormal fashion, they appear on the ECG as bizarre, wide complexes that appear much different from the normal beats.

at high risk for sudden death, those with paroxysmal supraventricular tachycardia or syncope, and those with persistent symptoms whose suspected arrhythmias have eluded detection by other means.

DECIDING TO TREAT

The development of electrophysiology studies has spurred the continuing improvement in treatments for heart rhythm disorders, but the ultimate decision as to whether or how to treat an arrhythmia still rests on an understanding of the whole patient. The patient's overall health, age, life-style, and tolerance of symptoms as well as the arrhythmia itself all weigh into the choice of therapy. Because of such considerations, two people with the same arrhythmia may well receive entirely different treatments. Some patients may not need any treatment at all, and can live long and comfortably with an irregular heart rhythm, confident that the occasional symptom does not signal a serious health problem. (See box, "Self-Help for Arrhythmias.") But because the symptoms do not tell

Self-Help for Arrhythmias

People can often slow down their own heart rates, and possibly suppress supraventricular arrhythmias, by controlling certain nerve impulses. This can be achieved in several ways: holding the breath, taking a slow drink of water, or bathing the face in cold water. Rubbing the neck may also help. If all of this fails, holding the nostrils closed and trying to blow through the nose (making the eardrums "pop") should provide some relief. Simply coughing may stop premature ventricular contractions (PVCs), those extra beats that cause palpitations or thumping in the chest.

Preventative measures include avoiding emotional distress and anxiety. Cutting down on stimulants such as caffeine may help, but an occasional candy bar, a couple of cups of coffee or tea a day, or an occasional caffeinated soda are generally safe to enjoy. Decongestants, often used in cold and allergy medications, can cause rapid heart rates. Also people should abstain from using cigarettes and alcohol because they may increase susceptibility to arrhythmias. With proper professional and self-care, most people with arrhythmias are not held back from living normal, productive lives.

the whole story, anyone who experiences the warning signs of a heart rhythm disorder should be sure to see a doctor.

In selected cases, electrophysiology studies can determine the cause of symptoms, such as fainting spells, or the need for a permanent artificial pacemaker. By administering antiarrhythmic drugs and attempting to induce arrhythmias, cardiologists can directly test the effectiveness of medications without waiting for spontaneous episodes to occur. This offers an advantage in devising safe, effective treatment, because not every antiarrhythmic drug is effective in every patient, and in some circumstances an antiarrhythmic drug may actually worsen the arrhythmia it is intended to suppress. (See Chapter 23.)

ANTIARRHYTHMIC DRUGS AND ARTIFICIAL PACEMAKERS

When used as an antiarrhythmic drug, digitalis, also known as digoxin (Lanoxin), slows impulse conduction through the atrioventricular node, thereby reducing the ventricular rate in order to treat atrial fibrillation or other supraventricular tachycardias.

Beta blockers are drugs used to inhibit the effects of hormones that cause the heart rate to increase. Beta blockers can also enhance effects of other antiarrhythmics. Propranolol (Inderal and others) is a commonly used beta blocker.

The effect of another class of drugs, calcium channel blockers, is similar to that of beta blockers. They change the electrical properties of heart tissues by inhibiting the flow of calcium in and out of cells. A small amount of calcium circulates constantly in the blood and regulates muscle contractions, among other functions. Diltiazem (Cardizem) and verapamil (Calan) are the primary calcium channel blockers used to treat arrhythmias. They slow the sinus rate, but not as effectively as beta blockers. They also slow conduction through the atrioventricular node. Calcium channel blockers, beta blockers, and digitalis are useful in treating atrial fibrillation and paroxysmal supraventricular tachycardias.

Quinidine (Quinidex, Quinora, and others) is a drug that works directly on the heart, as well as through the nerves that lead to heart muscles, to help stabilize irregular heartbeats. Procainamide (Procan), disopyramide (Norpace), and moricizine (Ethmozine) are synthetic drugs that have much the same uses as quinidine.

Antiarrhythmic drugs that work directly on the heart to suppress ventricular arrhythmias are tocainide (Tonocard) and mexiletine (Mexitil). They are often used in combination with other antiarrhythmic drugs. Flecainide (Tambocor) and propafenone (Rythmol) slow atrioventricular conduction and are effective against both supraventricular and ventricular arrhythmias. All of these antiarrhythmic drugs can worsen arrhythmias in some cases and are generally not prescribed unless careful testing has been done.

Amiodarone (Cordarone) is the most potent antiarrhythmic drug in use. In addition to suppressing virtually all types of arrhythmias, it acts as a beta blocker, an alpha blocker (blocks responses from the alpha-adrenergic nerve receptors), and a calcium channel blocker. Because of its many side effects, amiodarone is approved only for the treatment of serious arrhythmias that do not respond to other drugs. Researchers are seeking a less toxic form of amiodarone that may one day prove to be an antiarrhythmic agent with wider applications.

In some cases, instead of or in addition to drug therapy, a person will need an artificial pacemaker to correct an arrhythmia. Artificial pacemakers work in much the same way as the heart's natural pacemaker. They are small, surgically implanted units, about the size of a cigarette lighter, that use batteries to produce the electrical impulses that stimulate the pumping chambers of the heart. Tiny wires deliver the impulses to the heart muscle. Pacemakers are individually programmed to maintain a person's natural heart rate, and various types of pacemakers, pacing modes, and pacing rates are available to best suit individual needs.

Pacemakers are implanted while the recipient is under local anesthesia, but at least one day of hospitalization is required. Minor surgery is also necessary when the batteries run down and need to be replaced. (See Chapter 26 for more information about pacemakers.)

TREATMENT FOR SPECIFIC ARRHYTHMIAS

In the absence of other heart disease, the prognosis for sinus node dysfunction, the underlying cause for some slower heart rhythms, is good. When the symptoms of a slow heart rhythm are severe or debilitating, a pacemaker usually will help. Treatment of heart block is similar to that of sinus node disease. That is, patients with complete heart block usually require a pacemaker.

Treatment of atrial flutter and fibrillation is usually aimed at correcting the abnormal rhythm, but if this is not possible, medication, such as a beta blocker, digitalis, or verapamil, can be given to increase the degree of block between the atria and ventricle and slow the heart rate to within the normal range. Even though the heartbeat remains irregular, it is efficient enough to do its job. (People with Wolff-Parkinson-White syndrome who have atrial fibrillation, however, should not take digitalis or verapamil, because these drugs can paradoxically increase the heart rate and the likelihood of ventricular fibrillation.)

The prognosis depends on the overall health of the heart in which atrial flutter or fibrillation occurs. A decision to treat atrial flutter or fibrillation usually rests on how much the symptoms bother the patient. Paradoxically, slow heart rhythms may coexist with atrial flutter or fibrillation, a condition known as tachy-brady (fast-slow) syndrome, which can require treatment with both medicines and a pacemaker.

Chronic and distressing arrhythmias may be treated with electrical cardioversion. Cardioversion is used to treat atrial flutter and other arrhythmias, such as atrial tachycardia, atrial fibrillation, and ventricular tachycardia, when drug therapy fails. In this procedure, the patient is given a short-acting intravenous anesthetic, and an electrical current is delivered to the heart from a defibrillator through conducting paddles applied to the chest. The voltage varies according to the situation. The shock temporarily halts all electrical activity in the heart, allowing it to reestablish a normal heart rhythm by, in effect, starting over. When ventricular fibrillation occurs, electrical defibrillation is an emergency measure. The procedure is safe and effective.

Because atrial fibrillation may cause blood to stagnate in the atria, causing clotting, a physician may recommend an antiarrhythmic drug to maintain normal rhythm, a blood thinner (anticoagulant) to decrease the likelihood of clotting, or both. Though some studies suggest that an aspirin a day may decrease the risk of stroke associated with chronic atrial fibrillation, a more potent blood-thinning drug, such as warfarin (Coumadin), may be required.

People who experience paroxysmal supraventricular tachycardias (PSVTs) may require antiarrhythmic drugs, administered either at the time of an attack or on a daily basis. Accessory conducting pathways that mediate PSVTs may be surgically cut, preventing further arrhythmias.

A relatively new technique for treating this particular tachycardia, and especially Wolff-Parkinson-White syndrome, without surgery is called *radiofrequency catheter ablation*. In this procedure, a physician inserts a catheter into a blood vessel and threads it, under X-ray guidance, up to the area of the heart muscle where the accessory pathway is located. A mild current, produced by very-high-frequency alternating current—that is, radiofrequency current—is then transmitted from the catheter electrode tip to the site of the pathway. (This same current is the familiar "electric needle" used in various electrocautery procedures.) The resistance of the heart muscle to the current generates a small amount of heat. An increase of 10 degrees is all that is necessary to cause the death of the heart muscle cells in a very small area, about ⅕ inch in diameter. Once this occurs, the pathways can no longer conduct the extra impulses. The procedure produces little or no discomfort. It is done under mild sedation with local anesthesia, and the patient can return to normal activities within a few days.

Drug treatment aimed at suppressing premature ventricular contractions (PVCs) to prevent serious ventricular arrhythmias often fails to reduce the risk of sudden death. Prospects for effective treatments have brightened, however, with the recent development of electrophysiology studies and treatment programs that combine drug therapy with surgery and antiarrhythmic devices, such as implantable defibrillators. (See Chapter 26.) Individuals who have ventricular fibrillation or ventricular tachycardia (especially combined with fainting) should probably undergo full evaluation to determine the best treatment.

A newer and increasingly used option for treating life-threatening ventricular arrhythmias is the automatic implantable cardioverter-defibrillator (AICD). Unlike other types of treatment, this does not prevent arrhythmias but instead stops them within seconds. An electrode lead system is attached directly to the heart, leading to a pulse generator that is implanted under the skin in the upper abdomen. The pulse generator continuously monitors heart rate and rhythm through signals from the leads. When a tachyarrhythmia is detected, the pulse generator responds. It sends a series of up to five shocks via patch electrodes that are sewn directly onto the outside of the heart. This direct electric current should restore proper rhythm.

The automatic implantable cardioverter-defibrillator has proved extremely effective. The sudden death rate within the first year is 1 to 2 percent in patients who receive this device, compared with 20 to 50 percent for people who go untreated. The device is appropriate for people who have ventricular arrhythmias that cannot be controlled with drug therapy, but at present it can be implanted only in people who can withstand chest surgery.

Surgery, like ablation, has the potential to cure a person suffering from arrhythmias. This approach, however, should be taken only by people who have extremely serious arrhythmias that still occur despite antiarrhythmic medications, or by younger people who otherwise face a lifetime of drug therapy.

Surgery can provide a cure for atrial arrhythmias that occur when more than one electrical pathway exists; extra electrical pathways are destroyed or cut out. Traditionally people with Wolff-Parkinson-White syndrome are likely candidates for this surgery, although this now is accomplished most often with radiofrequency ablation. In the case of ventricular arrhythmias, sometimes the starting point for the abnormal impulses can be determined through electrophysiology testing and can be cut out, but the surgical mortality rate is 10 to 15 percent, and there may be recurrences in 20 to 30 percent of the cases. Often other necessary operations, such as coronary artery bypasses, are performed at the same time as antiarrhythmic surgery, and in some cases, part or all of an automatic implantable cardioverter-defibrillator system is attached as a backup. This eliminates the need for a second chest operation should the system be needed later.

CHAPTER 17

PERIPHERAL VASCULAR DISEASE

MICHAEL D. EZEKOWITZ, M.D., Ph.D.

Although the heart is the command center of the circulatory system, many medical conditions that afflict the heart may also or independently affect the network of arteries and veins that carry blood to and from the body's tissues. Such damage is generally referred to as peripheral vascular disease (PVD).

Arterial diseases may cause narrowing or blockage of vessels in the legs and other parts of the body distant from the heart (known as the *periphery*). Narrowing of the peripheral arteries happens in essentially the same way as narrowing of the coronary arteries. In coronary disease, the narrowing causes chest pain and, sometimes, heart attack. In peripheral arterial vascular disease, however, the most common symptoms are leg pains from decreased circulation. The veins, which send blood from the limbs and other tissues back to the heart, are also vulnerable to a variety of disorders that can cause blood clots to form or inflammation to develop.

HOW BLOOD CIRCULATES

The circulation of blood through the human body is divided into two interlocking systems: venous and arterial. Together, they keep a dynamic interchange of blood moving to and from the heart and lungs. (See Chapter 1 for a full explanation.)

Arteries carry freshly oxygenated blood from the heart to the rest of the body, starting in the central trunk artery, the aorta, which leads from the heart's main pumping chamber (the left ventricle). From the aorta, the arteries branch and divide into successively smaller vessels, and finally into tiny arterioles and capillaries that deliver oxygen to the body's tissues. Arteries are thick-walled and muscular; if an artery is cut, blood will spurt at high pressure and velocity with each beat of the heart. Arterial blood is scarlet, because it carries richly oxygenated red cells. Arteries such as the radial artery, located in the wrist near the thumb, are close to the surface of the body and are used to take the pulse.

Veins carry blood that has left much of its oxygen in the tissues back to the right side of the heart. It is then pumped into the lungs to pick up more oxygen. Compared to the flow of arterial blood, which is driven by the heart's powerful pumping, the flow of venous blood is relatively slow, returning from the lower body against the force of gravity. (A series of one-way valves inside the veins helps keep the blood from pooling or moving backward.) The flow of blood from a cut vein is slow and steady. Veins are thinner than arteries, and they appear bluish, because the blood they carry is low in oxygen.

The real work of the circulatory system—the exchange of nutrients for waste products—takes place in microscopic vessels called capillaries. These structures are as wide as a single cell and allow the dif-

Table 17.1
Diseases of the Veins

Diseases	Causes	Symptoms	Treatment
Blood clots (venous thrombosis)	Sluggish movement of blood (stasis) Damage to the lining of the vein Inflammation of the vein (phlebitis) Abnormal tendency to form clots (hypercoagulable state)	Sometimes none; sometimes shortness of breath; coughing up blood-tinged phlegm if clot moves to lung (pulmonary embolism); marked pain and swelling in one leg	Anticoagulant and blood-thinning drugs such as warfarin (Coumadin) and heparin; in repeated cases, insertion of a filtering device to prevent pulmonary embolism; bedrest for 3 to 5 days with legs elevated; elastic stockings worn below the knee; moist soaks and anti-inflammatory drugs such as aspirin or indomethacin (Indocin)
Chronic venous insufficiency	Complication following deep-vein clot	Swelling and discoloration of one or both legs	Same as for blood clot; knee-length elastic stocking indefinitely to prevent swelling
Inflammation of the leg veins (phlebitis), superficial or deep (see blood clots)	Infection or injury	Pain; redness; tenderness; itching; feeling of a firm cord in the calf or thigh	Anti-inflammatory drugs such as indomethacin (Indocin); analgesics such as aspirin; bedrest and leg elevation; anti-itch ointment such as zinc oxide; moist heat
Pulmonary embolism	Deep-vein clot moved to lungs	Sometimes none; sometimes chest pain that worsens upon inhaling; sandpaper-like sound heard through stethoscope; shortness of breath; coughing up blood; increased pressure in the lungs (pulmonary hypertension)	Clot-dissolving (thrombolytic) drugs such as urokinase (Abbokinase), streptokinase (Kabikinase or Streptase); anticoagulants such as warfarin (Coumadin) or heparin; in rare cases, surgery to remove the clot
Varicose veins	Backflow of blood in the superficial veins in the legs because of faulty valves; pressure from standing too long or during pregnancy; hormonal changes, during pregnancy, that dilate and relax veins	Sometimes none; sometimes pain; tingling or crawling sensation; unsightly appearance	Surgical removal; avoiding standing for long; wearing elastic or support stockings

fusion, or passage, of oxygen and nutrients into organs and tissues. The two sides of the circulatory system come together in these tiny vessels. The capillaries terminate in the smallest of veins, which in turn channel blood into the larger veins and back toward the heart through the largest veins, the inferior vena cava (from the lower body) and the superior vena cava (from the upper body).

DISORDERS OF THE VEINS

Blood clot formation in the veins (*venous thrombosis*) is the most common—and most threatening—medical condition involving the veins. It afflicts an estimated 5 to 6 million Americans every year. (See Table 17.1.)

The primary danger of a blood clot in the deep veins of the legs (see Figure 17.1) and abdomen is the possibility that a portion of the clot may break loose (embolus), which can travel to the lungs, where it can

Figure 17.1
A blood clot that forms in a deep vein in the leg or abdomen may travel through the bloodstream and lodge in the lung, a serious condition called pulmonary embolism. The arrows indicate the path of the blood clot.

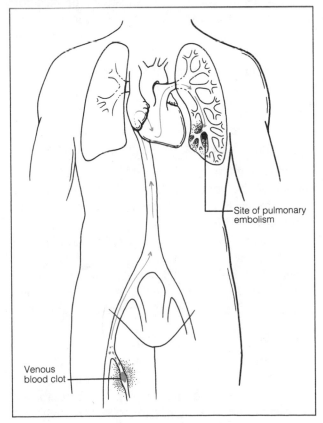

Site of pulmonary embolism

Venous blood clot

lodge in a pulmonary blood vessel. This is a serious condition called a *pulmonary embolus*, and if the blockage is large enough can be fatal. Blood clots in the superficial veins—those near the skin's surface—present little risk of embolization; they may cause localized pain and inflammation, but these symptoms can usually be treated with moist heat and medications such as aspirin. Clots in the deep veins in the calf are probably less threatening than clots in the deep veins above the knee, but, in either case, they must be treated aggressively.

Several conditions predispose a person to formation of blood clots in the veins. One is sluggish movement (*stasis*) of the blood in the veins of the limbs, especially the legs and feet. Damage to the lining of a vein, which may be caused by infection, injury, or trauma from a needle or catheter, can also be a factor. Inflammation of a vein (phlebitis), usually in the legs, is associated with clot formation as well. A third abnormality involves the blood's ability to coagulate too easily and form clots. This is called a *hypercoagulable* state. Injury to the inner lining of a vein causes platelets to congregate at the site, setting the stage for clotting when blood is sluggish or hypercoagulable.

Slow blood flow can be caused by any obstruction between the body's periphery and the heart. The massaging action of muscle contractions helps venous blood make its return trip; thus, a prime cause of slow blood flow is prolonged inactivity, which might occur, for example, as a result of a cast for a fractured bone in the lower extremity, extended bedrest after injury or illness, or even a long car or plane trip. On long trips, it is a good idea for someone who might be predisposed to getting a clot in a vein to get out of the car or stand up in the plane every hour and walk around for one or two minutes. This advice is especially good for obese people or those with diabetes, heart disease, heart failure, or other circulatory problems. Smokers are also very susceptible to clot formation and inflammation of the veins and arteries.

Other less common causes of sluggish blood flow include certain tumors and a buildup of fluid in the abdomen (ascites). A host of conditions, including some cancers, inherited abnormalities, and the aftermath of a heart attack or surgery, can increase the blood's tendency to clot.

A deep-vein clot may cause no symptoms; the first indication of its presence, in fact, may occur after it has traveled to the lung (pulmonary embolism), causing a person to cough up blood-tinged phlegm and experience shortness of breath and chest pain. The clot may also result in marked pain and swelling (edema) in one leg. Many other conditions, from joint diseases to heart failure, may cause pain or swelling in one or both legs. A carefully documented medical history and a few specific tests will usually lead to the diagnosis. Often a doctor can make the diagnosis merely by putting pressure on the calf or thigh muscle or flexing the ankle. If these maneuvers elicit a painful response, a deep-vein clot may likely be the culprit.

In most cases, the diagnosis must be confirmed using the test described below. The test considered the "gold standard" for diagnosing deep-vein clots is *contrast venography*. In this test, also called a venogram, a dye visible on an X-ray is injected into the veins of the feet; the patient is then tilted in various positions to facilitate blood flow from the lower veins to the heart, providing an X-ray image of the vein network. Venography is cumbersome and uncomfortable, and in a small percentage of tests, the results are questionable. The test also carries a small risk of infection or allergy to the dye. In many cases, the diagnosis can be made without this test.

Alternative tests include one in which blood flow in the legs is measured using a blood pressure cuff and two small electrodes. This quick technique, called *impedance plethysmography*, is useful for diagnosing clots above the knee. *Ultrasonography*, a completely noninvasive but relatively expensive technique, uses sound waves to form a picture of the veins and, in a variation called Doppler ultrasonography, measures blood flow. Other tests using radioactive isotopes may also be used. In one such test, called *platelet scintigraphy*, an injection of radioactively labeled platelets is used to locate clots and track their path through the veins over several days.

TREATMENT FOR VENOUS BLOOD CLOTS

After a venous blood clot has been discovered, a physician will first attempt to determine the underlying causes of abnormal clotting. Much of the time, the event causing the clot cannot be identified. However, clots that occur after long plane or car rides, surgery, or prolonged bedrest are relatively easy to explain. As a rule, immediate therapy consists of anticoagulant and blood-thinning medications such as warfarin (Coumadin) or heparin. The use of clot-dissolving (thrombolytic) drugs such as those now used to treat heart attacks is still considered controversial for clots in the veins, but may offer future promise. Lower doses of blood-thinning medications such as warfarin are usually continued for several months;

during this time, the blood's coagulation time must periodically be monitored (about every four weeks once it has stabilized) to guard against bleeding complications.

In patients who cannot take anticoagulants—for example, those with a bleeding ulcer or recent surgery patients—an umbrella-shaped filtering device may be inserted by catheter into the inferior vena cava, where blood from the legs is funneled back to the lungs, to prevent any major clots from reaching the lungs. This procedure usually is reserved for patients who have already experienced a clot or embolus to the lungs.

In addition to receiving medication, someone with a deep-vein clot should remain in bed during the acute attack (about three to five days), with legs elevated to prevent further swelling and facilitate venous blood flow. Moist heat and anti-inflammatory drugs such as aspirin or other, stronger nonsteroidal medications such as indomethacin (Indocin) may also be extremely helpful in controlling symptoms and aiding recovery. These should be used with care if in combination with anticoagulants. Once swelling improves, a firm elastic stocking should be worn *below* the knee whenever the person is out of bed. Most important, long periods of standing should be avoided.

In some people, a condition called *chronic venous insufficiency* may occur as a long-term complication following a deep-vein clot. It is characterized by swelling and discoloration of one or both legs. In these cases, a knee-length elastic stocking should be worn indefinitely to prevent swelling.

INFLAMMATION OF THE VEINS (PHLEBITIS)

The most common form of phlebitis is an inflammation of the superficial veins in the leg, usually caused by an infection or injury. The affected vein may appear reddened and feel like a firm cord in the calf or thigh. The condition is painful and is treated with moist heat and analgesics such as aspirin or some other nonsteroidal anti-inflammatory drug such as indomethacin (Indocin). Itching may be relieved by a nonprescription ointment containing zinc oxide.

The chief danger of phlebitis is an increased risk of clot formation and embolization, especially when it occurs in the deeper veins. Deep-vein phlebitis may cause the same symptoms as deep-vein thrombosis. There may be severe pain, tenderness, and fever.

VARICOSE VEINS

Normally, blood returns to the heart at a steady pace, helped along by exercise and by the veins' internal valve system. The valves act as one-way gates to prevent blood from pooling; they aid in moving blood against the force of gravity. If blood flow is too slow or the valves are damaged or ineffective, however, veins in the legs—especially superficial vessels in the lower legs—can swell, bulge, and twist into *varicose veins,* or varicosities. (See Figure 17.2.) Heredity of poorly functioning or absent valves seems to be a major factor. People who spend a lot of time standing are especially prone to varicose veins. Women may get them for the first time during pregnancy, because of pressure from the fetus on the veins in the abdomen (into which the leg veins drain) and hormonal changes that dilate and relax the veins.

Although varicose veins can cause pain or a sensation of tingling or crawling, they often produce no symptoms. However, they are considered unsightly. The condition can be corrected surgically in a procedure called "stripping," during which the varicose veins are simply tied off at intervals through skin incisions and pulled out from under the skin. (Nearby veins adapt by creating alternative pathways for the return of blood.) Alternatively, the varicosed veins

Figure 17.2
Varicose veins develop when the one-way valves in the superficial veins in the legs do not close properly, allowing blood to backflow and pool.

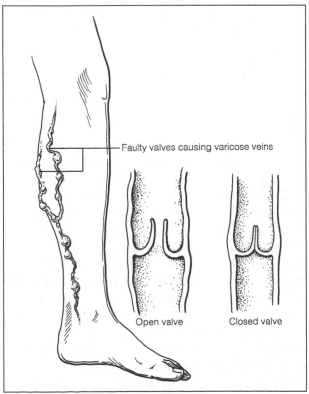

Faulty valves causing varicose veins

Open valve   Closed valve

may be injected with an irritating (sclerosing) substance, which causes them to shrink. Again, nearby veins assume the blood flow. Individuals with varicose veins should remain as thin as possible to reduce "back pressure" on the veins and should avoid standing for long periods of time. Elastic or support hose may provide some assistance to return blood flow, but tight garters, which impede circulation, should be avoided. Many people who have varicose veins do well and experience no limitations other than some swelling.

PULMONARY EMBOLISM

The closer to the heart that a clot is formed, the more likely it is to migrate to the lungs and form a pulmonary embolism. Such a clot may be fatal. It is also one of the most difficult causes of sudden death to diagnose. In some instances, there are no symptoms at all. In others, however, it may produce a variety of symptoms and signs, such as chest pain that worsens when a person inhales, a sandpaper-like sound heard through the stethoscope, shortness of breath, and coughing up blood. The embolism may resolve, leaving no permanent damage, but it can damage lung tissue or cause fluid buildup in the lung cavity. For instance, increased pressure on the right side of the heart over long periods of time may cause increased blood pressure in the vessels in the lungs, a condition known as pulmonary hypertension.

To diagnose a pulmonary embolus, a physician measures the levels of oxygen in the arteries and performs other tests to determine how well the lung is ventilated with air and supplied with blood. An obstruction to the lungs' blood supply, indicated by a lower percentage of oxygen in the blood, suggests the possibility of a clot. The diagnosis is confirmed by pulmonary angiography, in which the pulmonary artery is injected via a catheter with a dye so it will appear on an X-ray. The treatment for pulmonary embolus may involve clot-dissolving (thrombolytic) medication such as urokinase (Abbokinase) or streptokinase (Streptase), anticoagulants such as warfarin (Coumadin) or heparin, or other blood thinners; in rare cases, surgery is necessary to remove the clot.

PERIPHERAL ARTERIAL DISEASE

The coronary arteries that encircle and nourish the heart are the most common targets for the damage caused by atherosclerosis, the blockage of arteries with fatty deposits. However, atherosclerosis can affect arteries virtually anywhere in the body. When it occurs in the neck or the brain, it can cause a stroke. (See Chapter 18.) In the arteries supplying the legs, it can cause pain and, in a small minority of cases, tissue damage so severe it results in gangrene and amputation.

Atherosclerosis in the peripheral arteries is similar to that in the heart: Blood-borne fats, or lipids, infiltrate a damaged area of the vessel wall and cause further damage and thickening with the formation of a plaque. The inside passage of the artery becomes narrowed and may be blocked completely by a blood clot. This leads to *ischemia,* a condition in which arterial blood flow is impeded, resulting in too little oxygen being delivered to the tissue "downstream" from the narrowing or obstruction. The risk factors for arterial blockage in the periphery are identical to those for blockage in the coronary arteries, including high blood cholesterol, cigarette smoking, diabetes, and high blood pressure. Smoking is a particularly important risk factor for peripheral artery disease.

The classic symptom of peripheral arterial disease is crampy leg pain while walking, called *intermittent claudication.* Pain may worsen when a person walks faster or uphill. The pain usually stops when he or she rests. The cause is ischemia in the working muscles, a sort of "leg angina." (Angina pectoris, or chest pain, is usually caused by inadequate blood supply to heart muscle.) The pain of claudication is most often triggered by exercise, but may be brought on by other factors, including exposure to cold or certain medications, such as some beta blockers, that constrict blood vessels and decrease peripheral blood flow.

The location of the blockage determines the symptoms. If the obstruction is relatively low in the arterial branches supplying the legs, calf pain may be the result; higher blockage may cause thigh pain; and blockage higher than the groin (in the blood vessels in the abdomen) may also cause buttock pain and impotence.

When arteries are badly narrowed—or blocked altogether—leg pain may be noticed even when resting. At this point, the legs may look normal, but the toes may appear pale, discolored, or bluish (especially when the legs are dangling). Feet will feel cold to the touch. Pulses in the legs may be weak or absent. In the most severe cases, blood-starved tissues may actually begin to die. Lower-leg, toe, or ankle ulcers may occur, and in the most advanced cases, gangrene may result and necessitate the amputation of toes or feet.

Foot Care for People with Peripheral Vascular Disease

Poor circulation caused by peripheral vascular disease makes feet more vulnerable to injury and infection and slower to heal. For this reason, it is especially important to take proper care of the feet to avoid complications. Here are some tips:

- Inspect feet daily for calluses, ulcers, and corns.

- Wash feet gently each day in lukewarm water and mild soap (this can be part of a bath or shower); dry thoroughly but gently.

- If skin is dry, thin, or scaly, use a gentle lubricant or moisturizing lotion after bathing.

- To avoid fungal infection such as athlete's foot, use a plain, unmedicated foot powder.

- Cut toenails straight across and avoid cutting close to skin. If your eyesight or manual coordination is poor or you have trouble reaching your feet, have a family member or a podiatrist trim the nails.

- If you have calluses or corns, have them treated by a podiatrist. Avoid adhesive plasters, tape, chemicals, abrasives, or cutting tools.

- Wear sensible, properly fitted shoes; avoid high heels, open-toed shoes, sandals, and walking around barefoot. If any foot problems are present, such as bunions or hammer toes, have shoes specially fitted to avoid rubbing or blisters.

- Keep feet warm in cold weather with loose-fitting wool socks or stockings, but avoid using hot-water bottles or heating pads directly on feet. (Poor circulation can reduce sensation in the feet, making a burn more likely.)

However, such serious complications of peripheral arterial disease are uncommon.

Patients with poor circulation to the feet and toes should discontinue smoking if applicable, and pay particular attention to avoiding injury to those areas. Otherwise healing will be slower and infection more likely. (See box, "Foot Care for People with Peripheral Vascular Disease.") Feet should be kept warm, dry, and away from excessive heat (baths, heating pads), and avoid cutting toenails too short. Since peripheral arterial disease is more common in individuals with diabetes than in those with normal blood sugar, control of diabetes is important.

DIAGNOSIS AND TREATMENT

Other conditions, including various joint, muscle, and lower-back problems, can also cause a person to experience leg pain while walking. With peripheral arterial disease, however, the presence of typical symptoms—pain in the calf or thigh while walking that ceases upon stopping—and decreased pulses in the arteries in the feet are sufficient to make the diagnosis in most cases.

Decreased hair on the lower extremities indicates a chronic problem. Taking cuff measurements of blood pressure in the ankles or in other segments of the legs may help determine how much blood is getting to the feet. Tests may be performed before and after exercise. The diagnosis of peripheral arterial disease may be made using Doppler ultrasonography to see blood flow in the arteries, magnetic resonance imaging (MRI) to identify obstructions, or—most important—angiography. These procedures are expensive and are not necessary in most cases. Because angiography is an invasive procedure involving the injection of dye into the arteries, it is usually reserved for cases when surgery or angioplasty is a likely option. For example, in cases of severe claudication with evidence of poor circulation, discoloration, absent pulses, and cold extremities, angiography can determine the best course of treatment.

It has been estimated that 80 to 90 percent of patients with claudication will stabilize or improve with time. Perhaps 10 to 15 percent will require some type of interventional therapy; less than 3 to 5 percent will require amputation. In treating peripheral arterial disease, conservative measures should be given a fair trial before *any* invasive procedures are considered.

Several steps are essential: control of obesity and diabetes if present, the cessation of cigarette smoking (the majority of peripheral arterial disease sufferers are smokers), and adherence to a program of regular exercise, such as daily walking. Patients may typically be instructed to walk for a half hour to an hour a day, walking until the pain comes on, resting until it abates, then continuing to walk. Often such a walking regimen can increase the distance of pain-free walking, thanks to increased fitness and perhaps the development of alternate circulation paths through surrounding smaller vessels, called collateral circulation. Control of the risk factors for "hardening of the arteries," including elevated blood pressure and cholesterol, if present, is also extremely important.

Other forms of exercise, such as swimming or using an exercise bicycle, may also be helpful, particularly to people with other joint and muscle problems for whom strenuous weight-bearing exercise (such as jogging) could present a significant risk of injury. People with symptoms of peripheral arterial disease should consult a physician before taking up any new exercise program.

Anticlotting agents, such as an aspirin taken each day, and vasodilator drugs, such as hydralazine (Apresoline) or prazosin (Minipress), may be used to treat peripheral arterial disease. (Most of these medications, however, have not been proved effective.) An agent called pentoxifylline (Trental) is also available for the pain of claudication. (Beta blockers, often used for other cardiovascular conditions, may make peripheral arterial disease worse.) If these measures fail to halt peripheral arterial disease, and disability is severe or limbs are threatened, invasive techniques such as angioplasty or surgery may have to be used to open blocked arteries, but this is uncommon.

ANGIOPLASTY AND SURGERY

Balloon angioplasty is being used successfully to open blocked arteries in the legs of people with severe cases of peripheral arterial disease. The procedure, usually performed by a radiologist or cardiologist, is similar to that used in the heart. A balloon-tipped catheter is inserted through the skin and threaded through the arteries to the site of the blockage. When the balloon is inflated, it flattens the obstructing plaque against the artery walls and, ideally, widens the passageway for blood.

Balloon angioplasty is most successful on peripheral blockages that are relatively short and well-defined, rather than those that are long or scattered. For peripheral arterial disease, it has proved safe and effective for appropriately selected patients, offering the advantage of faster recovery time than that of bypass surgery. It usually requires only one to two days of hospitalization. However, in about 30 percent of all cases, the leg arteries become reclogged (called restenosis) within a year or two, and angioplasty or surgery may eventually be necessary again. In addition to balloon angioplasty, a variety of new catheter techniques are under investigation for use in the heart and the peripheral arteries, including devices that shave out plaques and laser tips that burn through them.

One surgical option for people with severe blockage involves opening the blocked vessel and stripping the plaque out, a procedure called endarterectomy.

Another is bypass surgery, in which a patient's own vein or a synthetic equivalent is grafted onto the blocked artery so that blood can flow around the obstructed area. The physician's thoughtful evaluation of an individual's profile as a surgical candidate is crucial in deciding upon the optimal treatment.

What makes an individual an appropriate candidate for angioplasty, surgery, or other procedures? As a rule, the potential benefits of intervention must clearly outweigh the risks. Patients with mild intermittent claudication are *not* candidates for surgery or catheterization. People with tissue damage or those who experience severe pain while at rest, however, may require opening of clogged arteries (revascularization) to avoid disability. Between these two extremes, individuals with severe intermittent claudication may benefit from angioplasty or even surgery if the blockages are of a type that can be readily corrected. (See Chapters 24 and 25.)

If major surgery is contemplated for peripheral vascular disease, a full cardiologic evaluation should be ordered. This is recommended because people with peripheral vascular disease may also have coronary artery disease, which may pose an additional risk that should be evaluated and treated appropriately.

AORTIC ANEURYSM

An aneurysm is a weakened area of a blood vessel wall that balloons outward and threatens to rupture.

Figure 17.3
In a dissecting aneurysm, the inner and outer layers of an artery separate, and blood pools between the layers, causing a swelling of the wall.

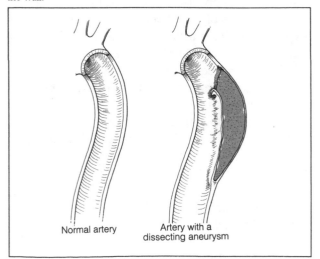

Normal artery   Artery with a
                       dissecting aneurysm

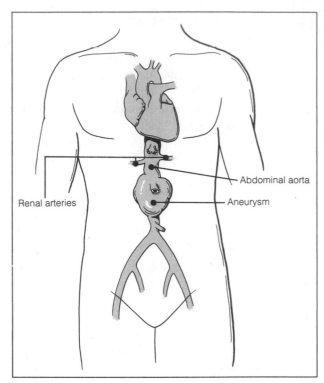

Renal arteries   Abdominal aorta
                                  Aneurysm

Figure 17.4
An aneurysm is the result of a weakening of an artery that causes it to balloon out. The most common site is in the abdominal aorta below the renal arteries.

In the aorta, the main artery leading away from the heart, such a rupture can have devastating consequences, flooding nearby tissues with blood and markedly reducing the supply of blood to the rest of the body, leading to possible immediate death if not treated promptly.

Aortic aneurysms generally fall into three categories. The walls of arteries consist of three tissue layers, with the middle muscular layer providing structural support. If an aneurysm forms as a result of damage to the middle layer, it is a *saccular aneurysm*. A *fusiform aneurysm* may form when the entire circumference of a section of the aortic wall is damaged. If the layers separate as a result of high blood pressure and blood is forced between them, causing the outer wall to swell, it is called a *dissecting aneurysm*. (See Figure 17.3.)

An aortic aneurysm may occur below the renal arteries that supply the kidneys, in the abdominal area (see Figure 17.4), or in the chest (thoracic) area at the arch of the aorta where it first branches off from the heart. The aneurysm is usually caused by atherosclerotic damage to the vessel wall, which weakens its structure. Hypertension may accelerate the process. It may also result from genetic or congenital conditions, such as Marfan syndrome, an inherited disease.

An aneurysm may cause no symptoms, or it may cause abdominal or chest pain. Large aneurysms can also produce more symptoms because they may apply pressure to adjacent blood vessels, nerves, and organs. In these cases, symptoms may include hoarseness, coughing, difficulty swallowing, or shortness of breath.

Perhaps most often, an aneurysm is detected as a result of a routine chest X-ray or when a physician palpitates the abdomen. Echocardiography, computed tomography (CT) scan, and magnetic resonance imaging (MRI) are techniques that can define the size and location of an aneurysm quite precisely. (See Chapter 10.)

The larger the aneurysm, the more likely it is to rupture. Surgical repair is usually imperative for large aneurysms or aneurysms that are expanding. For this reason, patients with small aneurysms are monitored regularly with full exams and imaging techniques. (Patients who spontaneously rupture the aneurysm usually die suddenly.)

Corrective surgery requires clamping the aorta and repairing the affected segment with a woven Dacron patch or graft. The strain on the heart that results when the aorta is clamped presents serious risks of its own in people with cardiovascular disease. For this reason, a person with significant associated coronary artery blockage should be carefully evaluated and may be advised to undergo coronary bypass surgery or angiography *before* the procedure to repair an aortic aneurysm.

OTHER ARTERIAL DISORDERS

RAYNAUD'S PHENOMENON

This vascular disorder is characterized by intermittent coldness, blueness, numbness, tingling, or even pain in the fingers and toes. (Usually it affects both hands simultaneously and the same fingers of each hand.) It is more common in women, who account for 60 to 90 percent of all cases, and those who are thin and high-strung seem to be most vulnerable. Caused by excessive constriction of the tiny arteries that nourish the fingers and toes (vasospasm), it may be triggered by a number of factors, particularly exposure to cold temperatures, emotional stress, smoking cigarettes, and activities such as swimming. When the hands are gradually warmed, normal color and sensation return, often accompanied by some redness and tingling as the blood flows back into tissues. People with this disorder should not apply too much heat to the affected fingers and toes; the use of moderate heat will be effective without the danger of tissue injury.

Raynaud's phenomenon may be associated with various connective tissue disorders, such as rheumatoid arthritis or lupus erythematosis, but in a majority of cases the underlying cause is unknown; when there is no other primary cause, the condition is known as Raynaud's disease.

Treatment of Raynaud's can be difficult and frustrating. Various approaches to drug therapy are under investigation, many of them directed at influencing the biochemical factors that constrict or relax the smooth muscles in the walls of the arteries. Although totally effective drug treatment remains elusive for many sufferers, many others are helped significantly with a calcium channel blocker such as nifedipine. The use of phenoxybenzamine (Dibenzyline), a medication that blocks the effects of adrenaline on blood vessels, may occasionally produce relief of symptoms. (Some beta blockers may aggravate symptoms.)

Usually, therapy consists of measures such as avoiding exposure to cold and wearing thermal gloves and thick socks. Because smoking causes blood vessel constriction, tobacco use should be discontinued. Biofeedback has had mixed results in relieving symptoms. Most individuals with the disease learn to live with it and, when possible, to avoid situations that cause it, but this cannot always be done.

Raynaud's disease doesn't usually cause tissue death, but over a long time, it may cause the skin of the fingers to become shiny and tight-looking, possibly with small ulcers caused by repeated ischemia. In advanced cases, the lining of the small arteries may thicken, and clotting may result, but this is rather rare. When Raynaud's phenomenon is caused by another disorder (such as lupus), effective treatment of the underlying condition may provide relief.

BUERGER'S DISEASE

This relatively rare condition, also called *thromboangiitis obliterans*, occurs overwhelmingly in men aged 20 to 40 who smoke cigarettes. (Only about 5 percent of all cases occur in women.) The disease causes inflammation in the small and medium-sized arteries and veins and eventually produces irreversible changes in the muscle walls of the blood vessels. It's a type of smoking-induced peripheral arterial disease, and the resulting ischemia can be so severe as to warrant amputation of fingers and toes. All smokers experience some degree of clamping down of the peripheral blood vessels (vasoconstriction). It is unknown why people with Buerger's disease experience this to such a severe degree. Genetic or autoimmune defects have been suggested as possible explanations for this condition.

Treatment consists of giving up smoking completely as soon as possible. Other measures may be taken to improve blood flow and treat tissue damage, but without the cessation of cigarette use, progression of the disease is likely.

LIFE-STYLE MEASURES

The well-publicized campaign to control cardiovascular risk factors has already made progress in reducing the toll from heart disease. Unfortunately, the effects of atherosclerosis on the rest of the cardiovascular system have received less attention. Anyone with peripheral arterial blockage, however, is suffering from essentially the same disease, and it is just as important for him or her to control high blood cholesterol, high blood pressure, diabetes, and obesity, and to stop smoking, as it is for the patient with heart disease. (Often, heart disease and peripheral arterial disease occur together—and one should be a warning that risk factors are present for the other.)

Too often, treatment of peripheral vascular disease has neglected to include alteration of life-style risk factors such as cessation of smoking, a low-fat and low-cholesterol diet, regular moderate exercise, weight control, maintenance of appropriate blood pressure, and control of diabetes. To prevent the recurrence or progression of symptoms, implementing these measures must be an integral part of any treatment plan.

CHAPTER 18

STROKE

LAWRENCE M. BRASS, M.D.

INTRODUCTION

Stroke is a form of cardiovascular disease affecting the blood supply to the brain. Also referred to as cerebrovascular disease or apoplexy, strokes actually represent a *group* of diseases that affect about one out of five people in the United States. When physicians speak of stroke, they generally mean there has been a disturbance in brain function, often permanent, caused by either a blockage or a rupture in a vessel supplying blood to the brain.

In order to function properly, nerve cells within the brain must have a continuous supply of blood, oxygen, and glucose (blood sugar). If this supply is impaired, parts of the brain may stop functioning temporarily. If the impairment is severe, or lasts long enough, brain cells die and permanent damage follows. Because the movement and functioning of various parts of the body are controlled by these cells, they are affected also. The symptoms experienced by the patient will depend on which part of the brain is affected.

Stroke is a major health problem in this country. Nearly 500,000 people in the United States have a stroke each year, and nearly a third of these people die during the first few months after their stroke. Of those who survive, about 10 percent are able to return to their previous level of activity, about 50 percent regain enough function to return home and carry on with only limited assistance, and about 40 percent remain institutionalized or require significant assistance in caring for themselves.

While the incidence of stroke has decreased a great deal over the past few decades, there is evidence that this trend may be leveling off.

Stroke is costly. The cost in human terms, to patients and their families, is impossible to estimate. The cost to the U.S. economy—in terms of medical care and lost income—amounts to over $25 billion each year.

Although stroke is often viewed as a disease of the elderly, it sometimes affects younger individuals. The incidence of stroke does increase with age, but nearly a quarter of all strokes occur in people under the age of 60.

Stroke patients are often cared for by neurologists, because of the complex nature of the symptoms caused by damage to the brain. However, strokes are very closely related to heart disease. Heart attacks (myocardial infarctions) and stroke are both caused by diseases of the blood vessels. They share many of the same risk factors, and modifying these risk factors may reduce the possibility of stroke. Many of the therapies used for cardiac disease show promise for some types of stroke. Finally, people who already have coronary disease may be at greater risk for stroke, and vice versa.

HOW THE BRAIN FUNCTIONS

To understand the signs and symptoms of stroke and why they can differ from patient to patient, it is necessary to understand a little about the brain and how it functions. There are literally thousands of possible symptoms that can result from a stroke, depending on which blood vessels and parts of the brain are involved. It is also important to realize that except for a brief period after birth, brain cells are unable to divide and form new cells. When brain cells die, they are not replaced. This is part of the reason for the limited ability of the brain to repair itself after injury, and why recovery from stroke is only partial in many cases. While someone who suffers a heart attack, for example, can lose 10 percent of heart tissue and still run a marathon, losing 10 percent of the tissue in certain parts of the brain can result in a devastating disability.

The human brain is the most complex structure known. It is composed of 100 billion nerve cells, called neurons; each neuron may connect to thousands of other brain cells. The trillions of connections are necessary for the integrative power of the brain. They also control body movements, interpret all sensations (hearing, vision, touch, balance, pain, taste, and smell), and mediate thought and language. Different areas of the brain control different functions. (See Figure 18.1.)

Although the brain represents only 2 percent of the body's weight, it uses about 25 percent of the body's oxygen supply and 70 percent of the glucose (sugar). Unlike muscles, the brain cannot store nu-

trients, and thus it requires a constant supply of glucose and oxygen. If the blood supply is interrupted for as little as 30 seconds, unconsciousness results; permanent brain damage may follow in as little as four minutes. The brain's high metabolic rate, sensitivity to changes in blood flow, and dependence on continuous blood flow are what can make strokes so dangerous. Figure 18.2 shows the major arteries supplying the brain.

The brain can be divided into three areas: *brain stem, cerebellum*, and *cerebrum*. The brain stem controls many of the body's basic functions, including breathing, chewing, swallowing, and eye movements. The major pathways from the cerebrum—the thinking part of the brain—also pass through the brain stem to the body. The cerebellum, attached to the back of the brain stem, coordinates movements and balance.

The cerebrum is divided into two hemispheres, left and right. In general, the left brain receives input (sensations) from the right side of the body and controls movement on the right side, so that a stroke in the right side of the brain will cause left-sided weakness. Conversely, the right brain controls the left side of the body.

Each side of the cerebrum is further divided into four lobes. The *frontal lobes* control motor function, planning, and expression of language. The *temporal*

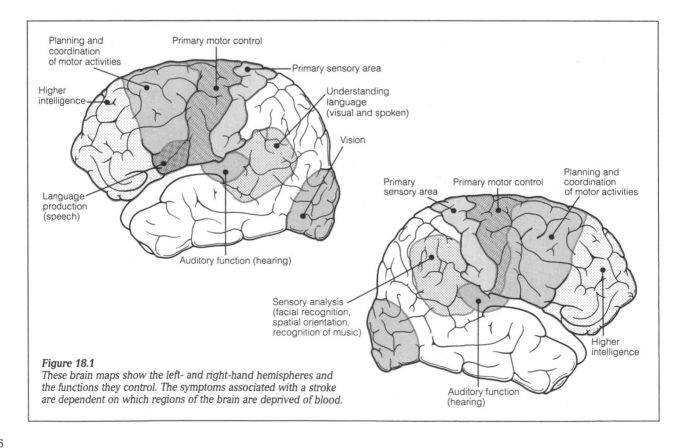

Figure 18.1
These brain maps show the left- and right-hand hemispheres and the functions they control. The symptoms associated with a stroke are dependent on which regions of the brain are deprived of blood.

YALE UNIVERSITY SCHOOL OF MEDICINE HEART BOOK

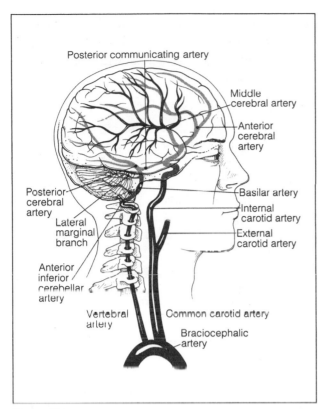

Figure 18.2
Shown are the major arteries feeding the brain. The carotid and its branches (anterior cerebral artery and middle cerebral artery) feed the front part of the brain and most of the cerebral hemispheres (top of the brain). The vertebral arteries join in the back of the head to form the basilar artery. These arteries and their branches supply the brain stem, cerebellum, and back parts of the brain.

lobes are involved with hearing, memory, and behavior. The *parietal lobes* interpret sensation and control understanding of language. The *occipital lobes* perceive and interpret vision. The right and the left sides of the cerebrum are not identical, but rather have specialized functions. In almost all right-handed people and most left-handers, the left brain is "dominant" and performs most language functions. The right side of the brain controls the abilities to understand spatial relations and recognize faces, as well as musical ability. It also helps focus attention.

RISK FACTORS AND STROKE PREVENTION

Given the devastating deficits often associated with a stroke, the need for prevention is obvious. Many of the risk factors for stroke (see box, "Stroke Risk Fac-

tors") can be treated or modified. Doing so may prevent an initial stroke or recurrent strokes, as well as decrease the risk of premature death, which is most often the result of coronary disease.

A number of stroke risk factors are the same as those for heart disease, although their relative importance varies. For example, a high blood cholesterol level is a much more significant risk for heart disease. This distinction is of little practical importance, because both coronary and stroke risk factors should be addressed in patients who are at risk for, or who have suffered, a stroke or a transient ischemic attack. (The latter, also called a TIA or a ministroke, is discussed later in this chapter.)

Three of the greatest risk factors for stroke—high blood pressure (hypertension), heart disease, and diabetes—often do not cause symptoms in their earliest stages. For this reason, it is important that all adults, but especially those with a family history of heart disease or stroke, have regular screening for

Stroke Risk Factors

Characteristics and life-style

Definite
Cigarette smoking
Excessive alcohol consumption
Drug use (cocaine, amphetamines)
Age
Sex
Race
Familial and genetic factors

Possible
Oral contraceptive use
Diet
Personality type
Geographic location
Season
Climate
Socioeconomic factors
Physical inactivity
Obesity
Abnormal blood lipids

Disease or disease markers
Hypertension
Cardiac disease
TIA
Elevated hematocrit
Diabetes mellitus
Sickle cell disease
Elevated fibrinogen concentration
Migraine headaches and migraine equivalents
Carotid bruit

these and other vascular risk factors. Routine check-ups should begin at age 20 and be repeated at least every five years, more frequently in later years or if warranted by the results of the initial screening. Blood pressure should be checked more frequently.

HIGH BLOOD PRESSURE

A major risk factor common to both coronary heart disease and stroke, high blood pressure is present in 50 to 70 percent of stroke cases, depending primarily on the type of stroke. The long-term effects of the increased pressure damage the walls of the arteries, making them more vulnerable to thickening or narrowing (atherosclerosis) or rupture.

There is no specific blood pressure reading that is considered normal, but rather a range. Most experts agree, however, that a reading greater than 140/90 mm Hg is abnormal, and anyone with such a reading should see a physician. But even mild elevations in blood pressure are associated with an increased risk for stroke. Sometimes mildly elevated blood pressure can be controlled by life-style modification, but medication is often needed. Although the patient may feel no different, control of blood pressure is associated with a marked decrease in the occurrence of stroke. (See Chapter 12.)

HEART DISEASE

Just as strokes are a strong risk factor for heart disease, heart disease is a strong risk factor for stroke, although only for one type of stroke, ischemic strokes. Heart disease is associated with stroke in two ways. First, damage to the heart (as, for example, from a heart attack) may make it more likely that clots will form within the heart. These clots can break loose and travel to the brain, causing a cardioembolic stroke. Heart disease and stroke are also associated because they are both manifestations of atherosclerotic disease in the blood vessels. If the blood vessels feeding the heart (the coronary arteries) are diseased, it is likely that arteries to the brain are also affected.

Patients with evidence of coronary artery disease, congestive heart failure, left ventricular hypertrophy (enlargement of the left side of the heart), disease of the heart valves, or arrhythmias (irregular heart rhythms) have a several-fold increase in the risk of stroke.

Several recent studies suggest that people with atrial fibrillation who take daily doses of either aspirin or warfarin (Coumadin) have a reduction of up to 80 percent in their risk of stroke. These findings suggest that an estimated 20,000 to 50,000 strokes might be prevented each year if all people with this condition had prophylactic drug treatment.

SMOKING

Smoking facilitates atherosclerosis and appears to be an independent risk factor for strokes that result from a clot. It also seems to be a risk for strokes that result from cerebral hemorrhage.

Men in Framingham, Massachusetts—a community studied extensively for cardiovascular disease—who smoked more than 40 cigarettes a day had twice the stroke risk of men who smoked fewer than 10. In a large Harvard Medical School study of women, the number of cigarettes smoked was found to be directly related to stroke risk. Women smoking more than 25 cigarettes a day had a 2.7 times greater risk of stroke from a clot or embolus and a 9.8 times greater risk of a hemorrhagic stroke. Data from both the Framingham Heart Study and the Honolulu Heart Study indicate that one can significantly reduce stroke risk by stopping smoking. Five years after they stop, ex-smokers have a stroke risk equal to that of non-smokers.

DIABETES

People with diabetes are at greater risk for stroke, just as they are for heart disease. Women with diabetes are at an even greater risk than men. High blood pressure compounds the risk. Although treatment of diabetes has not been conclusively shown to reduce risk, it is known that control of high blood sugar (hyperglycemia) can reduce the severity of cerebral damage during a stroke. For this and other reasons, diabetics should keep their blood glucose levels under strict control.

CHOLESTEROL

Studies have found a link between high blood lipid levels and atherosclerosis in cerebral arteries, but it is still unclear whether high cholesterol levels significantly increase stroke risk. They do, however, increase heart disease risk, so efforts should be made to reduce them.

OBESITY AND INACTIVITY

Obesity and a sedentary life-style are risk factors for stroke primarily because they increase the risk of high blood pressure, heart disease, and diabetes. They may also be independent stroke risk factors. Losing weight and following a moderate exercise regimen can help reverse these risks.

ORAL CONTRACEPTIVES AND ESTROGEN REPLACEMENT THERAPY

The role of oral contraceptives in stroke risk is still inconclusive, primarily because most research has looked at the effects of high-dose estrogen pills, and most women now use lower-dose preparations. Estrogen is believed to promote blood clotting; lower-dose estrogen preparations are thought to minimize this effect. Because studies have found no increase in current risk of stroke or heart attack in women who previously used oral contraceptives, it is believed that the pill does not promote atherosclerosis.

Several retrospective studies have suggested that oral contraceptive use is associated with an increase in stroke risk, while other studies have only found a significant risk of brain hemorrhage in women over age 35 who take the pill *and smoke*. Smokers who have migraine headaches and take oral contraceptives may be at a particularly high risk of stroke. Experts usually advise women who smoke not to use oral contraceptives—or better, to quit smoking.

In contrast, there is evidence to suggest that estrogen replacement therapy for postmenopausal women may slow the atherosclerotic process. In this group the use of estrogens may actually lower the risk of stroke (and heart disease).

HISTORY OF TRANSIENT ISCHEMIC ATTACKS (TIAs)

Researchers are learning that these "ministrokes" may be the most reliable warning of an imminent "full" stroke. Between 10 and 50 percent of strokes, depending on the type, are preceded by TIAs; if not treated, about one-third of all people who have a TIA go on to have a stroke within five years. TIAs are also indicators of potential coronary heart disease: Each year, 5 percent of those who have had at least one TIA have a heart attack. Anyone who has had a TIA should do whatever possible to reduce other risk factors. Drug therapy or surgery may be warranted to reduce the risk of subsequent TIAs, stroke, or heart attack.

HEREDITY AND FAMILY HISTORY

The chance of having a stroke is higher for people who have a family history of this disease. Part of the risk is due to inherited risk factors and part to family life-styles (eating and exercise habits, for example).

The presence of inherited risk factors does not mean that risk cannot be lowered. In one study, for instance, the hereditable risk for vascular disease was mostly due to a susceptibility to the effects of cigarette smoking. When cigarette smoking was eliminated, the hereditable effect was significantly lowered.

AGE

The risk of stroke rises significantly with age. After 55, it more than doubles with each passing decade. Each year, about 1 percent of people between ages 65 and 74 have a stroke—and 5 to 8 percent of people in that age group who have had a TIA go on to stroke.

Although risk associated with advancing age cannot be changed, it is an important factor in assessing stroke risk and planning preventive therapies.

AN EARLIER STROKE

Because the same factors that caused a first stroke are likely to cause a subsequent one, the risk of stroke for someone who has already had one is increased.

CAROTID BRUIT

A bruit is a noise made by turbulent flow in a blood vessel that usually can be heard only with a stethoscope. The most common cause is a narrowing of an artery because of atherosclerosis. Bruits tend to occur in the large arteries of the body, including the carotid artery in the neck. Even in patients without other symptoms, carotid stenosis (narrowing) and carotid bruits are associated with an increased stroke rate of 5 percent each year. Over the course of a lifetime, the cumulative stroke risk may be quite high.

The increased risk associated with the presence of a carotid bruit has prompted some physicians to recommend a surgical procedure called carotid endarterectomy to open the narrowing. Initial results of this procedure have proved disappointing in terms of preventing strokes. Patients with asymptomatic bruit should, if possible, be considered for referral to a medical center that has special expertise in cerebrovascular disease and is participating in a well-designed clinical trial.

OTHER RISK FACTORS

Other factors influence stroke risk, although to a lesser extent. These include an elevated hematocrit (number of red cells in the blood), geographic location (especially the southeastern United States, which is sometimes called the "stroke belt"), lower socioeconomic status, Type A personality (see Chapter 8), use of cocaine and amphetamines, and high alcohol consumption. Stroke deaths seem to occur more often during periods of extreme heat or cold.

TRANSIENT ISCHEMIC ATTACKS (TIAs)

A transient ischemic attack is a localized neurological problem caused by ischemia (decreased blood flow) that completely resolves within 24 hours. Most last only a few minutes. People who suffer a TIA often pass it off as nothing, especially when it goes away almost as quickly as it came. The more neurologists learn about the cause of TIAs, the more clear it becomes that a TIA presents a unique opportunity to prevent a stroke.

The importance of a TIA is not in its neurological symptoms—by definition, they disappear. Rather it is that a third of all patients will go on to have a stroke. TIAs represent about 10 percent of all cerebrovascular disease. Up to half of patients who suffer an ischemic stroke will report having had a TIA, and may never have sought treatment. TIAs also identify a group of people at high risk for heart attack. It is imperative that anyone who experiences a TIA consult a doctor for both neurological and cardiovascular evaluation. The key is to make the diagnosis and work to lower the risk.

The symptoms of a TIA are similar to those of a stroke—weakness or numbness on one side of the body, inability to speak or understand language, or lack of coordination—except they don't last as long. Any combination of the symptoms described for stroke, lasting more than a few seconds, should be considered as a possible TIA. (See box, "Common Warning Signs of Stroke and Transient Ischemic Attack.")

One additional common symptom of a TIA is transient monocular blindness, also called *amaurosis fugax* (flight of darkness). This is a brief change or distortion of vision in one eye that is often described as a misting, clouding, blurring, spottiness, or the sensation that a blind is being drawn down over the eye.

The evaluation of a patient for a TIA is similar to that for a stroke. Most patients will be hospitalized

Common Warning Signs of Stroke and Transient Ischemic Attack (TIA)

Because brain cells can die very quickly after a stroke, it is crucial to recognize warning signs of an impending stroke and get to a hospital quickly. Since the brain controls hundreds of activities, the range of stroke symptoms is broad. In spite of this, there are several common warning signs of stroke or TIA:

- Sudden weakness or numbness of the face, arm, and leg on one side of the body
- Loss of speech, or trouble speaking or understanding speech
- Dimness or loss of vision, particularly in only one eye or half of both eyes
- Sudden onset of blurred or double vision
- Unexplained dizziness
- Sudden onset of unsteadiness, lack of coordination, difficulty walking, or falling
- Sudden excruciating headache
- Recent change in personality or mental abilities, including memory loss

Although many of these symptoms can be caused by other diseases, the sudden onset of new neurological symptoms should prompt a person to seek immediate medical attention.

because of the concern of a subsequent stroke and the need for immediate treatment should one occur. Patients at low risk of stroke and those whose general medical condition precludes aggressive treatment may be followed on an outpatient basis.

The first step is to consider, and exclude, other disease that can mimic a TIA. (See box, "Conditions That Can Mimic a TIA.") Many of these diseases are serious neurological problems that also may require urgent treatment. After other diseases have been excluded, the physician will try to determine the mechanism of the TIA in order to help guide decisions about treatment. Most TIAs are due to either an embolus (blood clot) or restricted blood flow—often caused by a narrowing in the carotid artery. Brief TIAs (lasting less than 10 minutes) are commonly associated with carotid stenosis (artery narrowing), while longer-duration TIAs (lasting more than one hour) are more often caused by embolism.

If a TIA is due to restricted blood flow because of a carotid artery stenosis, surgery may be indicated.

Conditions That Can Mimic a TIA

Migraine
Seizure
Hypoglycemia (low blood sugar)
Other forms of stroke
Brain tumor
Arteriovenous malformation
Multiple sclerosis
Incipient syncope (fainting)
Orthostatic hypotension (low blood pressure)
Cardiac arrhythmia (irregular heartbeat)
Amnesia
Narcolepsy/cataplexy (disorders of excessive
    sleepiness)
Intracranial inflammation (e.g., brain infection)
Periodic paralysis
Pressure neuropathy (nerve compression)
Dizziness of uncertain cause
Anxiety
Hyperventilation
Labyrinthine (inner-ear) disease

If it is due to an embolus from the heart (as may occur with various abnormal heart rhythms), even if there is a carotid stenosis, surgery may not be appropriate. (For treatment options, see the discussion of long-term treatment of TIA and stroke elsewhere in this chapter.)

ISCHEMIC STROKE

There are two broad categories of stroke: *ischemic* and *hemorrhagic*. Ischemic strokes are caused by a lack of blood flow to the brain and account for about 70 percent of all strokes. (See Figure 18.3.) Hemorrhagic strokes, discussed later in this chapter, are caused by bleeding into the brain or adjacent tissues.

Within the category of ischemia, there are several subcategories of stroke. One common type, called *cerebral atherothrombosis* (also referred to as large artery disease), is caused by a clot (thrombus) that blocks blood flow in an artery. The narrowing leads to a low flow state referred to as *watershed (or distal field) ischemia*. (See Figure 18.4.) If the resulting lack of oxygen results in death of brain tissue and permanent damage, the term *cerebral infarction* is used.

Clots usually do not occur in healthy arteries, but tend to form at or adjacent to an area of a vessel damaged by atherosclerosis. In the atherosclerotic process, plaque—an amalgam of fatty substances, cholesterol, waste products of cells, calcium, and a blood-clotting material called fibrin—builds up as thick, irregular deposits on the inner lining of an artery. The irregular surfaces that plaque deposits create provide ideal places for clots to form and grow. In some cases, plaque deposits themselves can grow so large that they obstruct the opening (lumen) of the blood vessel and block the flow of blood. Surgery is often indicated to open these arteries.

Atherothrombic strokes are often preceded by TIAs, and they tend to occur at times when blood pressure is low—at night during sleep, or early in the morning before major activities start.

Another kind of ischemic stroke involving a clot is called a *cerebral embolism* or *embolic stroke*. This type is caused by a wandering clot (embolus) that forms in one part of the body, breaks loose (in whole or part), and travels in the bloodstream until it lodges in an artery in the brain or in a vessel leading to the brain. (See Figure 18.5.) Emboli can be formed from

Figure 18.3

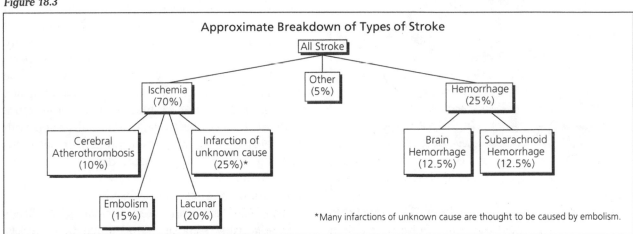

Approximate Breakdown of Types of Stroke

*Many infarctions of unknown cause are thought to be caused by embolism.

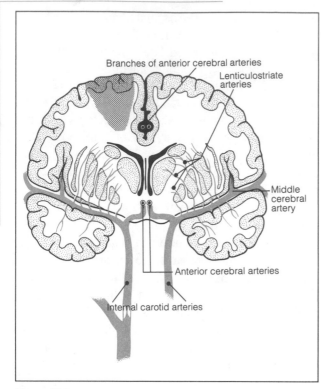

Figure 18.4
A watershed (or distal field) stroke is the result of narrowing of the large arteries feeding the brain.

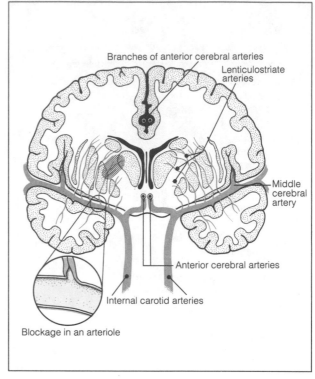

Figure 18.6
A lacunar stroke is the result of the complete blockage of an arteriole, the very small end of an artery that penetrates deep into the brain.

Figure 18.5
An embolic stroke is the result of a blood clot that forms in another part of the body and travels in the bloodstream until it lodges in an artery in the brain.

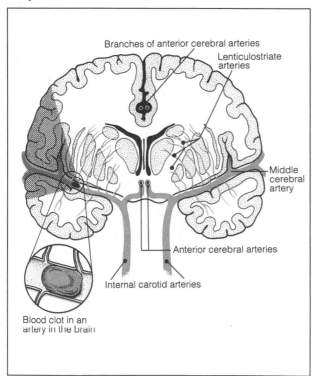

calcium, cholesterol, air, blood proteins, platelets, or by-products of an infection of the heart's inner lining (endocarditis). (See Chapter 15.) It is believed that most embolic strokes involve clots from the heart or the carotid arteries.

The most common cardiac conditions associated with emboli are atrial fibrillation, valvular disease, the presence of a prosthetic heart valve, endocarditis, congestive heart failure, and myocardial infarction. In atrial fibrillation, the two upper chambers of the heart (atria) quiver rather than beat effectively. Because blood is not pumped out of the atria (upper part of the heart) completely it tends to pool and form clots. One-third of all people with atrial fibrillation will have a stroke at some time, and the majority of these strokes will be embolic. Embolic strokes are probably the most common of ischemic strokes. (Many that have no proven cause are thought to be caused by embolism.) The use of anticoagulant drugs may help reduce the risk of clot formation—before or after such a stroke. (In fact, almost all people with atrial fibrillation should be on some form of long-term aspirin or anticoagulant drug therapy. See Chapter 23.)

The third form of stroke caused by blood clotting is called a *lacunar infarction* or *lacunar stroke*. These strokes are the result of occlusion (complete blockage) of arterioles, the very small ends of the arteries that penetrate deep into the brain. (See Figure 18.6.) The small size of the vessels sometimes makes lacunar strokes difficult to diagnose; in addition, some have no noticeable symptoms. There are, however, several classic syndromes that suggest the possibility of a lacunar infarction. The most common is a *pure motor stroke*, in which damage is confined to the main cabling system for motor signals from the brain to the spinal cord (internal capsule). As a result, the patient develops one-sided weakness without other symptoms. Similarly, a lacunar stroke in the thalamus (the main sensory relay center to the brain) can cause a *pure sensory stroke*. Surgery and the use of anticoagulant drugs do not appear to help a great deal in the short-term management of people with lacunar disease. Treatment concentrates on modification of long-term risk.

In spite of the most aggressive workup available in the 1990s, the mechanism of ischemic stroke remains unknown in over a third of all cases. Many of these cases of *infarction of unknown cause* appear to be due to embolism. Refinements in imaging technology and earlier evaluation of patients may help categorize these strokes better in the future.

At present, however, much can be determined by the specific symptoms and signs that a patient manifests. Defining the mechanism of a stroke can help determine prognosis, suggest appropriate therapy, and help the physician prepare the family for what to expect. For example, patients with lacunar stroke often recover their strength better than those who suffer other types; thrombotic strokes tend to worsen during the acute period before recovery begins; and embolic strokes are associated with a high rate of recurrence within the first few weeks.

HEMORRHAGIC STROKES

Hemorrhage accounts for about 20 to 25 percent of all strokes. In these strokes, blood seeps from a hole in a blood vessel wall into either the brain itself (intracerebral hemorrhage) or the space around the brain (subarachnoid hemorrhage).

BRAIN OR INTRACEREBRAL HEMORRHAGE

In this type of hemorrhagic stroke, blood leaks from small vessels at the base of the brain. Long-term exposure to high blood pressure is thought to weaken the walls of these small arteries, and eventually they burst. The term "cerebral" (meaning related to the part of the brain called the cerebrum) is also used.

About two-thirds of patients with an intracerebral hemorrhage have a history of hypertension; diabetes and atherosclerosis accelerate the damage. Other causes of bleeding into the brain include brain tumor, trauma, arteriovenous malformation (AVM), and stimulant drugs such as amphetamines and cocaine.

Intracerebral hemorrhage accounts for about 10 to 15 percent of all strokes. The onset of symptoms is usually acute, with severe headaches and decreased consciousness. Other symptoms depend on the size and location of the hemorrhage. One type of brain hemorrhage, *cerebellar* hemorrhage, is especially important to recognize because prompt evaluation, often followed by surgery, can be lifesaving. Cerebellar hemorrhage means bleeding into the cerebellum (rather than the cerebrum)—the part of the brain that coordinates movement and balance. Its symptoms usually include disequilibrium or dizziness, incoordination (especially trouble in walking), headache, nausea, and vomiting.

Treatment and prognosis of intracerebral hemorrhage varies with the size and location of the hemorrhage within the brain and the condition of the patient. A hematoma (blood that has clotted) near the surface may be easily evacuated (removed surgically), but deep bleeding may damage critical structures within the brain and pose a higher surgical risk. Whether surgery is performed or not, medical management centers on respiratory care, blood pressure management, and minimizing pressure within the skull. Seizures sometimes follow the hemorrhage, so anticonvulsant medications are often added to the regimen.

SUBARACHNOID HEMORRHAGE

Subarachnoid hemorrhage is usually caused by an aneurysm or a vascular malformation (described below). In addition to the damage caused by the blood shooting out of the artery, damage can be further worsened by the mass of blood pushing up against adjacent areas of the brain and blood vessels, or through secondary effects of the extruded blood on the brain's blood vessels (vasospasm).

The classic clinical feature of a subarachnoid hemorrhage is the sudden onset of an excruciating headache. It is often associated with a stiff neck, change in consciousness, nausea and vomiting, diffuse intellectual impairment, and seizures. Other symptoms may occur, depending on the location and size of the hemorrhage.

Patients with symptoms suggestive of a subarachnoid hemorrhage should have a CT scan, which will indicate the presence of blood in about 80 percent of cases. If the CT scan is negative or equivocal, a spinal tap (lumbar puncture) should be performed to look for evidence of bleeding.

ANEURYSM

An aneurysm is an outpouching in the wall of a blood vessel that forms at a point where the wall is weak. Although the weakness may be present at birth, the aneurysm usually forms and grows later in life. The outpouching may go unnoticed for years, or may suddenly rupture, in which case it can sometimes be fatal. The peak age range for an aneurysm rupture is between 40 and 60 years old. Aneurysms sometimes run in families; some are associated with other diseases. About a quarter of patients with one aneurysm will have additional ones.

The major impact of an aneurysm is the result of the rupture and bleeding, but the event may be followed in a few days by a secondary constriction of blood vessels, known as vasospasm. The vasospasm may be so severe that it impairs blood flow to the brain and causes a secondary ischemic stroke. Some advances have been made recently in treating vasospasm by using medications such as nimodipine (Nimotop), increasing the blood volume (usually done with intravenous fluids), or using medications to increase blood pressure.

An aneurysm can be treated surgically by placing a clamp at the base. The timing and type of surgery varies with the size and location of the aneurysm, the extent of the bleeding, and the neurological status of the patient. Under ideal circumstances, the surgery should be performed within 48 hours after the hemorrhage. This eliminates the risk of rebleeding. Surgery attempted five to ten days after a subarachnoid hemorrhage may cause, or worsen, vasospasm.

Occasionally an aneurysm will be found before it ruptures. It may be found because it is has pushed against important nerves or areas of the brain, causing pain or other symptoms, or because clots formed in the pouch of the aneurysm have traveled downstream and occluded a blood vessel, causing a TIA or stroke. Surgical clipping is usually recommended for unruptured aneurysms more than 10 mm (two-fifths of an inch) in diameter.

ARTERIOVENOUS MALFORMATION

An arteriovenous malformation (AVM) is a tangle of arteries and veins without the small vessels (capillaries) that normally connect the two. The walls of the vessels are often thin and have high rates of blood flow, conditions that predispose to bleeding. AVMs may produce symptoms by bleeding, putting pressure on structures within the brain, or shunting blood away from normal areas of the brain.

Small AVMs may not need to be treated, but when they are large or they cause significant symptoms, attempts should be made to obliterate them. This can be done surgically, by using radiation, or with a relatively new radiologic technique that delivers small pellets of glue that occlude the vessels leading to, and within, the AVM. Unfortunately many AVMs tend to recur.

Despite dramatic advances in our ability to diagnose the causes of intracerebral hemorrhages, the results of treatment remain disappointing. Mortality remains high, and problems in those surviving are often severe.

OTHER FORMS OF STROKE

In addition to the major causes of stroke described above, there are a number of other causes, including the two most common ones: cardiac arrest and hematomas adjacent to the brain. In cardiac arrest, the heart stops pumping blood or does not pump effectively, and the brain is deprived of both oxygen and glucose. Although the entire brain is affected, certain areas are more vulnerable. Memory and coordination are among the most frequent deficits after this type of stroke.

Hematomas—accumulations of blood that are the result of hemorrhage—sometimes occur in the outermost covering of the brain, the subdural or epidural layers. These are usually caused by injury, but may occur spontaneously, especially in the elderly. In this type of stroke, surgery can usually correct the problem by removing the clot, and may be lifesaving.

DIAGNOSING AND ASSESSING STROKE

Anyone experiencing symptoms of a stroke requires immediate medical help. Even if the ultimate diagnosis is not stroke, many diseases that can mimic a stroke are also medical emergencies.

If a physician cannot be contacted by telephone, the person should be taken to the nearest hospital emergency department at once. Many types of stroke require immediate treatment, and most of the promising new therapies for stroke are effective only if started within a few hours of the onset of symptoms.

A variety of diagnostic tools are available to the physician, from history-taking and trained observation to sophisticated radiologic imaging studies. The tests performed will vary with the type of stroke, its severity, and the planned therapies. Regardless of the tests used, the goals are the same: to exclude nonvascular reasons for the neurological symptoms and to pinpoint the cause, location, and extent of the stroke.

HISTORY AND EXAMINATION

Perhaps the most important diagnostic tool is the initial history and physical examination of the patient. Critical details about the medical history may have to be obtained from a family member if the patient is disoriented or unable to speak.

During the examination, the physician will test a variety of neurological functions: orientation, memory, emotional control, motor skills, tactile sensation, hearing, vision, and the ability to read, write, and speak. Using knowledge of brain anatomy and function, a neurologist can usually identify the area of the brain that is damaged by noting the specific symptoms. For example, difficulty with walking and balance is likely due to damage to the cerebellum. Specific deficits on one side of the body point to damage in the opposite cerebral hemisphere.

The general examination should also include a search for evidence of high blood pressure, coronary heart disease, or disease in other parts of the vascular system. Using findings from the history, neurological examination, and general examination, the physician will formulate an initial opinion about the location and type of stroke. Laboratory and radiological tests will then be ordered to help confirm or exclude the physician's initial suspicions.

LABORATORY TESTS

Tests are usually done on samples of blood, urine, and, occasionally, cerebrospinal fluid (fluid around the brain and spinal cord). They focus initially on excluding conditions that can mimic or worsen a stroke, such as infection or low levels of blood sugar. Screen-

ing may also be done for diabetes, elevated blood cholesterol, bleeding disorders, and abnormalities in blood proteins—risk factors for cardiac disease and recurrent stroke.

IMAGING STUDIES

Computed tomography (CT) scans and magnetic resonance imaging (MRI) are techniques that produce anatomic pictures of the brain. Computed tomography scans use multiple X-rays and computer reconstruction to create cross-sectional images of internal structures. Magnetic resonance imaging uses magnetic fields to create images. Each has advantages in different circumstances. Because these scans can delineate (and thus help exclude) such conditions as tumors, abscesses, and bleeding from trauma, they are often done early after a stroke. They can usually differentiate ischemic strokes from those that are due to bleeding.

The studies are often repeated several days after the onset of a stroke to determine its size and because the full extent of the damage may not be seen until then. If a patient's condition worsens, the tests may be repeated in order to help determine the cause of the deterioration.

Magnetic resonance devices are also capable of spectroscopically (based on spectrums of light) measuring chemicals within the brain. These measurements may be important in determining the mechanism of a stroke and the prognosis and best therapy for a particular stroke victim.

CARDIAC EVALUATION

An electrocardiogram (ECG) is usually the first step in a cardiac evaluation. An ultrasound examination (echocardiogram) of the heart may help pinpoint a source of an embolus.

ANGIOGRAPHY

Angiography involves the injection of a dye or contrast medium into an artery in order to study the blood vessels via X-ray pictures. It can be used to detect many of the abnormalities that cause stroke, including narrowing or occlusion of a blood vessel, embolus, atherosclerosis, dissections, arteriovenous malformations, and aneurysms.

Because angiography is an invasive technique, in that it introduces instruments and substances into the body, it may be associated with serious complications. These include inducing or worsening a stroke, allergic reactions to the contrast medium, and, very rarely, death.

Newer techniques using magnetic resonance imaging can be used to produce an angiogram noninvasively. As these images continue to improve in quality, they may replace conventional angiography.

ULTRASOUND

Ultrasound is a noninvasive technique that uses sound waves and their echoes to visualize structures and blood flow within the body. Two types of ultrasound are used in stroke diagnosis: carotid ultrasound (to measure flow in the carotid arteries) and transcranial Doppler (to measure flow in the intracranial arteries). Although the anatomical information it produces is not as precise as that obtained through angiography, ultrasound has the advantages of being painless and risk-free. It is often used to screen patients before invasive studies are done.

BLOOD-FLOW STUDIES

Blood-flow techniques—such as positron emission tomography (PET), single-photon-emission computed tomography (SPECT), and xenon inhalation—provide information on blood flow in the brain. These tests may show changes immediately after the onset of stroke symptoms, while computed tomography or magnetic resonance imaging may remain negative for several hours or days after a stroke.

The role of these tests is still being defined, and they are generally available only in large medical centers. They may be useful in determining the mechanism of a stroke (e.g., carotid stenosis) or determining prognosis early in the hospitalization.

STROKE TREATMENT

The primary goals of stroke treatment have changed, thanks to new drug therapy. Doctors now attempt to halt the progression of the stroke and to prevent recurrence. In years past, when it was believed that all brain cells died after about four minutes without blood flow, stroke was considered to be largely untreatable. Spurred on by observations in animals that at least partial recovery can occur after even an hour

of complete ischemia (lack of oxygen), researchers have discovered that regions of the brain with very minimal blood flow can survive—although they do not function normally—for several hours or perhaps days. These viable cells surrounding an infarct, called the "ischemic penumbra," are the focus of numerous experimental drug therapies aimed at restoring blood flow or preserving cell function.

As researchers learn more about the mechanisms of stroke, they are realizing that it is not simply a lack of blood flow that causes death of tissue; a progression of other processes (including inflammation and toxic buildup), called the ischemic cascade, may play an even greater role in causing lasting neurologic damage. Doctors believe that if they can interrupt this cascade, they may be able to prevent the devastating brain damage that was once the inevitable consequence of stroke.

TREATMENT OF ACUTE STROKE

Most treatment of stroke during the acute phase centers on maintaining fluids and electrolytes (chemical substances in the blood, such as sodium and potassium), avoiding low blood pressure (hypotension), and avoiding the secondary complications of stroke and paralysis. The latter includes pneumonia, urinary tract infections, muscle contractures, and pressure breakdown of the skin (bedsores). The physician will also attempt to anticipate and avert deterioration after a stroke. This will require constant monitoring and evaluation and may necessitate a number of laboratory tests.

Anticoagulant medications such as heparin are sometimes used to treat an acute ischemic stroke. While heparin does not dissolve existing clots, it can prevent the formation of new ones. Thus it may help prevent subsequent strokes, which occur in up to 20 percent of ischemic stroke cases.

Because heparin can increase some patients' tendency to bleed, its use is often restricted to those with the highest risk of recurrent stroke: patients with a progressing stroke, more than one TIA, or a cardiac source of embolism (often seen with myocardial infarction, atrial fibrillation, or valvular diseases). Related drugs known as heparinoids are now being evaluated and appear to be at least as effective, with a lower risk of bleeding.

Surgery is usually not used to treat an acute stroke, although it may be indicated for a hemorrhagic stroke (subarachnoid and brain hemorrhages) or a recent blockage of a carotid artery.

LONG-TERM TREATMENT OF TIA AND STROKE

After the acute phase of a TIA or stroke has passed, emphasis is placed not only on recovery and rehabilitation but also on preventing further vascular events, including ischemic stroke and myocardial infarction. Therapy may include modification of risk factors, drugs, or surgery, or a combination.

Risk factors are discussed earlier in this chapter. Treatment of high blood pressure and diabetes, along with smoking cessation, are probably the most important. The effects on stroke risk of modifying other factors—controlling weight, lowering cholesterol, and moderating alcohol intake—are not as well studied, but these modifications are generally recommended. Treatment of additional risk factors is best considered on an individual basis in consultation with a physician.

ANTIPLATELET MEDICATIONS

Platelets are cell fragments that circulate in the blood and play a key role in the formation of clots. Medications that inhibit platelet function, such as aspirin, lessen the tendency of blood to clot. Patients at high risk of stroke are known to benefit in several ways from taking aspirin daily. Aspirin therapy lowers the risk of stroke and stroke-related death.

Unfortunately, aspirin therapy is complicated by the fact that the optimal dose is unknown. If the dose is too low, the aspirin will not have an effect on the platelets; if it is too high, it may cause the blood vessel walls to release chemicals, resulting in the formation of more clots. Most authorities recommend between 325 and 1,200 mg aspirin per day (one to four tablets), a higher dose than that usually recommended to prevent a heart attack. More recent evidence suggests that doses as low as 80 mg per day may also have a protective effect.

Although aspirin has been shown to reduce the risk of stroke, it may not be appropriate for all patients. For example, it should not be used in patients whose blood pressure is not normal. Before beginning any treatment, even as simple as aspirin therapy, a patient should consult his or her physician. Aspirin should always be part of a larger program directed at all aspects of vascular disease prevention.

Ticlopidine, a relatively new antiplatelet medication, appears to be about 15 percent more effective than aspirin in reducing the risk of stroke in people who have had a TIA or minor stroke. This slight improvement in efficacy must be weighed against more serious side effects such as rash, diarrhea, and lowered white cell counts, and higher cost.

ANTICOAGULANTS

Like antiplatelet medications, anticoagulant drugs also interfere with the clotting mechanism, in this case by affecting the action of enzymes necessary for clotting. A commonly used anticoagulant is warfarin (Coumadin). Because it is a more powerful drug than aspirin, it is usually recommended only when aspirin therapy has failed or when it is clear that the source of the clots is the heart (e.g., when the patient has atrial fibrillation or has had a myocardial infarction or valvular heart disease).

Patients taking warfarin must be carefully monitored via periodic blood tests, known as prothrombin time tests, that measure the speed of clotting. Without monitoring, the dosage may be too low, increasing the risk of stroke, or too high, increasing the risk of bleeding complications. Patients also need to be aware that certain medications and foods (leafy green vegetables such as spinach and other foods high in Vitamin C) can alter the effectiveness of warfarin. However, dietary restrictions are not usually advised for patients on anticoagulants.

SURGERY

The goal in surgery is to provide a pathway for blood to get to the brain. This is most commonly done using a procedure known as carotid endarterectomy, in which a stenosis (narrowing) or ulceration of an atherosclerotic plaque in the carotid artery is removed.

Similar interim results were released in 1991 from two large studies of carotid endarterectomy. Participants in the study had experienced either a recent TIA or a nondisabling stroke, and each had a carotid-artery blockage of more than 70 percent. Participants who underwent endarterectomies showed a sixfold reduction in strokes, compared to those who did not have surgery. This dramatic result suggests that carotid surgery is likely to play a key role in the prevention of recurrent stroke in the coming years.

There are, however, several important points that should be made in interpreting these results. First, the carotid narrowing must be in a particular portion of the artery. For example, if a patient has a small stroke in the left brain hemisphere, this is not an indication for surgery on a narrowed right carotid artery. Secondly, these studies were carried out at leading medical centers that have low complication rates. Thus, the results suggest that carotid surgery, in the best of circumstances, reduces the risk of stroke. Whether this will hold true for all hospitals remains to be demonstrated. Finally, as physicians better understand stroke risk factors, it may be possible to use even more precise criteria to select patients for surgery. For example, even considering the group of people with the most severe carotid narrowing, there are many who will not have a stroke. Using risk stratification models and blood flow measurements, it may be possible to identify people who do not require surgery, even though they may have a carotid-artery blockage of more than 90 percent.

Despite the encouraging results of these two studies, there are still no answers for people with a carotid artery narrowing of less than 70 percent or for those who have not yet had a stroke or TIA. These questions are being investigated actively in clinical studies, and results should be available in the next few years.

Although conceptually appealing, the removal of a carotid stenosis is not without risk: There is a 10 percent complication rate across the United States. There is evidence to suggest that only medical centers where the complications and mortality rates are less than 6 percent should be performing the procedure.

Another way of providing blood to the brain is via a procedure known as extracranial-intracranial bypass, which involves connecting an artery from the scalp to one on the surface of the brain through a surgical opening in the skull. This procedure was recently tested in a large cooperative trial and was not demonstrated to be beneficial; it is not recommended at this time.

RECOVERY FROM A STROKE

Recovery after a stroke is dependent on many factors: the specific site of the brain injury, the general health of the patient, his or her personality and will, family support, and the care received. The best recovery is usually seen in a patient who has had a small ischemic stroke. Large subarachnoid hemorrhages pose the most difficult challenge for recovery. Nevertheless, there are few solid rules for prognosis, and each case should be considered on an individual basis.

Caring for a patient after a stroke is a multifaceted and often complex process. The care must include helping the patient recover from deficits (such as weakness of an arm or leg or an inability to speak clearly) and learn to function with any losses, dealing with the patient's emotional issues and those of the family, and preventing recurrent strokes.

REHABILITATION

In the immediate poststroke period, medical personnel care for the patient's physical needs in order to reduce the risk of complications. Patients who have difficulty swallowing, for example, may need to be fed intravenously until they are able to swallow water and food adequately. Most patients will be able to get out of bed for increasingly longer periods within two to three days and be able to leave the hospital in ten days to two weeks.

Planning for rehabilitation should begin as soon after the stroke as possible. Early attention to weak limbs can greatly improve the chances of a successful recovery. Simple measures such as frequent position changes while in bed and exercise of the paralyzed areas (including moving the arms and legs by physical therapists, nurses, and family members) can improve the circulation, maintain joint flexibility, maintain normal muscle tone, and get the family and patient involved in the recovery process. Physical therapy generally starts within four or five days after the stroke.

The rehabilitation process becomes more active as the patient becomes medically stable (usually within a day or two). Passive range-of-motion exercises, in which a family member, nurse, or physical therapist performs most of the movement, are replaced by active range-of-motion routines, in which the patient strives to regain strength in the affected limbs.

The efforts of the rehabilitation team also must focus on the mental aspects of recovery—not only to help patients overcome deficits in knowledge or memory, but also to help prepare them for the long recovery process and encourage them to lead lives as full as possible with the abilities they retain. It is important to keep in mind that many people have fought their way back from a stroke and continued to lead useful and fulfilling lives. Patients with the ability to make decisions should be included in family decision-making.

No program can succeed without a strong desire by the patient to be independent. Nevertheless, family involvement is also a key ingredient in a successful rehabilitation program. The family can provide a positive environment for the patient, nurturing the desire to be independent while reassuring the patient that he or she is still wanted, needed, and loved. Often giving a patient something to do, and to live for, is half the battle.

The family is also important because although most patients are able to leave rehabilitation facilities to return to their families, often they continue to have

Possible Consequences of Left- and Right-Brain Injury

Damage to the left side of the brain
Right-side paralysis
Speech and language deficits
Slow, cautious behavior
Memory problems related to language
Right-side neglect (less common than left-side; see below)

Damage to the right side of the brain
Left-side paralysis
Spatial-perceptual problems
Left-side neglect
Quick, impulsive behavior
Memory problems related to performance

some problems and their recovery process must continue at home. Family members should take as much of the responsibility for physical therapy at home as is practical. A nurse or physical therapist visiting the home for a few hours a week cannot alone provide the sustained encouragement and the level of activity needed to facilitate recovery.

Beyond the patient and family, rehabilitation is a team effort with input from physiatrists (rehabilitation physicians), neurologists, nurses, physical therapists, occupational therapists, speech therapists, and social workers. Their common goal is to help the patient and family achieve the maximal level of functioning possible.

Most stroke patients will need several types of therapy, described below, but the mix and amount of each will be tailored to the patient's needs and symptoms. Although symptoms of brain damage vary widely, some generalizations can be made. A common way of characterizing stroke injury is by the side of the brain affected. An injury to the right side of the brain that results in paralysis—temporary or permanent—will affect the left side of the body. Conversely, right-sided paralysis is the result of injury to the left side of the brain. Certain language problems and changes in behavior are also associated with left- or right-side damage. (See box, "Possible Consequences of Left- and Right-Brain Injury.")

PHYSICAL THERAPY

The primary objective of physical therapy is to help patients who are partially paralyzed learn to walk again. Starting slowly, the therapist will first work with the patient on simple exercises to increase range of motion and muscle tone. Once the patient is able to turn over and sit up unsupported, the therapist usually will have the patient try to start walking. A patient learns to walk while holding on to a bar for support, and then with the aid of a quadruped cane (one with a sturdy four-footed base) and, usually, ankle-foot braces for stability. An estimated 75 percent of all stroke survivors are eventually able to walk independently and will regain most of their ability by the end of the first month.

OCCUPATIONAL THERAPY

Although the ultimate goal is to help the patient resume some sort of employment, if possible, occupational therapy encompasses all aspects of everyday life. Occupational therapists help patients regain the muscular coordination necessary to perform basic activities such as dressing, bathing, and using the toilet. A patient who is paralyzed on one side is taught how to maneuver clothing using the able side of the body, and is advised about clothing styles—such as pullover rather than buttoned shirts—that are easiest to maneuver. Patients are taught how to use a wheelchair, and how to transfer from bed to wheelchair and vice versa. The occupational therapist will also advise the family about changes that can make a patient's move back home easier and safer: handrails in the bathtub and by the toilet, a raised toilet seat, and ramps in place of stairs, and widened doorways to accommodate a wheelchair, if one is still necessary.

SPEECH THERAPY

Two disorders that may occur after a stroke are *aphasia* (difficulty with language) and *dysarthria* (difficulty with articulation). Aphasia and dysarthria are not necessarily associated with a loss of the ability to think or understand.

Dysarthria is caused by weakness or paralysis of muscles in the face, mouth, neck, or throat. It can result in slow, labored speech, slurring of words, or a change in voice quality. Often the paralysis of the face muscles causes drooping of one side of the face and perhaps drooling.

Most stroke patients with left-brain injury have some degree of aphasia. It manifests itself in different ways in different patients; there may be difficulty making oneself understood, comprehending others' words, or reading, writing, or doing arithmetic. The complexity of the problem mirrors the complexity of the communication process, which involves on the one hand organizing thought, finding the words to express it, and producing the words, and on the other hand perceiving that someone wants to say something to you, following the words as they are spoken, and then comprehending the message in its entirety.

Aphasia may be equally frustrating for the patient and the family and friends, who may feel they can no longer communicate with the patient. Imagine waking up into a world where you mean to say one thing and something completely different comes out of your mouth, or one where your family seems to be speaking a foreign language that you cannot comprehend. This is what an aphasic patient may experience. But with the help of a speech therapist and a cooperative family, a stroke survivor has an excellent chance of regaining communication skills. If the patient is not able to produce speech specifically, that does not mean he or she cannot use and comprehend language in the larger sense of the word, which encompasses other communication tools such as gestures, movements, facial expressions, and noises.

A speech therapist should lay the groundwork while the patient is in the hospital, first working to obtain from the patient reliable (verbal or nonverbal) yes or no responses to questions. Then the therapist uses a variety of techniques, including repetition and pointing to pictures, to reestablish the fundamentals of language. In most cases, the knowledge of language hasn't been eradicated, and patients just need to regain their ability to recall what they have learned in the past. As with other memory losses, the patient will often regain ability to remember events that happened in the distant past, but will not be as able to remember things that happened in the very recent past—where he or she left a hat ten minutes ago.

ADJUSTING AFTER A STROKE

Rehabilitation may continue on an outpatient basis after the patient has returned home, and recovery may continue for months or even years. The most dramatic changes occur in the first three to six months or so; smaller changes may continue for long afterward.

There are no clear guidelines for how much activity benefits stroke patients and how hard to push them. They should be pushed hard enough to be challenged, but not so hard as to be continually frustrated.

Recovery from a stroke can be a painfully slow process. Both family and patient should take time to note successful efforts, and family members need to offer positive feedback, encouragement, and praise.

The stroke does not just happen to the patient—it happens to the family as well. Understanding how strokes can affect patients will make it easier for families to deal with the recovery process. Some of the major behavioral, cognitive, and emotional effects are discussed below.

APHASIA

The lack of ability to communicate may sometimes improve rapidly—within a few days or a week—but in many cases, recovery is a long process. The recovering aphasic patient needs stimulating and understanding companionship. In addition to helping these people feel loved and supported, engaging them in conversation and activity reinforces language skills. A patient who is left alone with little to do will progress much more slowly than one who is made to feel a part of the family, or has simple, arousing things to do, such as looking through a picture magazine.

Just as parents can grasp what toddlers mean when they gurgle or grunt or use made-up words, family members can often learn to understand the patient's limited, disjointed, or inappropriate speech during the first few weeks after the stroke. Patients may say "car" when they mean "couch," and may not realize that they are not being understood. They may use swear words that they never uttered before the stroke, or repeat the same word over and over. Family and friends can learn to speak slowly, use simple words and short sentences, and repeat them if necessary. A variety of computer software designed to help in language retraining is now available.

It is important for the family and friends neither to overestimate nor underestimate what the recovering patient understands. If the patient says yes or smiles and nods in agreement with something that is said, he or she may be responding to the speaker's facial expression or expressing pleasure about being spoken to. A speaker who consistently overestimates what the patient understands will become annoyed that the patient doesn't follow through and may decide that the patient is forgetful or uncooperative. Or the speaker may talk too much, thus overloading the patient and interfering with any understanding the patient may have. Unrealistically high expectations about what the patient should be able to do can be

Tips on Communicating with Stroke Survivors

When someone has difficulty speaking or finding the right words

- Help the patient point to the object he or she is trying to name, gesture the meaning of the word, or use other words to describe it.

- Respond positively to any nonverbal or verbal effort to communicate.

- Provide sentences to complete, such as "You said you're hungry for a ——?"

- Do not be bothered by slurred speech; accept the patient as he or she is every step of the way.

- Encourage talking as much as possible. The more words the patient uses, the more likely will be the recovery of speech.

- Work learning games into activities, such as asking the patient to name the foods he wants to eat, rather than using drills or doing obvious exercises like reciting the alphabet or counting.

- Write the name of an object in large letters as you show it to the patient.

- Once a patient learns a noun, such as "coffee," introduce the verb associated with it—such as "drink coffee," "drive car," "brush hair."

When someone has difficulty understanding speech

- Use short, concrete sentences, leaving out unnecessary words. For example, instead of saying "I'm going to go to the store now to buy some bread," say "Going, store, bread."

- Speak slowly and pause between sentences.

- Use visual aids such as pictures, or point to objects.

- Gesture as you speak.

- Keep background noise to a minimum when speaking.

- Do not shout.

- If the patient seems not to understand you, repeat or rephrase your request.

- Emphasize key words.

When someone has difficulty reading

- Buy simple books with large type and read them aloud to the patient until he or she is ready to try reading aloud.

- Show a picture of a written word.

- Underline key words.

- Gesture the meaning as the patient reads a difficult word.

When someone has difficulty writing

- The patient should start off printing very large letters, especially if paralysis means having to learn to write with the hand opposite from the one he or she is used to.

- Have the patient copy letters and words.

- Write words as you say them.

- Have an alphabet board visible when the patient is trying to write to help locate letters he or she is having difficulty recalling.

---

very frustrating for both patient and family. On the other hand, if the patient's cues that he or she *does* understand are missed, family members are less likely to continue to engage the patient in communication, which can have devastating effects on emotions and recovery. To avoid either extreme, family members need to be sensitive to nonverbal cues as well as verbal responses and to test understanding occasionally by saying something improbable and noting the patient's response. (See box, "Tips on Communicating with Stroke Survivors.")

OTHER NEUROLOGIC DEFICITS

Family members can also help lessen the impact of other neurologic-behavioral changes. If patients have difficulty remembering recent events, it is important to remind them of their recent successes in regaining functions. Patients with left-brain damage (with or without right-sided paralysis) are often slow, cautious, and disorganized when faced with an unfamiliar situation—even if their behavioral style was quite different before the stroke. Family members can help the patient by giving positive feedback for things done correctly. Patients with right-brain damage, on the other hand, tend to act impulsively and hastily; they are often poor judges of their own abilities and safety. Family members can help by reminding patients to take things slowly and carefully.

Some stroke patients suffer a loss of half of their visual field in each eye. Some patients, particularly those with right-brain damage, also have one-sided neglect: they do not compensate for their visual loss by turning their heads. Rather, they ignore everything—including objects and even sensations—on the side of the body where vision is impaired. Often a patient will not even recognize an arm or leg as being part of his body. People may have to approach patients from their unimpaired side in order to be noticed. Putting objects on the patient's good side—

such as clothes only on one side of the closet—can make management easier.

Deficits in spatial relations—judging the size, position, distance, or speed of objects, for example—are common among people with right-brain damage. This can create problems for self-care, making it difficult for a person to button a blouse correctly, steer a wheelchair without bumping into obstacles, read a newspaper without losing his or her place, or even sip soup from a spoon.

Other common, but not universal, problems that may occur following a stroke include:

- Poor concentration
- Poor judgment of time
- Disturbed sleep cycles
- Impaired memory
- Impaired judgment
- Loss of sexual desire
- Poor emotional control
- Depression

EMOTIONAL IMPAIRMENT

Often families and patient focus on the physical impairments after a stroke. These are readily apparent and easily understood. But the brain is also responsible for our thoughts and emotions. It is this aspect of damage after a stroke that is often the most difficult to deal with.

People who have recently suffered a stroke may have a loss of emotional control because of damage in the area of the brain that controls emotions. As a result, they may cry or laugh suddenly, often inappropriately, at times when they do not feel especially sad or happy. Some patients may become irritated and express anger with little provocation. Simply distracting the patient can often interrupt the emotional behavior.

On the other hand, true depression is not uncommon in stroke patients, whose lives have been changed drastically and who feel discouraged or hopeless. In part this can be a natural reaction to a devastating disease and the often slow and difficult recovery process. Often it is also caused by damage to areas of the brain and by neurochemicals responsible for mood and motivation. Signs of depression include excessive crying (which cannot be easily interrupted), fatigue, sleep and eating disorders, and loss of interest in activities. Support from family

members and an emphasis on the positive progress that has been made—without ignoring the existence of deficits—can be helpful. Antidepressant medications can be prescribed for patients whose downheartedness is hampering their progress.

Problems such as sexual dysfunction, loss of self-esteem, and difficulties in family relationships are best dealt with openly and with the help of trained medical personnel. These are important issues for quality of life following a stroke and should not be ignored. The important thing to remember is that many of these conditions can be helped. Sometimes just the knowledge that this is a common problem and that it is often self-limited is enough to get the patient and family back on track. In more serious cases, therapy (personal or family) and medications may be necessary. The key is to speak frankly and keep the physician and other health care personnel informed.

PHYSICAL ACCOMMODATIONS

Planning for returning home after a stroke may require some physical adjustments in the house. Many of these are simple and can be done by the family (rubber shower mats, soap enclosed in a cloth pouch to avoid slipping, handgrips, and removal of small scatter rugs); others may require more detailed planning and construction (ramps, lowered counters, high toilets, changing the height and location of light switches). Useful devices such as one-handed card holders, rocker knives, nonskid mixing bowls, and modified telephones can be purchased, often through specialized catalogs. These modifications are best planned in conjunction with occupational therapists and by sharing experience with other families through local support groups, such as stroke clubs.

TOWARD THE FUTURE

Several exciting approaches to stroke therapy are under investigation. All are in, or near, clinical testing in humans.

One investigational approach is thrombclytic therapy—the use of drugs such as t-PA (tissue plasminogen activator) to dissolve a clot and reopen the occluded vessel causing the stroke. This therapy has already proved successful in treating heart attacks and shows promising early results in stroke patients. The major drawback is an increased risk of bleeding.

Another approach is to route blood flow around the occlusion through small collateral vessels, after making these vessels larger by, for example, using vasodilating agents such as calcium channel blockers. An alternative is to lower the viscosity (thickness) of the blood (by, for example, adding plasma expanders) in order to make the flow through the small vessels easier.

Researchers are also attempting to determine the chemical reactions that lead to permanent damage during a stroke. Once these are understood, it may be possible to inhibit these harmful reactions selectively and lessen the damage. Calcium-channel-blocking drugs, already being used to treat other cardiovascular conditions, may help reduce the damage caused by a stroke.

Other drugs being investigated also work to protect the nerve cells. These include the NMDA-receptor blockers.

One of the newest areas of investigation is restorative neurology, which studies how the brain and nerves repair themselves after injury. Current medical wisdom says that in adults, nerve cells do not divide in order to create new cells, so that damaged brain cells cannot be replaced. This may be only partially true. While cell regrowth is not yet possible, it may be possible to influence how neurons communicate with each other after injury.

Nerve cells are "connected" to thousands of other nerve cells through connections called synapses, which change after injury to the brain. It appears that gangliosides, a class of molecules on the surface of neurons, help new synapses form. By giving stroke patients extra amounts of gangliosides, it may be possible to increase the number of synapses, permitting the brain to develop a wider variety of compensatory brain circuits and minimize the deficits. This therapy, now in clinical trials, would not change the size of the stroke, but could improve outcome for the patient.

SUMMARY

Neurology is on the verge of major breakthroughs in stroke treatment that hold promise for being able to drastically reduce the effects of stroke. But despite advances in treatment, prevention remains the most effective way of decreasing the national burden caused by strokes. Patients at risk must work with their doctors to reduce their likelihood of falling victim to a disabling stroke. Life-style changes and better management of high blood pressure have already been responsible, along with better treatment of strokes when they do occur, for a more than 50 percent decrease in stroke deaths over the past 20 years.

PART V

SPECIAL SITUATIONS

CHAPTER 19

WOMEN AND HEART DISEASE

LYNDA E. ROSENFELD, M.D.

INTRODUCTION

Heart disease in women is similar in many ways to heart disease in men. Like men, women can have high blood pressure and heart attacks. In fact, these are more prevalent in women than previously thought: Of the approximately 500,000 heart attack deaths each year, almost half occur in women, according to American Heart Association figures, and deaths from high blood pressure are at a similar ratio. Women can also suffer the same inborn (congenital) malformations, diseases of the heart valves, heart failure, and heart rhythm disorders as men.

Enough differences exist between male and female heart disease, however, to warrant consideration of the aspects that specifically apply to women. (See box, "Cardiovascular Disease in American Women.") These aspects include both uniquely female experiences with diseases such as atherosclerosis (hardening of the arteries) and hypertension, which affect both men and women, and uniquely female life experiences, such as pregnancy, which produce profound cardiovascular changes. Women have often been excluded from research studies about atherosclerosis; the perception has been that heart attack is more a male phenomenon, and researchers have feared that female subjects might become pregnant, which in the case of a drug study might cause injury to the unborn child. As a result, frequently cited facts about heart attack risk factors and treatments may apply more to men than women. The National Institutes of Health (NIH), however, has recently mandated that all researchers receiving NIH grants must now include women in their studies—or have a good reason for excluding them. The NIH has also created an office of Research on Women's Health. Thus in the future, more specific data should be available.

Cardiovascular Disease in American Women

- Between the ages of 45 and 64, one in nine women has some form of cardiovascular disease.

- One in three women above the age of 65 has some form of cardiovascular disease.

- Of the approximately 500,000 fatal heart attacks per year, almost half occur in women.

- Women who have a heart attack are twice as likely to die within the first two weeks as are men.

- Within the first year after a heart attack, 39 percent of women die compared with 31 percent of men.

The American Heart Association's Check-up Checklist for Women: Items to Discuss with a Doctor

____ Age

____ Race

____ Family history of heart disease, diabetes, cancer, other diseases

____ Blood pressure

____ Blood cholesterol, plus HDL and LDL cholesterol if appropriate

____ Blood triglycerides

____ Glucose tolerance (for people concerned about diabetes)

____ Ideal weight for age, height, and body type

____ Smoking behavior

____ Alcohol consumption

____ Response to stressful situations

____ Satisfaction with work and family life

____ Oral contraceptives

____ Estrogen replacement therapy (for postmenopausal women)

____ Dietary changes

____ Exercise routines

© 1989. American Heart Association. Used with permission.

WOMEN AND ATHEROSCLEROSIS (CORONARY HEART DISEASE)

Like men, women must consider heredity, age, race, blood pressure, blood cholesterol, and smoking as risk factors for coronary heart disease. (See Chapter 3.) However, women appear to be more affected by certain factors, such as smoking and diabetes, than are men. In addition, only women become pregnant, experience menopause, and are prescribed contraceptive pills and postmenopausal estrogens. These special considerations should be explored on an individual basis with a physician. (See box, "The American Heart Association's Check-up Checklist for Women: Items to Discuss with a Doctor.")

MENOPAUSE

For both men and women, the older the person, the more likely he or she is to develop heart disease.

Women, however, develop cardiovascular disease about ten years later than men. Heart attack is almost unheard of in young women, and in the age group 45 to 54, six times as many men as women have heart attacks. This difference may contribute to the reluctance of researchers to include women in heart attack studies of middle-aged individuals; many more people would have to be studied to prove whether or not a particular treatment was effective in women. By about age 60, though, women begin to catch up to men. (See Table 19.1.)

For women, risk increases gradually in the five to ten years after the female hormone estrogen begins to dwindle, around age 50. Researchers believe that estrogen, which regulates menstruation, protects women against heart attack by increasing a substance in the blood called high-density lipoprotein (HDL), which prevents blockages in the arteries. HDL carries cholesterol away from the arteries and out of the body. Premenopausal women have much higher levels of HDL cholesterol than men the same age. (See Chapter 5.)

Through a chain reaction of body chemicals, estrogen also keeps blood vessels from constricting and reducing blood flow to the heart muscle. Such a reduction in blood flow may cause chest pain, shortness of breath, and heart attack. Findings suggest that prostaglandins, hormones secreted by the uterus in

Table 19.1
Estimated Annual Number of Americans, by Age and Sex, Experiencing Heart Attack

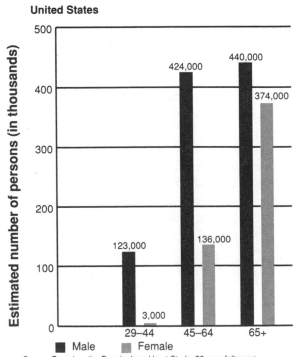

United States

Estimated number of persons (in thousands)

	29–44	45–64	65+
Male	123,000	424,000	440,000
Female	3,000	136,000	374,000

■ Male   ■ Female

Source: Based on the Framingham Heart Study, 26-year follow-up.

women of childbearing age, may also play a role in protecting women from heart disease. One of these substances helps to dilate blood vessels and prevents clotting.

When postmenopausal women take replacement estrogen, it seems to reduce their risk of heart attack by one-third to one-half. The majority of studies find that women who have never taken estrogen after menopause are at highest risk of heart attack; for women who have taken estrogen for the first ten years after menopause, the risk becomes moderate, and at lowest risk are women who have taken estrogen continuously since menopause. A Mayo Clinic research group estimates that giving estrogen to all women between the ages of 40 and 59 could reduce the number of women who experience heart attack by as much as 45 percent.

When menopause occurs naturally, the risk of a heart attack rises gradually; when it is caused by surgical removal of the ovaries (oophorectomy), heart attack risk rises more abruptly. One study showed that women who had an oophorectomy and had never taken replacement estrogen had about twice the risk of coronary heart disease as premenopausal women. After taking replacement estrogen, their risk returned to normal.

It is possible that estrogen will one day be a common preventive treatment for women at risk for heart attack, although doctors have to weigh this benefit against the possible increased risks of uterine and breast cancer associated with the use of this hormone. In addition, estrogen use among nonsmokers has been associated with an increased incidence of stroke. The results to date of several of these studies have been controversial; however, a very recent study, the Nurses' Health Study, suggests that the overall benefits of estrogen replacement therapy outweigh the risks. Yet, there is still a need for other well-controlled studies of progesterone (another female hormone) and/or estrogen therapy in postmenopausal women. (See box, "Pros and Cons of Estrogen Replacement Therapy.")

ORAL CONTRACEPTIVES

Oral contraceptives (OCs) contain estrogens, but the high-dose birth control pills of the past appeared to increase a woman's risk of heart attack; this may be related to the type and dose of estrogen used. In some women, oral contraceptives increased low-density lipoprotein ("bad" cholesterol), decreased high-density lipoprotein ("good" cholesterol), raised blood pressure and blood sugar slightly, and possibly in-

---

Pros and Cons of Estrogen Replacement Therapy

Pros:

- Prevents thinning of bones (osteoporosis).
- Relieves distressing symptoms of menopause, particularly hot flashes and vaginal dryness.
- May protect against heart disease (addition of progesterone may negate this benefit).

Cons:

- Increases risk of cancer of the lining of the uterus (endometrial cancer), except in women who have undergone a hysterectomy (addition of progesterone may decrease this risk).
- May accelerate growth of estrogen-dependent cancerous tumors; questionable effect on breast cancer.

Who Should Not Take Estrogen:

- Anyone with known or suspected breast cancer; anyone with known or suspected estrogen-dependent cancerous tumor(s)
- Anyone who is or suspects being pregnant
- Anyone with a history of blood clots associated with prior use of estrogen (risk is smaller than when using oral contraceptives)
- Anyone with undiagnosed abnormal genital bleeding
- Anyone with a history of stroke or heart attack

Possible Normal Side Effects (usually temporary):

- Breast tenderness
- Fluid retention
- Nausea
- Slight weight gain
- Vaginal bleeding

---

creased the ability of the blood to clot—especially in smokers. (See Chapter 6.)

Modern oral contraceptive formulations use lower doses and different forms of estrogen, and new studies hint that these oral contraceptives increase the risk of heart disease much less. In fact, some evidence indicates that lower doses of estrogen do not increase heart attack risk unless the woman smokes or has other risk factors. Similarly, a woman taking oral contraceptives is more likely to develop high blood pressure if she is overweight, has a family history of high blood pressure, or has mild kidney disease. (See Chapter 12.)

A woman on birth control pills should have her blood pressure checked about every six months, although her chances of developing high blood pressure as a result of using oral contraceptives are small. In a large study of oral contraceptive users, it was determined that although the average blood pressure rose somewhat (by 5 to 10 mm Hg), it remained within the normal range in the vast majority of women. In only a small percentage did it rise to levels of concern—above 140/90 mm Hg. Studies conflict as to whether the past use of a high-dose pill raises a woman's chance of cardiovascular disease.

Another reason that oral contraceptives may raise the risk of atherosclerotic heart disease is that they contain progestins, synthetic hormones that may raise LDL, lower HDL, and increase blood sugar. Some experts believe these changes are responsible for most of the risks.

SMOKING

Smoking is a major risk factor for heart disease in men, and it is probably the most significant risk factor in women, because it reduces a woman's two best protectors, estrogen and HDL. (See box, "Smoking as a Risk Factor for CHD in Women"; see also Chapter 6.) For every cigarette smoked, the risk of heart attack rises. Studies show that smoking one to four cigarettes a day doubles a woman's risk, and smoking more than 25 a day can raise it 5 to 15 times. Some researchers predict that if we ever have more women smokers than men smokers, heart attack will become a woman's disease—and that appears to be the direction in which our society is heading. Both men and women are quitting smoking, but women aren't quitting quite as fast as men. For the first time in the history of the Framingham Heart Study, more young women are smoking than young men. (The Framingham study is one of the few major epidemiologic studies examining coronary heart disease that has included women. It is a study of the entire community of Framingham, Massachusetts—several thousand people. The study began in 1939 and is still in progress.)

Fortunately, just as the risk of heart disease rises with every cigarette smoked, it falls with every cigarette left in the pack. As in men, the risk of heart attack is still higher in women who stopped smoking less than two years ago than in nonsmokers. By the time a woman has been an ex-smoker for two to three years, however, the increased chance of heart attack has dissipated. This is true even in women who have smoked for many years. Therefore, it is never too late

Smoking as a Risk Factor for Coronary Heart Disease in Women

The Nurses' Health Study reported the following:

- The number of cigarettes smoked per day was positively associated with the risk of fatal coronary heart disease, nonfatal heart attack, and angina pectoris.

- Even smoking one to four cigarettes per day was associated with a doubling of the risk of fatal and nonfatal CHD, and smoking 5 to 14 per day tripled it.

- The absolute effect of smoking is substantially increased when added to other risk factors.

to stop. Insurance companies have recognized this fact and will give standard policies to ex-smokers.

For women, smoking heightens the dangers of other risk factors. In one study, heart attack rates were higher in estrogen users who smoked cigarettes than in those who did not. An elevated blood cholesterol level also seems to raise the risk in smokers; exactly how much is not known. If a woman who smokes is also using oral contraceptives, she is up to 40 times more likely to have a heart attack than a woman who does not use either. In smokers, oral contraceptives aggravate other risk factors such as high blood cholesterol and high blood pressure. This does not mean a woman smoker should necessarily stop using oral contraceptives. It makes more sense to quit smoking, because its risks are much higher.

OBESITY

It has been known for years that obesity and heart disease go hand in hand in men. An eight-year-long study from Brigham and Women's Hospital in Boston indicates that for women, being even mildly overweight can increase heart attack risk dramatically, perhaps more than in men. For example, a woman 5 feet 4½ inches tall who weighs 137 to 145 pounds increases her risk by 30 percent over a woman the same height who weights less than 125 pounds. In women approximately 30 percent or more over ideal weight, 70 percent of all heart attacks could be traced to obesity. (Out of the 115,886 American women age 30 to 55 in the study group, there were 605 cases of some type of heart disease or heart attack, including 83 deaths.)

Researchers cannot explain exactly why obesity increases heart attack risk. A substantial portion of the risk is indirect—due to hypertension, diabetes, and other problems associated with obesity.

However, one subtlety that has been discerned is that a woman who follows the typical male weight gain pattern—heavy around the middle and shaped like an apple—has a higher risk of heart disease than a woman with a traditionally female pear shape. This is possibly because the sex hormones that influence blood fat levels also influence body fat distribution. It is believed that abdominal fat is more easily mobilized into cholesterol than fat from the hips or thighs. (A woman's waist measurement should be no more than 80 percent of her hip measurement.) Thus, "female-pattern" obesity may be a reflection of relatively higher female sex hormone levels, which, as noted earlier, may offer a degree of cardiovascular protection. Some of the risk associated with an "apple shape" may also be traced to cigarette smoking, which alters hormone levels and promotes male-pattern obesity.

CHOLESTEROL

A high cholesterol level is a well-known risk factor for atherosclerotic heart disease. (See Chapter 4.) However, many studies have shown this relationship to be less distinct in women than in men. The reason for this is that the total cholesterol level is a combination of the HDL and LDL levels, and for any given total level, women are more likely to have a higher HDL ("good" cholesterol) level than men. Many of these studies looked only at the total cholesterol level and not specifically at the amount of HDL cholesterol present.

TRIGLYCERIDES

Triglyceride is the chemical form in which much of the body fat exists at some point in the cycle of fat metabolism. It is usually measured along with LDL and HDL cholesterol to give a "lipid profile." However, the relationship between high triglyceride levels and heart disease is less clear-cut than that between high cholesterol levels and atherosclerosis. The Framingham Heart Study found that high triglyceride levels are related to a higher risk of heart attack in women but not in men. The reason is uncertain; researchers know that someone who has high triglycerides in the blood may also have high LDL and lower HDL cholesterol. High triglyceride levels are most commonly noted in obese people and in persons with

diabetes—two conditions more common in women than in men, and having an association with atherosclerotic heart disease.

CORONARY ARTERY SPASM

Factors relating to blood fats are usually the causes of atherosclerotic coronary artery disease; blockages are due to the buildup of fat deposits in the blood vessels. (See Chapter 11.) However, in the relatively few young women who have a heart attack or chest pains, other ailments such as coronary artery spasm, an abnormal contraction of the blood vessel that also causes reduced blood flow to the heart muscle, may be responsible for the damage.

DIABETES

A higher percentage of women than men have diabetes. In both sexes, diabetes is a risk factor for heart disease because high blood sugar speeds up hardening of the arteries and, thus, the development of heart disease. However, researchers have noticed differences between male and female diabetics. Diabetic women have lower HDL levels than diabetic men, and diabetes increases the risk of a second heart attack in women, but not in men. Researchers are still investigating the reasons for this. In addition, diabetes increases the risk of kidney disease and disease of the blood vessels, which may complicate treatment of coronary artery disease.

STRESS

As more and more women have entered the work force, researchers have wondered if the stress of working would harm their hearts. (See Chapter 8.) The Framingham study has shown that female clerical workers have a higher rate of heart attack than homemakers. The difference between these groups seems to be a psychological one: Clerical workers feel they have less control over their lives. This suggests that if women can work their way up the job ranks to managerial positions—which accord them more autonomy—they may maintain their lower heart disease rate. However, men under high pressure in these jobs may have a high heart attack rate. Unfortunately, upon reaching these jobs, women may also be more likely to eat high-calorie, high-cholesterol business dinners and perhaps to smoke, but they may be more likely to take advantage of company or insurance-covered physicals that will catch heart disease early.

Working women at all levels typically continue to have two jobs: their employment, and maintenance of a home and caring for children. Whether the stress related to these demands will have direct adverse effects is currently being investigated.

RESPONSE TO TREATMENT

Once a woman who is having a heart attack arrives at the hospital, she is slightly less likely to survive than a man. The differences are not great, however. About 1 percent fewer women than men survive balloon angioplasty, in which a small balloon is inflated inside the artery to crush a plaque; of those who do get through the procedure, more women than men have reclogging of the arteries, subsequent angina, and other complications. (See Chapter 24.) Bypass surgery is also more risky for women—up to two times more dangerous. In addition, after leaving the hospital following a heart attack, a woman is more likely to die of a heart attack than is a man. (See Chapter 25.) Black women do worse than white women both in surviving to leave the hospital and in survival over the long term. (See Chapter 22.)

This higher mortality may have several causes. Women may be less likely to pursue symptoms themselves, and they may be less likely to be referred for evaluation of symptoms. Perhaps more important, when they do finally have heart problems or are referred for tests, they are likely to be older than men, to have more advanced heart disease—and to have other diseases as well. A Yale study showed that the women who had heart attacks were more likely to have diabetes and hypertension. In a group of bypass patients at one hospital, women were an average of 68 years old, men 62. As a result, a woman is more susceptible to complications of her heart attack or its treatment.

The statistical differences in heart attack survival between men and women may actually relate not so much to sex as to size. In one study, body surface area was the strongest predictor of operative risk for bypass surgery. Women survived surgery about as well as men who were the same size. Size may be a factor for the simple reason that it may be harder to operate on a small artery than on a larger one.

Despite these facts, it is important to remember that overall, most women do well. According to the Minnesota Heart Survey, conducted in 1980, 92 percent of women with a heart attack survive hospitalization, 80 percent are still alive after one year, and 58 percent after four years.

BODY SIZE AND HEART ATTACK

Body size may also be a factor in why a heart attack occurs. One study found that a woman under 5 feet tall has a 50 percent greater chance of having a heart attack than a woman 5 feet 4 inches tall, although the total numbers in both groups of women were not great. Theories abound, the simplest being that a short woman's arteries clog more easily because they are small. Another is that shorter women may be more likely to carry their extra weight around the midriff, in the more risky "apple pattern." Finally, taller women have lower blood cholesterol than shorter women. This is not the case with men, and the reason for it is uncertain.

The idea that a small artery is likely to fill with plaque more quickly than a large one may also explain why more women than men (55 percent compared with 43 percent, in one study) complain of angina. It may explain, too, why each year thousands of women experience chest pain bad enough to lead them to coronary angiography, an X-ray of the heart and its vessels. (See Chapter 10.) However, one in five of these women is eventually told her arteries are perfectly normal and is referred to a gastroenterologist or psychiatrist, because some chest pain does relate to stomach acid, panic attacks, or anxiety. But researchers at the National Heart, Lung, and Blood Institute believe that in some women, vessels too small to be seen on a standard angiogram may be constricting or narrowing, causing their chest pain.

Most women with such microvascular (small-vessel) angina respond well to nitrates, medicines that dilate the blood vessels, and to calcium channel blockers, which prevent vascular spasm. (See Chapter 23.) These factors and the misconception that coronary artery disease is rare in women may also explain why women with chest pain and heart disease come to medical attention later than men.

PREVENTION

Stopping a heart attack before it ever starts is, of course, the treatment of choice. There are some measures that one can take before seeking medical help. (See box, "Self-Help in Promoting Heart Health.") The American Heart Association suggests that even men and women with no symptoms of heart disease should also have a resting electrocardiogram (ECG) done at ages 20, 40, and 60. In this painless test, technicians attach electrodes to the skin of the chest and limbs to monitor the heart's electrical characteristics. (See Chapter 10.)

Self-Help in Promoting Heart Health

- Quit smoking, and sit in no-smoking sections in public places.

- Exercise regularly.

- Maintain ideal weight.

- Cut the amount and kinds of fat and cholesterol in the diet.

- Have blood cholesterol checked at least once every five years.
   (Below 200 mg/dl is desirable, 200 to 239 mg/dl is borderline high, and 240 mg/dl or higher is too high.)*

- Monitor and control blood pressure.

- Take active steps to gain a sense of control in life.

*May not be significant if HDL levels are high.

Some physicians suggest that people who work in physically stressful jobs or have two or more major risk factors for heart disease should have an exercise electrocardiogram, given while running on a tread mill or exercising on a bicycle. This is called a stress test because it measures the heart's performance under the stress of exercise. Others, however, believe that this is not necessary other than in specific instances where unusual pain may be present or some other heart problem seems to exist.

During such a test, a young woman is far more likely to have a false positive result—a false indication of trouble—than a man is. Because there is a lower prevalence of the disease in women, any positive result has a greater chance of being false. Additionally, women's breasts sometimes make it more difficult to position the monitoring leads correctly. For a young, healthy woman with no family history of heart disease, the cost of an exercise ECG combined with the potentially confusing and anxiety-producing results may outweigh the benefit. A woman with symptoms or major risk factors should, however, have routine ECGs and a stress test. She may get more accurate results from a stress test combined with the use of a small amount of a radioactive material called thallium, or an echocardiogram, a sound-wave test of the heart. Such stress tests give more specific information about blood flow to various segments of the heart muscle.

The "gold standard" to determine the presence of coronary artery disease is angiography, a test in which dye is injected into the coronary arteries. The arteries' contours are then viewed via X-ray. Most patients, even some of those with chest pain, do not have to submit to all of these tests. (See Chapter 10.)

Studies on men have led experts to recommend that men at risk for heart attack or patients who have had a previous heart attack take aspirin every day to make a blood clot less likely. More recent studies examining aspirin's benefits in women have confirmed that the use of a baby aspirin or ½ a regular aspirin daily by women over age 50 is beneficial.

In women under age 50 with a strong family history of heart attacks at an early age, obesity, a smoking habit, or some other risk factor such as diabetes, it probably is a good idea to take one baby aspirin or one-half of a regular aspirin each day. This should not be done if blood pressure is high and uncontrolled or there is a history of stomach problems such as ulcers. The aspirin usually does no harm and may help prevent a heart attack, but each patient should check with her physician.

MITRAL VALVE PROLAPSE

Mitral valve prolapse (MVP) occurs when the valve between the left atrium (the upper heart chamber on the left side) and the left ventricle (the lower heart chamber on that side) contains excess tissue, buckles backward, and may fail to close properly. People with mitral valve prolapse usually show distinctive signs that a doctor will discover when listening to the heart. They have single or multiple clicks that change characteristically with body position (while squatting, sitting, or standing, for example) and may be associated with a heart murmur. The diagnosis can be confirmed by a simple sound-wave test—an ultrasound or echocardiogram.

This condition is more common in women than men by a ratio of at least two to one, but it is also more common in people with low body weight. So the increased prevalence in women may be explained by the fact that they tend to be smaller than men. A younger woman is more likely than an older woman to have mitral valve prolapse. Among the women in the Framingham Heart Study, 17 percent of women 20 to 29 years old had mitral valve prolapse compared to only 1.4 percent of women over 80. This may be because, as the ventricle dilates because of heart disease in old age, the excess tissue of the valve and, thus, the prolapse becomes relatively less apparent.

In addition to sex and size, heredity seems to be a factor in some cases of mitral valve prolapse. This leads one to believe that race may also be an indication, but no good studies have yet examined this issue. Scoliosis, "straight back," and other skeletal abnormalities and connective tissue diseases are also often linked with mitral valve prolapse. This is because in some patients with connective tissue disease, a weakness of the tissues may lead to stretching of the valve or disruption of the supporting tissues.

The majority of people with mitral valve prolapse have no symptoms and remain unaware of the condition, but other people report sticking chest pains, palpitations, awareness of irregular heartbeats, and panic attacks. The overall prognosis of mitral valve prolapse is excellent, and it is rarely fatal. However, mitral valve prolapse infrequently results in severe leakage of the valve and enlargement of the heart muscle (see Chapter 15), which requires valve replacement and, rarely, may cause a stroke. (Small blood clots that come from the abnormal valve may travel to the brain.)

Finally, endocarditis, an infection of the heart's inner lining or valves, occurs more often in people with mitral valve prolapse because infections can start more easily on a damaged valve. To reduce the risk of this complication, the mitral valve prolapse patient may need antibiotics before dental or surgical procedures or childbirth, especially if the valve is leaky.

Too often the patient with the "click syndrome" (MVP) is frightened by a physician and is led to believe that she has heart disease. It is important to emphasize that this finding occurs in normal healthy women who usually live long lives with no restrictions. If symptoms of palpitations or sticking chest pains are annoying, the use of small doses of beta blockers may alleviate them. (See Chapter 23.)

THE HEART AND PREGNANCY

Pregnancy normally brings about major changes in the circulatory system. Largely as a result of the hormones produced during pregnancy, blood volume increases by as much as 40 percent. This requires increased work by the heart. In the normal woman, the heart has enough reserve to accommodate this increased burden easily, but the heart of someone with underlying heart disease may not have sufficient reserve.

Mechanical factors are also important. When a pregnant woman lies on her back, her enlarged uterus can prevent return of blood from the legs—by compressing the vena cava—and thus reduce blood flow to the heart and the aorta, the major vessel that carries blood to the brain, abdomen, legs, and the rest of the body. This may cause light-headness. The pressure is relieved when the woman lies on her side rather than on her back. In addition, as the baby grows, it needs more and more oxygen and nutrients, and the mother's heart works harder to meet this demand until about ten weeks before delivery, when the demand diminishes a little. Before labor and delivery, the demand increases again.

During labor, heart rate rises with each uterine contraction and falls when the contraction subsides. In labor as in pregnancy, a woman can reduce the demand placed on her heart by lying on her side rather than on her back. As part of the increased demand is due to pain, anesthesia at the time of delivery can help as well. Local anesthetics such as the commonly used spinal anesthesia tend to reduce demand on the heart. With delivery and reduction of the large mass of the pregnant uterus, there is a sudden infusion of blood volume into the circulation, which may stress a weakened heart. This may be balanced by peripheral blood loss. It may take more than a week for the circulation to return completely to normal.

For a healthy woman, pregnancy and giving birth are of no more consequence to the heart than a bout of mild exercise. For a woman who has heart disease, however, they may be more of a challenge, and she should consult with her obstetrician and cardiologist before becoming pregnant. These experts can help her assess whether pregnancy is a good idea, because changes in pregnancy may be more dangerous in some conditions than in others. Today, most women who have heart problems can, with appropriate medical supervision, have safe pregnancies and healthy children.

Women with hypertension will have little trouble with pregnancy unless their blood pressure is very high—above 160/100—or if they have kidney trouble as well. Many physicians ask their hypertensive patients to monitor their own blood pressure at home. Blood pressure medication to be taken during pregnancy and before delivery will be carefully chosen. A woman with very high blood pressure may have to be hospitalized for a period during her pregnancy and will certainly receive antihypertensive and perhaps diuretic medication. A hypertensive woman

Common Heart Drugs: How Safe for the Pregnant Woman?

The list that follows represents the best information available at this time. Drugs that are considered safe may still produce some side effects. In all cases, the risks of medication must be weighed against the benefits, and all medications should be checked with your physician.

Anticoagulants (drugs to prevent clotting):

Acetylsalicylic acid (aspirin)	Not safe
Dipyridamole (Persantine)	Not safe
Heparin (Panheprin, Calciparine, Lipo-heprin, Liquaemin)	Considered safe but must be adjusted near term
Warfarin (Coumadin)	Not safe

Antihypertensives:

Atenolol (Tenormin)	Considered safe
Captopril (Capoten)	Not safe
Clonidine (Catapres)	Limited experience
Diazoxide (Hyperstat)	Limited experience
Diltiazem (Cardizem)	Relatively safe
Enalapril (Vasotec)	Not safe
Hydralazine (Apresoline)	Considered safe
Labetalol (Normodyne, Trandate)	Probably safe
Magnesium sulfate	Considered safe
Methyldopa (Aldomet)	Considered safe
Metoprolol (Lopressor)	Considered safe
Nadolol (Corgard)	Probably safe
Nifedipine (Procardia)	Relatively safe
Pindolol (Visken)	Probably safe
Prazosin (Minipress)	Limited experience
Propranolol (Inderal)	Considered safe
Spironolactone (Aldactone)	Limited experience
Timolol (Blocadren)	Probably safe
Verapamil (Isoptin, Calan)	Probably safe

Diuretics:

Chlorthalidone (Hygroton)	If used before pregnancy, may be continued
Ethacrynic acid (Edecrin)	Probably safe
Furosemide (Lasix)	Probably safe
Hydrochlorothiazide (Esidrix, Hydro-diuril, Oretic)	If used before pregnancy, may be continued
Metolazone (Zaroxolyn)	If used before pregnancy, may be continued

Nitrates (for angina):

Isosorbide dinitrate, sublingual and oral tablets (Isordil, Sorbitrate)	Probably safe
Nitroglycerin ointment (Nitro-Bid Paste, Nitrol)	Probably safe
Nitroglycerin patches (Transderm-Nitro, Nitro Dur, Nitro Disc)	Probably safe
Nitroglycerin sublingual tablets (Nitrostat)	Probably safe

Cholesterol- and triglyceride-lowering drugs:

Cholestyramine (Questran)	Considered safe
Colestipol (Colestid)	Considered safe
Gemfibrozil (Lopid)	Limited experience
Lovastatin (Mevacor)	Not safe
Nicotinic acid (also known as niacin)	Limited experience

Antiarrhythmic drugs[1]:

Amiodarone (Cordarone)	Limited experience
Digoxin (Lanoxin)	Considered safe
Disopyramide (Norpace)	Probably safe
Flecainide (Tambocor)	Limited experience
Mexiletine (Mexitil)	Limited experience
Phenytoin (Dilantin)	Not safe
Procainamide (Pronestyl, Procan SR)	Considered safe
Propranolol (Inderal and others)	Considered safe
Quinidine (Quinaglute)	Considered safe
Tocainide (Tonocard)	Limited experience
Xylocaine (Lidocaine)	Considered safe

[1]If used before pregnancy, may need to be continued. Most are not prescribed frequently in young women.

should never stop taking medication before consulting with her physician. (See Chapters 12 and 23.)

A cardiologist will also help a mother-to-be with heart disease decide whether she will need extra medication, should stay at the same dosage, or should decrease her current medication or stop it altogether. A woman with heart trouble may need to go on a regimen of new medication—for example, digitalis products, heart-strengthening medication, or diuretics. For some women with heart conditions, it may be better to go off a medication such as the blood thinner warfarin (Coumadin), as some medications are not recommended during pregnancy. Any woman taking heart medications should speak with her physician if possible prior to becoming pregnant. (See box, "Common Heart Drugs: How Safe for the Pregnant Woman?") In every case, doctors must weigh any negative effects of taking a medication against the concept that a healthy, stable mother will produce a healthier baby. Unfortunately, because most women do not need heart medications during pregnancy, experience with any given medication may be limited.

Many drugs are excreted in breast milk, and, as in pregnancy, it may be better to avoid drug therapy while nursing if possible. If it is not possible to discontinue medication, a woman should use the safest drug—for example, acetaminophen rather than aspirin, which can cause metabolic changes or a rash in the baby and can affect blood clotting in both mother and baby.

The cardiovascular changes and work of labor will be lessened if the baby is delivered by cesarean section before labor begins, but this must be weighed against the risks of surgery and the maturity of the baby. If labor has already begun, spinal and epidural anesthesia should stabilize heart output and blood pressure. Pregnant women with heart disease should be followed and, if possible, managed at centers with "high-risk pregnancy" programs in which obstetricians, obstetric anesthesiologists, cardiologists, and neonatologists can work together to achieve the best possible outcome for both mother and child.

PREGNANCY-INDUCED HEART DISEASE

Pregnancy can trigger a number of heart-related conditions. The normal circulatory and hormonal changes of pregnancy may cause women to become hypertensive for the first time, especially in the last three months. The hypertension usually disappears after delivery. When it does not, women should be sure to keep their blood pressure under control with medication, if necessary. At this time, a physician may also decide to look for secondary causes of the hypertension such as kidney disease.

When blood pressure rises during the last three months of pregnancy and is accompanied by swelling of the legs or the presence of protein in the urine, the condition is called *toxemia of pregnancy*. (See Chapter 12.) It is usually divided into two phases, *preeclampsia* and *eclampsia*. If the process is not controlled, eclampsia, or seizures, may result. Fortunately, this is extremely rare. Obstetricians routinely take blood pressure at every prenatal appointment and aggressively treat high readings.

It should be noted that because of dilated blood vessels in pregnancy, the blood pressure is lower during the first three months—about 100–110/65–80 mm Hg. If it rises above 130/85 in the second or third part of the pregnancy, this may actually represent a higher than normal pressure.

A condition that can result from childbirth is bacterial endocarditis. This is rare. It can occur in women with heart valve defects such as mitral valve disease (from rheumatic fever or mitral valve prolapse) and gets started when bacteria enter the bloodstream through bleeding sites that may occur during delivery. To prevent bacterial endocarditis, cardiologists often prescribe antibiotics at the time of delivery.

Another condition that can crop up near the time of delivery or soon after is *perinatal cardiomyopathy* —that is, heart muscle disease occurring around the time of birth. This abnormality of heart muscle function is also rare, and its cause is poorly understood. (See Chapter 15.) It may result in congestive heart failure and the buildup of fluid in the body.

CHAPTER 20

HEART DISEASE IN THE YOUNG

CHARLES S. KLEINMAN, M.D.

INTRODUCTION

Congenital heart defects are relatively rare; seriously debilitating heart abnormalities rarer still. Approximately 8 babies in 1,000—representing somewhat less than 1 percent of live births—have some form of cardiac malformation at birth. In only half of these babies is the abnormality severe enough to cause symptoms that could require medical or surgical treatment. It is believed that genetic factors may play a role in the cause of these defects, but the pattern of inheritance is generally unclear. In fact, in all but about 3 percent of cases the underlying cause of the abnormality cannot be identified.

New surgical procedures have been developed in the past few years that can treat defects in children who could once be offered only palliative therapy. Now all but the most severe anomalies can be successfully treated with either medication or surgery. In many cases, open-heart surgery is being replaced by less invasive techniques involving catheterization and balloon angioplasty.

Surgical procedures are being performed on progressively younger children, which has many long-term advantages for these patients. In the 1960s the average child undergoing surgery was of school age; today, about a third of all congenital heart disease cases are being corrected within the first week of life.

The trend reflects increased awareness of the signs and symptoms of congenital heart disease among general pediatricians and family practitioners, as well as the increased number of infants who are diagnosed prior to birth and to improved surgical and postoperative care.

Although congenital heart disease is the most common type of cardiac disease affecting infants and children, it is not the only type. Acquired heart diseases may also affect children, although fortunately the two most common forms of acquired heart disease in children, rheumatic fever and Kawasaki disease, are relatively rare. High blood pressure and high blood cholesterol (hyperlipidemia) are also found in children. Children whose families have either of these conditions are at higher than normal risk of developing them.

THE DEVELOPING HEART

The human embryonic heart begins to form from a single tubular structure in about the fourth week of pregnancy. Within the next four weeks, this tube gradually increases in length, and eventually a loop forms as the tube twists toward the right side. Next a wall, or septum, divides the heart into left and right chambers; soon there will be upper and lower chambers as well and four valves to keep blood flowing forward through these four chambers and out to all parts of the body.

It appears that multiple factors, including genetic and environmental ones, may interact to alter the formation of the heart during the first eight to ten weeks of development. A few specific environmental exposures during this critical period can cause structural abnormalities. These include exposure to certain medications (for example, anticonvulsant medications such as phenytoin, the dermatologic medication Accutane, and lithium salts), viruses (rubella, cytomegalovirus), parasites (toxoplasmosis), metabolic disorders (such as uncontrolled diabetes), and excessive alcohol consumption. Fortunately, exposure to these environmental factors does not always result in cardiac abnormalities.

To understand the nature of some congenital anomalies, it is helpful to understand a little about the fetal heart and how it works. Because the fetus uses the placenta, rather than the lungs, to obtain oxygen and to rid itself of carbon dioxide, the path of the blood flow before birth is different from what it will become afterward. To accommodate this, the fetal heart and circulation are somewhat different in structure from the mature heart. Two special blood vessels, the ductus venosus and the ductus arteriosus, and the foramen ovale, an oval-shaped hole in the atrial septum (the wall separating the upper chambers), allow this special circulatory pathway to operate. Normally, all three of these close spontaneously within hours to days after birth. (The normal path of circulating blood in the adult is described in Chapter 1.)

Because of the unique communications that exist within the fetal heart and the lack of dependence upon the lungs for respiration, it is possible for fetal hearts to develop with remarkable degrees of malformation without this causing difficulties for the fetus. Such abnormalities may become important only after the fetal circulation begins its transition to the newborn state, when the two sides of the circulation become separated from each other and the lungs and circulatory system attempt to function on their own.

Certain conditions or syndromes characteristically cause a constellation of related abnormalities in newborns; in these cases genetic abnormalities may cause specific malformations or other problems of more than one organ. For example, about half of babies with Down syndrome have cardiac malformations, and approximately 25 percent of them have an opening in the atrioventricular septum, the wall separating

the right and left atria and the ventricles. More than 90 percent of newborns with other genetic defects (trisomy 13 or 18) have ventricular septal defects. Newborns with other types of genetic abnormalities may have bicuspid aortic valves, aortic coarctation, atrial septal defects, or pulmonic stenosis. These abnormalities of the heart are frequent enough in such syndromes that when a newborn is suspected of having one of these genetic abnormalities, cardiac malformations should also be suspected, even if the baby is not yet showing signs or symptoms of heart disease.

THE FETUS WITH CONGENITAL HEART DISEASE

Clinical research over the past 15 years has made considerable progress in applying ultrasound imaging techniques to perform fetal echocardiography. This diagnostic technique makes it possible to view tiny fetal hearts in action and to diagnose some complex forms of cardiac structural malformation as early as the 16th to 20th week of pregnancy.

The use of fetal echocardiography has reassured many parents that their baby's heart is normal; for others, it has afforded an opportunity to know long before birth that there is a malformation. This, in turn, allows more time for counseling about possible care and future treatment for the baby. A small number of parents have elected to terminate pregnancies when extreme forms of heart disease have been diagnosed in the fetus, especially when these are associated with abnormalities of other organ systems or of the fetus's chromosomes.

Fetal echocardiography is a specialized technique that is not part of the standard ultrasound examination many women undergo during the first or second trimester of pregnancy. Perinatal cardiologists at Yale have advocated that a screening view of the four chambers of the fetal heart be included when any fetal ultrasound study is performed after the 16th week of pregnancy. Almost 90 percent of the severest cases of structural heart disease are suspected on the basis of such studies. Once a suspicion is raised, a more complete and specialized fetal cardiac examination should be performed, ideally involving a joint evaluation by a perinatal obstetrician and a pediatric cardiologist with experience in fetal cardiac imaging. This specialized exam, available at a number of major university medical centers throughout the country, is

Indications for Specialized Fetal Echocardiography

Specialized fetal echocardiographic studies may be recommended if previous test have shown any of the following conditions in the fetus, or if the mother has any of the following risk factors.

Fetal Conditions and Pregnancy Factors

Growth retardation
Hydrops (swelling of the fetus)
Heart rhythm disturbances
Structural abnormalities of other fetal organs
Abnormal appearance of heart on four-chamber screening exam
Abnormal location of heart in the fetal chest
Excessive amniotic fluid (polyhydramnios)

Maternal and Family Risk Factors

Mother has congenital heart disease.
Mother has taken any of these medications or substances:
    Anticonvulsants such as phenytoin (Dilantin)
    Isotretinoin (Accutane)
    Lithium
    Cocaine
    Excessive alcohol
Mother has any of these infections during pregnancy:
    Rubella
    Cytomegalovirus (CMV)
    Toxoplasmosis
    HIV
Mother has a metabolic disorder such as:
    Diabetes
    Phenylketonuria (PKU)
Congenital heart disease is present in a previous child, the father, or other relatives.
Genetic syndromes known to be associated with cardiac disease (e.g., tuberous sclerosis, Noonan syndrome, or Marfan syndrome) are present in the family.

appropriate when specific risk factors are present or suspected, which is the case in about 10 percent of pregnancies. (See box, "Indications for Specialized Fetal Echocardiography.")

DIAGNOSING HEART DISEASE IN INFANTS AND CHILDREN

When heart disease is suspected in a child, whether newborn or older, the pediatric cardiologist generally employs relatively standard techniques to establish a diagnosis. The evaluation begins with a history of the pregnancy and the child since birth, as well as detailed information about the family to determine if there is any family history of congenital heart disease or syndromes that may be associated with specific cardiac malformations. The rest of the evaluation will entail a physical examination and perhaps other diagnostic procedures.

PHYSICAL EXAMINATION

Regardless of how sophisticated diagnostic tests have become, a detailed history and a thorough physical examination remain key elements of a cardiac evaluation. Often the diagnosis can be suspected on the basis of these alone, although it may need to be confirmed, or the severity of the problem more precisely delineated, by further tests.

The pediatric cardiologist will listen carefully to the child's heart and lung sounds with a stethoscope, take the pulse in various locations, and check the blood pressure, using a special child-sized cuff. He or she will note the child's skin color and palpate (feel with the hands) the child's chest and abdomen as well as the internal organs. The doctor will also look for any evidence of swelling (edema), typically in the abdomen, eyelids, liver, and, in the older child, ankles. Also in older children, the doctor may check to see if the fingers and toes are bulbous at the ends and the nails curved. This condition, known as "clubbing," is an indication of insufficient oxygen reaching the extremities.

The physician will be able to detect a wide range of conditions by observing certain signs and symptoms. For example, in cases where a cardiac abnormality causes heart failure, an accumulation of fluid in the lungs often causes rapid and labored breathing. This congestion makes it more difficult to expand and deflate the lungs, and the infant may appear to be working harder than is normal to breathe. Such babies frequently feed poorly and therefore may be underweight. These infants have more severe types of congenital heart lesions, but fortunately, these are also less common.

In severe cases with serious congenital abnormalities, where there is congestion of the circulatory system, it is common for children to develop fluid accumulation in the liver. Parents sometimes become alarmed when it is noted that the liver is enlarged, fearing liver disease in addition to a circulatory problem. Actually, the problem is parallel to that often seen in elderly people with circulatory congestion who develop fluid accumulation in the feet, ankles, and legs at the end of the day. In young children, and especially in infants, who rarely stand, gravity does not make fluid accumulate in these areas. On the other hand, the liver of the newborn is covered with a capsule that stretches more easily than the capsule of an adult's liver. The liver, being a spongy organ with a generous blood supply, serves as a reservoir for the accumulated fluid.

In other instances, a child may have an anomaly that obstructs blood flow from the right ventricle to the pulmonary artery. If the abnormality is associated with a hole or shunt within the heart connecting the right and left sides (either ventricles or atria), oxygen-poor blood may find it easier to cross to the left side of the circulation than to pass through the obstruction to the lungs. This means that not enough blood will be sent to the lungs to pick up oxygen before being circulated to the body. Children with this condition often have a blue (cyanotic) cast to the skin and lips and tend to breathe deeply, in response to the central nervous system's detection of inadequate oxygen within the bloodstream.

The simple act of taking the blood pressure in the legs as well as the arms, in addition to taking the pulse at several points on the body, may reveal the possibility of another congenital anomaly, coarctation of the aorta. In children with this condition, the aorta is narrowed, usually between the arterial branches to the head and arms and the lower body. The pulses in the arms and neck may be easily detected, while pulses to the legs are decreased. For the same reason, the blood pressure in the arms may be high and the pressure in the legs lower.

The stethoscope is used to listen to the heart and to breath sounds over the lungs. The physician will listen to determine whether the child is able to move air in and out of both lungs, and may detect a bubbling sound (rales) that signifies severe congestion in the lungs. Fluid leakage into the lungs causes bubbles to form when the child's breathing causes air to pass into the fluid-filled areas.

When the cardiologist listens to the heart, he or she is listening to the sounds that correspond to the closure of the valves that separate the atria and ventricles (tricuspid valve on the right and mitral valve on the left). These valves close at the onset of the contraction of the ventricles (systole), during the period when blood is being ejected from the ventricles into the pulmonary artery and aorta. This is the first heart sound. When systole ends and the ventricles relax in order to refill with blood for the next contraction, the valves between the right ventricle and

pulmonary artery (pulmonic valve) and the left ventricle and aorta (aortic valve) close and produce in the second heart sound. Under normal circumstances the cardiologist can discern a splitting of this sound, because the pulmonic valve usually closes a fraction of a second after the aortic valve. If the movement of one of these valves is restricted, or in the extreme case that one valve has not formed, the cardiologist will detect only a single second heart sound.

A murmur or a swooshing sound heard through the stethoscope may be a clue that there is a cardiac lesion. Many families become quite concerned about the presence of a heart murmur, but more often than not it turns out to be inconsequential.

It is important to recognize that a murmur is not a specific disorder, but merely a sign; it is an extra sound that the physician hears in addition to the first and second heart sounds. The stethoscope detects the presence of vibrations in the structures beneath it. These vibrations are transmitted to the listener's ear and detected as noise. Keeping in mind that the heart functions as an elaborate pump that propels blood to various parts of the body, it is not surprising that vibrations may be created, sometimes even in the perfectly normally functioning heart and circulatory system. Many vibratory murmurs that are heard during childhood are "innocent," or "functional," murmurs that do not denote any structural abnormality. Many, if not most, children may be found to have such murmurs at some time or other during their development, and they require no specialized tests, treatment, or follow-up.

By determining the timing of the murmur and its quality, location, and distribution, the cardiologist should be able to determine whether a given murmur is innocent or whether it is being created by a valve leak, a hole between areas of the circulation, or an obstruction in a valve or artery.

While many patients may be evaluated using these classic diagnostic techniques and may not require further testing, in many cases some laboratory evaluations are advisable. In such cases the cardiologist usually follows a logical sequence, choosing the test that is most likely to supply the needed diagnostic information for a given suspected diagnosis. In most situations the cardiologist prefers to use the least invasive and least costly tests first.

ELECTROCARDIOGRAM (ECG)

This procedure involves the use of electrodes, placed in contact with the child's limbs and chest wall, which detect the electrical activity of the heart. The electrocardiogram is very useful for evaluating disorders of the heart rhythm as well as possible deficiencies in the delivery of blood and oxygen to the heart itself. The information may also suggest that the walls of the heart or its specific chambers are enlarged or thickened, although the echocardiogram (see below) can determine this more specifically. The test detects the heart's own electrical current and does not expose the patient to any form of energy, so there is neither risk nor pain involved.

CHEST X-RAY

The chest X-ray is useful in determining the exact size and location of the child's heart. In some complex forms of heart disease the heart may be displaced from its usual position in the left and center of the chest. The chest X-ray also provides important information concerning the amount of blood flowing to the patient's lungs and may detect the presence of fluid accumulation, pneumonia, or "air trapping" in the child's lungs. This procedure is painless, but does require that the child hold still (in some circumstances a special restraint may be needed). There is no pain, and the radiation exposure is minimal.

BLOOD TESTS

Blood tests may help assess the severity of certain types of congenital heart disease. In cyanotic heart disease, for example, where there is an inadequate blood supply to the lungs, the body's response is to increase the number of oxygen-carrying red blood cells, so that the same volume of blood will be able to deliver more oxygen to the tissues.

ECHOCARDIOGRAPHY (CARDIAC ULTRASOUND)

This painless test uses high-frequency sound waves to provide "sonar" pictures of the heart and great arteries. These cross-sectional views of the heart and its various internal structures give a complete picture of relative sizes of the structures and wall thicknesses of the heart and its attached blood vessels. Further, echocardiography can be used to assess the functioning of the ventricles and, with the addition of Doppler techniques, to measure blood flow patterns and velocities within the heart and blood vessels. This is the most valuable noninvasive test for obtaining anatomic detail in cases of congenital heart disease. (See Chapter 10 for more details.)

Although there is no risk from echocardiography itself, it does require that the child be still for long periods. This may require sedation or, in the case of transesophageal echocardiography (see below), even anesthesia, which carries a small risk of its own.

More recently, echocardiographic equipment has been modified to allow the transducer (the hand-held microphones that both transmit and receive sound waves) to be mounted on an endoscope (a tube-shaped apparatus) that can be passed into the patient's esophagus. This is useful for visualizing hearts in patients with large chests or chest deformities that make standard echocardiograms from the chest surface difficult. When necessary, transesophageal echocardiograms can be done in children if they are large enough to have an esophagus that can accommodate the endoscope. Transducers small enough to be used safely in infants are now being tested. At this point the most compelling indication for transesophageal echocardiography is in the operating room at the time of open-heart surgery. There it is used to evaluate cardiac anatomy just prior to heart surgery and to evaluate the anatomic and functional results of the surgery immediately afterward, before the patient is sent to recovery.

CARDIAC CATHETERIZATION

This procedure involves inserting a small-diameter cardiac catheter—a hollow, flexible tube—into a vein or artery and then advancing it under fluoroscopic control into various cardiac chambers and blood vessels. The physician carefully manipulates the catheter into the desired location and can then measure the blood pressure and flow in the various heart chambers and blood vessels. If a radiopaque dye is injected through the catheter, X-ray motion pictures called angiograms can be recorded. These movies demonstrate the blood flow through the normal and abnormal structures of the heart and are often ordered if cardiac surgery is being considered.

Cardiac catheterization (which is described in greater detail in Chapter 10) is a common diagnostic technique for coronary artery disease and other cardiac disorders in adults, and cardiac catheterization laboratories are available in many hospitals. It is essential, however, that pediatric cardiac catheterizations be performed in a *dedicated* pediatric cardiac catheterization laboratory by a team that includes physicians, nurses, and technicians specifically trained in pediatric techniques. The staff should also be able to provide extensive pre-catheterization counseling for both parents and patients, ideally augmented by written information geared to each level. If such counseling is unavailable or inadequate, parents should seriously question whether the particular facility being considered is a truly experienced pediatric cardiac center. Only a relatively small number of children with congenital heart abnormalities actually have to undergo cardiac catheterization.

SPECIFIC CONGENITAL MALFORMATIONS

The prognosis for children with most of the following congenital defects is good, and for some conditions it is excellent. Most will lead full, normal lives, although some will require surgical therapy and long-term monitoring, and in a few cases, activity (specifically, competitive sports) may have to be curtailed. Regardless of the extent of recovery, however, some of these children will have a lifelong increased risk of developing bacterial endocarditis. Fortunately, the risk can be significantly decreased by taking prophylactic measures. (See box, "Preventing Bacterial Endocarditis.")

PATENT DUCTUS ARTERIOSUS (PDA)

The ductus arteriosus is a shunt pathway in the fetal blood circulation that connects the pulmonary artery to the descending aorta. It provides a detour for fetal blood to bypass the lungs and travel instead to the placenta, where it receives oxygen. At birth, the umbilical cord is clamped, the infant begins to breathe through the lungs, and the duct is no longer needed. As the amount of oxygen in the blood increases, the body's production of prostaglandin E_1, a chemical substance that is thought to keep the ductus open, decreases. The duct closes functionally within hours after birth and permanently within the first few days of life.

In some newborns, however, this shunt does not completely close, a condition known as patent ductus arteriosus. Now, because of differences in pressure in the blood vessels, too much blood, rather than hardly any, travels to the lungs. Infants who are born extremely prematurely or those whose mothers had rubella (German measles) during pregnancy appear to be at higher risk for this condition.

In cases of patent ductus, the symptoms will depend upon the size of the duct opening as well as the age and degree of prematurity of the infant. If the

Preventing Bacterial Endocarditis

Children and adults with valve damage or congenital heart disease are particularly at risk of developing bacterial endocarditis, an infection of the endocardial tissue that lines the heart walls, valves, and blood vessels. Sometimes called infective endocarditis, this is a serious illness whose treatment requires intravenous antibiotics administered during a lengthy hospital stay.

Any situation—from simple teeth cleaning to complex surgery—that could result in bacteria entering the bloodstream potentially exposes the patient to this infection. Fortunately, the risk can be substantially reduced by consistent use of prophylactic antibiotics. The American Heart Association and American Dental Association recommend that antibiotics be administered an hour before and six hours following any procedure that is likely to result in exposure. This includes surgical procedures performed on any unsterile body parts—the mouth and upper respiratory, gastrointestinal, and genitourinary tracts.

Prophylaxis is recommended for all congenital cardiac malformations, with the exception of isolated *ostium secundum* atrial septal defect. Parents should discuss these preventive measures with their pediatrician, pediatric cardiologist, and dentist. Local chapters of the American Heart Association can supply free wallet cards detailing the recommended antibiotics and appropriate doses. (See Chapter 13.)

ductus is only slightly open, the amount of excess blood circulation to the lungs will be very small, and the only finding may be a characteristic continuous heart murmur, with no symptoms.

At the other end of the spectrum is the child with a completely open ductus arteriosus, which may literally flood the lungs and pulmonary blood vessels in early life. Such children usually become short of breath and show other evidence of pulmonary congestion, such as easy fatigue. They often have difficulty with feeding and may have delayed development. If the problem is not recognized promptly there may be chronic pulmonary infections as well.

Patent ductus may not be recognized initially in extremely premature infants, because many of them suffer hyaline membrane disease (the pulmonary disease of prematurity), which keeps them on a ventilator while their lungs mature. As the lung disease improves, however, the expected ability to be weaned from the ventilator does not materialize, because the lungs rapidly become compromised by increased blood flow and the accumulation of excessive fluid (pulmonary edema).

Surgery has been used for many years successfully to ligate, or tie off, a patent ductus. The surgery (described in Chapter 25) carries minimal risk and is recommended for all children who have this condition, even if the opening is small and the child has no symptoms. This is because patent ductus, however minor, carries a risk of developing endocarditis, a bacterial infection of the heart or blood vessels that bears a much greater risk for the child than does the surgery.

For premature infants, surgery can be avoided in many cases by administering medications such as indomethacin, which interfere with the body's production of prostaglandins and cause the duct to close spontaneously. Indomethacin is unlikely to be successful in full-term infants or older children, however, because the patency is usually due to an abnormal ductus arteriosus rather than delayed closure. In these cases, surgery is required.

In recent years a special technique has been developed for closing a patent ductus arteriosus under local anesthesia in the catheterization laboratory. This procedure uses a detachable, miniature umbrellalike device made of stainless steel covered with a Dacron mesh, the same material used for cardiac surgical patches. Under fluoroscopic guidance, it is advanced inside a catheter into the open ductus and released. It remains in place permanently and is quickly covered with the patient's own tissue. Although there is no risk of rejection and little risk to the procedure at all, it is still considered investigational by the Food and Drug Administration. Many experts believe it will soon become the treatment of choice for patent ductus in all but premature infants, replacing surgery.

SEPTAL DEFECTS

The cardiac septa are the walls within the heart that separate the right and left atria from one another, as well as the right and left ventricles from each other. Sometimes an infant is born with a hole in the septum, called either an atrial septal defect or a ventricular septal defect, depending on its location. Since intravascular pressures in the left heart chambers generally exceed those in the right, in cases of a septal defect without other complications, the blood will leak from the left into the right chamber; this is known as a left-to-right shunt.

VENTRICULAR SEPTAL DEFECTS

The ventricular septum consists of three distinct areas that fuse together to form a single, solid muscle wall. When there is a ventricular septal defect, some of the oxygen-rich blood within the left ventricle that is supposed to be pumped out to the body through the aorta is ejected through the defect directly into the right ventricle and then to the pulmonary artery, through which it goes to the lungs rather than into the aorta. If the defect is small, there may be no symptoms and the only sign may be a loud (but harmless) murmur. The defect may ultimately close by itself or remain open with no real damage to the heart or pulmonary circulation.

If the defect is large, on the other hand, the amount of blood that recirculates through the pulmonary circulation may be great. The lungs may become congested, leading to shortness of breath and, in many cases, failure to gain weight adequately.

In the case of a large defect, the increased amount of blood returning to the heart from the lungs means that the left side of the heart also becomes overburdened. In order to provide adequate blood flow to the body, the heart pumps harder than normal and the heart rate and the force of contractions are increased. This may lead to an enlargement of the heart. The increased flow and pressure in the lungs may eventually lead to damage to the pulmonary blood vessels. If the heart is not able to sustain this extra work, the child may go into heart failure, which can lead to a backup of blood in the veins and accumulation of fluid in the lungs and other body tissues.

A newborn with a ventricular septal defect often will not develop a full set of symptoms for several days or weeks, because the left-to-right shunt is dependent upon the drop in pulmonary resistance that does not occur until some days after birth. The most compelling problems involve respiratory distress and growth failure. Medications may be used to help the heart and lungs to compensate for the extra burden that the ventricular defect and shunt place upon them. Digoxin and diuretics are most commonly prescribed, as well as vasodilators. If medical therapy is unsuccessful, or if the amount of blood flow into the lung or the blood pressure within the pulmonary vessels remains elevated for several months, surgery is recommended to close the defect with a patch. (See Chapter 25 for description.) In situations where there is only one hole, surgery is almost always successful.

Many ventricular septal defects, including some that are large enough to cause symptoms in the newborn period, tend to narrow spontaneously or even close completely. If the defect has not completely closed by the time the child is 5 to 7 years old, it is not likely that it will. On the other hand, in the absence of a significant overcirculation to the lungs, enlargement of the heart, or increase in pulmonary artery pressure, the mere presence of a ventricular septal defect does not warrant surgical treatment.

ATRIAL SEPTAL DEFECTS

Like the ventricular septum, the atrial septum forms during the embryonic development of the heart. Defects may develop at a number of locations in the wall (see the later discussion of atrioventricular canal defect). Most commonly, the defect involves the foramen ovale, an oval-shaped hole in the wall that is present in all children during the fetal period but closes spontaneously soon after birth. If the foramen ovale is larger than it should be or if the flap of tissue that usually closes it is displaced or deficient, the hole may remain after birth. Such a problem is referred to as an *ostium secundum* defect.

In most patients with atrial septal defects, symptoms are rare during childhood. While children with large atrial left-to-right shunts are often thin, neither respiratory symptoms nor severe growth failure is common. If anything, there may be a heart murmur, but it may not be evident until the child's second year. In itself, the murmur is not a problem, but it should be monitored periodically.

With the passage of years, however, these low-pressure shunts at the atrial level result in gradual enlargement of the right atrium and ventricle. It is not unusual for adults with this defect to develop symptoms related to cardiac rhythm disturbances such as atrial fibrillation or, later on, evidence of congestive heart failure. (See Chapters 14 and 16.)

Perhaps 25 percent or more of atrial septal defects diagnosed incidentally because a murmur is heard or through echocardiography done during infancy will close spontaneously. When the child reaches 2 or 3 years of age, most atrial defects that are producing clinical signs (enlarged right heart, substantially increased pulmonary blood flow), although not necessarily symptoms, should be repaired. This is because spontaneous closure after this age is highly unlikely and there is a risk of symptoms in later life.

Traditional surgical repair for an atrial septal defect, involving a Dacron patch, is both safe and effective. Even more promising is a new clamshell-like double-umbrella device that can be implanted under local anesthesia via a catheter procedure (similar to the one described in the earlier discussion of patent ductus arteriosus). Although the device is still considered investigational, it is expected to be approved by the Food and Drug Administration and ultimately to replace open-heart surgery in more than half of atrial septal defect repairs. The treatment of the other forms of atrial septal defect requires surgery in all cases. (See Chapter 25.)

ATRIOVENTRICULAR SEPTAL DEFECT (CANAL DEFECT)

This defect, also called an atrioventricular septal defect, is usually quite complex, and can be partial or complete. The complete defect, which is more common, involves the portion of the heart where the atrial septum (the wall vertically dividing the heart's upper chambers) meets the ventricular septum (separating the heart's lower chambers), as well as the valves—mitral and tricuspid—that divide these chambers horizontally. Partial defects may involve only the lower portion of the atrial septum (called *ostium primum* atrial septal defect and usually associated with a mitral valve defect) or, rarely, may involve only the ventricular septum, with or without a mitral valve abnormality.

The effect of the complete canal defect is a large hole spanning both the upper and lower parts of the septum and the presence, in place of two discrete mitral and tricuspid valves, of one large valve that spans both sides of the defect. The defect is compounded by the fact that this rudimentary valve does not always close properly, so that some of the blood flows back, or regurgitates, into one of the upper chambers. These defects usually result in an excessive amount of blood flowing to the lungs (a large left-to-right shunt) early in life, which produces severe symptoms of congestion and pulmonary hypertension. Infants with this congenital defect are often emaciated because of the hard work required to breathe and the consequent inability to take adequate nourishment. Their lips and fingernails may appear blue (cyanotic) if they have severe pulmonary edema.

Atrioventricular septal defect is often associated with Down's syndrome: Approximately 25 percent of children born with this syndrome have the defect, while approximately 50 percent of children with the defect have Down's syndrome.

Surgical intervention for atrioventricular septal defect is usually required within the first few months of life, regardless of the presence of Down's syndrome, because medical management is rarely able to prevent severe congestive heart failure. Without surgery, there is usually irreversible damage to the walls of the pulmonary blood vessels. (See Chapter 25.)

SEMILUNAR VALVE STENOSIS (AORTIC STENOSIS, PULMONARY STENOSIS)

The semilunar valves are the aortic, which lies between the left ventricle and the aorta, and the pulmonic, separating the right ventricle from the pulmonary artery. They are so named because their leaflets (flaps of tissue at their openings) are shaped like crescent moons. Stenosis, or a narrowing of the opening, may occur in either of these valves because they are thicker than normal or because they have deformed or fused valve leaflets.

In a child with pulmonary stenosis, the right ventricle must pump more vigorously to send sufficient blood to the lungs to be oxygenated. As a result, its muscular walls may become enlarged, thickened, and less efficient. If the stenosis is severe, the child may tire rapidly from any sort of exertion. An infant with severe stenosis may appear quite cyanotic and need immediate treatment—the hormonelike substance prostaglandin E_1, followed by balloon valvuloplasty (see below). If the impairment is only slight, treatment may not be necessary, but the child should be monitored for any indication that the condition is worsening.

In cases of aortic stenosis, the narrowed entrance to the aorta makes it more difficult for oxygenated blood to reach the body, and it may result in severe changes in the muscle of the left ventricle, gradually resulting in congestive heart failure. These babies are often found to have scarred and dilated left ventricles, in which case the prognosis is quite poor. At the other end of the spectrum are children with mild stenosis who may have no symptoms at all (although a heart murmur may be present), nor require treatment.

Although surgery has been the traditional treatment for children with either of these conditions, most newborns who have a severe obstruction in either valve now receive balloon dilation valvuloplasty. In this procedure, a balloon-tipped catheter is threaded through an artery or vein into the heart to the center of the valve. The balloon is then inflated, stretching the valve's opening.

Balloon valvuloplasty for the pulmonary valve has been very successful, and at Yale and other institutions it has completely replaced surgery for both newborns and older children. In contrast to the con-

dition in adults, aortic balloon valvuloplasty has a promising outlook, although it may carry a risk of the development of valve insufficiency (also a risk with traditional surgery), in which the valve does not close properly and blood "leaks" backward.

Children who undergo surgical or balloon valvuloplasty of the aortic valve need to be followed throughout life, because there is a tendency for the valve to calcify and degenerate, along with recurrent stenosis or progressive insufficiency or both. A complete surgical replacement of the valve may ultimately be required.

COARCTATION OF THE AORTA

This is a constriction, or narrowing, of a section of the aorta, the main artery carrying blood from the heart to the body. It increases pressure in the arteries closest to the heart, those serving the head and arms, while circulation to the legs remains poor.

In the newborn, coarctation may not be evident for as long as a week—until the ductus arteriosus closes. In some cases this is accompanied by a sudden obstruction to blood flow from the left ventricle, and may lead to acute heart failure and shock. Such infants may need respiratory support and will require medical treatment with prostaglandin E_1, which may help reopen the ductus. Other drugs may be given to improve cardiac contraction, but ultimately, surgery will be needed.

Coarctation may also be associated with other cardiac malformations, including ventricular septal defects and aortic or mitral valve abnormalities. Infants with these multiple anomalies are often quite ill, and require aggressive medical and surgical treatment.

Surgery involves either removing the constricted section of the aorta completely, patching it with a synthetic material, or creating a patch from a section of artery from an arm. In approximately a third of surgical repairs in newborns the coarctation recurs, regardless of the type of surgery. Recurrent lesions may be manageable using balloon angioplasty.

Occasionally coarctation may not be diagnosed until later in childhood. This almost invariably is associated with hypertension in the upper body that had not been detected earlier. If the condition is severe, the child may tire quickly, have headaches, leg cramps, and a pale appearance, and develop slowly.

For children, surgery (described above) is still routinely performed, but balloon angioplasty techniques are being refined and may ultimately replace surgery. In this case, a balloon-tipped catheter is advanced into the aorta and the balloon inflated until it stretches the areas of constriction.

The prognosis for infants and children who have surgery is quite good. Without repair, hypertension can become severe. It also appears that the older the patient at the time of repair, the higher the likelihood that he or she will have persistent hypertension.

CYANOTIC CONDITIONS

Children with certain types of congenital anomalies have a cyanotic appearance: a blue tinge to the mucous membranes, particularly evident in the lips and the finger- and toenail beds. This is a result of lower than normal amounts of oxygen in their systemic blood (the blood that circulates from the heart to all parts of the body except the lungs). In these children, defects that result in right-to-left shunting allow blood from the veins (after it has delivered its oxygen to the cells) to mix with oxygenated blood in the arteries. Such children may have obstructions to blood flow to the lungs combined with communications (holes) within the heart that allow the right-to-left shunt. A third type of defect, transposition of the great arteries, results in systemic venous blood returning directly to the aorta, because the aorta is abnormally connected to the right ventricle, while the pulmonary artery arises from the left ventricle. (See discussions of specific conditions below.)

Children who have deep cyanosis tend to be "hyperpneic"—that is, their central nervous system response to low levels of oxygen results in deep breathing, but it is generally unlabored. This is in contrast to children with left-to-right shunts, who, because of excess fluid in the lungs, have very labored (dyspneic) breathing.

TETRALOGY OF FALLOT

The most common cause of cyanotic congenital heart disease, tetralogy of Fallot is classically described as having four basic components: a ventricular septal defect, pulmonic stenosis (narrowing), an aorta that is unusually positioned above the ventricular septal defect, and thickening of the right ventricular muscle. In actuality, there is one primary problem with cardiac malformation: the upper portion of the ventricular septum aligns incorrectly, resulting in the presence of a large ventricular septal defect under the aorta. This is positioned in such a way that the aorta appears to arise from both the left and right ventricles. The misaligned septum narrows the outlet

from the right ventricle to the pulmonary artery, resulting in pulmonary stenosis. Because the blood flow into the pulmonary artery is obstructed, the oxygen-poor blood entering the right ventricle finds it easier to enter the aorta and body than to enter the pulmonary artery.

Infants with this defect usually develop symptoms at an early age; cyanosis may be apparent shortly after birth. Toddlers may tire easily or even faint as a result of normal exertion.

Tetralogy of Fallot is very amenable to complete surgical repair (described in Chapter 25), and children who have this operation before school age can lead relatively normal lives. Recent evidence, however, indicates that those who undergo surgery very early seem to have better heart function than children who undergo surgery at a later age. Further, palliative shunts (temporary holding measures) have been shown often to result in inadvertent scarring and deformation of the pulmonary arteries, making subsequent surgery more difficult.

TRANSPOSITION OF THE GREAT ARTERIES

In transposition of the great arteries the aorta arises from the right ventricle, while the pulmonary artery arises from the left ventricle, instead of the reverse. The result is that blood that has already been oxygenated returns to the lungs for more oxygen, while blood lacking oxygen is circulated to the body. Without some immediate way for these two parallel circulations to mix, the infant will not survive. Ironically, what allows survival is another defect, either patent ductus arteriosus or an atrial or ventricular defect, that provides a path for some oxygenated blood to reach the body's tissues.

Until fairly recently, only infants with a second defect were able to survive. With the advent of an interventional catheterization procedure called balloon septostomy, this pathway can be created on an emergency basis. A balloon-tipped catheter is threaded through a vein into the right atrium, across the foramen ovale, into the left atrium, and then forcefully withdrawn until the inflated balloon tears a small flap of tissue, resulting in the production of an atrial septal defect.

The septostomy is only a temporary measure to provide oxygen to the body. It must be followed by surgery to correct the physiology permanently. The most recent procedure used to repair the defect is an arterial switch, in which the aorta and the pulmonary artery are retransposed with the coronary arteries reimplanted to restore normal blood flow. Although patients who undergo this procedure seem to have a much better prognosis than those who receive the atrial switch developed some 30 years ago, the long-term results of the procedure remain to be seen.

PERSISTENT TRUNCUS ARTERIOSUS

This extremely rare condition is the result of a misalignment of the ventricular septum. The pulmonary arteries appear to arise as branches from the ascending aorta ("truncus"). Although this condition is considered a form of cyanotic heart disease because the circulating blood has less oxygen than normal, infants with this condition seldom appear cyanotic. They do develop an extremely heavy overcirculation of blood to the lungs and are usually quite ill with congestive cardiac failure. The extra work these infants must do just to breathe makes it difficult for them to feed, and many fail to develop properly. Some of these infants develop severe insufficiency (leakage) of the valve that controls the origin of the truncus, a rare condition that can be fatal.

The prognosis for children with this defect has improved considerably in recent years with the advent of surgery for complete repair in early infancy, rather than early palliative procedures with later repair. Early surgery helps prevent severe malnutrition and pulmonary vascular damage. The condition usually requires another operation prior to starting school, and perhaps one or two further open-heart procedures in later childhood or early adulthood.

Some infants with persistent truncus arteriosus are found to have deficiencies in calcium metabolism (known as hypoparathyroidism) and cellular immunity (thymic aplasia), and they may be at risk for unusual infections.

TRICUSPID ATRESIA

Atresia refers to the complete absence of an opening in a body organ. In tricuspid atresia the valve that allows blood to flow directly from the right atrium to the right ventricle is absent. This anomaly is usually found in conjunction with an atrial septal defect, which does allow the blood to leave the right atrium. In infants with tricuspid atresia, the systemic venous blood (returning to the heart after delivering oxygen to the body) crosses the atrial septum through the defect into the left atrium, where it mixes with oxygenated blood. This oxygen-deficient mixture then flows through the mitral valve and enters the left ventricle to be pumped out to the body, resulting in cyanosis.

In some cases, the great arteries arise normally—the aorta from the left ventricle and the pulmonary artery from the right ventricle, which is usually hypoplastic (underdeveloped). In such cases there is a ventricular septal defect as well, and the pulmonary valve, which allows blood to flow from the right ventricle to the pulmonary artery, is usually stenosed (narrowed). If the ventricular septal defect is large, the child may have excessive blood flow to the lungs, leading to congestive heart failure. If the pulmonary valve is narrowed or if the ventricular septal defect spontaneously closes, the child will develop cyanosis.

In other cases, the great arteries are transposed (see earlier discussion), producing increased pulmonary blood flow and leading to congestive heart failure, or there may be pulmonic stenosis, resulting in substantial cyanosis.

Early surgery is necessary to ensure that blood flow is as normal as possible, even though the procedure at this point is only palliative. To maintain or increase blood flow to the lungs and relieve the cyanosis, septostomy with a balloon (see the earlier discussion of transposition of the great arteries) or blade is used to enlarge or keep open the atrial septal defect. Alternatively, surgery may be performed to create a palliative shunt between pulmonary and systemic circulations to increase blood flow to the lungs until a type of surgery called a Fontan procedure can be done. Although the Fontan procedure is not a true repair, it is the best long-term solution available at this time. It has been in use for many years and allows the child to grow up with a reasonably normal, although somewhat restricted, range of activities. Long-term monitoring by a pediatric cardiologist will be required.

On the other hand, if there is too much blood flow to the lungs, resulting in severe congestive cardiac failure, the condition may be treated medically with digoxin and diuretics. If this proves unsuccessful, surgery may be used to place a constricting band around the pulmonary artery until more permanent surgery can be attempted.

PULMONARY ATRESIA

In this congenital anomaly there is no pulmonary valve to allow blood flow from the right ventricle into the pulmonary artery. Newborns with this condition are usually quite cyanotic (blue in appearance), because not enough blood reaches the lungs to become oxygenated. Some of the blood that should flow from the right atrium into the right ventricle instead is shunted across an opening in the septum into the left atrium. The blood that reaches the left atrium mixes with oxygenated blood from the lungs, and this oxygen-deficient mixture is circulated throughout the body, producing the symptoms of cyanosis.

Some blood does manage to reach the lungs because it flows through the ductus arteriosus, a passageway that is present during the fetal period that connects the pulmonary artery to the descending aorta. This duct usually begins to close within hours after birth, worsening the cyanosis, unless prostaglandin E_1 is administered to keep it open until surgery can be performed.

The prognosis for pulmonary atresia represents a broad spectrum, depending upon the size of the right ventricle and the pulmonary arteries. If the right ventricle is very small and thick-walled, the long-term effectiveness of surgical repair is questionable. If it is slightly larger but unable to act as a pump, a Fontan procedure (described in Chapter 25) may be used to circumvent it by creating a connection directly from the right atrium to the pulmonary arteries. If the ventricle is of adequate size, it may ultimately be included in the circulation after surgery. To increase the size of the pulmonary arteries, balloon angioplasty may be required.

Children with pulmonary atresia will require long-term follow-up by a pediatric cardiologist, even when surgery is completely successful.

TOTAL ANOMALOUS PULMONARY VENOUS CONNECTION

This rare cyanotic condition involves an anomalous (out-of-place) return of oxygenated blood via the pulmonary veins from the lungs. Oxygenated blood from the lungs, rather than returning to the left atrium, flows instead through the anomalous vein directly to the right atrium or to veins returning to the right atrium. There it mixes with unoxygenated blood, and some of the mixture flows through a defect in the atrial septum and out through the aorta to the body. If the connections are narrow, this may obstruct vein return from the lungs and lead to severe pulmonary edema and cyanosis. The rest of the mixture flows into the right ventricle and travels to the lungs through the pulmonary artery. Surgery to patch the atrial septal defect and connect the pulmonary vein to the left atrium is generally successful if performed in early infancy.

HYPOPLASTIC LEFT HEART SYNDROME

This is potentially the most serious of congenital malformations, with the poorest prognosis. Fortunately,

it is relatively rare. In its mildest form, it includes a moderately small left ventricle with a mild degree of obstruction; at its most severe, the left ventricle is very tiny, underdeveloped, and completely isolated from the rest of the heart and circulation because both the mitral and the aortic valves are missing (a condition called atresia). Such infants may seem normal for the first several days, because the ductus arteriosus has not yet completely closed and it provides a route for systemic circulation. Blood flows from the pulmonary artery, through the ductus arteriosus, into the aorta.

Once the ductus arteriosus closes, the newborn develops shock and ultimately fatal multiorgan failure. Survival depends on maintaining the patency of the ductus arteriosus with the hormonelike substance prostaglandin E_1 until definitive surgery can be performed. The most common surgery for this disorder (discussed in Chapter 25) must be considered, at best, innovative therapy that still borders on clinical investigation. Called the Norwood procedure after the physician who developed it, it is a staged operation that results initially in the infant living with a single (right) ventricle. A rudimentary aorta is constructed at the expense of the pulmonary artery, and a shunt is established to connect the systemic circulation to the pulmonary artery. This procedure is followed some months to years later by a Fontan operation, which is essentially only palliative. Current overall survival rates are in the range of 40–50 percent.

The alternative is neonatal cardiac transplantation. (See Chapter 25.) This is quite innovative, bordering on clinical experimentation, and experience is limited, but initial survival statistics are encouraging, as are midterm results. Whether, in the long term, transplant complications will require retransplantation is not yet known.

Both approaches have promise and should be offered to the families of all infants born with the severe form of hypoplastic left heart syndrome. At present, however, many families who are faced with this tragedy in the absence of encouraging survival rates appear to choose an expectant course of management, providing compassionate pain relief while allowing nature to run its course.

HIGH BLOOD PRESSURE

In adults, the cause of high blood pressure is discovered in less than 10 percent of cases. In these instances (known as secondary hypertension), the cause may be an abnormality of another organ, such as the kidney, or it may even be the result of a congenital heart condition, such as coarctation of the aorta. Secondary hypertension is significantly more common in children than in adults. Sometimes the underlying cause can be remedied and the blood pressure will drop to normal. The earlier high blood pressure is noted, the more likely it is that a specific cause will be found. Primary, or essential, high blood pressure accounts for the other 90 percent of cases.

For all people over age 18, high blood pressure is defined as a reading of 140/90 or more when taken several times over a period of weeks. (See Chapter 12 for information on measuring blood pressure.) For children, these numbers are lower. For example, a pressure of 130/85 would be considered high for a 12-year-old boy or girl. (See Table 20.1.)

Although somewhat under 3 percent of all children are found to have high blood pressure, the condition may be more serious if it starts in childhood and goes undetected for many years. Blood pressure should be measured as part of each child's annual physical. If it is elevated, it should be checked again within several weeks or months, preferably in a setting in which the child is relaxed and comfortable. This is especially important if either of the child's parents or another close relative has high blood pressure. At least once, the child's blood pressure should be measured in the legs as well as the arms.

If a child is found to have high blood pressure, it can sometimes be lowered with simple measures. If the child is overweight, losing the excess weight should be the first step. Ideally, this should be accomplished through exercise as well as calorie reduction. Exercise is not only an important habit to establish for life-long health, but it can have an effect on blood pressure, in addition to helping to control weight.

Reducing the amount of salt in the diet may be helpful. Salty snacks such as potato and other chips, pretzels, and salted popcorn are some of the foods that boost sodium consumption. Unfortunately, these may not be easy for some children to give up. Parents need to be sure that are plenty of substitutes—fresh fruit, vegetables, and juice—readily available. Cereal (without the sugar frosting) is a good food for nibbling that need not be limited to breakfast. (See Chapters 5 and 12 for additional information.)

If the blood pressure is very high or resistant to these changes, medication, such as diuretics or angiotensin-converting enzyme (ACE) inhibitors, may have to be considered.

In all cases of elevated blood pressure in children under the age of 8 to 10, some additional studies (such as X-rays of the blood vessels to the kidneys) should be done. In children often a specific cause will be found, and it can usually be treated.

HIGH BLOOD CHOLESTEROL (HYPERLIPIDEMIA)

High blood cholesterol levels, like high blood pressure, can be found in children as well as in adults. In a small number of children, perhaps 1 to 2 percent, this is a result of a genetic abnormality called familial hypercholesterolemia, and the levels can be very high. Another 13 to 14 percent have elevated cholesterol readings unrelated to genetics. The typical high-fat American diet may be one of the underlying causes.

The long-term danger of high levels of cholesterol in the blood is the development of atherosclerosis, a condition in which the inner walls of the arteries thicken and become narrowed and irregular. The process starts when excess cholesterol, a fatlike substance, hardens into plaque and is deposited on the artery walls. Atherosclerosis is a major cause of coronary heart disease.

Some pediatricians and pediatric cardiologists recommend that all children have a blood cholesterol test by the time they enter school, while others feel this is only necessary for children at special risk. At the very least, children with a family history of elevated cholesterol or early heart disease (under age 65) should have an initial test by age 5, with follow-up tests every few years. A ten-year follow-up is probably sufficient for children with normal levels and no family history.

Blood (serum) cholesterol is measured in milliliters

Table 20.1
Upper Limits of Normal Blood Pressure in Children
(These numbers are approximate.)

Age	Pressure
Up to 6	110/75
6 to 10	120/80
11 to 14	125/85
15 to 18	135/85–90

per deciliter of blood, ml/dl. For children, an ideal level is 150 ml/dl or less (compared to 200 ml/dl in adults). A child found to have elevated cholesterol should be treated by diet first. A heart-healthy diet recommended by Yale, the American Heart Association, and many other organizations calls for no more than 30 percent of calories from fat and no more than 300 milligrams of cholesterol. (See Chapter 5.) This is a general recommendation for healthy adults and children age 2 and over (under age 2, more fat is needed for development).

If the child's cholesterol is greatly elevated, it may be necessary to restrict fat and cholesterol further. This decision is best made in consultation with a pediatrician or pediatric cardiologist. A registered dietitian may be a useful resource for helping the entire family find practical ways to have a healthy diet.

Exercise can also be helpful in controlling cholesterol by raising the level of high-density lipoprotein (HDL), considered the beneficial form of cholesterol. If diet and exercise are unsuccessful in lowering a very high level (for a child, this is above 250 ml/dl), drugs may have to be used.

RHEUMATIC HEART DISEASE

Rheumatic fever has been almost eradicated in the United States in the past three decades, but recently it seems to have reappeared in several communities. Although outbreaks have traditionally been higher among urban children of lower socioeconomic status, the most recent cases have been seen primarily in suburban and rural middle-class children.

Rheumatic heart disease is the end result of rheumatic fever, which follows about 1 percent of cases of acute streptococcal (strep) infection of the throat. Rheumatic fever may be an exaggerated response of the immune system in which the body produces substances to fight off the strep infection that are toxic to its own cells instead.

The symptoms of rheumatic fever, which usually develop within two weeks but may not appear for several months, include fever, skin rash, swelling of the joints, and involuntary twitching of muscles (chorea). In about a third of cases there is inflammation of the heart tissue and valves. In other cases, symptoms may be vague, such as generalized fatigue, and go unrecognized. Most cases occur in children aged 5 to 15, although adults are occasionally affected.

The fever that gives this disease its name may last up to two weeks and be accompanied by arthritis-like pains in the joints. The pain may migrate from one joint to another and be accompanied by redness and inflammation. A lacy rash called erythema marginatum may also be present, as well as rapid, involuntary twitching and jerking of the muscles. If there is heart involvement, the child may be short of breath, tire easily, and have a poor appetite. If the physician finds heart enlargement and a murmur, chest X-rays, an electrocardiogram, and possibly an echocardiogram will be ordered to confirm rheumatic heart disease.

Rheumatic fever is treated primarily with bed rest and a number of medications, depending on the symptoms. Aspirin or steroids such as prednisone or cortisone may be prescribed for joint pain and possible inflammation of the heart. Diuretics or a sodium-restricted diet may be necessary to reduce excess work by the heart caused by fluid retention. Sedatives or tranquilizers may be used to relieve muscle twitching.

Children who have had rheumatic fever are at risk of recurrence and are usually given prophylactic antibiotics to prevent this. Prophylactic antibiotics are also recommended before any surgery or other procedure that is likely to involve blood, especially for those who have rheumatic heart disease. This therapy helps reduce the risk of developing endocarditis, a bacterial infection of the heart valves or heart lining.

The dramatic declines in rheumatic fever have been due to better detection and to treatment with antibiotics. Prevention depends upon prompt treatment. A culture should be taken of any sore throat that comes on suddenly and is accompanied by a fever, which may be as high as 104°F. Other symptoms may include headache, nausea, vomiting, and abdominal pain. The culture will determine whether the sore throat is caused by a virus or a bacterium and, if so, which type. (Rheumatic fever can only be caused by group A hemolytic streptococcus.) Strep throat, regardless of which type of bacterium caused it, can be treated effectively with penicillin or other antibiotics; there is no effective treatment for viral sore throat.

KAWASAKI DISEASE (MUCOCUTANEOUS LYMPH NODE SYNDROME)

Kawasaki disease is a rare acute inflammatory disease of children that is thought to be the result of infection, possibly viral, although a responsible agent has not been identified. Each year in the United States approximately 1,500 children develop this inflammation of the mucous membranes and lymph glands, and 98 percent of these children recover. In about one out of five cases there is cardiac involvement, primarily the formation of aneurysms (outpouchings in the vessel walls) in the coronary arteries. Some patients may have myocarditis, pericarditis, and hepatitis. The 2 percent mortality is related to coronary arterial aneurysms and thrombosis.

The incidence of Kawasaki disease appears to be rising, but this may only be because of better recognition and reporting. The disease itself has only been identified in the past 20 years or so. Incidence is highest in Japan and among Asian children in other countries, including those in Hawaii. It is not limited to Asian children, but incidence appears to be lower among Caucasians. Boys, for unknown reasons, seem to develop Kawasaki disease twice as often as girls. The infection primarily affects children under 10, 80 percent of whom are under 5.

The symptoms are varied and uncomfortable, including a sudden high fever (102°F., spiking to 104° or 105°F.); a deep red rash that may mimic hives, scarlet fever, or measles; swollen hands and feet that sometimes have dark red or purple blotches on the palms and soles; bulbar conjunctivitis (red eyes); swollen lymph nodes, particularly on one side of the neck; and inflammation of the mouth, with a strawberry appearance to the tongue and swelling and cracking of the lips. There may also be a stiff neck, diarrhea, or abdominal pain. About 40 percent of the children will develop painful but temporary arthritis, or swelling of joints, especially in the legs.

The acute phase lasts several days to a week, with symptoms subsiding as soon as the fever disappears. In two to three weeks, the skin on the hands and feet may peel. Treatment is aimed at ameliorating the symptoms and may require hospitalization. Aspirin may be given to reduce fever and inflammation, but a large single intravenous dose of gamma globulin seems to shorten the acute inflammatory phase of the disease and appears to cut the risk of aneurysm by more than half.

Long-term cardiac complications, if there are any, may be seen as early as two weeks after the onset of the disease. Aneurysm formation and abnormalities of heart function are usually best diagnosed by echocardiography. In approximately one-half of patients whose aneurysms remain after the acute phase of the disease has resolved, these aneurysms will disappear within two years. It is unclear, however, how many of these children will ultimately develop coronary occlusions and have cardiac symptoms.

In some cases coronary angiography, for diagnosis and prognosis, may be warranted. Long-term antithrombotic aspirin therapy is recommended for coronary artery aneurysm follow-up care, or coumadin if the aneurysm is uncommonly large. In rare cases, patients ultimately require coronary artery bypass surgery, and some go on to develop myocardial infarctions.

SUMMARY

Most children with cardiac problems who are encountered in 1991 have some form of congenital heart disease. Only about half of the 8 cases of congenital heart disease in 1,000 liveborn children require any form of treatment.

The 1980s witnessed remarkable improvements in surgical management techniques, including the widespread use of cardiac transplants that accompanied the introduction of cyclosporin for immunosuppression. Transplants are now used in the management of complex structural disease in children and newborns. In addition, the 1980s witnessed the development of a technique for treatment of the hypoplastic left heart syndrome.

The 1990s offer the promise of more successful interventional catheterization techniques to ameliorate obstructed blood vessels, and to provide definitive procedures for the closure of intracardiac shunts, without need for open-heart surgery.

The development of new high-resolution and high-speed imaging systems shows promise that may allow MRI and CAT scanners, in tandem with ultrasound scanners, to make cardiac imaging more precise and less invasive than in the past.

The advances that have been made in fetal cardiac imaging have given birth to subspecialty care of the fetus with congenital heart disease. It is likely that future developments will include the introduction of prenatal catheterization and surgical techniques aimed at repair of the malformed fetal heart.

When parents are confronted with the fact that their newborn child has congenital heart disease, there is often a period of disbelief and denial, which is a normal response to learning bad news. Unfortunately, in some of the most severe cases of congenital heart disease, parents may be called upon to make important management decisions, the consequences of which they and other members of the family may live with for many years to come. These decisions are often made in an extremely emotionally charged atmosphere at a time when reasoned decisions may be difficult. The newborn "management team" must try its utmost to provide accurate information to the parents regarding diagnosis, management options, and prognosis (short- and long-term) to allow the parents the best opportunity to make informed decisions.

CHAPTER 21

HEART DISEASE IN THE ELDERLY

LAWRENCE H. YOUNG, M.D.

INTRODUCTION

The elderly represent the fastest-growing segment of the American population. By the year 2000, it is estimated that people over age 60 will account for more than 15 percent of all U.S. citizens; those over 80 will constitute about 4 percent, or some 10 million Americans. Clearly, the nation's efforts to prevent and effectively treat heart disease must include older Americans and take into account their special needs and concerns.

Any discussion of heart disease in the elderly must begin by defining just what "elderly" means in the context of cardiovascular health. When does old age begin? There are various criteria: chronological age, or the number of years one has lived; physiologic age, including the presence or absence of diseases of old age; and, of course, mental acuity.

As medical progress continues to lengthen expected life spans, the concept of "elderly" has shifted upward. Although there is no clear-cut threshold of old age, for purposes of medical classification physicians tend to define "elderly" as beginning in the range of 65 to 70. In practice, however, treatment decisions are based not on age alone but on a person's entire medical profile and mental outlook—both of which may be "young" or "old" for a particular chronological age.

HOW THE HEART GROWS OLD

As a person ages, the heart undergoes subtle physiologic changes, even in the absence of disease. (See box, "Physiologic Changes in the Aging Heart and Blood Vessels.") The muscles of the aged heart may relax less completely between beats; as a result, the pumping chambers (ventricles) become stiffer and may work less efficiently, especially if specific cardiac diseases are present. In old age, the heart also may not pump as vigorously or as effectively as it once did. The older heart also becomes less responsive to adrenaline and cannot increase the strength or rate of its contractions during exercise to the same extent it could in youth. We all come to realize that although a 50- or 100-yard dash was easy when we were 20, it is extremely difficult as we get older—the heart just can't get enough blood out to muscles to supply them with adequate oxygen.

The rate of this change or decline in cardiovascular function varies greatly among individuals. In an otherwise healthy person, the decline is not likely to be of great importance, but when another condition, such as coronary artery disease or a valve disorder, affects the heart, these age-related changes may compound the problem or its treatment.

The vascular system, too, experiences gradual changes over the decades. The walls of the arteries

Physiologic Changes in the Aging Heart and Blood Vessels

The Heart

- Muscle relaxes less between beats (becomes stiffer).
- May not pump blood as efficiently.
- Is less responsive to stimulation by the nervous system.
- Is less able to increase strength of contractions during exercise.
- Walls may thicken.

The Blood Vessels

- Walls become less elastic.
- Reflex that maintains blood pressure upon standing up may become slower.

Note: Despite all of these changes, most older individuals function quite well unless a specific heart muscle or valvular disease is present.

tend to lose their elasticity and stiffen, even without internal blockage from fatty deposits (atherosclerosis). Commonly, this may lead to a specific kind of high blood pressure among older people called isolated systolic hypertension (discussed below).

Cardiovascular disease—including coronary heart disease, hypertension, heart valve disease, and rhythm disorders—becomes increasingly common with advancing age. (See box, "Types of Cardiovascular Disease More Common in the Elderly.") By the

Types of Cardiovascular Disease More Common in the Elderly

- Isolated systolic hypertension
- Orthostatic hypotension
- Heart failure
- Aortic stenosis
- Mitral annular calcification
- Complete heart block
- Sick sinus syndrome
- Atrial fibrillation
- Stroke

age of 80, for example, 20 percent of Americans have symptomatic coronary heart disease. The changing role of various risk factors over time is discussed in this chapter, as are the arguments for making so-called life-style changes to prevent or slow the progression of coronary heart disease in old age. Heart problems in old age may affect quality of life, length of life, or both. While coronary heart disease is the leading cause of death in elderly Americans, it and other problems—such as rhythm disturbances and valve dysfunction—are also important because of the symptoms they present: for example, chest pain, as well as fatigue, shortness of breath, or fainting.

HYPERTENSION: UNSAFE AT ANY AGE

High blood pressure is more common with advancing age, and so are its associated complications, of stroke, kidney disease, heart attack, and heart failure. By the seventh decade of life, close to half of all Americans have hypertension, usually of unknown cause. (Chapter 12 presents a general discussion of the diagnosis and treatment of hypertension.)

Elderly people should have blood pressure measured annually, and high levels (generally defined as 160/90 mm Hg and above) should be treated. The notion has long persisted that a certain degree of high blood pressure is a normal part of the aging process, and may even be necessary to pump sufficient blood to vital organs. More recently, however, convincing evidence has been gathered that hypertension in the elderly is *not* benign. Even in old age, lowering elevated blood pressure can save lives. Control of hypertension may not be achieved as readily as in younger patients, but even so, partial treatment can lower the rate of potentially serious complications, a conclusion backed up by well-documented evidence from several long-term research studies.

How aggressively should high blood pressure in the elderly be treated? In general, lowering even mildly elevated blood pressure is potentially beneficial, and perhaps of greatest benefit for people with other kinds of cardiovascular disease. For those with no other heart disease, a trial of diet modification, moderate exercise, and (if indicated) smoking cessation and weight loss may be sufficient to lower blood pressure and reduce other concomitant risks.

On the other hand, highly restrictive or rigid programs of diet or exercise for the elderly are inadvisable and unlikely to succeed.

If antihypertensive drug therapy is prescribed for an older person, he or she will probably need to visit the doctor for regular checkups to monitor the results. It is important that the patient report any possible side effects; in most cases, they can be controlled or eliminated by adjusting the dosage or the type of medication used. (Medication should not be abruptly stopped, since that may, under certain circumstances, cause blood pressure to rebound to high levels.)

Even among those with normal blood pressure, some degree of light-headedness or dizziness is not unusual in older people, especially upon arising from a sitting or lying position. This condition, called *orthostatic hypotension* (position-related low blood pressure), is caused by a slowing of the body's reflexes that maintain blood flow from the heart to the brain and other organs in an efficient manner. Medication for high blood pressure can worsen this tendency—another reason that careful monitoring of therapy is important. Many physicians prefer to start older patients on a lower dosage of medication and increase the dosage more gradually than they might with younger patients.

For a majority of older people, a simple treatment regimen with small doses of a diuretic or other drug, such as a beta blocker, calcium channel blocker, or ACE inhibitor, will be sufficient to lower blood pressure to a safe range with few, if any, unpleasant side effects. In prescribing a drug to lower blood pressure, the physician must also consider other medications a patient is taking, other medical problems that may be present, and what financial limitations, if any, may affect a person's ability to afford medication. (Some types of antihypertensive drugs are significantly more expensive than others.) If the doctor doesn't inquire about these factors, the patient should not hesitate to discuss his or her concerns.

A special type of high blood pressure that is more common in elderly people is called *isolated systolic hypertension.* In this condition, only the upper, or systolic, reading in the two-part blood pressure reading is elevated (for example, 160/70 or 200/80). The systolic reading represents a recording of the pressure exerted against the arterial walls when the heart contracts and pumps blood out; the lower, or diastolic, number represents the arterial pressure between heartbeats. In younger people with hypertension, both the upper and lower readings are likely to be elevated. But as the arterial system stiffens with age, the systolic pressure alone may be elevated to

as high as 200 mm Hg or more during ejection (pumping) of blood from the heart.

Elevated systolic pressure is a known risk for cardiovascular disease. The value of lowering it has recently been proved by a major study called the Systolic Hypertension in the Elderly Program (SHEP). Yale was one of the major participating centers in this study. Treating isolated systolic hypertension can now be recommended to reduce the incidence of stroke, heart attack, and heart failure. When other symptoms of heart disease (such as angina) are also present, it may be even more important to lower the systolic pressure than if no symptoms are present.

Another condition resulting from high blood pressure, especially in old age, is *left ventricular hypertrophy,* or thickening of the heart's main pumping chamber, the left ventricle. After many years of pumping against heightened resistance, the heart enlarges under strain and its walls begin to thicken. This condition bodes ill for the heart's future health; it may eventually lead to heart failure, as the heart works harder to fill with blood or eject it. Drugs are the primary treatment for hypertension with left ventricular hypertrophy. In general, many drugs—including ACE inhibitors, calcium channel blockers, and beta blockers—can prevent or sometimes reverse hypertrophy; calcium channel blockers may be used to enhance the hypertrophic heart's relaxation between beats. Effective treatment will reduce heart size in about half of people with high blood pressure and enlargement of the left side of the heart.

CORONARY HEART DISEASE

Coronary heart disease is the leading killer of older people; half of all heart attack victims are over 65. While men have markedly higher rates of coronary heart disease in middle age than do women, women's rates of coronary disease begin to rise sharply after menopause; ultimately their rates are about equal to those of men.

In the past few decades, efforts to prevent coronary heart disease have centered primarily on so-called premature heart disease—blockage of the coronary arteries that occurs in middle age. The very term implies that some degree of coronary blockage is a natural consequence of aging. But this isn't necessarily so. In some cultures, where the average blood cholesterol and blood pressure is lower than in many industrialized societies, the prevalence of coronary heart disease among the elderly is not nearly as great.

The perception of heart disease in old age as virtually inevitable has thus given way to a more intervention-minded approach that seeks to prevent heart disease and preserve heart function—and overall health and well-being—as long as possible, or at least as long as seems reasonable.

Coronary heart disease may be manifested as reversible episodes of myocardial *ischemia*, characterized by chest pain (angina) or shortness of breath, or by a more severe form, a heart attack, in which inadequate blood flow leads to the death of heart muscle and scar formation. In older patients, heart attacks often result in more complications and longer hospital stays, with slower and more difficult recoveries. Heart failure and rhythm changes may be more frequent in this age group.

So-called silent heart attacks—those occurring without the classic symptoms of chest pain—are more likely in old age, especially in diabetic individuals. Instead of causing the typical crushing chest pain or pressure, a heart attack may announce itself with a symptom such as "heartburn," shortness of breath, fainting, or confusion; in some cases, the symptoms are few or none. Older people accustomed to minor illnesses and discomforts may also be less likely to notice or complain of such vague symptoms. The elderly, and those who care for them, should be aware of these atypical warning signs of a heart attack and seek prompt evaluation. Evidence of heart damage may be detected on an electrocardiogram or echocardiogram.

It is not surprising that the treatment of coronary heart disease may involve a somewhat different set of considerations in a 75-year-old than in a 45-year-old. Prophylactic administration of lidocaine, an antiarrhythmic drug used to prevent ventricular rhythm changes, may not be given initially in the elderly, because this drug tends to produce confusion or other side effects in older patients. Thrombolytic therapy —medication to dissolve blood clots obstructing flow to the heart—may be used when the physician judges its benefit to outweigh the risk of bleeding in an elderly person, but it must be used with caution. Treatment decisions may also reflect differences in patients' expectations in terms of physical activity; some patients may accept physical limitations with advancing age more readily than others.

The management of angina may also differ. Older patients may be more willing to accept some degree of angina rather than undergo surgery or other intervention. The elderly may be more prone to dizziness and other side effects of anti-anginal medications than younger people, and further, they may not tolerate them as well. This may be especially true with nitroglycerine derivatives. Beta blockers also tend to slow the heart more in older people. This is not a cause for concern unless the rate decreases to less than 50 beats a minute and symptoms of weakness or dizziness occur.

HEART VALVE DISORDERS

The four valves that perform the vital function of keeping blood flowing properly through the heart's four chambers are subject to a broad range of malfunctions (discussed in detail in Chapter 13). Certain types of valve disorders are far more common among the elderly. Some can be treated effectively with medications, regardless of age; others will not respond to medication but can be treated surgically, an option that may merit consideration if symptoms interfere with the activities of daily life.

The most common valvular problem in old age is aortic valve disease. The aortic valve is the gateway for blood pumped from the left ventricle to the rest of the body. *Aortic sclerosis* refers to the process of thickening and stiffening (fibrosis, or scarring) in the valve. It affects up to a third of all elderly people. The valve itself, however, may continue to function adequately for years, with nothing more than a heart murmur heard by the physician on examination with the stethoscope. The murmur is caused by turbulence of blood passing through the valve.

In *aortic stenosis*, the aortic valve becomes narrowed and blocked by hard, calcified deposits. This condition is present in about 4 percent of all elderly people. Severe aortic valve stenosis can cause fainting (because of impaired blood flow to the brain across the narrowed valve); heart failure (when the heart's muscle becomes unable to pump blood in a forward direction through the too-small opening); and chest pain (because of increased work and a lack of sufficient oxygen reaching heart muscles).

Aortic stenosis can usually be diagnosed from the physical exam, but echocardiography is a key technique used to assess the severity of this and other valve abnormalities. Surgical replacement of the aortic valve is an accepted and often highly successful treatment in elderly as well as younger patients. In patients who are otherwise healthy, valve replacement (using either a specially treated heart valve from a pig or an artificial valve) may return the heart's function to normal or near-normal.

In addition to valve replacement surgery, newer, nonsurgical options are sometimes considered for opening up a narrowed aortic valve. *Aortic valvuloplasty*, in which a balloon-tipped device is threaded through the heart and opened to expand the diseased valve, may be recommended for individuals who are at especially high risk for surgery. At present, however, this procedure has had limited success and is not very widely recommended. Surgery is a much more effective treatment for long-term relief. In the absence of other complicating medical factors, aortic valve replacement can be achieved at an acceptable, albeit somewhat higher, risk than in younger people. The decision concerning surgery must, however, take into account the total condition of the patient.

Another valvular problem seen almost exclusively in the elderly is *mitral annular calcification*, or calcification of the ringlike support structure around the mitral valve. The resulting malfunction usually causes either blockage of the valve or blood to leak back (regurgitate) into the atrium from the ventricle. The condition is seldom severe, and typically does not require surgical correction.

Older people with a valvular problem such as aortic stenosis, or even mitral valve prolapse, are more prone to *endocarditis*, or infection of the heart valves. The infection-causing bacteria may enter the bloodstream from infection in other sites, such as the urinary or gastrointestinal tract, or from the normal mouth during dental work. Prompt treatment for infection and the use of prophylactic antibiotics before dental work and other procedures with a risk of infection are especially important for people with valvular heart disease.

RHYTHM DISORDERS AND PACEMAKERS

Problems with the heart's rhythm and the electrical system that governs it can occur at any age, but are more common in old age. Rhythm abnormalities, or *arrhythmias*, may cause no symptoms, or they may be sensed as slow or missed beats, "flutters," palpitations, light-headedness, dizziness, or fainting. The heart's rhythm may be too slow (*bradycardia*) or too fast (*tachycardia*). (See Chapter 16.)

SLOW RHYTHM DISORDERS

Among elderly people, slow rhythms are a chief concern. In old age, the electrical system that carries the signal to trigger the heart's timely contractions may run into trouble at several points in its pathway of specialized tissues.

"Sick sinus syndrome," unusual in younger people, is a relatively common cause of rhythm disturbance in the elderly. No relation to the sinuses in the head, this syndrome refers to the *sinus node*, a specialized patch of electrically active tissue that acts as the heart's internal pacemaker. This "on-board computer" may malfunction after decades of trouble-free service, because of disease of the heart muscle or for no known reason. As a result, the heartbeat may slow down—in some cases, to a rate below 35 or 40 beats a minute, which will cause the blood pressure to fall to very low levels. Fatigue, confusion, malaise, and fainting may follow. Drug therapy for high blood pressure or coronary heart disease with one of the beta blockers or, less commonly, with a calcium blocker may sometimes precipitate symptoms in patients with this syndrome. Symptomatic sick sinus syndrome may have to be treated by implantation of an electronic cardiac pacemaker, which often affords immediate and striking improvement of symptoms.

Rhythm problems can also crop up in other parts of the heart's electrical system. The wear and tear of age on the electrical conducting fibers can cause a condition called *heart block*, in which the impulses fail to travel efficiently between the atrium and the ventricle; the ventricle may be triggered irregularly or not be triggered to contract at all, and as a result, the individual may faint. Minor types of heart block can be present for many years without symptoms, but if the patient has severe heart block accompanied by fainting, a pacemaker may be necessary.

Pacemakers are being continually refined and improved to handle a wide range of rhythm disorders. Pacemaker implantation is generally considered a low-risk procedure even for elderly patients, and is done under local anesthesia. The small risk entailed is justified by what is often a marked relief of disturbing or disabling symptoms.

FAST RHYTHM DISORDERS

The atria, the heart's upper chambers, may give rise to an excessively rapid and irregular rhythm called *atrial fibrillation*. This condition, which affects up to 5 percent of the older population, is generally not dangerous and can be controlled with medication.

Occasionally, the patient will require a procedure called cardioversion—very brief anesthesia and an electrical shock to correct this rhythm. In some cases in the elderly, the restoration of regular rhythm does not last long and fibrillation recurs. Patients with atrial fibrillation are at increased risk of developing blood clots in the heart that may embolize (travel) and block blood vessels elsewhere in the body (for example, in the brain, causing a stroke). This risk is somewhat higher in the elderly; for some patients, anticoagulant medications or aspirin may be prescribed to thin the blood and lower the risk of stroke.

Ventricular arrhythmias, those originating in the heart's lower chambers, are particularly likely after a heart attack or in the presence of heart failure. These arrhythmias are usually minor but, when prolonged, may lead to light-headedness, dizziness, or fainting spells, and can occasionally be quite dangerous. Severe ventricular arrhythmias (such as ventricular tachycardia) may require intensive therapy with anti-arrhythmic drugs or occasionally the implantation of an internal electrical device called a cardioverter defibrillator to shock the heart should a dangerous arrhythmia occur.

CARDIAC DIAGNOSIS: CONCERNS FOR THE ELDERLY

Elderly people with symptoms suggestive of heart diseases undergo essentially the same diagnostic process as younger patients. Much can be learned from the medical history, physical examination, and electrocardiogram. In many cases, noninvasive tests will also be used. Echocardiography and nuclear scans may help to reveal more information about the heart's structure and function. In specific cases, the use of cardiac catheterization or other invasive testing is necessary to guide treatment or provide a blueprint for surgery or angioplasty. However, judgment must be employed when considering elderly people for invasive testing, particularly if a patient is too frail to undergo surgery or other intervention without great risk.

The increased range and effectiveness of noninvasive cardiac testing has been a boon to elderly patients. Echocardiography, in which sound waves are bounced off the heart's internal structures, has great value in confirming valve disease and other malfunctions. Holter monitoring, using a portable electrocardiograph testing device generally worn for 24 hours, helps pinpoint rhythm disturbances under conditions of daily living.

The exercise stress test, a standard procedure in diagnosing and assessing the severity of coronary heart disease, may prove difficult for older patients who are unable to walk rapidly on a treadmill because of arthritis, decreased muscle strength, or other medical problems. Even at a very low workload, however, the electrocardiogram taken during a stress test may document the occurrence of myocardial ischemia or arrhythmias and yield valuable information.

Thallium, a radioisotope, is sometimes injected into a vein in minute amounts to assess blood flow through the coronary arteries to different areas of the heart during exercise. For those older patients unable to exercise, a drug (either dipyridamole or adenosine) can be used to mimic the effect of exercise on the heart during the thallium scan.

Elderly patients with significant angina that has not responded to various medical therapies may be tested by *coronary arteriography*, in which a catheter is threaded through an artery to the heart. An X-ray-opaque dye is released into the coronary arteries to directly visualize the interior channel of the vessels. While complications from this procedure are low, as a rule such tests are performed only when the patient is a candidate for further intervention such as surgery or balloon angioplasty. Cardiac catheterization is also performed in patients with severe valve disease, in anticipation of corrective surgery. (See Chapter 10 for more detailed information on diagnostic tests.)

TREATMENT OF THE ELDERLY

The issues surrounding treatment decisions for older people are complex, and involve many more factors than age alone. Physician and patient should decide together on an individualized treatment plan, based on overall health, life-style, and expectations.

In some situations, such as the repair of a seriously malfunctioning valve or severe and uncontrollable chest pain, surgical intervention may be the only option. But in other cases, the physician may often try more conservative methods, including different types of medications, before recommending surgery or other invasive treatments. In the elderly, some cardiac procedures or surgery may not necessarily prolong life, but they may improve its quality through the relief of symptoms such as chest pain, fainting, and weakness. Occasionally, the decision may literally be a matter of life or death, or of the preservation of a patient's ability to function independently.

Procedures such as balloon angioplasty and coronary bypass surgery, which aim to open or circumvent blocked coronary arteries, are considered relatively safe for many older persons. However, no invasive treatment is without risk of complications.

Angioplasty, for example, may be complicated in the elderly by the increased difficulty of threading the catheter past vascular blockage in the legs; complications such as bleeding or clots are also more common in older patients. More diffuse blockage and calcification of the vessels may make opening a blockage with the balloon more difficult. A careful assessment of whether an older person is a good candidate for such intervention is essential.

As surgical techniques have improved, cardiac surgery has been performed with increasing success in the elderly. Even in octogenarians, the risk of not surviving coronary bypass surgery is now as low as 5 to 10 percent in elective (nonemergency) operations, and as low as 15 to 20 percent for emergency procedures. In a typical patient aged 40 to 50, the risk is closer to 1 percent, so the *relative* risk rises significantly with age. Nonetheless, the *absolute* risk for older patients is still modest when weighed against the consequences of forgoing surgical treatment when needed.

Older patients should, however, expect longer hospitalizations after surgery than younger patients, and a somewhat more arduous recovery. Elderly patients who have multiple medical conditions—and, especially, multiple heart problems—fare least well. They are more prone to complications such as pneumonia and other infections, kidney or bladder problems, poor appetite, and, sometimes, confusion or depression. They require meticulous care from the medical staff and encouragement from their families—not just in the period right after surgery, but during convalescence and cardiac rehabilitation as well. Occasionally, postoperative problems may persist for months.

It is essential for the physician and patient's family to respect the elderly patient as an individual. Some people desire minimal medical intervention in old age, regardless of the consequences, and accept the limitations of age-related diseases; others will wish to take whatever measures are available to maintain an active life as long as possible. Both approaches are valid, and should be discussed thoughtfully by medical personnel, the patient, and his or her family.

ISSUES IN DRUG TREATMENT

Because of metabolic changes, the elderly are more likely to experience side effects from many drugs, and dosages may require more delicate adjustment. (See box, "Drugs and the Elderly.") Complicated dosage schedules may present difficulty; poor vision, arthritic hands, and memory loss may also make it hard for some elderly people to follow a medication regimen. Economic issues increasingly are having an impact on decisions regarding drug treatment. It is not uncommon for a patient who requires three different cardiac medications to pay several hundred dollars a month—a sum that may be impossible on a fixed income. Newer, more expensive drugs are not necessarily better; patients should not be afraid or ashamed to discuss the issue and the cost with their doctors.

RISK FACTOR MODIFICATION: BETTER LATE THAN NEVER?

Data from the Framingham Heart Study and other population studies have shown that most cardiac risk

Drugs and the Elderly

Slower metabolism and other physiologic changes in the aging body may cause drugs to act differently in elderly patients than in younger ones. The following are some of the cardiovascular drugs to which the elderly may be more sensitive. Many of these drugs can still be used, but the dosage must be adjusted accordingly.

- High blood pressure medication may produce dizziness and orthostatic hypotension, especially the vasodilators, diuretics, or some of the calcium blockers.

- Dizziness from anti-anginal medications (especially nitroglycerin derivatives) is also more common.

- Toxicity from digitalis (used in heart failure) may be more common.

- The use of anticoagulant drugs (to prevent clots) may result in bleeding more readily and is dangerous in people who are unsteady and subject to frequent falls.

- Beta blockers tend to slow the heart more.

- Intravenous lidocaine may cause more confusion.

factors continue to exert their influence in old age. Although few research trials on risk factor intervention have included significant numbers of elderly people, there may be benefit to corrective measures that do no harm at virtually any age.

BLOOD PRESSURE

As mentioned, controlling blood pressure in old age has been proved to reduce the risk of stroke. Two large studies demonstrate a reduction in coronary heart disease complications and heart failure in patients treated with medication. Control of blood pressure is critical in patients who have active coronary heart disease and symptoms of angina, or who experience a heart attack. Reducing the amount of work that the heart has to do, by lowering blood pressure, reduces the need for oxygen and helps to alleviate symptoms.

SMOKING

In population studies, smoking has produced confusing results in terms of its importance as a cardiac risk factor among the elderly. It appears to be a greater statistical risk for those under 65, but this may be because older smokers die at such increased rates from other causes, such as lung cancer; this fact may mask to some extent the real impact on coronary heart disease. The deleterious effects of smoking probably continue regardless of age. Smoking may promote easier clotting of the blood and affect the ability of the heart muscle to take up oxygen from the bloodstream; cigarettes are therefore especially dangerous for older people with lung disease or angina.

OBESITY

The worst impact of excess weight in old age may be the added strain on the heart, lungs, and vascular system; diabetes may also be more difficult to control. In older people with symptomatic heart disease who might be candidates for surgery, obesity may significantly increase the risk of the procedure.

LACK OF EXERCISE

A sedentary life-style has been shown to be a preventable cardiac risk. In old age, it is probably too late to undo the results of a lifetime of inactivity—but it's not too late to begin mild exercise, such as a daily walk, with almost immediate benefits in terms of overall physical condition and well-being. With or without heart disease, older people will feel better if they become—or remain—active, provided such activity is done in moderation with the advice of a physician. There is some evidence that it will promote mental acuity as well.

DIABETES

The incidence of non-insulin-dependent (Type II) diabetes rises with age, and this disorder compounds other cardiac risk factors in elderly people. Many factors that help control diabetes, such as weight control and exercise, do the heart a favor as well.

CHOLESTEROL AND THE ELDERLY: HOW REAL A RISK?

Is high blood cholesterol a risk factor for heart disease in the elderly, as it has proved to be for younger people? And, if so, does lowering cholesterol levels in older people help them lead longer or healthier lives? These two questions are difficult to answer, for some of the reasons discussed more fully in Chapter 4. Older people as a group have higher rates of coronary heart disease than younger people, making it seem logical that cholesterol control might benefit this group the most. Yet studies of risk factors have shown that blood cholesterol is a weaker predictive factor of heart disease in the old than in the middle-aged.

Does this mean that older people needn't be concerned about their blood cholesterol levels? Not necessarily. There is some evidence that not only high total cholesterol but particularly high levels of "bad" (LDL) and low levels of "good" (HDL) lipoprotein components are indeed risk factors for older people. Data gathered by the Framingham Heart Study have shown that elevated blood cholesterol may increase heart disease risk for those as old as 80. However, treating cholesterol disorders in the elderly, whether by diet or drugs, has been studied little. At this point, there are no data showing that such treatment prolongs life in this age group.

How to treat high cholesterol in the elderly, then, should depend on the degree of cholesterol abnormality plus an individual's overall risk factor and health profile. In general, an older person with symptoms of heart disease is a more logical candidate for cholesterol lowering (to prevent progression of the disease) than a person with no apparent coronary heart disease and few other risk factors.

For example, an active, otherwise healthy person in his or her late 60s who has just undergone a coronary artery bypass graft would be well advised to keep blood cholesterol low, to keep the new coronary bypass grafts "clean" (without atherosclerosis) as long as possible. (In people with high cholesterol levels, bypass grafts are particularly prone to clogging, or closure.) On the other hand, a person at age 80 with various other medical problems is probably not a candidate for sweeping dietary changes or, most especially, a course of cholesterol-lowering medication.

At any age, cholesterol lowering should start with the most conservative measures, such as dietary modification, moderate exercise, and weight loss when needed. In older people, whose nutritional status is more likely to be inadequate, dietary changes should be monitored to avoid doing more harm than good. Older people need foods that are digestible, affordable, and convenient, and prefer foods that are familiar. They don't need to abandon red meat or eggs completely, for example, and should not be expected to make sweeping alterations in their daily diet. The indications for cholesterol-lowering drug therapy in the elderly are still uncertain at this point, given the need for long-term therapy and the incidence of inconvenient side effects from some of the more affordable prescribed drugs.

SUMMARY

By the time a person reaches 65, his or her heart has done an astounding amount of work. The adult heart beats more than 100,000 times a day, pumping roughly 2,000 gallons of blood through 60,000 miles of blood vessels every 24 hours. The strongest muscle in the body, the heart at 65 still has the capacity for many more years of service. Nevertheless, natural physiologic changes in old age will somewhat lessen its efficiency. The aging heart (as well as the blood vessels) becomes less elastic, so it is not able to relax as completely between beats. The heart's walls thicken, especially in the pumping chambers, and it may enlarge in size. The heart also becomes less responsive to stimulation by adrenaline, so it isn't able to "gear up" for exercise by increasing the strength and rate of contractions.

Physiologic changes in the heart and blood vessels make the elderly more prone to certain types of cardiovascular disease. These include isolated systolic hypertension, orthostatic hypotension, heart failure, certain valve disorders (particularly of the aortic valve), and certain rhythm abnormalities, particularly bradycardias, or slow rhythms.

The outlook for most of these conditions is excellent. Many can be treated by medication, while others are helped by surgery or pacemakers. In mild cases, life-style changes may be enough. In many cases, drug treatment is successful and preferred over surgery or other invasive therapy. This is primarily because the risks associated with these procedures are somewhat higher in the elderly, especially those with other health problems, and because the recovery period is usually longer. Drugs may affect the elderly differently from younger patients, however, and care must be taken to achieve the right dosage and type of drug or combination of drugs.

Although life-style changes made in old age may no longer have the same impact on reducing the risk of heart disease, some—such as regular exercise and smoking cessation—can positively affect the quality of life. Maintaining an appropriate body weight is important. Control of high blood pressure, whether by life-style changes, medication, or both, is also important in maintaining health. All patients should maintain a prudent low-fat diet, in order to reduce blood cholesterol. However, the case for aggressive treatment of high cholesterol is not as strong. In the absence of symptoms of coronary artery disease, it may not be justified. However, for people who already have heart disease, especially those who have had bypass surgery, it may be beneficial.

CHAPTER 22

RACIAL AND ETHNIC DIFFERENCES IN HEART DISEASE

ADRIAN OSTFELD, M.D.

INTRODUCTION

Despite its decline in the past few decades, cardiovascular disease remains the leading killer of Americans, regardless of race or ethnic background. While minorities—African-Americans in particular—may suffer as often as whites from heart disease and stroke, they do not seem to share equally in the medical progress against these conditions.

Lack of research on minority populations makes difficult any generalizations about racial and ethnic differences. The data gathered on heart disease among African-Americans, for example, constitute only a small fraction of that available on whites, at the time of this writing. It is expected that the National Institutes of Health will shortly undertake to provide new information on this issue.

Within the African-American population, the impact on health of regional, socioeconomic, and other distinctions has yet to be adequately explored. As for other ethnic groups, such as Hispanics or Asians, even less is known. Limited research has been done on Hispanics, and what little has been done varies. Mexican-Americans in Texas, for example, differ in

many ways from Cubans in Florida, who in turn are different from Puerto Ricans on the East Coast. Data from one Hispanic group, then, cannot be used to draw conclusions about the others.

QUESTIONS IN SEARCH OF ANSWERS

In 1984, a group of leading epidemiologists (scientists specializing in the comparison of disease rates among different population groups) outlined the most important gaps in knowledge of heart disease in U.S. minorities. These questions are guidelines for present and future research:

- Do rates of coronary heart disease in African-Americans differ from those in U.S. whites, independent of the effects of known risk factors?

- Specifically, do African-American men have lower heart disease rates than white men? If so, can this be explained by higher levels of HDL cholesterol ("good" cholesterol) or higher levels of physical activity in African-American men than in white men?

- How valid are the data that suggest significantly higher rates of heart disease in African-American women than in white women? If the data are valid, is greater obesity among blacks the cause?

- Is socioeconomic status a risk factor for coronary heart disease among African-Americans? If so, is its effect independent of other known risk factors such as smoking and high blood pressure?

- What are the reasons for the higher rates of high blood pressure—particularly severe high blood pressure—in African-Americans than in whites? (See Figure 22.1.)

Figure 22.1
Estimated Percent of Population with Hypertension by Race and Sex, U.S. Adults Age 18–74

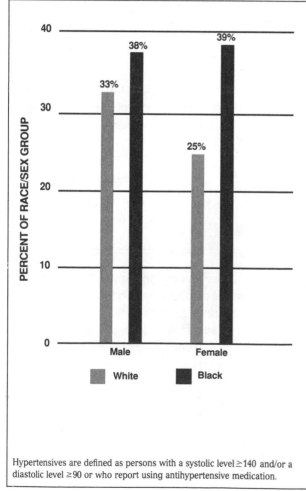

Hypertensives are defined as persons with a systolic level ≥140 and/or a diastolic level ≥90 or who report using antihypertensive medication.

Source: National Health and Nutrition Examination Survey II, 1976–80.

HEART DISEASE: A DIFFERENT PICTURE?

In 1980, African-Americans constituted about 11.5 percent of the U.S. population. The prevalence of coronary heart disease (CHD)—that is, the number of people who have coronary heart disease during a given year divided by the total number of people at risk for it (30 million in this case)—among African-Americans in the United States is similar to that among whites.

African-Americans may have somewhat different forms of coronary heart disease, such as a higher rate of "silent" (undetected) heart attacks in which no obvious symptoms are reported. They also may show certain types of electrocardiographic abnormalities more often than whites. Although the chances of having a heart attack are similar among African-Americans and whites, in African-Americans a heart attack is more likely to be fatal.

Death rates from both heart attack and stroke have declined in the past 25 years among both blacks and whites in the United States, probably because of a combination of better prevention, detection, and treatment of certain risk factors and the attacks themselves. However, African-Americans have lagged in comparison to whites in the *rate* of that decline. (See Table 22.1 and Figure 22.2.)

Although the death rates from diseases of the heart have declined for African-American men and women, the drop has been less than in white Americans. In 1988, the last year for which there is published information, African-American heart disease death rates were much higher than those in whites.

Table 22.1
Racial Differences in Death Rates from Heart Diseases, Age-Adjusted

Race and Sex	Deaths per 100,000 resident population				
	1970	1980	1986	1987	1988
All groups	253.6	202.0	175.0	169.6	166.3
White male	347.6	277.5	234.8	225.9	220.5
Black male	375.9	327.3	294.3	287.1	286.2
White female	167.8	134.6	119.0	116.3	114.2
Black female	251.7	201.1	185.1	180.8	181.1

Source: National Center for Health Statistics, National Vital Statistic System.

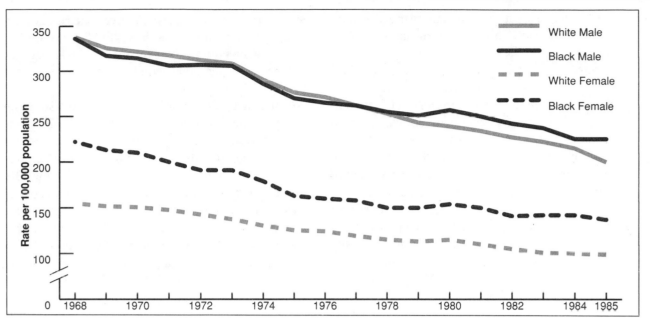

Figure 22.2
Rate of Coronary Heart Disease for All Ages, United States, 1968–1985

Source: National Center for Health Statistics, National Vital Statistic System.

In attempting to analyze the meaning of such trends, researchers first try to determine whether coronary heart disease occurs more or less often in minority groups and whether the disease itself is more severe. Also under scrutiny are the accepted risk factors for coronary heart disease. High blood cholesterol, smoking, and hypertension were identified as risks through research on overwhelmingly white populations, but they may not have the same effect on the heart health of other ethnic groups in the United States.

Possible reasons for variations include different risks for minorities, reduced access to medical care or limited ability to pay for it, and the possible stresses produced by disadvantage in education, jobs, and housing. The effects of "multiple jeopardy," in the form of negative environmental, social, and economic conditions early in life, may be reflected in the fact that African-Americans have higher levels of sickness, disability, and death than whites in every age group. There may also be genetic differences that could account for some varying disease patterns.

RISK FACTORS: HOW AFRICAN-AMERICANS COMPARE

Although some cardiovascular risk factors may be the same or less threatening in the African-American community, others are more marked. For instance, high blood pressure and diabetes may be even more important coronary risks for African-Americans than for whites, and African-American women are at particularly high risk of obesity (which can lead to both high blood pressure and diabetes).

Rates of high blood pressure are the most important difference yet documented between African-Americans and whites. Not only do more African-Americans have high blood pressure, but they also suffer disproportionately from its adverse health effects.

As a rule, African-Americans and whites seem to have roughly equivalent levels of total and LDL ("bad," or artery-clogging) cholesterol. African-Americans, however, have been shown in some (but not all) studies to have higher levels of HDL or "good" cholesterol, which may serve to offset some of the risk from other factors, such as hypertension. Whether HDL really cancels out or modifies other risks among African-Americans, though, is unproved, and, of course, this does not appear to protect African-Americans from an increased incidence of strokes or kidney failure as a result of hypertension.

Smoking appears to have the same devastating effects on the cardiovascular system of African-Americans and whites. In past decades, smoking was believed to be less common among African-Americans, and those who did smoke were believed to use fewer cigarettes than white smokers. More recent data indicate a rising proportion of African-American smokers as quitting rates increase faster among whites than African-Americans. High alcohol consumption is another risk for high blood pressure and stroke; available data indicate that African-Americans are more likely to be heavy drinkers (or total abstainers) than whites.

Obesity is a known risk for African-American women from middle age onward and may contribute significantly to the increased presence of hypertension. Excess weight has also been shown to be an independent risk factor for heart disease, regardless of other and possibly related risks like diet or lack of physical activity. One study found that 50 percent of African-American women aged 24 to 55 were obese (defined as 20 percent or more above desirable weight), compared to 22 percent of white women in the same age group. (Racial differences in obesity between African-American and white men are negligible.) In a 1982 survey done in New Haven, Connecticut, the average older African-American woman was about the same height as the average older white woman, but weighed 17 pounds more—a significant added burden for the heart and vascular system. Because African-American women report consuming fewer calories on average than white women, the possibility exists that a metabolic difference may contribute to their obesity.

Statistics on African-American/white differences regarding physical activity and type of diet are conflicting and confusing. Traditionally, it was believed that African-Americans were more active physically than whites because of their greater likelihood of having jobs that involved hard physical labor. This perception may be outdated.

Data on diet patterns by race are also somewhat inconclusive. The high-fat, high-salt diet of rural Southern African-Americans is no longer the standard; as African-Americans have become urbanized, their diet has more and more come to resemble that of other Americans. Some differences remain, however. Dietary surveys and market research suggest that African-Americans do not consume as much milk as whites, partly because of their higher rates of lactose intolerance, a condition that makes it difficult to digest milk sugar. African-Americans also are more likely to eat salty snacks and cook with hard (saturated) fats such as lard.

It seems logical that the effects of poverty might serve to erode good nutrition, even with government support programs; the kinds of "heart-healthy" diets often promoted by health authorities include large amounts of lean meat and fish, fresh fruits and vegetables, and complex carbohydrates, foods that may prove too expensive for many African-Americans.

Diabetes mellitus, another established risk for heart disease in whites, strikes African-Americans even harder and may raise their cardiac risk accordingly. African-Americans make up 15 percent of all Americans who have diabetes; their prevalence rate of the disease per 1,000 people is about 32, compared to about 24 for whites. In both races, diabetes is more common with advancing age, and in most studies it is more common among women than men. But in all adult age/sex categories, diabetes is 33 percent higher among African-Americans than among whites. According to government statistics for 1979 to 1981, the rate of diabetes in African-American men was 16 percent higher than in white men, but the rate in African-American women was 50 percent higher than in white women. The high prevalence of obesity among African-American women is believed to account for at least some of these disparities. Diabetes is also a frequent companion to other cardiovascular risks, such as hypertension.

THE MEANING OF RACE

An enduring controversy in the study of racial health differences centers on the role of race itself, versus other factors closely linked to race—economic position, community stability, and life outlook. Is race nothing more than a set of genetically transmitted characteristics, such as skin color? Or is race, for the purposes of public health discussions, a more complex entity involving socioeconomic status, education, life-styles, beliefs, and culture?

How to separate these factors from purely genetic ones in evaluating medical research remains a difficult task. Confounding the issue is the changing effect of race over time—both positively (as in civil rights and occasional socioeconomic gains) and negatively (as reflected in urban ills like rising rates of crime, AIDS, and drug abuse). Furthermore, many African-Americans are descended at least in part from persons of both European and Native American ancestry, making genetic hypotheses tenuous.

The well-being of African-Americans has improved over the past half century, but remains significantly below that of whites. Life expectancy for both races has risen, but a gap persists.

To isolate the health effects of past and continuing inequality is difficult indeed. Are African-Americans more prone to die from heart disease because the disease follows a different and more severe course among them, or because they are exposed to more risk factors, or because they have poorer access to medical care? Is health behavior by African-Americans a contributing factor? Investigators warn that these open questions, combined with the available statistics on minority health, make it unwise to attempt any sweeping generalizations about African-Americans and cardiovascular disease until more research has been completed.

THE MEANING OF ETHNICITY

The study of heart disease among various ethnic groups is complicated by many variables, not the least of which are diet and life-style changes undergone by many minority group members as they assimilate, over several generations, into the American "melting pot." This process of assimilation may have positive implications for overall health, such as increasing affluence that allows better access to medical care and more adequate nutrition. But cardiovascular disease is a disease of affluent, industrialized societies, and minorities who partake of America's characteristic diet, rich in fat and animal protein, and sedentary lifestyle may find their low "native" heart disease rates on the rise.

For example, one landmark study of the effect of diet on blood cholesterol and coronary heart disease compared Japanese people in Japan with Japanese who had moved to Hawaii and San Francisco. The Japanese have a typically low dietary intake of total fat, saturated fat, and dietary cholesterol, reflected in their low levels of blood cholesterol and low rates of coronary heart disease (the lowest, in fact of any industrialized nation). As the immigrant groups changed over to a typically American diet, however, their blood cholesterol levels and coronary heart disease death rates came to resemble the American average. Despite their similar genetic backgrounds, differences in environment—diet in particular—made them more "American" than "Japanese" in relation to heart disease.

While data are lacking, it is probable that many other ethnic minorities undergo changes in cardiovascular risk profile, not only when they enter American life, but as they make their way up the ladder of economic and social progress. The Chinese diet in China, for example, was shown in recent research to be very low in fat and cholesterol (and high in complex carbohydrates such as rice and vegetables) in many regions and associated with low rates of heart disease. But Chinese food as prepared and consumed in most American restaurants is high in fatty meats that are less available to poorer, rural populations and emphasizes high-fat, high-calorie methods of preparation such as double-frying.

The diet of many Mediterranean countries, such as Italy and Greece, is associated with a relatively low rate of coronary heart disease, but it is unknown whether this protection has carried over into American life among families of Italian and Greek descent.

It does seem true, however, that while people who migrate from a country with low rates of heart disease to a country with higher rates may experience an increase in heart attacks, they still maintain a lower rate than natives of the new country. This has been reported in the cases of Norwegian-Americans and Yemenite Jews who migrated to Israel.

Many aspects of life-style and health among ethnic groups await further examination, including the effects of stress, alcohol use, levels of "good" and "bad" (HDL and LDL) blood cholesterol, and blood pressure. Some populations do seem genetically prone to obesity; but the easy availability of high-calorie foods in the United States, combined with almost universal access to television (with its combination of inactivity and junk-food advertising), make the impact of American life hard to separate from inherited susceptibility to weight gain and its associated risks. Some heart disease risks, including obesity and smoking, have been shown to *decrease* with a rise in education level and socioeconomic status—suggesting that after a certain period, the risks linked to America's abundance may recede because of conscious behavioral change.

THE UNSOLVED CHALLENGE

The high rate and severe toll of high blood pressure among African-Americans remain a public-health priority. Because high blood pressure (hypertension) is the main cause of stroke, the best way to examine the effects of high blood pressure is to look at the death rates from stroke. (See Table 22.2.) Although death rates have fallen appreciably in recent years, the rates for African-Americans are nearly double those for whites.

Various theories about this difference between the races propose that the real answer may lie in a combination of factors. Lower socioeconomic position

Table 22.2
Racial Differences in Death Rates from Stroke,
Age-Adjusted

Race and Sex	Deaths per 100,000 resident population				
	1970	1980	1986	1987	1988
All groups	66.3	40.8	31.0	30.3	29.7
White male	68.8	41.9	31.1	30.3	30.0
Black male	122.5	77.5	58.9	57.1	57.8
White female	56.2	35.2	27.1	26.3	25.5
Black female	107.9	61.6	47.6	46.7	46.6

Source: National Center for Health Statistics, National Vital Statistic System.

and less education have tended to lead to higher blood pressure in either race, but do not explain all the differences. In studies that weeded out the statistical effects of income and education, the race gap in hypertension remained. According to 1977 data on 159,000 adults gathered by the federally supported Hypertension Detection and Follow-up Program, African-Americans were almost twice as likely as whites to have hypertension even after adjusting for age, weight, and education.

Physiologic factors have been studied for clues to African-American hypertension. It is possible that the levels of hormones regulating blood pressure (via the sympathetic nervous system) may differ somewhat between African-Americans and whites. The role of certain nutrients in the diet has been examined in regard to high blood pressure, and some evidence suggests African-American/white differences.

DIET AND LIFE-STYLE

An excess of dietary sodium has been implicated as a suspect in raising high blood pressure, at least in those individuals sensitive to its effects on the vascular system. While dietary surveys show that African-Americans consume about as much sodium as whites in this country, research suggests that African-Americans may excrete sodium from their bodies more slowly and be more likely to retain it—characteristics that may increase blood pressure.

Another nutrient with a possible role in blood pressure is potassium. A low intake of potassium or a high ratio of sodium to potassium in the body may contribute to hypertension. African-Americans do appear to consume less potassium than whites, a factor that may increase their sensitivity to the effects of salt. New research has also suggested a role for calcium in modifying blood pressure, and some dietary data also point to a lower calcium intake among African-Americans because of their increased prevalence of lactose (milk sugar) intolerance and reduced milk intake.

The role of stress in high blood pressure among African-Americans is intriguing. Tension or stress does not cause hypertension—at least not directly—in any racial group. Stress causes temporary rises in blood pressure, but *essential hypertension*—the constant elevation of blood pressure—is usually of unknown cause. There is, however, preliminary evidence suggesting that constant exposure to stress, such as that experienced by disadvantaged individuals in high-crime urban areas, may contribute to eventual sustained elevation of blood pressure.

Investigators have also continued to explore the so-called Type A hypothesis, which holds that time-driven, overly ambitious people with high levels of hostility may have an increased risk of heart disease. While no specific research has been performed on Type A behavior in African-Americans, it is reasonable to assume that the effects of racial prejudice and socioeconomic disadvantage could lead to a hostile attitude and behavior pattern in some people.

In a 1973 study by Ernest Harburg, Ph.D., people living in "high-stress" areas of Detroit (characterized by poverty, broken families, and crime) had higher blood pressure levels than residents of low-stress neighborhoods, with the association stronger among African-Americans than whites. Harburg also investigated the effects on blood pressure of an emotional response to being treated unfairly. Higher blood pressures were measured in those individuals who were most likely to hold anger in or feel guilty about showing it. As might be expected, men living in high-stress areas had higher levels of suppressed hostility. In another study, the higher the level of social instability in a given county (measured by yardsticks like single-parent families and men in prison), the higher the death rate from stroke.

An "active coping style" against formidable odds, a trait termed "John Henryism" by Sherman A. James, Ph.D., a researcher at the University of Michigan, is being investigated. According to folklore, John Henry was an African-American steel driver—that is, a tunnel driller—who challenged a steam-driven machine in a battle of speed and strength.

John Henry beat the machine, but then died of exhaustion. The response of African-Americans to residual disadvantage in every area of American life, James and some other scientists suggest, is likewise an intense and determined approach that musters few resources against great odds—and may take its toll in ways yet to be fully determined.

GENETIC THEORIES

Finally, scientists—who have traditionally been wary of racial and genetic theories in regard to the practice of medicine—have been cautiously examining possible explanations for African-American hypertension in light of the circumstances under which the African-American population came to the Americas. Perhaps, some speculate, the brutal conditions aboard slave ships led to the survival of only those individuals whose bodies were best adapted to conserving vital minerals such as sodium when food and water were scarce. The descendants of these survivors might then have passed along these traits in the form of salt-conserving kidneys. This could predispose African-Americans to high blood pressure, even under more favorable life conditions.

High blood pressure is most serious for blacks in the Western Hemisphere, although many blacks have blood pressure levels more like those of American whites. The blood pressure of rural African-Americans is lower than that of blacks living in African cities. This may, however, be related to a change in diet or a weight gain. Even urban African blacks, however, have lower blood pressures than their urban American counterparts.

Physiologic differences may also affect the success or failure of hypertension treatment in African-American communities. It appears, for example, that African-Americans respond better to treatment with diuretics, such as hydrochlorothiazide (Esidrix or Hydrodiuril), a first-line agent of antihypertensive drug therapy. African-Americans do not respond as easily to another class of blood-pressure-lowering agent, the ACE inhibitors, such as captopril (Capoten). (See Chapter 23.)

Drug treatment of other ethnic groups may also have results that differ from those in whites. There are some data suggesting that Chinese people are more sensitive to the effects on blood pressure and heart rate of propranolol (Inderal and others), one of a group of drugs called beta blockers that are commonly used to treat angina and high blood pressure.

The results of public health efforts within the African-American community to detect and control hypertension have met with some success. Extensive screening programs have been conducted through churches and other community institutions. But much remains to be done. According to several studies, African-Americans are less likely to have their high blood pressure under medical control. Young African-American males in particular have proved difficult to reach, and health authorities continue to explore nontraditional routes for spreading the message.

THE GAP BETWEEN DIAGNOSIS AND TREATMENT

Data have shown that African-Americans are less likely to receive diagnosis and treatment in the same manner as whites once they show symptoms of coronary heart disease. Reasons for this are complicated.

According to a 1982 review, medical treatment of high blood pressure produces greater decreases in illness and death rates among African-Americans than whites, and greater efforts must be made to get more African-Americans under effective treatment. Access to medical care, and the ability to pay for it, are major concerns that may influence treatment in minority groups. In a 1989 survey, African-Americans were about twice as likely as whites to receive medical care in hospital clinics, emergency rooms, and other facilities with poor continuity of care (for example, patients are likely to see a different doctor on every visit).

Two researchers, Mark B. Wenneker, M.D., and Arnold M. Epstein, M.D., in a study of discharge data from Massachusetts hospitals in 1989, reported that white patients underwent significantly more angiography (to diagnose blockages in the coronary arteries) and more than twice as many bypass operations and angioplasty procedures (to clear blocked arteries). The differences, the researchers acknowledged, could stem from African-Americans having less severe heart disease than whites, or to a stronger tendency to refuse high-tech treatment options.

A very recent study of hospitals in New York State confirmed that African-Americans are less likely to have angiography, bypass operations, and angioplasty. It also showed that differences in severity of heart disease could not account for the lesser rates of these procedures in African-Americans. Other studies have confirmed the disproportionately low use of coronary bypass and angioplasty in African-American patients with heart disease. There is also evidence that African-Americans are less likely to agree to such procedures, which may reflect a continuing distrust by some African-Americans of the medical establishment.

Better preventive health services, broader health insurance coverage, and improved continuity in the management of cardiovascular disease could lower deaths and disability in minority communities. Meanwhile, research specifically directed at African-Americans and other ethnic groups is needed in order to direct the continuing efforts most appropriately.

PART VI

METHODS OF TREATMENT

CHAPTER 23

CARDIOVASCULAR DRUGS

LAWRENCE S. COHEN, M.D., LAWRENCE DECKELBAUM, M.D.,
JONATHAN ISAACSOHN, M.D., FORRESTER A. LEE, M.D.,
CRAIG A. McPHERSON, M.D., MARVIN MOSER, M.D.,
and LYNDA E. ROSENFELD, M.D.

INTRODUCTION

When people are diagnosed with heart disease, they may be treated in several different ways. Controlling risk factors that can be managed—cutting down on fat and cholesterol and quitting smoking—will be the first changes they will have to make. (See Chapter 3.) Exercise will become part of their lives, if possible. Drug therapy may be the next course of action.

The variety and scope of cardiovascular drugs have increased tremendously in the past few decades, and new drugs are being approved annually. In the 1950s, effective oral diuretics became available. These drugs dramatically changed the treatment of heart failure and hypertension. In the mid-1960s a class of agents called beta blockers was discovered. This led to major changes in physicians' ability to treat patients with hypertension or angina pectoris. Calcium channel blockers and ACE inhibitors became widely used in the 1980s, and they, too, have allowed patients with hypertension, heart failure, and coronary artery disease to be treated more effectively. The development and use of thrombolytics, the "clot busters," have revolutionized our ability to treat patients having a heart attack.

The decade of the 1990s holds even greater promise as the powerful tools of genetic engineering produce new and even more effective drugs to prevent and treat patients with heart disease.

Initially, a person on drug therapy may have to try different drugs to find the one that is the most effective and has the fewest side effects. People with other health problems or physical characteristics may find one type of drug to be more useful than another. (See box, "Factors in Choosing Certain Cardiovascular Drugs.") More than one drug may be used at a time. Once a dose has been established, combination drugs may be used—two or more drugs are combined into a single pill. Whatever the possibilities, a person and his or her physician will have to work together to find the right therapy, whether it is a drug that has been around for 50 years or one that has just become available. A well-informed patient will have a better sense of the treatment process and will be a better consumer when the time comes to purchase the drugs. (See box, "Shopping Around for Prescription Drugs.")

Cardiovascular drugs can be divided into several categories, each of which is discussed below. The listings here are alphabetical by drug families. (See box, "Therapeutic Drug Categories," for listing by disease entities.)

Factors in Choosing Certain Cardiovascular Drugs

For African-Americans	Calcium channel blockers and diuretics are most effective. ACE inhibitors and beta blockers can be made more effective by combining with a diuretic.	For people who have had a stroke or ministroke	Drugs that may cause a decrease in standing blood pressure (orthostatic hypotension), which can result in fainting spells, should probably be avoided or taken with great care. These include alpha blockers such as prazosin (Minipress) or drugs like guanethidine (Ismelin).
For people over 60	Calcium channel blockers and diuretics are generally most effective. Avoid drugs that may cause depression (centrally acting drugs). Those who take guana-drel (Hylorel), guanethidine (Ismelin), doxazosin mesylate (Cardura), prazosin (Minipress), or terazosin (Hytrin) must be careful when standing up quickly; fainting because of low blood pressure (orthostatic hypotension) could result.	For people with a heart rate slower than 50 (bradycardia)	Beta blockers, diltiazem (Cardizem), and verapamil (Calan, Isoptin, Verelan) should be avoided.
		For people with a history of depression	ACE inhibitors, alpha blockers, diuretics, vasodilators, and drugs like guanethidine (Ismelin) do not worsen or provoke depression. Centrally acting drugs such as clonidine (Catapres), methyldopa (Aldomet), and especially reserpine (Serpasil) should be avoided; they may cause or exacerbate depression.
For people who experience episodes of severely rapid heartbeats (tachycardia)	The drugs of choice may be a beta blocker or verapamil (Calan, Isoptin, Verelan). If this is not effective, combining with a diuretic may help, but certain blood potassium levels must be monitored in order to detect any harmful decrease.		
For people who experience migraines	Beta blockers or calcium channel blockers may help.	For people with angina pectoris	Beta blockers or calcium channel blockers are especially effective and may be combined with a potassium-sparing diuretic. Drugs that cause rapid heartbeat, such as vasodilators, should be avoided or taken with a beta blocker.
For people who experience sexual dysfunction	ACE inhibitors, alpha blockers, calcium channel blockers, or vasodilators may be preferable to other antihypertensive drugs.		
For people who have had a heart attack	Beta blockers protect against a second heart attack, making them the drugs of choice. If blood pressure needs to be further controlled, a combination of thiazide and potassium-sparing diuretics may be added to the regimen.	For people with asthma or chronic lung disease such as emphysema	ACE inhibitors and diuretics are acceptable. Calcium channel blockers may protect against asthma that is provoked by exercise. Beta blockers should be avoided.

For people with diabetes	ACE inhibitors may have beneficial effects on the kidneys, and alpha blockers are usually well tolerated. Beta blockers should be used with care; they can sometimes mask symptoms of insulin shock. Beta blockers and diuretics may adversely affect blood glucose levels, but this is not common or important in most instances. Potassium-sparing diuretics should be used with caution by people with kidney disease.	For people with kidney failure	Loop diuretics such as furosemide (Lasix) or bumetanide (Bumex), metolazone (Diulo, Mykrox, Zaroxolyn), and vasodilators such as minoxodil (Loniten) may be especially useful. Potassium-sparing diuretics and drugs like guanethidine (Ismelin) should be taken with care.
For people with elevated cholesterol levels	People who take beta blockers or diuretics should have their blood chemistries checked periodically.	For people with osteoporosis (thinning of the bone)	Potassium-sparing and thiazide diuretics may help preserve bone structure.
		For people with Raynaud's phenomenon (white fingers or toes in cold weather)	Beta blockers should be avoided. ACE inhibitors, calcium channel blockers, diuretics, methyldopa (Aldomet), prazosin (Minipress), and reserpine (Serpasil) may be used.
For people with gout	Diuretics should be avoided or taken with care; they can provoke an acute attack.	For pregnant women	Beta blockers, hydralazine (Apresoline), and methyldopa (Aldomet) appear to be safe and effective. Obstetricians are often reluctant to use diuretics.
For people with heart failure	ACE inhibitors may be especially effective. Alpha blockers, diuretics, and vasodilators may also have beneficial effects.	For young people	Beta blockers may be most useful but also may decrease exercise performance in some individuals.

Shopping Around for Prescription Drugs

People who are on long-term drug therapy may have an unavoidably large fixed expense, but they can make sure they get the most for the money. Here are some suggestions.

- Ask your physician if it is possible to substitute a generic for the brand name. The generics are often less expensive.
- Call several pharmacies that are close to home, and compare prices.
- Take notice of factors other than price. Is the service better at one pharmacy? Are the staff more courteous? Are they able to answer all questions?
- Investigate drug plans that come with health insurance, or check with your state's drug assistance program. Organizations such as the American Association of Retired Persons (AARP) have drug purchase programs that offer good prices and delivery service.

In the end, the goal is to get the best drug at the best price while enjoying the benefits of good service and continuity of care.

Therapeutic Drug Categories

Drugs to treat angina	Beta blockers, calcium channel blockers, nitrates	Drugs to treat high blood pressure (hypertension)	ACE inhibitors, alpha blockers, alpha and beta blockers, beta blockers, calcium channel blockers, centrally acting drugs, combination drugs, diuretics, peripheral adrenergic antagonists, vasodilators
Drugs to treat blood clot disorders	Anticoagulants		
Drugs to treat heart failure	ACE inhibitors, combination drugs, diuretics, digitalis drugs	Drugs to treat high cholesterol	Cholesterol-lowering agents
Drugs to treat heart rhythm disorders (arrhythmias)	Antiarrhythmic drugs, anticoagulants (for atrial fibrillation), beta blockers, calcium channel blockers, digitalis drugs	Post-heart attack drugs	Anticoagulants, thrombolytics, and antiplatelets; beta blockers
		Post-heart valve replacement drugs	Anticoagulants

ALPHA-ADRENERGIC BLOCKING DRUGS (ALPHA BLOCKERS)

These drugs work through the autonomic (automatic) nervous system by blocking nerve receptors that are called alpha receptors. Alpha receptors normally promote constriction of the arterioles. Blocking constriction promotes dilation of vessels and lowers blood pressure as well as reducing the work of the heart in some situations. Alpha-blocking drugs also inhibit the actions of one of the adrenal hormones, norepinephrine, that raise blood pressure as part of the fight-or-flight response.

Alpha blockers are usually prescribed along with other blood-pressure-lowering drugs, such as a beta-blocking drug and/or a diuretic. In general, alpha blockers are not as effective for initial therapy as some of the other blood-pressure-lowering medications. There are now several medications available that combine the effects of blocking both the beta and alpha receptors.

EXAMPLES OF ALPHA BLOCKERS

Generic names (trade names): doxazosin (Cardura)
   prazosin (Minipress)
   terazosin (Hytrin)

How supplied: doxazosin—tablet (1 mg, 2 mg, 4 mg, 8 mg)
   prazosin—capsule (1 mg, 2 mg, 5 mg)
   terazosin—tablet (1 mg, 2 mg, 5 mg, 10 mg)

Available as generic: prazosin—yes
   doxazosin, terazosin—no

Description: Prazosin is an alpha blocker, antihypertensive, and vasodilator that has been available since 1975. Terazosin also blocks alpha receptors, which causes blood vessels to dilate. Doxazosin, available since early 1991, is the most recently introduced of these three.

Effects: They lower high blood pressure and may reduce the workload of the heart in heart failure.

Possible side effects: One major side effect of alpha blockers is a drop in blood pressure when a person stands up abruptly (orthostatic hypotension); this can result in dizziness or fainting. This may also occur if the person drinks alcohol, stands for long periods of time, exercises, or is exposed to hot weather. Care must be taken to avoid sudden changes in position, especially when first taking the drugs. Other side effects that are less common include nausea, headache, and palpitations.

Approximate cost: for bottle of 100,
doxazosin—average wholesale price, $.06***;
1 mg, $63.06***;
2 mg, $63.06***; 4 mg, $66.21***;
8 mg, $69.52***
prazosin—1 mg, $32.59 to $45.37 (generic, $14.63 to $31.17); 2 mg, $42.99 to $60.53 (generic, $19.13 to $38.69)
terazosin—2 mg, $77*

Dosage: doxazosin—1 mg to 16 mg once per day
prazosin—2 mg to 15 mg per day divided into two or three doses
terazosin—1 mg to 5 mg per day

Notes:

• Diuretics increase the blood-pressure-lowering effect of these drugs.

• Excessively low blood pressure may develop in people who are also receiving a beta blocker such as propranolol.

• Unlike some other antihypertensives, prazosin does not slow heart rate and may actually increase it.

• Terazosin may act to relax bladder outlet muscles.

EXAMPLE OF ALPHA AND BETA BLOCKERS

These may occasionally be used as initial therapy in hypertension. They are most often used if other medications are not effective.

Generic name (trade names): labetolol (Normodyne, Trandate)

How supplied: tablet (100 mg, 200 mg, 300 mg), injection (5 mg/ml in 20 ml or 40 ml vials and 4 ml or 8 ml prefilled syringes)

Available as generic: no

Description: It is an alpha and beta blocker introduced in 1984. Reduces the rate and force of the heartbeat and widens arteries to increase the flow of blood.

Effect: Lowers elevated blood pressure and relieves angina.

Possible side effects: Nausea and indigestion; these usually subside with long-term use. Less frequent effects are cold hands and feet, temporary impotence, and nightmares. Dizziness may occur initially or as dosage is increased.

Approximate cost: for 100 100-mg tablets, $24–33*

Dosage: 200 mg to 800 mg per day (300 mg per day if injected)

Notes:

• Labetolol should be used with caution by people with lung problems, asthma, or diabetes.

• Monoamine oxidase inhibitors (MAOIs) may cause a severe rise in blood pressure when taken in conjunction with labetolol.

• Cimetidine (Tagamet) may increase effect of labetolol.

ANGIOTENSIN-CONVERTING ENZYME (ACE) INHIBITORS

These drugs act to prevent production of a hormone, angiotensin II, that constricts blood vessels. They belong to the class of drugs called vasodilators—drugs that dilate blood vessels, an effective way to lower blood pressure. ACE inhibitors first became available in the early 1970s and are now commonly used to treat several heart conditions.

ACE inhibitors improve blood flow to various organs and decrease the workload on the heart in heart failure. In addition to dilating blood vessels, ACE-inhibiting medications may produce some beneficial effects indirectly by preventing the abnormal rise in hormones associated with heart disease, such as aldosterone. Aldosterone acts on the kidneys to retain salt and water. Some of these effects remain unproved.

ACE inhibitors are widely used to treat high blood pressure, or hypertension, a major risk factor for cardiovascular disease. Used alone or in combination with other drugs, ACE inhibitors have also proved effective in the treatment of congestive heart failure. They interfere with excessive constriction of blood vessels that occurs during heart failure, allowing the heart to distribute blood more effectively to all body organs. ACE inhibitors are among the few medications that have been shown to prolong patients' lives in addition to treating the symptoms of heart failure.

Although their relatively high cost may be a drawback for many people, ACE inhibitors may be among the first-choice drugs for hypertensive patients with diabetes or heart failure. They may also be an appropriate alternative for patients who suffer impotence from beta blockers and other medications. They are less effective in African-Americans than in whites. They are most effective when combined with small doses of a diuretic, and this is available in a combination drug. A dry hacking cough is a common side effect.

EXAMPLES OF ACE INHIBITORS

Generic names (trade names): captopril (Capoten)
   enalapril (Vasotec)
   lisinopril (Prinivil, Zestril)

How supplied: captopril—tablet (12.5 mg, 25 mg, 50 mg, 100 mg)
   enalapril—tablet (2.5 mg, 5 mg, 10 mg, 20 mg)
   lisinopril—tablet (5 mg, 10 mg, 20 mg, 40 mg)

Available as generic: no

Description: Captopril was the first of the ACE inhibitors. They block the agent that constricts blood vessels by interfering with a chain of chemical reactions called the renin-angiotensin system. This improves the flow of blood. ACE inhibitors also prevent an abnormal rise in hormones associated with heart failure, such as adrenaline and aldosterone.

Effects: They dilate the blood vessels and improve the flow of blood, thus lowering high blood pressure, relieving vascular muscle spasm, and reducing the workload of the heart.

Possible side effects: Common side effects are dizziness or weakness, loss of appetite, a rash, itching, a hacking, unpredictable cough, and swelling.

Approximate cost: for 100 tablets,
   captopril—12.5 mg, $45.87 to $64.83; 25 mg, $54.99 to $76.79; 50 mg, $75.17 to $108.49
   enalapril—5 mg, $77 to $99*
   lisinopril—10 mg, $60.50 to $66*

Dosage: captopril—12.5 to 37.5 mg per day starting dose; 75 to 150 mg per day maintenance dose; must be taken at least twice a day
   enalapril—2.5 mg or 5 mg to 30 mg per day
   lisinopril—5 mg to 30 mg once daily

Notes:

- Cimetidine (Tagamet) may increase side effects and decrease captopril's effectiveness.
- For people with certain kidney abnormalities, ACE inhibitors may further disrupt kidney function.
- Should probably not be taken along with potassium-sparing diuretics.

ANTIARRHYTHMIC DRUGS

These drugs correct an irregular heartbeat and slow a heart that is beating too fast. "Poisons in small doses are the best medicines," wrote a physician in 1789, "and useful medicines in too large doses are poisons." This general principle of sound pharmacology holds especially true for antiarrhythmic drugs. The compounds used to treat heart rhythm disorders are potent medications. Regardless of the type of antiarrhythmic drug, patients should never take more than prescribed. Conversely, because the effectiveness of these drugs depends on maintaining the optimum level of medication in the blood, the patient should be sure to take them according to the physician's instructions. (See Chapter 16.)

Each of the antiarrhythmic drugs may be used to treat many different rhythm disorders, and two patients taking the same medication do not necessarily have the same problem. Many patients tolerate antiarrhythmic medications quite well, but all of these drugs may cause side effects, so patients should promptly report any new sensations, symptoms, or difficulties to the doctor.

Although the vast majority of patients benefit from antiarrhythmic drugs, heart arrhythmias may paradoxically worsen in 5 to 10 percent of patients. For that reason and the fact that the more serious heart rhythm abnormalities occur in sick patients, antiarrhythmic drugs are often first given in the hospital, so the effects on heart rhythm can be carefully monitored. These may be measured by an electrocardiogram, Holter monitor, telemetry, and/or electrophysiology studies. Most of the time, however, these drugs can be continued safely without hospitalization.

The heart's response to a given medication may change over time, making regular follow-up visits essential. Changes in treatment regimen, either to relieve side effects or to increase effectiveness, are common. Because different antiarrhythmic drugs may interact in undesirable ways, patients should make sure that any doctor prescribing a new medication knows about any other antiarrhythmic drugs that have already been prescribed.

EXAMPLES OF ANTIARRHYTHMICS

Generic name (trade name): amiodarone (Cordarone)

How supplied: tablet (200 mg)

Available as generic: no

Description: It is the most potent antiarrhythmic agent in use. Acts as a beta blocker, alpha blocker, calcium channel blocker, and antihyperthyroid.

Effects: Suppresses all types of arrhythmias.

Possible side effects: Most serious side effect is lung inflammation. Also causes liver inflammation, muscle degeneration and weakness, loss of balance, and slow heart rate. Skin may become more susceptible to sunburn and may take on a blue-gray discoloration. Paradoxically, amiodarone can cause both thyroid underactivity—with symptoms of fatigue, intolerance to cold, constipation, and weight gain—or hyperthyroidism—characterized by sleeplessness, heat intolerance, sweats, weight loss, and rapid heart rate. Other side effects are rash, weight loss, nausea, constipation, dizziness, fainting, palpitations, and changes in vision.

Approximate cost: for 60 200-mg tablets, average wholesale price, $139.39**

Dosage: 200 mg to 600 mg per day

Notes:

• Because of its many side effects, amiodarone is approved only for the treatment of serious arrhythmias that do not respond to other drugs. Researchers are seeking a less toxic form of amiodarone that may one day prove a highly beneficial antiarrhythmic agent.

• Doses of digitalis drugs or warfarin-type anticoagulant drugs should be reduced in conjunction with amiodarone.

Generic name (trade name): digoxin (Lanoxin)

How supplied: tablet (0.125 mg, 0.25 mg, 0.5 mg), capsule (0.05 mg, 0.1 mg, 0.2 mg), elixir (0.05 mg per ml, 60-ml bottle), injection (0.5 mg in 2 ml, 0.1 mg in 1 ml)

Available as generic: yes

Description: It is a digitalis drug extracted from the leaves of the foxglove plant.

Effects: Relieves heart failure and corrects some abnormal heart rhythms.

Possible side effects: Side effects are tiredness, nausea, loss of appetite, confusion, vision disturbances, and palpitations.

Approximate cost: for 100 tablets, 0.125 mg, $5.59 to $8.63; 0.25 mg, $5.99 to $10.19

Dosage: 0.125 mg to 0.25 mg per day for adults; reduced dosage for children based on weight and age

Notes:

• Check with doctor before combining with any other medication. There are numerous drug interactions.

• People taking digoxin should be monitored because an effective digoxin dose may be near the toxic dose.

Generic name (trade name): disopyramide phosphate (Norpace)

How supplied: capsule (100 mg, 150 mg) and extended-release capsule (100 mg, 150 mg)

Available as generic: yes

Description: It is a synthetic drug that reduces the force of the heartbeat (similar to procainamide and quinidine).

Effects: Corrects some abnormal heart rhythms, particularly rapid heartbeats.

Possible side effects: Its most serious side effect is weakening of heart contractions in hearts that are already mildly to moderately weak. Dry mouth is common, constipation can occur, and men can sometimes have difficulty urinating. (These three can often be reversed by giving a drug called pyridostigmine [Mestinon] as well.) Low blood sugar has also been noted, and certain forms of glaucoma may become worse.

Approximate cost: for 100 100-mg capsules, average wholesale price, $45.20**; for 100 100 mg extended-release capsules, average wholesale price, $54.45**

Dosage: 100 mg three to four times per day

Notes:

• Phenytoin (Dilantin) and rifampin (Rifadin, Rifamate, Rimactane) may reduce the effect of disopyramide.

• People with diabetes should use disopyramide with caution.

• Disopyramide has drug interactions with drugs having anticholinergic effects, such as a belladonna and phenobarbital mix (Donnatal) or propantheline bromide (Pro-banthine).

Generic names (trade names): flecainide (Tambocor)
propafenone (Rhythmol)

How supplied: flecainide—tablet (50 mg, 100 mg, 150 mg)
propafenone—tablet (150 mg, 300 mg)

Available as generic: no

Description: These are highly potent drugs used only for serious ventricular arrhythmias that fail to respond to other medications and never in patients with a history of heart attack or congestive heart failure.

Effects: Suppresses vigorous potentially dangerous ventricular arrhythmias.

Possible side effects: May worsen some arrhythmias, weaken cardiac pumping, slow heart rate, or increase blood sugar. May cause fever, rash, liver inflammation, confusion, loss of concentration, dizziness, a metallic taste in the mouth, or changes in vision.

Approximate cost: for 100 capsules or tablets, flecainide—50 mg, average wholesale price, $48.66**
propafenone—150 mg, average wholesale price, $59.16***; 300 mg, average wholesale price, $107.34***

Dosage: flecainide—100 mg to 200 mg twice a day
propafenone—150 mg to 300 mg three times a day

Notes:
- Never used in patients who have already had a heart attack.
- Drug interactions are minimal.
- May decrease the effectiveness of a permanent pacemaker, requiring an increase in the pacing threshold.
- Digoxin levels should be reduced in conjunction with flecainide.

Generic name (trade name): lidocaine (Xylocaine)

How supplied: injection (50-mg and 100-mg prefilled 5-ml syringes, 100-mg 1-ml ampules, 100-mg/ml 5-ml ampules, or in larger vials for intravenous infusion)

Available as generic: yes

Description: Introduced in 1949, lidocaine is a powerful local anesthetic and antiarrhythmic when given by injection or intravenous infusion.

Effects: Controls abnormal heart rhythms, particularly after heart attack, during heart surgery, or after an overdose of digitalis drugs.

Possible side effects: Side effects are infrequent but may include anxiety or restlessness, confusion or memory loss, nausea or vomiting, twitching or tremors, shallow breathing, or seizures.

Approximate cost: 50-mg prefilled 5-ml syringe, average wholesale price, $79.09***; 100-mg prefilled 5-ml syringe, average wholesale price, $82.65***

Dosage: varies

Generic name (trade name): mexiletine (Mexitil)

How supplied: capsule (150 mg, 200 mg, 250 mg)

Available as generic: no

Description: It is a local anesthetic and antiarrhythmic that came into use in the 1980s. Related to the drug lidocaine.

Effects: Suppresses ventricular arrhythmias.

Possible side effects: Fever, rash, lower blood platelet count, liver inflammation, nausea, confusion,

loss of concentration, dizziness, tremors, and changes in vision may occur.

Approximate cost: for 100 150-mg capsules, average wholesale price, $57.95**

Dosage: 150 to 300 mg three to four times per day

Notes:
- Adverse effects can be reduced by taking the drug with meals.
- Drug interactions are minimal.

Generic name (trade names): procainamide (Procan SR, Pronestyl, Pronestyl SR)

How supplied: capsule or tablet (250 mg, 375 mg, 500 mg), sustained-release tablet (250 mg, 500 mg, 750 mg, 1,000 mg), injection (100 mg/ml in 10ml vial or 500 mg/ml in 2-ml vial)

Available as generic: yes

Description: It is a synthetic antiarrhythmic, anesthetic-type drug in use since 1951.

Effects: Corrects some abnormal heart rhythms, especially a too rapid heartbeat in the ventricles. Also used in the treatment of Wolff-Parkinson-White syndrome. (See Chapter 16.)

Possible side effects: Fever, rash, liver inflammation, weight loss, nausea, confusion, and loss of concentration may occur. Prolonged use of procainamide can cause drug-induced lupus, especially in people who metabolize the drug slowly (a tendency that can be determined with a blood test). Can result in a positive lupus blood test. Symptoms of lupus, an autoimmune syndrome, are fever, joint pain, low blood counts, and inflammation of the linings of the lungs or heart (felt as chest pain on deep inhalation).

Approximate cost: for 100 500-mg tablets, generic, $12.83 to $20.97

Dosage: short-acting, 250 mg to 750 mg every four hours; sustained-release, 500 mg to 2,000 mg every six hours

Notes:
- Procainamide can depress white blood cell counts, increasing the risk of infection.

Generic name (trade names): quinidine gluconate (Duraquin, Quinaglute Dura-Tabs, Quinalan Sustained-Release)
quinidine sulfate (Quinidex Extentabs)

How supplied: quinidine gluconate—tablet (sustained-release 324 mg, 330 mg)
quinidine sulfate—tablet (200 mg, 300 mg), extended-release tablet (300 mg), capsule (325 mg)

Available as generic: yes

Description: Used since 1918, this is one of the oldest antiarrhythmics. It is derived from the bark of the South American cinchona tree.

Effects: It controls many different abnormal heart rhythms, especially those that are fast or irregular.

Possible side effects: Diarrhea is the most common side effect. In rare cases, may cause a drop in blood platelets, causing bruises or bleeding. Other possible effects are fever, rash, dizziness, and ringing in the ears.

Approximate cost: quinidine sulfate—100 200-mg tablets, generic, $10.67 to $16.43

Dosage: 200 mg to 400 mg three to four times per day

Notes:

- Digoxin dosage should be cut in half if taken with quinidine.
- Quinidine may increase bleeding if taken in conjunction with warfarin (Coumadin).
- Phenobarbital and rifampin reduce the effect of quinidine.

Generic name (trade name): tocainide (Tonocard)

How supplied: tablet (400 mg, 600 mg)

Available as generic: no

Description: It came into use in the 1980s and is related to lidocaine.

Effects: It suppresses ventricular arrhythmias.

Possible side effects: Most significant common side effects are weight loss, nausea, and tremors. Other less common effects are fever, rash, depressed white blood cell count, liver inflammation, confusion, loss of concentration, dizziness, and disturbances in vision. About 0.1 to 0.2 percent of patients suffer lung inflammation, a potentially serious side effect.

Approximate cost: for 100 400-mg tablets, average wholesale price, $75.20**

Dosage: 200 mg to 600 mg three times per day

Notes:

- Collectively, tocainide's more serious side effects have discouraged its use as a frontline drug.

ANTICOAGULANTS, ANTIPLATELETS, AND THROMBOLYTICS

These drugs are sometimes referred to as "blood thinners," but this term is not truly accurate. They inhibit the ability of the blood to clot—preventing clots from forming in blood vessels and from getting bigger. Under a number of different circumstances, it becomes necessary to stop clotting. Anticoagulants, antiplatelet agents, and thrombolytics each have specific indications and uses.

Any patient who has had a heart valve replaced with a mechanical valve (see Chapter 13) requires lifelong oral anticoagulants in order to prevent clots from forming on the valve. Patients who develop atrial fibrillation (see Chapter 16) may require anticoagulants; clot formation in the left atrium is a potential hazard of this rhythmic disturbance. Oral anticoagulants are prescribed for patients who develop thrombophlebitis, an inflammation of the veins in the legs or pelvis. (See Chapter 17.) One of the dangers of this condition is the development of blood clots that may travel to the lungs and cause pulmonary emboli. Lastly, some patients who have a serious heart attack involving the front surface of the heart are prescribed an anticoagulant to prevent clots from forming on the inner lining of the scar.

Heparin is an anticoagulant that is administered intravenously when rapid anticoagulation is necessary. All patients undergoing open-heart surgery are treated with heparin while their blood is being oxygenated by the heart-lung machine. At the end of the operation, medication is given to reverse the effects of heparin. (See Chapter 11.)

When a person first develops thrombophlebitis, heparin is often used because its action is almost immediate. It also is used in people who have had a heart attack and have been treated with thrombolytic therapy. Keeping the affected artery open often requires vigorous anticoagulation.

Aspirin is not an anticoagulant but has a profound effect on a component of the blood called platelets—blood cells that stick together and cause clots to form. Platelets are important in blood clotting and are in large part responsible for allowing us to stop bleeding when we cut ourselves. Platelets are also in part responsible for the formation of a clot in a coronary artery—a phenomenon that initiates many heart attacks. Because of aspirin's ability to inhibit the clotting action of platelets, it is designated as an antiplatelet and is frequently prescribed in patients who have recovered from a heart attack, in order to prevent clots from forming in the veins used for coronary bypass surgery.

The most recent and exciting class of drugs that are useful for people with heart attacks are the thrombolytic drugs. These agents are given intravenously as soon as possible with the goal of dissolving the offending clot within a coronary artery. A patient having a heart attack can be helped considerably if the clot can be dissolved before it causes permanent, debilitating damage. The three most commonly used thrombolytics are t-PA, streptokinase, and APSAC. They are generally used only in hospitals or in emergency situations.

EXAMPLES OF ANTICOAGULANTS, ANTIPLATELETS, AND THROMBOLYTICS

Generic name (trade names): acetylsalicylic acid or aspirin (Alka-Seltzer, Anacin, Ascriptin, Bayer, Bufferin, Easprin, Ecotrin, St. Josephs, Zorprin)

How supplied: tablet (81 mg, 325 mg, 650 mg), capsule (325 mg, 650 mg), rectal suppository (325 mg, 650 mg)

Available as generic: yes

Description: It is a nonnarcotic analgesic and antiplatelet used since 1899.

Effects: Helps prevent blood clots. Also treats pain, fever, arthritis, colds, menstrual cramps, headaches, and joint and muscular aches.

Possible side effects: Indigestion is the most common side effect.

Approximate cost: Varies greatly. Generic may cost only pennies per pill. Shop around for best over-the-counter drug values.

Dosage: to inhibit clotting, 81 mg to 325 mg per day

Notes:

- Aspirin can cause Reye's syndrome, a rare brain and liver disorder that usually occurs in children.
- Aspirin may increase the effect of other anticoagulant drugs.

Generic name (trade name): dipyridamole (Persantine)

How supplied: tablet (25 mg, 50 mg, 75 mg)

Available as generic: yes

Description: It is an antiplatelet and antianginal drug first introduced in the late 1970s.

Effects: Helps keep blood clots from forming in people who have just had a heart attack, heart surgery, a stroke, or a heart valve replacement (usually given with aspirin or warfarin).

Possible side effects: Adverse effects are rare, but may include nausea, headache, flushing, dizziness or faintness, or rash.

Approximate cost: For 100 tablets, 25 mg, $26.17 to $36.39 (generic, $4.97 to $11.13); 50 mg, $40.87 to $65.99 (generic, $9.13 to $16.87)

Dosage: 75 mg to 400 mg per day

Note:

- Dipyridamole may increase the effect of other anticoagulants.

Generic name (trade names): warfarin (Coumadin, Panwarfin)

How supplied: tablet (1 mg, 2 mg, 2.5 mg, 5 mg, 7.5 mg, 10 mg)

Available as generic: yes

Description: Warfarin is the prototype oral anticoagulant. It and some drugs related to it have been used for nearly 50 years.

Effects: Prevents blood clots, especially in the leg and pelvic veins where blood flow is at its slowest. Also used in people with atrial fibrillation or after a heart valve replacement.

Possible side effects: Excessive bleeding is the most common adverse effect. Nausea or vomiting, loss of appetite, abdominal pain or diarrhea, rash or bruising, and hair loss are also possible.

Approximate cost: For 100 5-mg tablets, $48.29 to $61.13 (generic, $28.33 to $37.37)

Dosage: 15 mg on the first day of treatment, 10 mg on the second, and 2.5 mg to 7.5 mg per day thereafter

Note:

- Interacts with a variety of drugs. Check with your physician and pharmacist.

BETA-ADRENERGIC BLOCKING DRUGS (BETA BLOCKERS)

These drugs probably reduce blood pressure by reducing the output of blood from the heart (or perhaps by blocking the production of angiotensin). They were first introduced in the United States in the 1960s to treat angina and to lower blood pressure. Specifically, they block responses from the beta nerve receptors. This serves to slow down the heart rate and to lower blood pressure.

Beta blockers also block the effects of some of the hormones that regulate blood pressure. During exercise or emotional stress, adrenaline and norepinephrine are released and normally stimulate the beta receptors—sensors that transmit messages to the heart to speed up and pump harder. By blocking the receptors, beta blockers act to reduce heart muscle oxygen demands during physical activity or excitement, thus reducing the possibility of angina caused by oxygen deprivation.

Beta blockers may be prescribed as the initial drugs to lower blood pressure, or they may be given along with a diuretic or other antihypertensive drug. In general, beta blockers are more effective in younger patients. Because they relieve angina, they may be the drug of choice for people who have this problem along with high blood pressure. Beta blockers also damp heart rate increases caused by stress, exercise, or anxiety. Stage performers occasionally take them to combat the heart palpitations, voice cracking, or fine tremors of the hands that may be associated with stage fright.

For reasons that are not fully understood, African-Americans do not seem to respond as well as whites to beta blockers, although there are exceptions. Because beta blockers may actually constrict peripheral blood vessels, they generally are not recommended for people with circulatory problems in their hands or legs. They also are not prescribed for people with asthma. Their use tends to result in a spasm of the bronchial tubes in the lungs of susceptible persons.

Most patients tolerate beta blockers well, especially if they are administered in low doses along with a diuretic or other antihypertensive drug. The effects of beta blockers are particularly complemented by nitrate therapy for angina.

EXAMPLES OF BETA BLOCKERS

Generic names (trade names): acebutolol (Sectral)
  atenolol (Tenormin)
  metoprolol (Lopressor)
  nadolol (Corgard)
  pindolol (Visken)
  propranolol (Inderal)
How supplied: acebutolol—capsule (200 mg, 400 mg)
  atenolol—tablet (50 mg, 100 mg), injection (0.5 mg/ml, 10-ml ampule)
  metoprolol—tablet (50 mg, 100 mg), injection (1 mg/ml, 5-ml ampule)
  nadolol—tablet (20 mg, 40 mg, 80 mg, 120 mg, 160 mg)
  pindolol—tablet (5 mg, 10 mg)
  propranolol—tablet (10 mg, 20 mg, 40 mg, 60 mg, 80 mg, 90 mg), sustained-release capsule (60 mg, 80 mg, 120 mg, 160 mg)
Available as generic: acebutolol, atenolol, metoprolol, nadolol, pindolol—no
  propranolol—yes
Description: Acebutolol, atenolol, and metoprolol are cardioselective (acting mainly on the heart as opposed to both heart and lungs) beta blockers that were first introduced in 1985, 1981, and 1978 respectively. Nadolol was introduced in 1980. Pindolol is one of the newer beta blockers. Propranolol was introduced in 1968 and was the first beta blocker to be available in the United States.

Effects: They treat hypertension, angina, some abnormal heart rhythms, palpitations, and tremors caused by overactivity of the thyroid gland, and anxiety such as stage fright. May protect the heart from further damage after a heart attack. May help prevent migraine headaches.

Possible side effects: Lethargy and cold hands and feet because of reduced circulation may occur. Also may cause nausea, nightmares or vivid dreams, and impotence. May also precipitate asthmatic attack.

Approximate cost: For 100 tablets or capsules,
  acebutolol—200 mg, average wholesale price, $58.21***; 400 mg, average wholesale price, $77.40***
  atenolol—50 mg, $66.59 to $92.99; 100 mg, $107.37 to $147.99
  metoprolol—50 mg, $35.97 to $53.37; 100 mg, $61.57 to $83.99
  nadolol—40 mg, $73.99 to $103.33
  pindolol—5 mg, average wholesale price, $54.48***; 10 mg, average wholesale price, $69.60***
  propranolol—20 mg, $27.77 to $45.93 (generic, $10.47 to $17.43); 40 mg, $38.27 to $56.57 (generic, $12.69 to $23.27); 80 mg long-acting, $70.60 to $93.73 (generic, $41.23 to $57.87)
Dosage: acebutolol—200 mg to 600 mg per day
  atenolol—25 mg to 100 mg per day
  metoprolol—50 mg to 150 mg per day
  nadolol—40 mg to 160 mg per day
  pindolol—10 mg to 40 mg per day
  propranolol—40 mg to 240 mg per day
Notes:
- None of the beta blockers should be used by asthmatics or people with chronic lung disease.
- Beta blockers should be used with caution in insulin-dependent diabetics and people with peripheral vascular disease.

Altogether, there are about 10 beta blockers currently on the market in the United States, including betaxolol (Kerlone), carteolol (Cartrol), penbutolol (Levatol), and timolol maleate (Blocadren). For more complete information on these less commonly prescribed or newly released medications, consult your physician or pharmacist.

CALCIUM CHANNEL BLOCKERS

Calcium plays a central role in the electrical stimulation of cardiac cells and in the mechanical contraction of smooth muscle cells in the walls of arteries. Calcium channel blockers are relatively new synthetic drugs that work by blocking the passage of calcium into the muscle cells that control the size of blood vessels. All muscles need calcium in order to constrict; by preventing the muscles of the arteries from constricting, blood vessels open up (dilate), allowing blood to flow through them more easily. Blood pressure is reduced.

Calcium channel blockers are effective in initial treatment of high blood pressure in about 30 to 40 percent of patients with hypertension. They may be added to a diuretic or other antihypertensive medication. They are generally well tolerated (even by people with asthma), but they are more costly than diuretics or beta blockers. Thus, many doctors still recommend that other drugs be tried first.

EXAMPLES OF CALCIUM CHANNEL BLOCKERS

Generic name (trade name): diltiazem (Cardizem)
How supplied: tablet (30 mg, 60 mg, 90 mg, 120 mg), sustained-release capsule (60 mg, 90 mg, 120 mg)
Available as generic: no
Description: It is a calcium channel blocker and antianginal drug, introduced in 1984.
Effects: Reduces the frequency of angina attacks and lowers blood pressure.
Possible side effects: Headache, nausea, tiredness, ankle swelling, dizziness, and rash can occur.
Approximate cost: for 100 tablets, 30 mg, $31.99 to $43.69; 60 mg, $49.63 to $65.43; 90 mg, $67.57 to $88.63
Dosage: 60 mg to 240 mg per day

Generic names (trade names): nicardipine (Cardene)
nifedipine (Procardia, Procardia XL)
How supplied: nicardipine—capsule (20 mg, 30 mg)
nifedipine—capsule (10 mg, 20 mg), extended-release tablet (30 mg, 60 mg, 90 mg)
Available as generic: no

Description: Nicardipine is one of the more recently introduced calcium channel blockers. Nifedipine is a calcium channel blocker and antianginal and antihypertensive drug introduced in 1982.
Effects: They help relieve anginal pain and prevent attacks, reduce blood pressure, and help improve circulation in the limbs.
Possible side effects: May cause redness of face and neck, headache, palpitations, dizziness, nausea, low blood pressure, ankle swelling, and rash.
Approximate cost: for 100 tablets,
nicardipine—20 mg, $44 to $49.50*
nifedipine—10 mg, $40.27 to $57.13; 20 mg, $79.97 to $111.37; 30 mg XL, $92.99 to $118.23; 60 mg XL, $164.63 to $215.89
Dosage: nicardipine—60 mg to 120 mg per day
nifedipine—30 mg to 120 mg per day

Generic name (trade name): nimodipine (Nimotop)
How supplied: capsule (30 mg)
Available as generic: no
Description: It is a calcium channel blocker, available since 1989, that is used to treat people who have had a burst blood vessel in the head (known as subarachnoid hemorrhage or ruptured aneurysm). (See Chapter 18.)
Effects: It may help relax constricted blood vessels (known as vasospasm), a condition that can lead to a recurrence of stroke.
Possible side effects: Dizziness or lightheadedness, headache, nausea, fast heart rate, skin rash, or swelling of the lower extremities may occur.
Approximate cost: for 100 30-mg capsules, average wholesale price, $480.19***
Dosage: 60 mg, every four hours for 21 consecutive days

Generic name (trade names): verapamil (Calan, Isoptin, Verelan)
How supplied: tablet (40 mg, 80 mg, 120 mg), sustained-release tablet (180 mg, 240 mg), capsule (120 mg, 240 mg), sustained-release caplet (180 mg, 240 mg), injection (5-mg/ml and 10-mg/ml ampules, 5-mg/2ml and 10-mg/4ml vials)
Available as generic: yes
Description: It is a calcium channel blocker, antianginal drug, and antiarrhythmic drug introduced in 1981.
Effects: Suppresses some arrhythmias, helps prevent anginal attacks, and reduces high blood pressure.

Possible side effects: Excessively slow heart rate, low blood pressure, headache, swelling of feet, and constipation may occur.

Approximate cost: for 100 80-mg tablets, generic, $19.87 to $32.69

for 100 240-mg SR capsules, $100.37 to $136.67

Dosage: 120 mg to 360 mg per day

CENTRALLY ACTING DRUGS

Drugs in this category act on the brain centers to reduce nerve impulses that constrict blood vessels. Vessels open up (dilate); they may also cause the heart to beat more slowly.

Centrally acting drugs are not widely used in initial treatment of high blood pressure; instead, they are given along with a diuretic or other antihypertensive drugs when these drugs alone do not produce an adequate reduction in blood pressure.

EXAMPLES OF CENTRALLY ACTING DRUGS
(Central Alpha-Adrenergic Agents)

Generic names (trade names): clonidine (Catapres, Catapres-TTS)

guanabenz (Wytensin)

guanfacine (Tenex)

How supplied: clonidine—tablet (0.1 mg, 0.2 mg, 0.3 mg), 7-day transdermal patch (0.1 mg/day, 0.2 mg/day, 0.3 mg/day)

guanabenz—tablet (4 mg, 8 mg)

guanfacine—tablet (1 mg)

Available as generic: clonidine—yes

guanabenz, guanfacine—no

Description: These are antihypertensives that reduce the stimulatory nerve impulses from the brain to the heart.

Effects: Lower blood pressure.

Possible side effects: Drowsiness or sedation, constipation, dry mouth, headache, dizziness or weakness, rash, depression, ankle swelling, cold hands, and impotence may occur.

Approximate cost: for 100 tablets,

clonidine—generic, 0.1 mg, $11.73 to $25.27

guanabenz—4 mg, $44 to $46.20

guanfacine—1 mg, average wholesale price, $45.47***

Dosage: clonidine—0.1 mg to 1 mg per day

guanabenz—4 mg to 24 mg per day divided into two doses

guanfacine—1 mg to 3 mg per day

Note:

• Clonidine also may minimize withdrawal symptoms during smoking cessation or alcohol detoxification and may relieve hot flashes that occur during menopause.

Generic name (trade name): methyldopa (Aldomet)

How supplied: tablet (125 mg, 250 mg, 500 mg), suspension (50 mg/ml in a 473-ml bottle)

Available as generic: yes

Description: It was introduced in the 1960s and is still a widely used antihypertensive.

Effects: It lowers blood pressure.

Possible side effects: Dizziness or lightheadedness, drowsiness, headache, dry mouth or stuffy nose, swelling of ankles or feet, tiredness or weakness, fever, depression, and liver inflammation may occur.

Approximate cost: for 100 tablets, generic, 250 mg, $12.13 to $20.47; 500 mg, $23.47 to $38.37

Dosage: 250 mg to 1,000 mg per day divided into two doses

Note:

• Methyldopa may be suitable for treating high blood pressure in women during late pregnancy.

CHOLESTEROL-LOWERING AGENTS

To determine whether drug treatment for a blood cholesterol problem is necessary, the level of blood cholesterol must be measured. If it is over 200 mg/dl, your doctor may wish to repeat the test for confirmation and to perform additional measurements of the levels of HDL and LDL cholesterol (the "good" and "bad" components) and triglycerides (blood fats).

There is some question whether or not the new limits of cholesterol levels for defining risk are appropriate for elderly people or those with no other risk factors for heart disease. The reduction in life expectancy may not be of significance, for example, if the cholesterol level of a 70-year-old man or woman is 260 or 270, unless other factors are present.

The first step in treatment for elevated blood cholesterol is a diet low in saturated fat and cholesterol. Other measures may also be recommended, including loss of excess weight, regular moderate exercise, smoking cessation, and reduction of excessive alcohol intake. In general, drug therapy is prescribed to reduce elevated levels of cholesterol or other blood fats *only* after several months of dietary modification alone have failed to do the job adequately.

How high a level of blood cholesterol warrants drug therapy? This is a decision made by the physician, based on a person's individual health profile—including age, overall health status, cardiovascular risk factors, history of heart disease, and many other factors.

Remember, cholesterol-lowering medication is considered an adjunct to dietary modification, not a replacement for it. If a person on drug therapy for high blood cholesterol continues to eat a high-fat, high-cholesterol diet, the effects of the medication may be undermined or undone. Once drug therapy for elevated blood cholesterol is begun, the therapy may have to be continued indefinitely. This is why the decision to begin cholesterol-lowering drug therapy calls for careful consideration.

Drugs that lower cholesterol do so in various ways and have differing effects on the various components of total blood cholesterol (including HDL and LDL cholesterol and triglycerides). An individual's "lipid profile," or the levels of various fats in the bloodstream, helps determine which drug or drugs to prescribe. (Sometimes physicians use the ratio of total to HDL cholesterol, or of LDL to HDL, in assessing risk and determining a course of treatment.) Other factors in drug selection include cost, side effects, convenience, safety, effectiveness, and impact on cardiovascular risk as shown in clinical trials.

EXAMPLES OF CHOLESTEROL-LOWERING AGENTS

Generic names (trade names): cholestyramine (Questran, Questran Light)
colestipol (Colestid)

How supplied: cholestyramine—powder (carton of 60 9-gm packets or can of 378 gm)
colestipol—granules (box of 30 5-gm packets; bottle of 500 gm)

Available as generic: no

Description: These drugs, called bile acid sequestrants, work in the intestine to bind bile acids, which are then excreted. This stimulates the liver to remove more LDL cholesterol from the blood in order to manufacture more bile acids. The medications are in powder form and must be taken mixed with water or some other liquid such as orange juice. They are available in packets or in bulk, with a scoop equal to one packet.

Effects: Total cholesterol may be reduced 15 to 20 percent on an average regimen. However, these drugs do not reduce triglycerides and, in fact, may raise them in some people.

Possible side effects: Constipation, bloating, heartburn, nausea, vomiting, headaches, and interference with absorption of other drugs may occur. Many people are unable to tolerate dosages high enough to produce the desired effect.

Approximate cost: cholestyramine powder—$63.74 per carton of 60 packets**; $27.92 per can (378 gm)**
colestipol—$27.99 per box of 30 packets**; $62.29 per bottle (500 gm)**

Dosage: 2 to 4 packets or scoops twice daily; most effective when taken with meals

Notes:

- May interfere with absorption of several drugs, including thiazide diuretics, digoxin, warfarin, beta blockers, thyroid medications, and antibiotics. Patients taking any of these drugs may be advised to take them one hour before or several hours after a dose of bile acid sequestrant.
- To decrease the possibility of constipation, increase intake of fluids and dietary fiber. If constipation still occurs, ask the physician about taking a psyllium-based stool softener or other laxative.
- With a long record of safety and effectiveness, these drugs are listed among the first choices for cholesterol-lowering therapy. Inconveniences include the gritty powder form of the medication and the common side effects of constipation and other gastrointestinal disorders.

Generic name (trade name): gemfibrozil (Lopid)

How supplied: capsule (600 mg)

Available as generic: no

Description: This drug, which belongs to a class of agents known as fibric acids, works by breaking down a component of blood cholesterol called very-low-density lipoprotein (VLDL).

Effects: Gemfibrozil is prescribed to lower elevated levels of blood triglycerides and to increase HDL. However, the drug may also cause a moderate reduction in LDL cholesterol. Thus, it may be indicated for individuals who have very low levels of HDL cholesterol in addition to high total or LDL cholesterol levels.

Possible side effects: Muscle aches or weakness, abdominal pain or discomfort, diarrhea, and nausea may occur.

Approximate cost: for 100 600-mg capsules, $88.23 to $122.17

Dosage: 600 mg twice daily (most effective when

taken 30 minutes before morning or evening meals)

Notes:

- Gemfibrozil may increase the effect of warfarin and other anticoagulant drugs; if you take an anticoagulant drug, your physician may need to readjust the dosage.
- Offers convenience and relative lack of side effects; however, increases chance of developing gallstones or liver dysfunction.
- Another drug in this class, fenofibrate (Lipidil), may soon be available in the United States.

Generic name (trade name): lovastatin (Mevacor)
How supplied: tablet (20 mg, 40 mg)
Available as generic: no
Description: The drug restricts the liver's production of cholesterol by inhibiting the action of an enzyme called HMG-CoA reductase. As the liver synthesizes less cholesterol, it absorbs more LDL ("bad") cholesterol from the bloodstream.
Effects: May lower LDL cholesterol by 30 to 40 percent. At higher doses, it may moderately decrease triglycerides and increase HDL cholesterol as well.
Possible side effects: Headache, rash, muscle ache or weakness, dizziness, lightheadedness, cataracts, and liver function abnormalities may occur.
Approximate cost: for 100 20-mg tablets, $167.63 to $215.27
Dosage: 20 mg to 80 mg
Notes:

- Lovastatin causes relatively few side effects in most people. However, as a newer drug, it has a shorter track record of safety than some other agents.
- It is possible that lovastatin may cause liver dysfunction or cataracts. For this reason, liver function tests every six to eight months and annual eye examinations may be recommended for people taking the drug.
- Other drugs in the category of HMG-CoA reductase inhibitors that may become available in the future include simvastatin (Zocor), pravastatin (Pravachol), and fluvastatin (LoChol), pending FDA approval for prescription use.

Generic names (trade names): nicotinic acid, niacin (Nia-Bid, Niacels, Niacor, Niaplus, Nicolar, Nicobid, Slo-Niacin)
How supplied: tablet (100 mg, 250 mg, 500 mg), sustained-release capsule (250 mg, 500 mg, 750 mg), timed-release preparation (125 mg, 250 mg, 500 mg)
Available as generic: yes
Description: Nicotinic acid, a B vitamin, works in the liver in a manner that is still unclear.
Effects: It lowers triglycerides and LDL cholesterol; raises HDL cholesterol.
Possible side effects: Itching, rash, or flushing of the skin, gastrointestinal distress, dizziness, lightheadedness, and rapid heartbeat may occur.
Approximate cost: for 100 500-mg tabs, $43.52** (Generics may be a fraction of the cost of brand names. Shop around for best over-the-counter drug values.)
Dosage: 500 mg to 1,000 mg or more, three times a day (usually taken with meals). Dosage usually starts low (for example, 100 mg three times a day) and increases slowly over several weeks to minimize side effects.
Notes:

- It can be purchased without a prescription, but should not be taken as a cholesterol-lowering medication unless prescribed by a physician. At the high doses necessary to lower cholesterol, niacin is as powerful as any prescription drug, and should be monitored accordingly for effects and side effects.
- It is safe and effective, but often causes side effects, particularly flushing and itching at the outset of therapy. This can be minimized by taking aspirin once a day; ask your physician. At high doses, liver function abnormalities may occur; periodic testing of liver enzymes, blood sugar, and uric acid may be necessary.
- Skipping doses may increase side effects when the drug is next taken. If you stop taking the drug for more than two days, ask your physician about restarting at a lower dose.
- Sustained-release form occasionally has caused severe liver damage, even at low doses (500 mg).

Generic name (trade name): probucol (Lorelco)
How supplied: tablet (250 mg, 500 mg)
Available as generic: no
Description: Probucol works in the bloodstream to alter the makeup of LDL cholesterol, causing it to be removed more quickly from the blood.
Effects: It lowers total and LDL cholesterol, but it also may lower beneficial HDL cholesterol. May inhibit the oxidation of LDL cholesterol and thus help keep it from being deposited in artery walls.

Possible side effects: Indigestion, diarrhea, headache, rash, and insomnia may occur.

Approximate cost: for 120 250-mg tablets, $65.82**; for 100 500-mg tablets, $94.86**

Dosage: 500 mg twice daily

DIGITALIS DRUGS

Like many drugs, digitalis was originally derived from a plant, in this case the foxglove. Digitalis has the primary effect of strengthening the force of contractions in *weakened* hearts, but it is *not* a cardiac vitamin that can make a strong heart stronger. It is also used in the control of atrial fibrillation. The most commonly used digitalis products are digoxin and digitoxin.

Physicians and folk healers have used digitalis preparations for more than 200 years to treat various ailments. The major benefits of foxglove extracts in patients with heart disease were believed to be a result of their ability to control abnormally fast heart rhythms. At the turn of the 20th century, however, it was recognized that digitalis improves the function of the failing heart independently of its effects on the heart rhythm.

The drug penetrates all body tissues and reaches a high concentration in the muscle of the heart. Its molecules bind with cell receptors that regulate the concentration of sodium and potassium in the spaces between tissue cells and in the bloodstream. These two minerals determine the level of calcium—a potent stimulator of heart contractions—within muscle cells. Digitalis preparations act by increasing the amount of calcium supplied to the heart muscle and thus enhancing its contractions.

Digitalis drugs also affect electrical activity in cardiac tissues. They control the rate at which electric impulses are released and the speed of their conduction through the chamber walls.

These two actions determine the two major uses of digitalis drugs in heart disease—treatment of heart failure and control of abnormal heart rhythms.

Digitalis preparations are a major class of drugs used in the treatment of heart failure. By increasing the force of heart contractions, they increase the amount of blood pumped with each beat. The improved pumping capacity offsets the mechanisms that lead to the enlargement of the failing heart. A more efficient heart pumps more effectively, reducing the tendency for fluid retention and tissue congestion.

When patients with heart failure start taking digitalis, their symptoms improve significantly, particularly the breathlessness that results from congestion of fluids in the lungs. Digitalis drugs also reduce swelling in the legs, alleviate fatigue as blood and oxygen are delivered more effectively to body organs, and increase the person's overall capacity to perform daily activities and exercise.

Digitalis may be given on a short-term basis in acute heart failure or over a long period of time to treat chronic heart failure. Physicians usually prescribe digitalis together with diuretics, which further promote removal of fluids from body tissues. Newer classes of drugs, particularly ACE inhibitors, are now also combined with digitalis and diuretics in the treatment of heart failure.

The availability of other heart failure medications allows physicians to prescribe digitalis drugs at doses that are less likely to produce serious side effects. However, digitalis remains the standard against which the effectiveness of new heart failure therapies is measured.

Digitalis drugs can be used to treat disturbances of the heartbeat, particularly the abnormally rapid contractions of the atria referred to as atrial or supraventricular arrhythmias (especially atrial fibrillation). The drugs restore the normal heartbeat either by interrupting the abnormal rhythm or by slowing down the rapid beats to a rate at which effective and coordinated heart contractions are possible.

EXAMPLES OF DIGITALIS PREPARATIONS

Generic name (trade names): digoxin (Lanoxicaps, Lanoxin)

How supplied: tablet (0.125 mg, 0.25 mg, 0.5 mg), capsule (0.05 mg, 0.1 mg, 0.2 mg), elixir (0.05 mg per ml, 60-ml bottle), injection (0.5 mg in 2 ml, 0.1 mg in 1 ml)

Available as generic: yes

Description: It is a digitalis drug extracted from the leaves of the foxglove plant. It slows the heart rate so that each beat is more effective in pumping blood.

Effects: It treats heart failure and corrects some abnormal heart rhythms.

Possible side effects: Some side effects include tiredness, nausea, loss of appetite, and disturbances in vision.

Approximate cost: for 100 tablets, 0.125 mg, $5.59 to $8.63; 0.25 mg, $5.99 to $10.19

Dosage: 0.125 mg to 0.25 mg per day for adults; reduced dosage for children based on weight and age; up to 3 times a day to start and then once daily

Notes:

- Check with doctor before combining with any other medication. There are numerous drug interactions.
- People taking digoxin must be carefully monitored, because an effective digoxin dose may be near the toxic dose.

Generic name (trade names): digitoxin (Crystodigin, Purodigin)
How supplied: tablet (0.05 mg, 0.1 mg)
Available as generic: yes
Description: A digitalis drug from the foxglove plant, it strengthens the force of the heart's contractions.
Effects: See digoxin.
Possible side effects: See digoxin.
Approximate cost: for 100 0.05-mg tablets, average wholesale price, $2.68***, 0.1-mg tablets, average wholesale price, $4.32***
Dosage: 0.05 mg to 0.2 mg per day; every 6 to 8 hours for first few doses, then once daily

Note:

- See digoxin.

DIURETICS

Diuretics, commonly referred to as water pills, lower blood pressure by increasing the kidney's excretion of sodium and water, which in turn reduces the volume of blood. These are among the older antihypertensive agents, having been introduced for use in the United States in 1957. They are still widely used, either alone or in conjunction with other antihypertensive drugs. Diuretics are also highly effective in the treatment of heart failure.

There are several types of diuretics, which are classified according to their site of action in the kidney. The thiazide diuretics work in the tubules (the structures that transport urine in the kidneys).

The loop diuretics are more potent than the thiazide diuretics. They are so named because they work in the area of the kidney called the loop of Henle. They are usually prescribed when a thiazide diuretic proves insufficient or for patients with heart failure or compromised kidney function.

A third class, the potassium-sparing diuretics, work in the area where potassium is excreted. They

prevent the excessive loss of potassium that sometimes occurs with the thiazides. They are most often given in conjunction with a thiazide or loop diuretic.

Diuretics are highly effective, generally well tolerated, and less expensive than most other antihypertensive medications. They were the medications used in all of the long-term hypertension treatment studies that demonstrated a marked decrease in strokes and heart failure.

EXAMPLES OF THIAZIDE DIURETICS

Generic name (trade name): chlorthalidone (Hygroton)
How supplied: tablet (25 mg, 50 mg, 100 mg)
Available as generic: yes
Description: It is a thiazide diuretic introduced in 1960. It removes excess water and sodium from the body.
Effects: It reduces fluid retention in people with heart failure, kidney disorders, liver disease, or premenstrual tension, and it lowers blood pressure.
Possible side effects: Although uncommon, lethargy, cramps, rash, or impotence may occur. Some of these effects may be caused by loss of potassium and may be avoided by including a potassium supplement or potassium-sparing agent in the regimen.
Approximate cost: for 100 tablets, generic, 25 mg, $8.87 to $18.07; 50 mg, $9.77 to $18.47
Dosage: 12.5 mg or 25 mg to 50 mg per day
Notes:

- If potassium loss is excessive and digitalis drugs are also being taken, the side effects of those drugs may be increased.
- It interacts with lithium to cause lithium toxicity.
- It may prevent calcium kidney stones or help prevent osteoporosis.
- It may cause uric acid level or glucose level in blood to increase (leading to or aggravating gout or diabetes, respectively). It may also adversely affect lipids.

Generic name (trade names): hydrochlorothiazide (Esidrix, Hydrodiuril, Oretic)
How supplied: tablet (25 mg, 50 mg, 100 mg)
Available as generic: yes
Description: It is a thiazide diuretic introduced in 1958. It removes excess water and sodium from the body.
Effects: It reduces fluid retention in people with heart failure, kidney disorders, liver disease, or pre-

menstrual tension, and it lowers blood pressure.

Possible side effects: See chlorthalidone.

Approximate cost: for 100 tablets, generic, 50 mg, $3.67 to $7.59

Dosage: 25 mg to 50 mg per day

Notes:

- See chlorthalidone.

Generic name (trade names): metolazone (Diulo, Mykrox, Zaroxolyn)

How supplied: tablet (0.5 mg, 2.5 mg, 5 mg, 10 mg)

Available as generic: yes

Description: It is a thiazide diuretic. See chlorthalidone.

Effects: See chlorthalidone.

Possible side effects: See chlorthalidone.

Approximate cost: for 100 0.5-mg tablets, $35.20*

Dosage: 2.5 mg to 10 mg per day

Notes:

- Metolazone is longer-acting than most thiazide diuretics.
- See chlorthalidone.

EXAMPLES OF LOOP DIURETICS

Generic name (trade name): bumetanide (Bumex)

How supplied: tablet (0.5 mg, 1 mg, 2 mg), injection (0.25 mg/ml 2-ml ampules or 0.25 mg/ml 2-, 4-, and 10-ml vials)

Available as generic: no

Description: It is a short-acting loop diuretic.

Effects: It reduces fluid retention resulting from heart failure, liver disease, or kidney disorders, and it lowers elevated blood pressure. In emergencies, it relieves fluid retention in the lungs.

Possible side effects: See chlorthalidone.

Approximate cost: for 100 1-mg tablets, $31.27 to $43.39

Dosage: 0.5 mg to 2.5 mg per day divided into two doses

Notes:

- Larger doses may be required for people with kidney disease.
- See chlorthalidone.

Generic name (trade name): furosemide (Lasix)

How supplied: tablet (20 mg, 40 mg, 80 mg), oral solution (10 mg/ml, 60-ml or 120-ml bottle), injection (10 mg/ml, 4-ml or 10-ml prefilled syringes, ampules, or vials)

Available as generic: yes

Description: It is a short-acting loop diuretic that has been in use for more than 20 years.

Effects: See chlorthalidone.

Possible side effects: See chlorthalidone.

Approximate cost: for 100 tablets, 20 mg, $9.87 to $17.69 (generic, $6.17 to $11.53); 40 mg, $13.89 to $22.37 (generic, $6.53 to $12.27)

Dosage: 20 mg to 40 mg per day divided into two doses

Notes:

- Larger doses may be required for people with kidney disease.
- See chlorthalidone.

EXAMPLES OF POTASSIUM-SPARING DIURETICS

Generic name (trade name): amiloride (Midamor)

How supplied: tablet (5 mg)

Available as generic: yes

Description: It is a potassium-sparing diuretic that is rarely used alone.

Effects: Combined with thiazide or loop diuretics, it treats high blood pressure and fluid retention resulting from heart failure or liver disease.

Possible side effects: If excessive potassium is retained, muscle weakness and numbness may result. The drug also can cause upset stomach, lethargy, or rash.

Approximate cost: for 100 5-mg tablets, average wholesale price, $37.76***

Dosage: 5 mg to 10 mg per day

Note:

- It should not be taken in conjunction with lithium.

Generic name (trade name): spironolactone (Aldactone)

How supplied: tablet (25 mg, 50 mg, 100 mg)

Available as generic: yes

Description: It is a potassium-sparing diuretic introduced in 1959, and it is rarely used alone.

Effects: Combined with thiazide or loop diuretics, it treats elevated blood pressure and fluid retention resulting from heart failure, liver disease, or a kidney disorder (nephrotic syndrome).

Possible side effects: If too much potassium is retained, muscle weakness and numbness may result. Nausea and vomiting are fairly common. Side effects may also include diarrhea, lethargy, irregular menstruation, breast enlargement in men, impotence, or rash.

Approximate cost: for 100 tablets, 25 mg, $10.03 to $17.13

Dosage: 25 mg to 50 mg, given 3 to 4 times per day

Note:

• Interacts with lithium and digoxin.

Generic name (trade name): triamterene (Dyrenium)

How supplied: capsule (50 mg, 100 mg)

Available as generic: no

Description: It is a potassium-sparing diuretic introduced in 1964 that is rarely used alone.

Effects: See spironolactone.

Possible side effects: If too much potassium is retained, muscle weakness and numbness may result. It also can cause upset stomach, lethargy, or rash.

Approximate cost: for 100 capsules, average wholesale price, 50 mg, $28.50***; 100 mg, $35.85***

Dosage: 50 mg to 100 mg per day

Note:

• All of the potassium-sparing diuretics are available in combination tablets with thiazide diuretics. Examples include Dyazide and Maxzide, which combine triamterene and hydrochlorothiazide, or Moduretic, which combines amiloride and hydrochlorothiazide. These and other diuretic combinations are among the most commonly used medications in the treatment of hypertension. See section entitled "Combination Drugs" near the end of this chapter.

NITRATES

The oldest and most frequently used coronary artery medications are the nitrates. Nitrates are potent vein and artery dilators, causing blood to pool in the veins and the arteries to open up, thus reducing the amount of blood returning to the heart. This has the effect of decreasing the work of the left ventricle and lowering the blood pressure. Nitrates may also increase the supply of oxygenated blood by causing the coronary arteries to open more fully, thus improving coronary blood flow. Nitrates effectively relieve coronary artery spasm. They do not, however, appear to affect the heart's contractions.

EXAMPLES OF NITRATES

Generic name (trade names): nitroglycerin (Deponit NTG, Minitran, Nitro-Bid, Nitrogard, Nitroglyn, Nitrol, Nitrolingual, Nitrong, Nitrostat, Transderm-Nitro, Tridil)

How supplied: sublingual (dissolves under tongue) tablet (0.15 mg, 0.3 mg, 0.4 mg, 0.6 mg); controlled-release buccal (dissolves in the cheek) tablet (1 mg, 2 mg, 3 mg); controlled-release oral tablet (2.6 mg, 6.5 mg); controlled-release swallowable capsule (2.5 mg, 6.5 mg, 9 mg, 13 mg); ointment (2 percent or 15 mg per inch in 1-gm, 3-gm, 20-gm, 30-gm, or 60-gm tubes); oral metered-dose spray (0.4 mg/spray in 14.49 gm/200-dose container); skin patch (0.1 mg/hour, 0.2 mg/hour, 0.4 mg/hour, 0.6 mg/hour)

Available as generic: yes

Description: This antianginal drug and vasodilator was introduced in the late 1800s.

Effects: Temporarily relieves and prevents anginal pain.

Possible side effects: Headaches, flushing, and dizziness may occur.

Approximate cost: For 100 tablets or capsules, average wholesale price, 0.4 mg SL, $3.94***; 1 mg to 3 mg buccal, $16.09 to $19.32***; 2.6 mg to 6.5 mg controlled-release oral, $4.95 to $5.40***; 2.5 mg to 6.5 mg controlled-release capsule, $7.81 to $7.88***

for a 2 percent, 60-gm tube of ointment, $4.50 to $8***; for 14.49 gm/200-dose container of oral spray, $15.88***; for 30 skin patches, 0.2 mg/hour, $36.24***

Dosage: 2.6 mg to 27 mg per day (oral tablets); 0.15 mg to 0.6 mg per dose (sublingual); 1 mg to 2 mg per dose (buccal); 1 to 2 inches of 2 percent ointment per dose, or one skin patch daily

Notes:

• Nitroglycerin interacts with antihypertensive drugs to lower blood pressure.

• Nitroglycerin cannot be stored for long periods of time without losing its effectiveness.

• Nitroglycerin skin patches should be used intermittently to avoid the development of tolerance to the drug. Leaving the patch off overnight is usually sufficient.

Generic name (trade names) isosorbide dinitrate (Dilatrate-SR, Iso-Bid, Isordil, Sorbitrate, Sorbitrate SA)

How supplied: Sublingual (dissolves under the tongue) tablet (2.5 mg, 5 mg, 10 mg); chewable tablet (5 mg, 10 mg); swallowable tablet (5 mg, 10 mg, 20 mg, 30 mg, 40 mg); controlled-release tablet (40 mg); controlled-release capsule (40 mg)

Available as generic: yes

Description: It is a nitrate vasodilator and antianginal drug introduced in the late 1970s; it is a longer-acting form of nitroglycerin.

Effects: It relieves and prevents angina.

Possible side effects: Headaches, flushing, or dizziness may occur. Less frequently, fainting may occur.

Approximate cost: for 100 tablets, generic, 5 mg, $3.89 to $9.29; 10 mg, $4.73 to $10.77; 20 mg, $6.19 to $13.17

Dosage: for relief of angina, 5 mg to 10 mg per dose; for prevention of angina, 40 mg to 160 mg daily

Notes:

- Alcohol and other antidepressants may further lower blood pressure.
- Unlike nitroglycerin, isosorbide dinitrate can be stored for long periods of time without losing its effectiveness.

PERIPHERAL ADRENERGIC ANTAGONISTS

These drugs, which are among the older antihypertensive agents, lower blood pressure by inhibiting the release of adrenaline or by blocking its effect on the nerve endings. Dilation of blood vessels results. They have a sedating effect at high dosages. This remains a major drawback to the continuing use of the drug to treat high blood pressure. This is the least expensive of all the antihypertensive medications, and, in combination with a diuretic, is effective in lowering blood pressure.

EXAMPLE OF PERIPHERAL ADRENERGIC ANTAGONISTS

Generic name (trade name): reserpine (Serpasil)

How supplied: tablet (0.1 mg, 0.25 mg)

Available as generic: yes

Description: This is the oldest drug in this category. It is derived from the rauwolfia plant.

Effects: It lowers moderately high blood pressure. It is rarely used by itself; usually used with a diuretic.

Possible side effects: Drowsiness, diarrhea, nausea, dry mouth, dizziness, headache, depression, muscular aches, temporary impotence, weight gain, and rash may occur.

Approximate cost: for 100 tablets, average wholesale price, 0.1 mg, $5.19***; 0.25 mg, $8.81***

Dosage: 0.1 mg to 0.5 mg per day

Notes:

- Reserpine is a component of several combination drugs. See the section entitled "Combination Drugs."
- The rauwolfia plant has been used in India and other Asian countries for many years as a sedative.
- Reserpine is also used for some psychiatric disorders.
- The drug should not be used by people with a history of mental depression.
- The use of reserpine in conjunction with digitalis drugs or quinidine may cause abnormal heart rhythms.

OTHER VASODILATORS

As their name indicates, these drugs lower blood pressure by opening up or dilating arteries, thereby facilitating blood flow through them. Vasodilators are rarely used as initial therapy and are usually prescribed along with other drugs such as a beta blocker and a diuretic. Some produce a very rapid reduction in blood pressure, especially when administered by injection. Thus, they may be useful in treating a hypertensive crisis. For chronic use, several office visits may be needed to fine-tune the dosage. Side effects may be annoying, and lowering of blood pressure may be less when these drugs are used as initial treatment.

EXAMPLES OF MISCELLANEOUS VASODILATORS

Generic name (trade name): hydralazine (Apresoline)

How supplied: tablet (10 mg, 25 mg, 50 mg, 100 mg), injection (20 mg/ml, 1-ml ampule)

Available as generic: yes

Description: It is an antihypertensive and vasodilator introduced in the 1950s.

Effects: It lowers moderately to severely high blood pressure.

Possible side effects: Side effects include nausea and vomiting, headaches, dizziness, and irregular heart beat. Less frequently, loss of appetite, rash, flushing, or joint pains will occur. Prolonged use of hydralazine can cause drug-induced lupus, especially in people who metabolize the drug slowly (a tendency that can be determined with a blood test). Symptoms of lupus, an autoimmune syndrome, are fever, joint pains, low blood counts, and inflammation of the linings of the lungs or heart (felt as chest pain on deep inhalation).

Approximate cost: for 100 tablets, 25 mg, $4.03 to $7.43; 50 mg, $5.73 to $10.23

Dosage: 50 mg to 100 mg daily, generally up to a maximum of 200 mg daily

Generic name (trade name): minoxidil (Loniten)
How supplied: tablet (2.5 mg, 10 mg)
Available in generic: yes
Description: This antihypertensive and vasodilator is never used by itself; it is usually used with a diuretic and other drugs.
Effects: In combination, it controls dangerously high blood pressure and pressure that is rising very rapidly.
Possible side effects: It increases hair growth, especially on the face, back, etc.; other common side effects are fluid retention and shortness of breath. It can cause tiredness, dizziness or lightheadedness, nausea, headache, or rash.
Approximate cost: for 100 10-mg tablets, $71.50 to $82.50*
Dosage: 5 mg to 20 mg per day
Notes:

• It is always prescribed with a diuretic and often with a beta blocker.
• Because of its side effect of increasing hair growth, it is now available in a solution to treat baldness (Rogaine).

COMBINATION DRUGS

When a person begins drug treatment for heart ailments, his or her physician must first determine the correct dose of the particular drug or drugs that are most effective. Cardiovascular drugs often work best in combination, so the physician may prescribe several different combinations and different doses before achieving optimal results.

In some cases, drugs that are commonly prescribed together are available in a single pill, which may, in some cases, be less expensive than its separate components. Convenience is a major advantage to combination therapy: If a person is on a long-term

regimen including two or three drugs in dosages that are available in a single medication, the physician may prescribe the combination drug to save the person time and effort in his or her daily routine. It should be stressed, however, that combination drugs are usually not prescribed for initial drug therapy.

Some examples of combination drugs now available are listed below. Further information is available by finding each component in other sections of this chapter.

EXAMPLES OF COMBINATION DRUGS

Generic name (trade name): amiloride/ hydrochlorothiazide (Moduretic)
How supplied: tablet (5 mg/50 mg)
Description: It is a potassium-sparing diuretic/ thiazide diuretic.
Approximate cost: for 100 tablets, $38.50*

Generic name (trade name): atenolol/chlorthalidone (Tenoretic)
How supplied: tablet (100 mg/25 mg, 50 mg/25 mg)
Description: It is a beta blocker/thiazide diuretic.
Approximate cost: for 100 tablets, 50 mg/25 mg, $81.73 to $112.29

Generic name (trade name): captopril/ hydrochlorothiazide (Capozide)
How supplied: tablet (25 mg/15 mg, 25 mg/25 mg, 50 mg/15 mg, 50 mg/25 mg)
Description: It is an ACE inhibitor/thiazide diuretic.
Approximate cost: for 100 tablets, 25 mg/15 mg, $63.80 to $66*

Generic name (trade name): clonidine/ chlorthalidone (Combipres)
How supplied: tablet (0.1 mg/15 mg, 0.2 mg/15 mg, 0.3 mg/15 mg)
Description: It is a centrally acting drug/thiazide diuretic.
Approximate cost: for 100 tablets, 0.1 mg/15 mg, $27.50 to $49.50*

Generic name (trade names): chlorthalidone/ reserpine (Demi-Regroton, Regroton)
How supplied: tablet (25 mg/0.125 mg, 50 mg/0.25 mg)
Description: It is a thiazide diuretic peripheral adrenergic agonist.
Approximate cost: for 100 tablets, average wholesale price, 25 mg/0.125 mg, $92.59***; 50 mg/0.25 mg, $105.50***

Generic name (trade name): enalapril/
hydrochlorothiazide (Vaseretic)
How supplied: tablet (10 mg/25 mg)
Description: It is an ACE inhibitor/thiazide diuretic.
Approximate cost: for 100 tablets, $88 to $93.50

Generic name (trade name): hydralazine/
hydrochlorothiazide (Apresazide)
How supplied: capsule (25 mg/25 mg, 50 mg/50
mg, 100 mg/50 mg)
Description: It is a miscellaneous vasodilator/
thiazide diuretic.
Approximate cost: for 100 capsules, average
wholesale price, 25 mg/25 mg, $32.83***;
50 mg/50 mg, $49.06***; 100 mg/50 mg,
$59.77***

Generic name (trade name): hydrochlorothiazide/
reserpine (Hydropres)
How supplied: tablet (25 mg/0.125 mg,
50 mg/0.125 mg)
Description: It is a thiazide diuretic/peripheral
adrenergic antagonist.
Approximate cost: for 100 tablets, average
wholesale price, 25 mg/0.125 mg, $22.83***;
50 mg/0.125 mg, $35.61***

Generic name (trade names): labetolol/
hydrochlorothiazide (Normozide, Trandate
HCT)
How supplied: tablet (100 mg/25 mg,
200 mg/25 mg, 300 mg/25 mg)
Description: It is an alpha- and beta-blocking drug/
thiazide diuretic.
Approximate cost: for 100 tablets, average
wholesale price, 100 mg/25 mg, $33.21***; 200
mg/25 mg, $48.72***; 300 mg/25 mg, $64.83***

Generic name (trade name): lisinopril/
hydrochlorothiazide (Zestoretic)
How supplied: tablet (20 mg/12.5 mg, 20 mg/25 mg)
Description: It is an ACE inhibitor/thiazide diuretic.
Approximate cost: for 100 tablets, average
wholesale price, 20 mg/12.5 mg, $87.24***;
20 mg/25 mg, $88.32***

Generic name (trade name): methyldopa/
hydrochlorothiazide (Aldoril)
How supplied: tablet (250 mg/15 mg, 250 mg/25 mg,
500 mg/30 mg, 500 mg/50 mg)
Description: It is a centrally acting drug/thiazide
diuretic.
Approximate cost: for 100 tablets, generic,
250 mg/25 mg, $16.83 to $29.47

Generic name (trade names): propranolol/
hydrochlorothiazide (Inderide, Inderide LA)
How supplied: tablet (40 mg/25 mg, 80 mg/25 mg),
long-acting capsule (80 mg/50 mg, 120 mg/
50 mg, 160 mg/50 mg)
Description: It is a beta blocker/thiazide diuretic.
Approximate cost: for 100 tablets, 40 mg/25 mg,
$33*; for 100 long-acting capsules, 80 mg/50
mg, $55 to $60.50*

Generic name (trade name): reserpine/hydralazine/
hydrochlorothiazide (Ser-Ap-Es)
How supplied: tablet (0.1 mg/25 mg/15 mg)
Description: It is a peripheral adrenergic antagonist/
vasodilator/thiazide diuretic.
Approximate cost: for 100 tablets, generic, $7.57 to
$12.63

Generic name (trade name): spironolactone/
hydrochlorothiazide (Aldactazide)
How supplied: tablet (25 mg/25 mg; 50 mg/50 mg)
Description: It is a potassium-sparing diuretic/
thiazide diuretic.
Approximate cost: for 100 tablets, generic,
25 mg/25 mg, $10.03 to $17.13

Generic name (trade name): triamterene/
hydrochlorothiazide (Dyazide, Maxzide)
How supplied: tablet (37.5 mg/25 mg, 50 mg/25 mg,
75 mg/50 mg)
Description: It is a potassium-sparing diuretic/
thiazide diuretic.
Approximate cost: for 100 tablets,
Dyazide—$24.37 to $35.49
Maxzide—$54.47 to $80.73
generic—75 mg/50 mg, $17.73 to $28.07

CHAPTER 24

CORONARY ANGIOPLASTY AND INTERVENTIONAL CARDIOLOGY

MICHAEL W. CLEMAN, M.D.

INTRODUCTION

Patients with severe coronary artery disease have traditionally been treated first with drug therapy and then, if necessary, with coronary artery bypass surgery. In the past decade, so-called interventional cardiology devices—angioplasty, atherectomy, lasers, and stents—have opened new vistas for successful treatment of heart disease symptoms with techniques that are far less invasive than traditional surgery. Rather than constructing a new route for blood flow, as in bypass surgery, these procedures open or widen existing ones. For patients in whom cardiovascular drugs are not effective, they offer a major advantage of being performed under local anesthesia, which greatly hastens recovery and as a result lowers cost.

Atherosclerotic plaque is the culprit that creates candidates for these therapies, by virtue of narrowing the coronary arteries. Within the walls of the arteries, plaque deposits containing cholesterol, connective tissue, and calcium, as well as arterial muscle cells, intrude into the vessels. The plaque deposits ultimately cause stenosis, a narrowing of the lumen, or inner orifice of the blood vessels, which limits the space available for blood circulation and, consequently, the amount of blood delivered to the heart muscle.

Over time, as this process continues, the reduced delivery of blood means that the heart muscle does not get enough oxygen. This condition, called ischemia, may trigger chest pain, or angina pectoris —a major indicator of coronary artery disease. Approximately 6 million Americans suffer from angina, which can range in severity from mildly annoying to the feeling of a viselike grip in the chest that radiates to the left shoulder, left arm, or jaw. Angina attacks are most often provoked by physical exertion, when the heart needs more oxygen than it does at rest.

Sometimes a diseased coronary artery becomes totally blocked by a blood clot, and a heart attack ensues. If the ischemia has been silent—without pain—the heart attack may be the first indication that there is advanced atherosclerosis. Whatever the sequence of events, severely narrowed arteries require treatment, either to lessen the pain or to prevent an initial or a subsequent heart attack. (See Chapter 11.)

BALLOON ANGIOPLASTY

Increasingly, balloon angioplasty (technically called percutaneous transluminal coronary angioplasty, or PTCA) has replaced or has been combined with coronary bypass surgery to open blocked coronary arteries. As its name implies, the procedure actually uses a miniature balloon which, when inflated inside a coronary artery, compresses plaques against the artery walls and cracks them to widen the channel through which blood can flow.

The angioplasty procedure was developed by the late Dr. Andreas Gruentzig, who performed the first human procedure at the University of Zurich, Switzerland, in the fall of 1977. The technique was adopted quickly in the United States, where doctors in New York and California performed the first angioplasties simultaneously in March 1988. From then on it was adopted rapidly, growing from 2,000 procedures performed in 1979 to more than 227,000 in 1988.

The advantage of the angioplasty procedure for physicians is that it is a faster and less invasive method to treat atherosclerotic plaque buildup. Angioplasty patients experience a quicker and less painful recovery. The procedure requires only a two- to three-day hospital stay and recuperation time is minimal. Coronary artery bypass surgery, which involves opening the chest cavity, requires several hours under general anesthesia and necessitates a week or two in the hospital, followed by several weeks more of recuperation for a patient to mend completely at home. (See box, "Advantages and Disadvantages of Angioplasty.")

IDENTIFYING ANGIOPLASTY CANDIDATES

Although balloon angioplasty sounds like the ideal therapy for patients with angina that does not respond to medication, it is not right for everyone. For example, a patient with triple vessel disease—that is, blockages in three or more coronary arteries—is generally a better candidate for bypass surgery. Angioplasty is more appropriate for a person who has significant blockage of only one or two arteries that causes recurrent angina and restricts his or her daily

Advantages and Disadvantages of Angioplasty

Advantages	Disadvantages
Can be performed under local anesthesia.	Generally used only for single- or double-vessel disease.
Recovery is shorter and less painful compared to surgery.	Is less efficient if there are many points of stenosis in a single artery.
Less expensive than surgery.	May not be effective if plaque is calcified (hardened).
May be feasible for patients unable to withstand surgery.	Restenosis rate is 25–35 percent with first procedure; may have to be repeated.
There is no noticeable scar.	Cannot be used if occlusion is located in area not reachable with catheter.

activities. Angioplasty may be suitable for a person who experiences angina during mild to moderate exercise. It may also be appropriate for a person with silent ischemia who has had a heart attack and is subsequently found to have one or two significantly narrowed vessels. Finally, angioplasty may be suitable for a patient who has had reclosure of a saphenous vein or left internal mammary artery graft used for previous coronary bypass surgery.

The ideal—though by no means the only—candidate for angioplasty has a single, well-defined obstruction in the left anterior descending, left circumflex, or right coronary artery; good heart function (pumping quality) as shown on diagnostic tests; angina that cannot be controlled by drugs and that affects quality of life; and good general health that would not be expected to pose complications for the procedure. Sometimes two dilations may be done in a single vessel if it is narrowed in two places in close proximity.

The presence of coronary heart disease does not automatically qualify a candidate for angioplasty. To begin with, not all plaques respond to the angioplasty technique. Lesions vary in their size, location, and composition; some are too long or much too calcified —hardened by age—for angioplasty. Some lesions are out of reach of a balloon-tipped catheter.

In other instances, the guide wire used to thread the balloon catheter into the vessel may be unable to penetrate hardened plaque that has completely clogged (occluded) the artery. Or the patient may have so many stenoses that bypass surgery would restore much more blood flow than would an angioplasty.

THE PROCEDURE

Angioplasty is performed in a cardiac catheterization laboratory. (See Figure 24.1 A-E.) Before the procedure begins the patient is usually given a sedative and will receive local anesthesia at the site of the femoral artery in the groin where the balloon catheter

is introduced. To start the balloon procedure, the operator makes a small incision and inserts a hollow, Teflon-coated guide catheter through the femoral artery and, using a fluoroscope to visualize the path, threads it up toward the heart into the particular coronary artery that contains the blockage. The cardiologist will first confirm the size and location of the obstructions by using the dye to outline the arteries, a procedure known as coronary angiography. (See Chapter 9.)

Another catheter, tipped with an inflatable balloon, is then inserted into the guiding catheter and

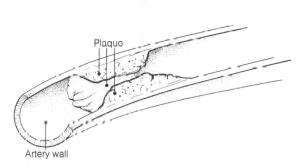

Figure 24.1A
This diagram of an opened artery shows a large buildup of plaque.

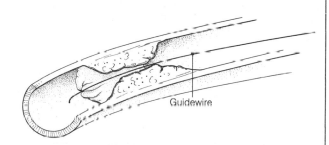

Figure 24.1B
A thin, flexible guidewire is threaded through the coronary artery to go beyond the obstruction.

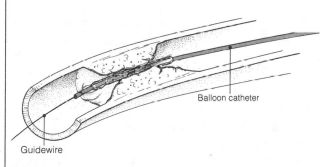

Figure 24.1C
Next, the catheter containing the deflated balloon is inserted over the guidewire.

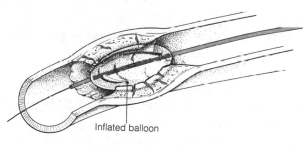

Figure 24.1D
The balloon is then inflated (usually several times), compressing the lesion and pushing it back against the arterial wall.

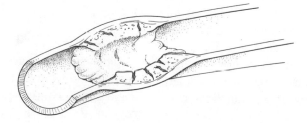

Figure 24.1E
The balloon and catheter are removed, leaving the widened channel.

moved to the point where blood flow is thwarted by a plaque. The plastic balloon itself is tiny and sausage-shaped. Once inflated it will span the width of a normal artery—anywhere from 1/10 to 2/10 inch. A flexible wire (a "bumper" guide wire) extends beyond the deflated balloon tip and is used to navigate the twists and turns of the arterial tunnels of the human body. Once the catheter reaches the site of the blockage, the surgeon looks for an opening in the obstruction through which to pass the balloon. If the plaque has calcified, this may require probing. The deflated balloon is then moved forward over the guide wire, into position next to the lesion in the artery. Dye may be injected through the balloon so that the operator can gauge the exact location of the lesion, its nature, and its severity on X-ray, and then follow the progress through the procedure.

At the site of each lesion, the physician uses a hydraulic device to suck any air out of the balloon. Then, using a mixture of contrast dye and saline (sterile salt water), it is inflated several times for 30 to 120 or more seconds each time. Each inflation blocks the blood flow and squeezes the lesion back against the arterial wall to restore or enlarge an open channel. The balloon effectively stretches out the blood vessel like an injection mold.

While the plaque isn't removed, the balloon pressure compresses and imbeds it into the wall rather than leaving the lesion loosely attached to the wall.

Upon completion of the procedure, the entire catheter system is pulled out and another angiogram is performed to confirm the results. The small incision is generally closed by direct compression without stitches and the patient is usually sent to the coronary care unit or other special holding area for special observation. After one or two days of observation, the patient will be able to leave the hospital and return to a full range of activities.

A physician will usually follow the patient with periodic exercise stress testing. In selected cases, particularly if there are residual or recurrent symptoms, a repeat angiogram may be recommended in the following months to see how well the procedure holds up. More than 90 percent of angioplasty patients have a good immediate result, defined as an arterial channel that is at least 50 percent open. For the patient, the most obvious indication of this result is the freedom from chest pain.

COMPLICATIONS

Like all surgical and interventional procedures, angioplasty poses the possibility of complications. A small percentage of patients experience abrupt closure of the artery during the procedure. This may happen because the artery goes into spasm, is split by the catheter, or is occluded by a blood clot. The physician will reinflate the balloon to open the artery when this happens. But if this fails, or the artery closes after the angioplasty has been completed, emergency bypass surgery may be needed.

About 3 percent of all angioplasty patients experience a heart attack during the procedure—which may then require emergency bypass surgery. Usually this happens when the artery involved in the procedure closes. However, a heart attack may be triggered by a smaller arterial branch snapping shut because the angioplasty has dislodged a blood clot. If the vessel is small, it is unlikely that emergency surgery will be needed.

The mortality rate for angioplasty in a single vessel is very low, about 0.1 percent (compared to 1 to 2 percent for bypass surgery).

The major problem of angioplasty is the relatively high rate of restenosis, or renewed blockage. Roughly a third of all patients will experience a recurrence of arterial narrowing within the first six months following the procedure. Many kinds of restenosis may occur. Hyperplasia is an overgrowth of cells that is thought to be mediated in part by the body's response to injury—in this case, the cracking of the artery walls during the angioplasty procedure itself. Or the atherosclerotic lesion may grow up again and incorporate a blood clot. But once a patient passes the six-month mark successfully, the likelihood of plaque building up in that particular spot in that artery is much smaller.

The prescription for restenosis generally is another angioplasty. It could take as many as three or four procedures to maintain the patency of the arterial channel.

LASER ABLATION

Angioplasty using a laser instead of a balloon has been developed over the past decade and may prove to be a useful supplement to the treatment of coronary artery disease. Indeed, lasers are increasingly used in conjunction with the balloon technique. It should be noted, however, that laser angioplasty remains an experimental procedure and is available at only a few research centers.

The procedure is similar to that of balloon angioplasty, except that the laser catheter is tipped with a metal probe or a fiber optic probe heated by a light beam, which melts through fatty lesions—both stenoses (narrowings) and occlusions (blockages). The laser procedure in some cases surpasses the balloon in its ability to melt away calcified lesions as well.

Generally physicians use a guide wire with a balloon to attack hard plaque first before using a laser. Contrary to popular belief, the laser does not vaporize plaque in a puff of smoke. Rather, the laser ablates, or removes, the lesion layer by layer. The laser homes in and eradicates tiny areas of plaque. The plaque is converted into gaseous products and microscopic particles.

The laser procedure is a delicate one, requiring the surgeon to focus the laser energy on lesions without creating a hole in the wall of artery or making a mechanical puncture. To make laser ablation more effective and safer, researchers still have to perfect the guide wires and the mechanism's overall flexibility for taking the tight corners of the coronary arteries. The equipment will also have to be made more compatible with vascular tissue, so as not to induce spasm or encourage deposition of fibrin (a blood-clotting substance).

A number of different types of lasers are under investigation, but the cool excimer laser appears promising. It delivers energy at an average temperature of 40°C. to avoid cooking or burning the surrounding tissue with short pulses of energy. Others under review include continuous wave laser radiation, such as that emitted by Nd:YAG or CO_2 lasers. These ablate plaque without thermal (heat) damage to the nearby wall.

STENTS

Another way to attack the narrowing of coronary blood vessels is to use a mechanical apparatus called a stent. These tiny metal "scaffolds" are inserted and erected in a collapsing artery to keep it open in a manner similar to the way construction workers might use supports to prop up a collapsing tunnel.

Stents can be used in a variety of medical situations. During angioplasty, they are employed as secondary supports to hold a vessel open while the physician presses back lesions, thus preventing abrupt closure. Stents are also a stopgap measure for patients who aren't immediately medically fit for surgery. That is, the stent may provide temporary pat-

ency (opening) of an artery when a patient who has undergone angioplasty turns out to need an emergency coronary artery bypass graft. Thus, the stent may assist in preventing a heart attack and allow the bypass surgery to be done as an elective rather than an emergency procedure.

The problem of restenosis following angioplasty or laser ablation has galvanized interest in intravascular stents. They can be useful in controlling dissection of the vessel walls after balloon angioplasty or another coronary intervention. Stents provide the means to "tack up" intimal debris (the cells and deposits that accumulate on the intima, the inner surface of the blood vessel walls) and to seal off a tear in the blood vessel wall that may result from angioplasty.

After balloon angioplasty, a stent can be delivered inside a catheter to the site of earlier blockage and expanded within the arterial lumen. The size of a spring in a ballpoint pen, the stent has metal wires that imbed themselves within the intima, the innermost of the three layers of a blood vessel.

A variety of stent designs have been developed. They have received varying degrees of acceptance by the medical community. The Palmaz-Shatz stent is one of the more popular ones. It is a flexible stainless steel tube that appears meshlike. The device is ½ inch long, is as narrow as a piece of spaghetti, and weighs as little as a straight pin.

The potential for developing thrombi (blood clots) is ever present when there has been an injury to the arterial lining. However, successful application of a stent requires a certain amount of clotting, because endothelium cannot grow on bare metal. The cells require a thin layer of fibrin and thrombus (clotting material), and the Shatz stent configuration best allows for the development of fibrin and thrombus together. The stent is completely covered by native blood vessel cells in two to three weeks. The wires themselves become embedded within these cells, which proliferate at the site of implantation.

The use of stents is still in the experimental stage in the United States, and further study is required to determine risks to patients. Very little is known about the long-term effects of putting metal devices in coronary arteries. Patients may need anticoagulation drug therapy for a short time after stent delivery. Researchers must determine whether blood clot formation at the stent site will be a problem and whether stents actually reduce the incidence of restenosis after angioplasty.

Research conducted recently in Europe showed poor results (commonly complete reocclusion or significant restenosis) with one particular type of stent, the Wall stent. Newer models, however, especially those impregnated with chemicals that are intended to retard clot formation, may prove more effective. Clearly, more study is needed.

ATHERECTOMY

Another experimental approach to reopening narrow coronary vessels is atherectomy. This procedure uses a rotary device—a high-speed cutting drill mounted on a catheter—that literally shaves off plaque from an artery wall. The main reason for using an atherectomy device is to traverse small and tortuous coronary arteries that are difficult to navigate with thin angioplasty guide wires alone.

A variety of device designs are under review by the medical community. One type, the Auth Rotablator, uses a high-speed oblong burr that may range in diameter from 1.25 to 4.5 millimeters. Imbedded in the bit are fine diamond abrasive particles that whir at up to 120,000 revolutions per minute to finely ablade the tissue. A flexible driveshaft allows for the passage of a stainless-steel guide wire with a flexible spring tip. The wire moves ahead and can be steered independently from the shaft and the burr, which do not start rotating until the guide wire reaches the plaque in a selected artery.

Once the Rotablator is in place, its operation is similar to that of a dentist's drill. Compressed air or nitrogen powers a turbine to deliver rotational energy to the burr through the driveshaft. The air pressure controls the speed of the burr's rotation. During rotation, sterile saline runs through the catheter sheath to cool the entire system.

The atherectomy device is delivered to the site of the blockage via a catheter, in the same way as the balloon device in conventional angioplasty. Once the device is in place and the drill is turned on, it is allowed to reach a certain rate of rotation before the abrasive tip is advanced over the guide wire. When the physician feels the plaque resist the drill, the tip is successively pulled back and then thrust out again to maintain high-speed rotation. The drill is withdrawn once it punctures the lesion.

Before the rotational device and guide wire are completely withdrawn, dye is injected to verify the quality and success of the procedure. If the stenosis is still sizable, balloon angioplasty may be performed to improve the result.

Grinding plaque in this way has its limits. One concern is that not all the debris (atheroma) will be captured from the far side of the blockage by suctioning the blood around that area, and that this debris may flow through the bloodstream to collect in a smaller artery and cause blockage. Researchers using the Auth Rotablator report that the debris is usually too small to clog capillaries. Other atherectomy devices are designed to capture and hold the atheroma protruding into the vessel in a capsule until it is removed.

The main difference between atherectomy and balloon angioplasty lies in the methods by which they dispatch the plaque in artery walls. Angioplasty splits the plaque and stretches the vessel wall. Atherectomy removes sections of diseased intima and leaves a polished surface devoid of plaques. Compared to laser angioplasty, atherectomy carries a lesser risk of perforation, because the device affords greater control. Also, an atherectomy device can remove calcified lesions while a laser angioplasty usually cannot.

VALVULOPLASTY

Just as atherosclerotic buildup in coronary arteries can be relieved with angioplasty, a heart valve that becomes clogged or narrowed by calcium can be opened by a procedure called valvuloplasty. The valvuloplasty procedure, developed over the last decade, involves opening the valve with a larger balloon-tipped catheter, which is then inflated to press back the calcium in the valve or to correct the anatomical deformity that has caused the narrowing.

All four heart valves are subject to this treatment. Mitral stenosis is a condition in which the mitral valve, which controls blood flow from the left atrium (upper chamber) to the left ventricle (lower chamber) of the heart becomes narrowed, so that blood flow is diminished. In adults, it is most commonly the result of a previous bout of rheumatic fever. Mitral valvuloplasty appears to be relatively successful, producing a restenosis rate of less than 10 percent within the first year.

The aortic valve controls blood flow from the left ventricle to the aorta, the blood vessel that carries blood from the heart to various parts of the body. When the aortic valve is affected by stenosis, or narrowing, surgical valve replacement remains preferable, because the disease is a degenerative one, diagnosed increasingly in older patients. Putting in an artificial valve provides a more favorable outcome than trying to widen the passage. Indeed, restenosis rates for aortic valvuloplasty hover at 50 percent. In some cases, however, the procedure is used to increase blood flow temporarily in aortic valve patients until they are strong enough to undergo surgery for a new valve. Tricuspid and pulmonic stenosis are quite common but can be treated safely and effectively with balloon valvuloplasty. The short-term and long-term success rates are similar to that seen with mitral valvuloplasty. (For additional information, see Chapter 25.)

HEART SURGERY

JOHN C. BALDWIN, M.D., JOHN A. ELEFTERIADES, M.D., and GARY S. KOPF, M.D.

INTRODUCTION

Mankind has long recognized the heart as vital to sustaining life—often romanticizing it as the repository of the soul and the seat of the emotions—but we did not have the ability to repair it surgically until a relatively short time ago. Open-heart surgery seems so commonplace now that it is sometimes difficult to remember that it was not widely available until the mid-1970s. Curiosity and experimentation, however, have existed for centuries.

Although the first successful operation on the living heart was not until the middle of this century, the recorded history of open-heart surgery goes back as far as about 400 B.C., when Greek physicians provided an account of the workings of the aortic and pulmonary valves. A second-century-A.D. Greek physician, Galen of Pergamon, who was an active dissector of human cadavers, described the heart in detail, but with some notable inaccuracies that were not cleared up until the writings of Andreas Vesalius in 1534.

It was not until the pioneering work of William Harvey, the 17th-century English physician, that blood circulation and the role of veins and arteries were understood. Prior to Harvey's famous dissertation, *De Mortu Cordis*, it was generally thought that the blood ebbed and flowed like whimsical tides, controlled by the consumption of food.

The first recorded successful heart surgery performed on a living human being was in 1896, when a Frankfurt physician sutured a wound in the heart

of a young German soldier. Great strides have been made in this field of surgery since the removal of shell fragments from the hearts of American soldiers in World War II and the first repairs of inborn (congenital) abnormalities in 1945.

Surgical technique in the early 1900s was far more advanced than the ability to keep patients alive. Ability to operate, however, was limited by the inability to operate on a heart that was still beating.

The difficulty of operating on a beating heart was not resolved until the mid-1950s and early 1960s. In early experiments, scientists found they could stop and restart the heart, but this left less than three minutes in which to operate before irreparable brain damage occurred. Philadelphia's John Gibbon was one of the doctors working on a solution: a machine that would take over the circulation of the blood. His first model was tested in animal experiments in 1931, but it was not until 1953 that Gibbon was able to perform a successful operation on a human patient using total cardiopulmonary bypass.

Taking over the blood circulation involves far more than simply pumping blood. The machine has to resupply the oxygen that the body's cells have removed from the red blood cells and pump the blood at sufficient pressure to supply all the organs in the body, without damaging the white or red blood cells or the platelets carried by the circulating blood.

It was not until the mid-1970s that the machines became sufficiently sophisticated to achieve safe, widespread use. Today's bypass machines can maintain the patient's circulation for many hours without serious side effects. Nevertheless, cardiothoracic sur-

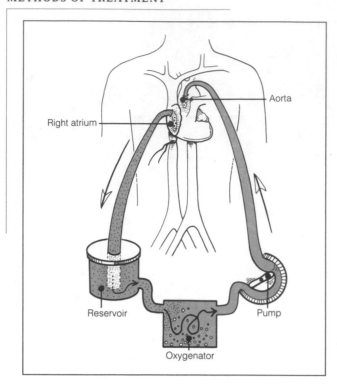

Figure 25.1

The heart-lung machine takes blood from the patient's heart to a reservoir from which it travels through a series of thin-walled membranes. These membranes allow oxygen to enter the red blood cells. After impurities are filtered from the blood, it is pumped to the aorta for distribution to the body.

geons seek to keep operating time to a minimum in order to reduce even the small chance of ill effects.

The cardiopulmonary bypass machine (popularly known as the "heart-lung machine") works as follows (see Figure 25.1). Blood is passed along a tube from the patient's heart (usually from the right atrium) to a pump that pushes blood through a series of thin-walled membranes that duplicate the lung's method of allowing oxygen to enter red blood cells. The oxygenated blood is passed through a series of fine-meshed filters to trap any impurities. The blood is then redirected to the aorta, the body's largest artery, where it is distributed to the arteries around the body.

The other technical innovation that allowed doctors to operate on the heart for an extended period of time was the introduction of safe preservation techniques, using extremely cold temperatures (hypothermia), for a heart that has been stopped. In the late 1950s, Dr. Norman Shumway showed that the heart's demand for oxygen could be considerably reduced and the heart muscle cells preserved if the heart was immersed in a cold salt (saline) solution.

During today's heart operations, three methods of hypothermia are combined: cooling of the entire body by cooling the blood in the heart-lung machine,

immersing the heart in cold saline, and injecting a cold solution of potassium directly into the heart. The high concentration of potassium instantly stops the heart's electrical activity. By slowing down the heart muscle's demand for oxygen, the surgeon is able to preserve heart muscle (myocardial) cells for as long as six hours. The enhanced techniques of cell preservation have also made it possible to preserve a donor heart for cardiac transplantation during long-distance transport.

OPEN-HEART SURGERY

A description of a coronary artery bypass operation is somewhat representative of other types of heart surgery that follow similar patterns, although there is obviously some variation, depending on the particular surgery. A primary difference between coronary artery bypass and most of the other surgeries is that the heart chambers are *not* opened in bypass surgery—as they would be for valve replacement, for example. Surgery in which the heart's chambers are entered always carries some additional risk; this is primarily due to the increased possibility of air entering the heart, and surgeons take extra care to avoid this.

Once a physician has determined that surgery is necessary, the preparation begins. (See box, "Before and After Open Heart Surgery: What to Expect for Adults.") On the morning of surgery, the patient is given a mild tranquilizer to reduce any anxiety related to the operation. Electrodes connected to an ECG monitor are then attached to the patient's back to allow constant monitoring of the heart's electrical activity during the operation. Following the administration of a local anesthetic, intravenous (IV) lines are inserted into the veins of the arm or wrist. These IV lines allow the anesthesia team to administer anesthetics directly into the bloodstream and to replenish body fluid with salt solution. One of these lines is threaded up the vein all the way to the vena cava (a large vein near the heart) to allow administration of medication directly to the heart. Another IV line allows measurement of the pressure and oxygen level in the arteries.

A special balloon-tipped catheter, known as the Swan-Ganz catheter, is inserted into a neck vein and threaded down into the cavity of the right heart and through the right ventricle; blood flow carries it

Before and After Open Heart Surgery: What to Expect for Adults

Before having open heart surgery, the patient will meet with the cardiothoracic surgeon, who will already have reviewed the tests (such as films from the angiography) and will explain the results of these tests, what the surgery entails, the benefits the patient can expect from surgery, and, especially, the risks of surgery. This meeting provides the patient a chance to voice fears, ask questions, and perhaps look over the angiogram film to develop a better understanding of why the operation is necessary. The hospital where the surgery is to take place will most likely provide easy-to-follow literature on the particular surgery and informative meetings for the whole family to discuss pre- and postoperative care.

Approximately two weeks before the surgery, the patient may be instructed to stop taking any medications that might affect the ability of the blood to clot, including aspirin, dipyridamole (Persantine), and warfarin (Coumadin). The patient should continue taking beta blockers and calcium antagonists if he or she is on them and can continue use of nitrates to relieve chest pain. The day before the operation, the patient will be expected to check into the hospital and again undergo a battery of tests—chest X-ray, ECGs, blood tests, urinalysis—even though he or she may recently have had all these tests. This is an important step to make sure that there has been no change in the status of the patient's health and to ensure that no small but important detail has been omitted. The patient will be asked about medications and alcohol, cigarette, and recreational drug use. It is vital that the answers be forthright and complete, as any of these substances can adversely affect the healing process.

The night before the surgery, the patient will be asked to shower in order to reduce the bacteria on the skin. No food will be allowed after midnight, because anesthesia is safer on an empty stomach. The anesthesiologist will usually visit the patient the night before in order to explain what the anesthesia does and how the anesthesia team takes care of the patient's breathing with the respirator. The chest area will be scrubbed clean and washed with an antiseptic solution, and body hair will be shaved where necessary.

On the morning of the surgery, the person will be given a mild tranquilizer to reduce anxiety about the operation. Monitoring electrodes will be attached, and local anesthetic will be administered before placement of intravenous lines. Catheters (thin tubes) that perform such duties as collecting urine and monitoring blood pressure are inserted. The first few seconds of the administration of the general anesthetic should be the last part of the operation the patient remembers.

After the surgery, the patient is taken to the intensive care unit (ICU), where specialized nursing care is available around the clock and sophisticated instruments monitor the heart's electrical activity, blood pressure, temperature, and other vital signs. The patient's family will generally be allowed to visit at this time, although the patient will be groggy from the anesthetic and unable to speak because of a tube in the windpipe (endotracheal) that helps the person breathe with a respirator. The ICU experience can be disorienting, as there is little to differentiate day and night, and the patient will drift in and out of consciousness. The nurses are specially trained in communicating by touch and signboard, and they will do everything possible to make the patient comfortable.

Each person recovers at his or her own speed, and much depends on the nature of the surgery. In most cases, the patient will be taken off the respirator the morning after surgery, and the catheters and intravenous lines will be removed within two days. The patient can then hasten his or her recovery by following the guidelines for inflating the lungs (by sucking on a special lung-exercising device) and by making an effort to become mobile, especially by walking. (See Chapter 28 for more information on cardiac rehabilitation.)

---

through the pulmonic valve into the lung or pulmonary artery. The Swan-Ganz catheter provides an accurate reading of the pulmonary arterial blood pressure (based on the pressure at the tip of the balloon) and indicates how well the heart is functioning. A sensitive temperature probe at the tip of this catheter can also tell the surgical team how well blood is circulating.

A Foley catheter is inserted into the patient's bladder before the operation. The amount of urine collected by this catheter is a sign of how well the patient's kidneys are functioning and whether the kidneys are receiving sufficient oxygenated blood.

Anesthetic agents are then administered directly into the veins. These agents have three functions: to block pain and induce drowsiness, to relax the muscles and prevent the person from moving and jerking during the operation, and to cause temporary amnesia so the person is not disturbed by a detailed recollection of the operation. The anesthesiologist carefully monitors the patient's vital signs throughout the operation, adjusting the dosage of medications and anesthetics appropriately.

Once the patient has been anesthetized, a tube (endotracheal) is inserted into the patient's windpipe. The tube connects to the respirator—a bellows-like instrument that performs the work of breathing for the patient. Another tube (nasogastric, or NG) is also inserted to collect stomach fluids that might otherwise nauseate the anesthetized patient.

An anticoagulant, heparin, is also administered at the start of the operation. This "blood-thinner" prevents clots, or emboli, from forming and helps to protect the patient from a stroke. The effects of the heparin will be reversed at the end of the operation by the administration of another drug, protamine, that encourages coagulation.

Once the patient has been prepared, the surgeons begin. For open-heart surgery, the chest is cut open at the midline of the breastbone (sternum) and the breastbone is separated. The chest is then gradually pried open with special retractors to reveal the lungs and, between them, the tough sac of tissue (the pericardium) that protects the heart.

If the internal mammary artery (an artery that supplies blood to the chest wall) is to be used for bypass grafting, at this time it will be gently separated from the chest wall. During the opening of the chest, another surgeon will have been working on the patient's legs to remove several usable lengths of a vein (approximately 20 centimeters, or 8 inches, for each bypass). These lengths of vein are about the diameter of a drinking straw. Later in the operation, the surgeon will take each in turn and sew one end into a tiny hole punched into the aorta and attach the other end to a coronary artery, thereby providing the bypass pathway around each narrowing in the coronary arteries. (See Figure 25.2.)

Once the sac covering the heart has been opened, the surgical team sets up the heart-lung machine. Several plastic tubes are hooked up to the machine. When it is clear that the heart-lung machine is providing adequate circulation, the aorta is clamped, and the heart is stopped with an injection of cold potassium solution directly into the aorta. The outside of the heart is also bathed in a cold salt solution to further induce hypothermia. The patient is now on total bypass; his or her blood circulation has been completely taken over by machine. The surgeons now can attach the bypassing vessels. (Or, if this is an operation other than a coronary bypass, the chambers of the heart can be opened and the appropriate surgery performed.)

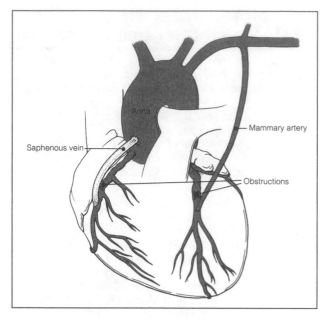

Figure 25.2
This illustrates the two main types of coronary bypass grafts: saphenous vein and internal mammary artery. On the left, a section of saphenous vein from the leg is sutured between the aorta and a coronary artery, bypassing the blockage. The left internal mammary artery, normally found in the chest, is redirected to bypass another blockage.

Once the direct surgery on the heart has been performed, the aortic clamp is removed, and the blood is gradually warmed. The heart may begin beating by itself, or the surgeon uses a brief shock to restore electric activity. Pacemaking wires are placed to allow electrical control of the heart rate. When the heart supports its own blood circulation again, the patient can be taken off the heart-lung machine, any bleeding can be stopped, and incisions can be closed. After the patient is taken off the bypass machine, protamine is injected to reverse the effects of the heparin by restoring the normal clotting ability of blood, and the patient is transferred to an intensive care unit.

CORONARY ARTERY BYPASS SURGERY

In the last few years, coronary artery bypass grafting has become not only the most common heart operation, but also one of the most frequently performed surgical procedures. In 1988, 320,000 bypass operations took place in the United States. The procedure has become so entrenched that it is easy to forget the first such operation was performed as recently as

1967, at the Cleveland Clinic, when Dr. Rene Favaloro used a vein from a leg to bypass a blocked coronary artery. The basic operation has remained much the same, but improvements in surgical technique, in heart preservation during heart-lung machine use, and in the understanding of when and how to also use an artery from the chest wall as a graft have led to longer-lasting grafts, reduced death rates, and increased ability to provide relief for older and sicker patients.

This surgery is usually elective (except for the emergencies that may occur during a threatened heart attack), and the patient often plays a large role in deciding both when and whether to have the operation. By the time most patients are considering the operation, they will have experienced symptoms of heart disease and already have made life-style changes and been treated with medication.

It is useful to distinguish between surgery that is required based on the location of blockage in an artery (anatomic indications) and surgery that is done to improve the heart's function and relieve symptoms (functional or symptomatic indications). Anatomic indications are determined by cardiac catheterization and other tests. Currently, coronary angioplasty may provide an effective alternative to surgery in certain instances. (See Chapter 24.)

Several types of artery narrowing call for surgery. The left main branch of the coronary arteries is a short section leading from the aorta (like the main trunk of a tree) that divides into the circumflex and left anterior descending arteries. If the left main branch is narrowed or constricted (stenotic), it is of particular concern, because the blood supply to much of the heart could be suddenly reduced. People with untreated left main artery disease have an approximate death rate of 50 percent over a five-year period.

The other major artery, which also divides into smaller branches, is the right coronary artery. It supplies blood mainly to the right side of the heart and the underside of the left ventricle. When this artery becomes narrowed or blocked, it is usually not as serious as when the left arteries are affected; surgery is usually not necessary if right artery blockage is the only major problem.

Triple-vessel disease refers to significant (greater than 70 percent) narrowing of the interior of all three coronary arteries. Without coronary bypass, patients with triple-vessel disease have a relatively poor prognosis, particularly if heart function is reduced.

Patients who have suffered damage to the muscle of the main pumping chamber from a heart attack may also be considered candidates for coronary artery bypass surgery. This chamber, the left ventricle, plays a crucial role in pumping arterial blood to the rest of the body (including the coronary arteries themselves), so its efficiency must be maintained. Left ventricle efficiency is usually determined by the amount of blood squeezed out with each beat (the ejection fraction). Coronary artery bypass surgery is advisable when this becomes reduced to a less than adequate level.

Choosing surgery to improve function or relieve symptoms is a more subjective decision; the person's own feelings about life-style restriction may be an important criterion. When chest pain (angina) occurs with unusual frequency or at rest, despite continuing use of medication, surgery may be strongly urged: These symptoms are often warning signs of an impending heart attack. However, some patients with less serious angina that may not actually be getting worse may also opt for surgery, as they may be intolerant of the medications or of the restrictions imposed upon their work and leisure activities.

The principle of coronary artery bypass surgery is to provide a new blood supply for sections of the heart muscle whose own supply of arterial blood is restricted by a blocked artery. The conduit that supplies the new route for blood can be a section of a vein that has been removed from the leg (saphenous vein) and attached to the aorta and the coronary artery to bypass the narrowed section. Another possible conduit source is an artery called the internal mammary artery, a blood vessel that usually supplies blood to the chest wall. There is strong evidence that a bypass using a section of this artery is less susceptible to becoming blocked in the future. Only 60 percent of grafts using a vein are still open after ten years as opposed to more than 90 percent of grafts using an artery.

Surgery using internal mammary artery grafts takes slightly longer because the detaching and reattaching process is more complicated, so there was some early resistance to their use. Nearly all bypass surgery patients who have multiple grafts now have at least one using the internal mammary artery. There are, however, some reasons to avoid using it; these will be considered by the surgeon.

It should be noted that internal mammary artery grafts are often performed in conjunction with saphenous vein grafts. Surgeons believe that providing more new conduits to replenish the blood supply increases the chances of a successful long-term outcome. This is the reason for triple, quadruple, and even quintuple bypasses (referring to the number of new conduits created). The number of bypass grafts does not necessarily indicate the severity of the disease. Too often, patients are led to believe that a quadruple or triple bypass implies that they may have a terrible condition. This is not true. Several of the blockages bypassed may have been relatively "minor" ones.

The patient who has received a coronary artery bypass graft can expect considerable relief from symptoms, and, in many cases, increased lifespan. It should be remembered, however, that the graft vessels are subject to fatty blockage at an increased rate, so care must still be taken to reduce the risk factors that caused the original blockage. (See Chapter 3.) The surgery sets the disease back to an earlier stage; it does not "cure" atherosclerosis. A certain number of patients—especially those whose original bypass surgery occurred more than ten years ago—will find that they are candidates for a second bypass (or "re-op"). This second bypass operation carries only slightly more risk than the first and is an important option for people whose grafts have become constricted and whose symptoms have recurred.

Newer and better surgical techniques now allow surgeons to operate safely and effectively on some people who only a few years ago might have been considered too old or too sick for surgery.

VALVE REPLACEMENT

The heart's valves perform the vital function of maintaining blood flow in the correct direction. The *mitral* valve directs the flow of blood from the left atrium into the left ventricle, and the *aortic* valve allows blood to pass from the left ventricle into the aorta. The *tricuspid* and *pulmonary* valves perform the equivalent tasks on the right side, but are under considerably less pressure than the valves on the left side and—although they may suffer from similar disorders—are less likely to be so severely impaired as to require surgery. (See Chapter 13.)

Problems with the heart valves and their functioning can be of two kinds: narrowing (stenosis), when the valve opening is constricted and blood flow reduced, and regurgitation, when some of the blood leaks back into sections of the heart from which it has just been expelled because the valve leaflets do not close properly. A poorly functioning valve in which the leaflets neither open nor close properly may cause both problems.

While poorly functioning valves most often can be

detected by listening with a stethoscope, a definitive diagnosis of valve disease usually requires such tests as X-rays and an echocardiogram. The decision to operate and correct a valve abnormality will depend on whether the condition is life-threatening and to what extent it has affected the person's life-style. Most problems with valve disease are not of an urgent nature, and the decision does not have to be rushed.

The exception is when the valve opening between the aorta and the left ventricle is blocked (aortic stenosis), which surgeons consider an urgent problem if symptoms occur (such as chest pain, faintness, and shortness of breath) and if the narrowing is severe. About 50 percent of such patients die within four years without surgery. When the aortic valve does not close properly (aortic insufficiency), the decision to operate depends on the degree of damage that shows up on various tests and on whether the person has symptoms. (Less active people may be willing to curb their activity—thus reducing demand on the heart—in order to keep their symptoms to a minimum and avoid surgery.) Poorly functioning aortic valves can result in enlargement of the left ventricle, a condition that must be monitored carefully.

When the valve opening between the upper and lower chambers of the left side of the heart (mitral valve) becomes severely blocked (mitral stenosis), it usually requires surgery. Because the narrowing of the valve opening may cause blood to back up into the lungs, careful monitoring of symptoms such as shortness of breath is required, and surgery may be called for to prevent serious heart failure. When the mitral valve closes improperly (mitral insufficiency), the desirability of surgery is usually determined by how severely the symptoms affect the patient's lifestyle and how well they can be controlled by medical treatment.

Heart valve disease can be surgically treated in three ways: Constricted openings can be enlarged with a balloon catheter; the injured valve can be surgically reconstructed; or the valve can be replaced, either with an artificial valve or with a healthy valve from a pig's heart.

A balloon catheter can be used to alleviate mitral stenosis in some cases. (See Chapter 24.) Mitral valve problems associated with rheumatic fever usually occur because the leaflets stick together. Sometimes simply opening the leaflets enough to separate them from each other is all that is required to solve the problem. To accomplish this, the balloon catheter is threaded through the valve. When it is in place, the balloon at the tip of the catheter is inflated gently until it enlarges the opening. This procedure is rarely an option for aortic stenosis, except in people whose life expectancy is limited because of other diseases. Balloon dilation is not effective, and there is a risk that the calcified leaflets will break off and enter the bloodstream, causing a stroke.

Surgical repair can be performed on the mitral valve, particularly to relieve mitral insufficiency. The procedure followed is the same as for other forms of open-heart surgery. The heart is stilled and the left atrial chamber opened, then the leaflets are reconstructed to allow the valve to close properly. If the leaflets of the mitral valve have become stuck together as the result of rheumatic fever, the surgeon can separate them and suture any damaged edges to ensure that they close efficiently. The advantage of this surgery is that there is no new valve to wear out, nor does the patient ordinarily have to follow a regimen of blood thinners as he or she would with a mechanical heart valve replacement.

Artificial valves have been in use since 1952, when Charles Hufnagel successfully replaced a patient's aortic valve with a caged-ball artificial valve. Some mechanical valves are of the "tilting disk" variety, while others are of the "ball-and-cage" variety. (Figures 25.3A–C show some commonly used artificial valves.) The latter consist of a metal ring covered in Dacron and a thin metal cage. Inside the cage is a ball, which exactly fits the dimension of the ring. Blood flowing in the correct direction moves the ball away from the ring towards the cage and flows by uninterrupted. When the blood begins to flow in the opposite direction, it pushes the ball back into the ring, creating a tight seal that prevents leaking. The tilting disk valves work somewhat along the principle of a hinged door that is opened due to pressure from one side and shut tightly due to pressure from the opposite side. Mechanical valves make a clicking noise with each heartbeat, but the patient usually can not hear this.

Valve replacement is performed during open-heart surgery. Artificial valves are carefully sutured or sewn into the ring surrounding the valve opening, completely replacing the natural valve. (See Figure 25.3D.) Approximately 80 percent of patients who survive the first postoperative year are able to return to normal activity, even though they may previously have been severely restricted by breathlessness from heart failure or by fainting spells and angina. The downside of the operation is that it carries with it a 5 percent mortality risk (somewhat higher than for coronary artery bypass surgery), partly because of the possibility of a stroke caused by loosened calcium

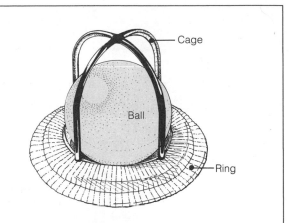

Figure 25.3A
There are two major types of mechanical valves: tilting disc and ball-and-cage. The Starr-Edwards (brand name) model shown here is a ball-and-cage valve. When blood flows forward, the ball is pushed to the top of the cage. When blood flow ceases, the ball falls back on the ring and seals the valve closed.

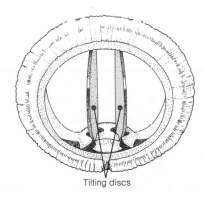

Figure 25.3B
The St. Jude's (brand name) bileaflet model is a tilting disc valve. If blood flows in the wrong direction, the discs close, much like a hinged door, sealing the vessel opening.

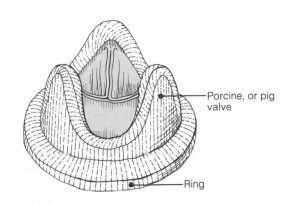

Figure 25.3C
A Carpentier-Edwards mitral valve model. This is a porcine valve, or pig valve, mounted on a synthetic ring.

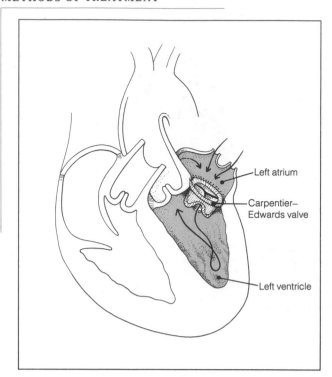

Figure 25.3D
A Carpentier-Edwards model replacing the mitral valve in the heart. The arrows indicate the direction of blood flow.

deposits or air bubbles entering the bloodstream (the latter being a risk in any open-heart surgery). Convalescence may also be prolonged, especially for older people.

An alternative to mechanical valves is the use of valves from pigs. There is currently some debate as to which replacement valves are most suitable, the synthetic ones or those obtained from pig hearts. The patient should carefully weigh the advantages and disadvantages of each, recognizing that technical circumstances may occasionally require the surgeon to use one or the other.

The synthetic valves have the advantage of durability; they may often last a lifetime. On the rare occasions that a mechanical valve does fail, it may do so suddenly and cause the heart to fail. A disadvantage is that the patient will have to follow a lifetime regimen of anticoagulants such as warfarin (Coumadin) to prevent blood clots from forming around the mechanical parts. Taking anticoagulants also places some restrictions on the patient's activity; contact sports or other activities that could result in bruising or internal bleeding usually have to be avoided. Patients also have to be more careful to avoid infections that might form on the new valve surface. Antibiotics have to be taken before the patient undergoes procedures such as dental work.

Valves taken from pig hearts do not ordinarily require the patient to take anticoagulant medication for more than six to eight weeks following surgery. The disadvantage of these replacement valves is that they do wear out and may have to be replaced after about ten years. They wear out gradually, so there is little risk of a sudden episode of heart failure. It should be noted that valve tissue does not cause rejection problems as seen with heart transplantation. Recent studies have shown that the natural valve compares favorably with the artificial valve over a ten-year period; patient longevity may even be enhanced. When comparing the statistics, people should bear in mind not just the length of time a valve will last, but also the problems of infection and anticoagulant drug therapy.

SURGERY FOR HEART RHYTHM DISORDERS (ARRHYTHMIAS)

Arrhythmias are disturbances in the heart's electrical conduction system, which controls both the sequence and the frequency of heartbeats. These can take the form of harmless "palpitations" or become present as a sign of injury or disease. Irregular or rapid rhythms generally originate in two areas: the ventricles (the lower part of the heart) or the supraventricular areas (the upper part of the heart). Ventricular arrhythmias commonly occur as extra beats and are generally of no importance. In people who have had heart attacks with tissue damage, however, a sustained run of extra beats can be serious. Between the dead muscle and the normal muscle is an unstable "border zone" from which extra beats may arise. If they occur in sequence and at a rapid rate (ventricular tachycardia) or as rapid, irregular, and uncoordinated beats (ventricular fibrillation), urgent treatment is required.

Many people with a history of ventricular tachycardia or fibrillation come to the surgeon after having experienced near "sudden death" and resuscitation. If these arrhythmias have been recurrent and are not controlled by medical therapy (see Chapter 16), further studies may be necessary. Cardiac catheterization and the use of an electric probe may help to locate a problem in the heart muscle. The surgeon then cuts out unstable areas that are causing the arrhythmia. The operation has a mortality rate of around 12 percent, but it is effective in preventing these serious arrhythmias from recurring. This type of procedure is necessary only in a very small number of patients with severe arrhythmias. In certain patients with arrhythmias and additional problems such as angina, the surgeon may also place an implantable defibrillator (AICD) at the time of bypass surgery. (See Chapter 26.)

Arrhythmias can also occur in people who are born with extra conducting pathways. The impulse from the atria short-circuits the normal pathway and activates the ventricle sooner than normal. The short-circuiting is detectable on an electrocardiogram. The most common type of abnormal pathway result is Wolff-Parkinson-White (WPW) syndrome, in which an additional conducting pathway bypasses the atrioventricular (AV) node, which separates the atria from the ventricles. The AV node normally acts as a regulating block for electrical impulses passing from the atrium to the ventricle, and the additional pathway can allow abnormally frequent electrical signals from the atria to set up arrhythmias in the ventricles.

Patients with Wolff-Parkinson-White syndrome are, for the most part, young and have otherwise normal hearts. Most of them have few symptoms, but may experience episodes of rapid heartbeats, some of which may be severe. The syndrome was formerly treated with medication, which was not completely effective in preventing recurring arrhythmias. Today, if symptoms are recurrent and severe, the extra conducting pathway can be removed during open-heart surgery. This operation provides a cure, and the mortality rate during surgery is low.

REPAIR OF ANEURYSMS

An aneurysm is a severe weakening in the wall of an artery or organ. The weakened area balloons out. In addition, the bulging area may either press on and disrupt the function of other vital organs or burst and hemorrhage.

There are two kinds of aneurysms that may directly affect the heart: left ventricular aneurysm and aortic aneurysm. Left ventricular aneurysms may appear following a heart attack (myocardial infarction, or MI). This is a relatively uncommon occurrence. It is a bad sign, because it indicates that a lack of oxygen has caused extensive damage to the muscular wall of the left ventricle. Surgeons operate on left ventricular aneurysms if they are accompanied by arrhythmias, congestive heart failure, or blood clots. The operation

is performed through the area of the heart attack, and the surgeon seeks to remove or repair the weakened area of the ventricle wall. This operation allows the ventricle to function more effectively (although heart muscle that has been destroyed cannot be restored) and can usually give the person a reasonable life expectancy.

An aneurysm in the aorta may be surgically repaired by replacing that section with a prosthetic graft, usually made of Dacron. This surgery can also have decent results, but it carries a mortality risk of approximately 10 percent.

HEART TRANSPLANTS

The idea of replacing a diseased heart with a healthy one has long fascinated surgeons. The earliest heart transplant was carried out in 1905 at the University of Chicago. Doctors successfully implanted a heart into a dog's neck; a beat was sustained for several hours. The first demonstration of the possibility that a transplanted heart could completely take over the circulation was made by a Russian physician in the 1950s.

Transplants in which the transplanted heart is placed in the normal anatomical position and the diseased heart removed were soon recognized as being desirable. The first such transplants were done in the early 1960s using animals. In 1964, a dying 67-year-old man's defective heart was replaced with that of a chimpanzee; a beat was sustained for a few hours. Three years later, Christiaan Barnard became a worldwide celebrity as the first surgeon to successfully transplant a heart from one human being to another.

These initial attempts were dampened by poor survival rates for the patients. Several more advances were required before heart transplantation became a truly viable method of treatment in the early 1970s.

PATIENT SELECTION

Careful selection of transplant recipients has led to an improvement in the success of these operations and in the more effective use of the limited pool of available donor organs. A recipient of a heart transplant should be someone who is less than 60 years old (there is no lower age limit), who is suffering from end-stage congestive heart failure (see Chapter 14) with severe symptoms, and for whom survival without the transplant is extremely limited. The main causes of this type of severe heart failure are coronary artery disease (see Chapter 11) and heart muscle disease (see Chapter 15), although some transplants are now being done for congenital heart disease (see Chapter 20).

A transplant is usually not advised when another major systemic disease exists, such as a malignancy, lung disease, collagen vascular disease (such as lupus), or insulin-requiring diabetes mellitus.

Rigorous criteria for donor selection have also greatly increased the success of heart transplantation. The suitable donor has to be less than 35 years of age and to have sustained brain death (usually from cerebral trauma, for example a head injury or stroke) with no evidence of chest injury. Signs of infection, a history of cardiac illness, or prolonged use of cardiopulmonary resuscitation would rule out the donor's organ.

When a donor heart that meets these criteria becomes available, the next step is to match it promptly with an appropriate recipient. Matching is now done through regional organ banks, and the donor organ is flown to the hospital where the recipient is concurrently being prepared to receive it. Matching is done on the basis of blood type, and there is a general requirement that the donor be approximately the same size or larger than the recipient. The reason for the latter requirement is to avoid exposing the donated heart to the increased blood pressure requirement that is present in a larger person.

THE OPERATION

When an appropriate donor/recipient match has been made, based on careful screening techniques, the donor's chest is opened. The heart is carefully examined for previously unrecognized injury, is cooled, and then is removed from the chest. It is particularly important that the correct protocol for the donor operation be followed carefully.

The recipient is also carefully prepared for surgery; the surgeons try to time the use of the heart-lung machine with the arrival of the donor organ. The recipient's heart is not removed in its entirety—some portions of the atria, or thin upper chambers, are preserved. (See Figure 25.4A.)

Transplanting only part of the heart greatly simplifies the operation. The main sections that need replacing are the ventricles (whose muscular walls do most of the heart's work), the valves, and only part of the atria. (See Figure 25.4B.)

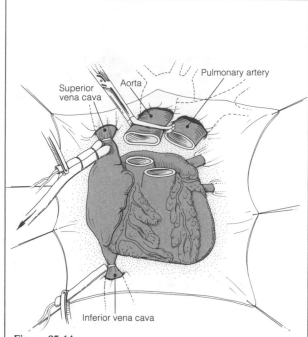

Figure 25.4A
Before a heart transplant, a heart-lung machine will take over the patient's blood circulation, and the major arteries and veins leading to the heart must be clamped off.

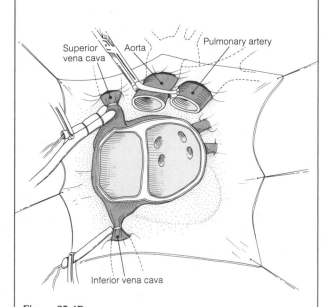

Figure 25.4B
The diseased portion of the heart is then removed.

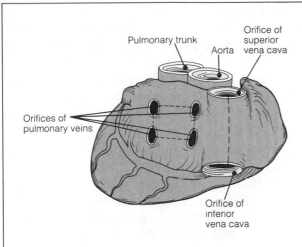

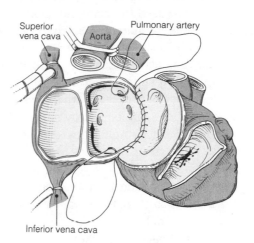

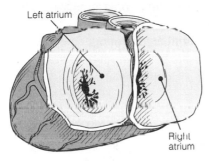

Figure 25.4C
The donor heart has been prepared for the transplant and is kept cool throughout the operation.

Figure 25.4D
The donor heart is affixed to the remaining heart tissue.

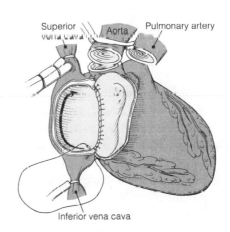

Figure 25.4E
The aorta and the pulmonary artery are reattached.

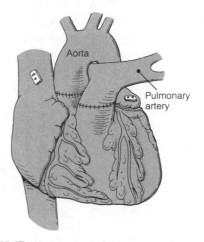

Care is taken throughout the operation to keep the donor heart cool and to keep air from being trapped in the heart chambers. (See Figure 25.4C.) When the connections are complete (see Figures 25.4D–F), the patient's new heart is gradually warmed and resuscitated, then taken off the bypass machine. As in most other forms of heart surgery, atrial and ventricular pacing wires are attached to the outside of the heart to allow for rapid treatment of any rhythm disturbances after the chest has been closed.

Two major issues are of concern after surgery: preventing and diagnosing the possible rejection of the donor heart by the recipient's body, and avoiding infections. The high mortality and failure rate of heart transplants in the late 1960s arose largely from a lack of knowledge in properly managing these potential difficulties.

Graft rejection results when the body's immune system recognizes the donated organ as an alien substance and begins attacking and trying to destroy the "intruder." Because perfect matching of donated tissue with the recipient's tissue is simply not feasible for these kinds of operations, the immune system needs to be suppressed. The discovery of cyclosporine (Sandimmune), a drug that originated in a soil

Figure 25.4F
Once the connections are complete, the transplanted heart is gradually warmed, and the patient is taken off the heart-lung machine. Bloodflow through the heart is restored.

mold from Norway (dug up by a vacationing researcher), has increased the ability to suppress certain aspects of the immune system that may cause graft rejection, while still allowing the body to maintain its defenses against infection. Cyclosporine, even in small doses, mainly suppresses one kind of immune cell (T-cell lymphocyte), whereas earlier immunosuppressant medications unnecessarily suppressed a broader range. T-cell lymphocytes are important components of the system that tends to surround and get rid of foreign substances. Cyclosporine is generally taken in combination with other immunosuppressant drugs—such as a steroid medication called prednisone (Deltasone) and azathioprine (Imuran)—so smaller doses of each medication can be used.

Improved methods of diagnosing rejection have also led to better long-term management of the body's immune response. Effective testing is essential, because the clinical signs of rejection are generally unreliaise: The patient may complain of malaise or have a low-grade fever, but often there are no discernible symptoms. Rejection of the new heart cannot be reliably diagnosed using an electrocardiogram. Cardiac biopsy, performed under local anesthesia by passing a biopsy instrument through a vein and into the heart, is required to allow microscopic study of the tissue. If rejection appears to be taking place, the dosage of cyclosporine can be increased and then lowered again to normal levels once the patient has improved.

Heart transplantation has come to be an effective and beneficial option for some patients who, without the surgery, would have lived for only a few months at best. Approximately 85 percent of patients are still alive after the first year and 65 percent after five years, and complete rehabilitation occurs in about 87 percent of the patients. Patients must be followed very closely after transplantation: Routine clinic visits are necessary with regular biopsies scheduled in order to detect rejection. In addition, cardiac catheterization and coronary angioplasty may be performed annually to assess the condition of the heart and coronary arteries.

HEART AND LUNG TRANSPLANTS

Transplanting both the heart and one or both lungs is becoming more common for seriously ill patients. Recipients for the double transplant may have sufficiently high blood pressure in their own lungs to cause the failure of a donor heart, or they may be patients suffering from end-stage lung disease with associated heart failure. Distant procurement of lungs has only recently become possible, because the lungs have an extreme sensitivity to oxygen deprivation (ischemia). Lungs can now be maintained for up to six hours outside the body by a new technique of preservation.

The combined heart-lung transplant has a higher mortality than the heart transplant alone, but better preservation of donated organs and improvements in postoperative care have made this an option for selected patients. While technically feasible in many patients, transplantation of a heart or heart and lungs is a major, serious operation with a long period of convalescence. It is a clearly desirable option for only a small number of younger people with advanced, nontreatable heart and lung disease.

PEDIATRIC HEART SURGERY

Approximately 10 percent of the cardiac surgery in this country is performed on infants and children. Problems requiring this surgery are almost exclusively congenital in nature—the children are born with heart defects. (See Table 25.1.) This is in contrast to cardiac surgery performed on adults, which is predominantly for problems acquired during their lifetime, such as coronary artery disease.

Congenital defects vary from straightforward problems, such as a "hole" in the heart, producing mild symptoms or none at all, to complicated malformations that result when a good portion of the heart has failed to develop. Normally, these lead to life-threatening situations. Depending on the heart defect, there are two common conditions that may arise. Children who have more than the normal amount of blood flow to the lungs as a result of a defect may suffer from congestive heart failure. This often causes difficulties in eating, lack of weight gain, rapid breathing, and sweating. A large hole between the left and right main chambers of the heart (ventricles) can produce this.

On the other hand, children with blockage resulting in less blood flow to the lungs may suffer from blueness of the skin (cyanosis). Although they may gain weight and grow well, they are cyanotic because of the low level of oxygen in their blood. These children are often physically limited, and they can suffer from complications such as infections and blackouts.

There are many different congenital heart defects, some of which are quite rare. More common defects account for the majority of clinical problems. It must be remembered that each individual case is unique and may have mitigating factors that require special consideration or treatment.

When there are one or more holes in the wall that separates the right atrium from the left atrium, the child has an *atrial septal defect*. This results in some shunting of blood from the left side (high-pressure side) of the heart to the right side (low-pressure side) through the hole. This is called a "left-to-right shunt." There is increased blood flow to the lungs, but pressure in the lungs generally remains low, and the child usually shows no symptoms. The problem is most often diagnosed when a heart murmur is discovered or when there has been an increase in heart size (noted on an electrocardiogram or chest X-ray). While the defect may not produce symptoms in the child, if the hole is large enough it may cause heart enlargement, heart failure, or heart rhythm disorders over the years, significantly decreasing the normal life span.

If surgery is considered necessary, it is usually performed electively when the child is between the ages of 2 and 4. (See box, "Before and After Open Heart Surgery: What to Expect for Children.") The holes most often can be closed with a suture, but if they are particularly large, a small patch made from the patient's own pericardial (outside wrapping of the heart) tissue or a Dacron patch can be used. The operation provides a complete cure, and it is extremely rare for the holes to open up again. Antibiotic treatment to prevent infection need not be required for more than a few months after the operation, and the patient should be able to lead a full and active life. A recently developed catheterization procedure that is still considered investigational by the Food and Drug Administration shows promise in treating atrial septal defects. See Chapter 20 for more information.

When there is a hole in the septum, or dividing muscle, between the right and left ventricles, the defect is called *ventricular septal defect*. As with the atrial septal defect, a considerable amount of blood is pumped back into the low-pressure right ventricle (left-to-right shunting). This condition may exist without symptoms for many years. When they do occur, symptoms can include breathing difficulties and congestive heart failure as a result of the large amounts of blood filling and congesting the lungs.

If the opening is large and the infant is very small and ill, a band may be placed around the pulmonary artery to restrict blood flow into the lungs and pre-

Before and After Open Heart Surgery: What to Expect for Children

Most children who require open-heart surgery are admitted to the hospital the day before surgery. They undergo the usual preoperative tests, such as an electrocardiogram (ECG), chest X-ray, and blood work. The children are familiarized with the hospital setting, and the parents are introduced to the staff and setting of the intensive care unit (ICU). Surgery usually lasts several hours, depending on the complexity of the operation. After surgery, the child will be taken either to a cardiothoracic intensive care unit or a special pediatric intensive care unit.

For simple procedures, children may be discharged from the hospital four to five days after the operation. More complex procedures entail a longer stay of ten days or more. Once home, the children can be treated much as always— although care should be taken not to put stress on the surgical incisions until full healing has taken place. In children, it takes a month for the breastbone (sternum) to heal fully. Obviously it is difficult to restrict the activities of infants or young children, and all that is usually required is that parents themselves limit their contact with the incision area. Parents should also ensure that the children understand the need to take prescribed medications regularly, and, if the child is being treated with blood thinners such as warfarin (Coumadin), to avoid activities that might result in bruising. Continued follow-up after discharge and close communication with physicians are essential for good results.

vent heart failure. Complete repair is then carried out within the first year or two of life, when the band is removed. This course of action is becoming less common; even in very young infants, repair as a first step is considered optimal.

The holes are closed, usually with a small patch of Dacron or Gore-Tex rather than the sutures that are used to close atrial septal defects. The long-term results are very good once the hole is closed, and cure is essentially complete. Postoperative complications are uncommon, but they can include heart rhythm irregularities or the presence of a small residual hole.

The most common form of cyanotic congenital heart disease is *tetralogy of Fallot*. Even so, it is relatively rare. The syndrome includes four abnormalities: a large ventricular septal defect; a displacement of the aorta to the right side so that blood without adequate oxygen enters it from the right ventricle; a

Table 25.1
Corrective Surgery for Congenital Heart Defects

Defect	Description	Surgery	Prognosis
Atrial septal defect	One or more holes in the wall that separates the right and left atria	Hole(s) closed with a suture or a small patch made from the patient's own tissue or from Dacron.	Operation provides a complete cure; extremely rare for holes to open up again.
Ventricular septal defect	A hole in the septum between the right and left ventricles	Hole(s) closed with a small patch of Dacron or Gore-Tex.	Cure is essentially complete; rare complications are heart rhythm problems or small residual septal defect.
Tetralogy of Fallot	A large ventricular septal defect, a displacement of the aorta so blood with low oxygen enters it from the right ventricle, a thickened right ventricular wall from increased pressure, and partial blockage of the pathway from the heart to the lungs	Ventricular septal defect closed and blockage of blood flow removed from between the right ventricle and the lungs.	Good long-term results; minority experience right-heart failure or heart rhythm disorders requiring additional surgery or continued medication.
Transposition of the great arteries	Transposition of aorta and pulmonary artery	Most common operation for past few years is arterial switch operation (ASO), in which the aorta and pulmonary artery are reconnected at the proper locations, and the coronary arteries are switched as well.	Short-term results are good; it is too soon to know long-term results.
Congenital valve disorder	A deformity of any of the heart's four valves, most commonly aortic valve constriction or narrowing (stenosis)	Valve is opened and repaired and/or replaced with a mechanical valve when child is large enough to accommodate valve of available size.	Results with mechanical valves are good, but anticoagulant medication must be taken indefinitely.
Complete atrioventricular canal	A central defect connecting all four chambers in the central part of the heart with only one large common atrioventricular valve	Atrial and ventricular septal defect is closed, and two valves are created from the one valve.	Results are generally good; significant number of patients need valve repair or replacement later.

Defect	Description	Surgery	Prognosis
Tricuspid atresia	A severely underdeveloped right side of the heart (usually with only one adequately sized ventricular chamber)	Fontan procedure diverts all the venous blood return from the body directly into the lungs, bypassing the pumping chambers and returning to the lungs to the one good ventricle to be pumped out.	Does not provide cure but seems to offer long-term relief from cyanosis and heart failure; children require careful lifelong follow-up; long-term consequences remain to be seen.
Hypoplastic left heart syndrome	A severely underdeveloped left side of the heart, including the ventricle and ascending aorta	Norwood procedure creates new outflow for heart and shunt to provide blood to lungs until child is old enough to undergo Fontan-type procedure; other option is cardiac transplant.	Results are encouraging in both cases; however, long-term effects of immunosuppressive drugs on growth and development not understood.
Patent ductus arteriosis	A blood vessel that fails to close after birth and continues to connect the aorta and pulmonary artery	Abnormal connection is closed with small, metal clip; does not require open-heart surgery.	Provides a complete cure.
Coarctation of the aorta	Narrowing of the aorta	Constriction removed through reconstruction of aorta.	Some patients have recurrence of coarctation, but it can be repaired by a balloon dilation procedure in a cardiac cath lab.

thickened right ventricular wall resulting from the increased pressure inside the right ventricular cavity; and partial blockage of the pathway from the heart to the lungs (pulmonary artery).

The symptoms of tetralogy of Fallot are different from those of a simple ventricular septal defect because of the effects of the other complications; blood flow does not increase in the lungs and cause heart failure. Instead, there is a right-to-left shunt of blood —blood without adequate oxygen travels from the right ventricle out the aorta. Not enough blood passes through the pulmonary artery to receive oxygen from the lungs, so children with this defect are often intensely cyanotic; they appear blue from lack of oxygen. Under certain conditions, such as stress, this oxygen deficiency may suddenly become much worse. This results in "cyanotic spells," which can be serious. Urgent surgery of some kind is necessary.

If an infant has severe symptoms at an early age, placement of a temporary shunt may be required to provide more blood flow to the lungs. The long-term corrective procedure involves open-heart surgery, including two steps: closing the hole between the two ventricles and opening up the artery from the right ventricle to the lungs. The long-term results of the operation are good; most patients grow normally and have normal lives. A minority of patients have difficulties later in life with heart failure or heart rhythm disorders and may require additional surgery or continued medication.

A very rare congenital defect in which the aorta and pulmonary artery are switched is called *transposition of the great arteries*. The aorta is connected to the right ventricle instead of the left ventricle, and the pulmonary artery is connected to the left ventricle instead of the right ventricle. So blood that contains a great deal of oxygen that normally should go into the arteries of the body via the aorta is instead pumped back into the lungs. Blood with less oxygen ends up in the liver, brain, kidneys, and so on. These infants are often severely cyanotic.

This transposition can be corrected, but that requires a complicated surgical procedure that sometimes has less than satisfying results. However, newer surgical approaches to correcting this rare abnormality appear promising.

An infant can be born with a deformity of any of the heart's four valves, but the most common *congenital valve disorder* is aortic constriction or narrowing (stenosis). In this defect, the aortic valve may be small or poorly developed (hypoplastic), or the leaflets may be thickened. The decision on how early to operate depends on the extent of the narrowing and the symptoms. During the operation, the valve will be opened and repaired, if possible; otherwise, it will have to be replaced. There currently are no artificial valves small enough for very young infants, so valve reconstruction has to be done in these cases, with possible replacement at a later stage. Children frequently require placement of mechanical valves, because valves from pig hearts tend to harden rapidly with calcium deposits when placed in someone so young. Mechanical valves require that children take anticoagulant medication indefinitely to keep blood clots from forming in the valves.

A defect seen in children with Down syndrome is a *complete atrioventricular canal*. In this disorder, instead of two separate atrial-ventricular valves—the mitral on the left and the tricuspid on the right—there is only one large common atrioventricular valve. These children may require several complicated operations to correct this major defect.

In extremely rare cases, infants are born with a severely underdeveloped right side of the heart (usually with only one ventricular chamber instead of two). The defect is referred to as *tricuspid atresia*. A variety of problems can result, and the infant may be either cyanotic or experiencing heart failure, depending on the amount of blood flow to the lungs. One or more procedures will be required to relieve symptoms during infancy; the nature of these will depend on the physiology of the individual defect.

Usually at about age 2, the patient can undergo a Fontan procedure, an operation first performed in the early 1970s, which involves diverting all the venous blood return from the body directly into the lungs, thus bypassing the pumping chambers. Blood then returns from the lungs to the one good ventricle, where it is pumped out to the body. Consequently, the one ventricle does the work of two: pumping the blood through the arterial system and then through the lungs in series. Although this operation does not really cure the defect, it appears to offer the best long-term relief available to children with only one heart pumping chamber. The operation does relieve cyanosis and heart failure. These children, however, do require careful lifelong follow-up, and the long-term consequences of the operation remain to be determined.

The vast majority of children with *hypoplastic left heart syndrome*—another rare abnormality that consists of a severely underdeveloped left heart, including the ventricle and ascending aorta—die within the first week after birth. Two recent surgical approaches have had encouraging results, however. One is the Norwood procedure, which does not provide a cure but does allow children to grow enough to undergo a Fontan-type operation. The Norwood procedure creates a new outflow for the heart, using the pulmonary artery, and creates a shunt to provide blood flow to the lungs.

The other approach to these babies is heart transplant shortly after birth. Early results are encouraging, but the long-term effects of the necessary drugs (which repress the immune system and fight rejection) on growth and development in children are not well understood. However, with these two approaches, there is some hope for these infants who otherwise cannot survive.

Two other more common congenital problems, easily treated surgically, are *patent ductus arteriosis* and *coarctation of the aorta*. A patent ductus arteriosis can be treated with a simple surgical procedure that does not require open-heart surgery. The ductus arteriosis is a blood vessel that connects the aorta and the pulmonary artery while the child is still in the womb. Its purpose is to allow blood to bypass the lungs, because they are not functioning before birth. Blood flows from the right side of the heart to the pulmonary artery directly to the aorta and out to the body. In a few cases, this vessel fails to close normally within a few days after birth and remains open or "patent." Blood then flows into the lungs and may cause heart failure. The defect usually can be treated successfully in the newborn period with medicine or a simple surgical procedure in which the abnormal connection is closed with a small metal clip, applied through an incision in the left side of the chest.

Coarctation of the aorta refers to a congenital narrowing of the aorta after it leaves the heart. This obstructs and reduces blood flow to the rest of the aorta, the arms, legs, kidneys, and other vital organs. This condition also causes a rise in the blood pressure near the blockage (in the arms). The constriction is removed by surgical reconstruction of the aorta. Normal circulation is restored. High blood pressure, which may become permanent, is common in patients who have not been treated early enough, but when it is adequately treated in childhood, the hypertension is most often relieved eventually. Some patients may have a "recurrence" of coarctation later in life. This can often be repaired by a balloon dilation procedure done in the cardiac catheterization laboratory. (See Chapter 24.)

Children with coarctation usually have no symptoms early in life. An elevated blood pressure, heart murmur, diminished pulses in the legs, or poor development of the lower extremities may suggest the diagnosis.

SPECIAL CONSIDERATIONS IN PEDIATRIC HEART SURGERY

Like all heart surgery, this area is highly specialized and should be performed only in medical centers by surgeons who devote a large part of their professional careers to the treatment of congenital heart disease. Availability of experts in pediatric cardiology, pediatric anesthesia, and pediatric intensive care is essential to the successful outcome of these operations. Technological advances in all these areas have led to lower mortality and better long-term success rates.

CHAPTER 26

PACEMAKERS AND ANTITACHYCARDIA DEVICES

WILLIAM BATSFORD, M.D.

INTRODUCTION

The heart's natural pacemaker is an electrical timing device that controls the rate of the heart's muscular contractions, enabling the heart to pump blood under the wide range of demands encountered in daily life, from sprinting for a taxi to sleeping late on a Sunday morning. Everyone's heart speeds up or slows down under different conditions and may on occasion appear to flutter or skip a beat. These palpitations are almost always minor and transitory. However, sometimes the heart's electrical system malfunctions and serious rhythm disorders result. These cardiac arrhythmias can be debilitating and even life-threatening, but the ready availability of artificial pacemakers and the recent advent of implantable defibrillators have revolutionized their treatment. Today, physicians can help patients with electronic devices that directly counteract these serious rhythm disturbances. (See Chapter 16.)

Implantable electronic devices have been developed to treat both abnormally slow heart rates (bradycardias) and excessively rapid heart rates (tachycardias). Such rhythm disorders arise because of disruptions in the normal production or transmis-sion of electrical impulses within the heart. The heart's natural pacemaker is the sinus node (SN), located in the upper right atrium near the point where blood returning from the head and limbs reenters the heart. Specialized cells in this node emit electrical impulses at the rate of about 70 per minute. These impulses spread throughout the atria and travel to the ventricles via the atrioventricular node (AV node). This electrical system ensures that the impulses reach the right part of the heart at the right time and at the right pace, coordinating the contraction of the heart muscle so that it can pump effectively.

When the sinus node fails to generate impulses, or transmission is blocked in some part of the electrical system, an abnormally slow heart rate can result. Assuming that this bradycardia is not the side effect of a medication or produced by some other reversible condition, the most likely cause is disease in the sinus node, the AV node, or some other part of the conduction pathway. If the patient is experiencing symptoms and the heart rate is extremely slow (below 45 or 50), the condition may be markedly improved by an artificial pacemaker. There are, however, many people who function normally with slow heart rates of 40–50 and evidence of some degree of heart block. Pacemakers should be reserved for those with symptoms and advanced degrees of block.

331

PACEMAKERS

Since their introduction in the 1960s, pacemakers have steadily shrunk in size and grown in sophistication, yet the basic principles of their operation remain the same. The job of the pacemaker is to maintain a minimum safe heart rate by delivering to the pumping chambers appropriately timed electrical impulses that replace the heart's normal rhythmic pulses. The device designed to perform this life-sustaining role typically consists of a power source about the size of a silver dollar (containing the battery), control circuits, and wires, or "leads," that connect the power source to the chambers of the heart. The leads are placed in contact with the right atrium or the right ventricle, or both. They allow the pacemaker to sense and stimulate in various combinations, depending on where the pacing is required. (See box, "The Pacemaker Alphabet.")

The Pacemaker Alphabet

Pacemakers are often referred to by a three-letter code that denotes how and where they operate.

- The first letter tells which heart chamber can be paced (controlled by the pacemaker). The letter may be A for atrium, V for ventricle, or D for dual (both).

- The second letter denotes the chamber in which the pacemaker is able to sense a natural impulse. This letter may also be A, V, or D.

- The third letter tells whether the pacemaker's response to sensing an impulse is to inhibit or trigger an impulse, or both. The letter may be I for inhibit, T for trigger, or D for dual.

The majority of pacemakers are either one of two types, VVI or DDD. In the VVI, known as a demand pacemaker, the first V means that it is the ventricle that is paced, the second V means that it is in the ventricle that the natural impulse is sensed, and the I means that the pacemaker inhibits its own impulse whenever it senses a natural impulse. In the DDD (known as a universal pacemaker), the first D means that it is either the atrium or the ventricle that is paced, or both, the second D means that it is in either the atrium, the ventricle, or both that the natural impulse is sensed, and the third D means that the pacemaker either inhibits or triggers an impulse, depending on what it has sensed.

A physician will prescribe a pacemaker with a pacing mode and rate that is best suited to the patient's needs, taking into account the patient's age and activity level, as well as the nature and degree of malfunction.

DEMAND PACEMAKERS

A ventricular demand pacemaker, which aids a patient who has a slow ventricular rate caused by blockage of the electrical impulses to the ventricles, employs the most basic pacing mode; the device consists of a pacemaker with a single lead to the right ventricle. "Demand" signifies that the device will provide impulses only when they are needed.

The pacemaker is individually programmed to maintain the patient's natural, intrinsic ventricular rate, which usually falls between 50 and 70 beats per minute. If the patient is completely dependent upon the pacemaker, the rate might be set as high as 80 to 90 beats per minute to meet the demands of daily exertion. If the pacemaker senses that the ventricles are being stimulated at their normal pace, then it does not deliver an impulse. Otherwise the pacemaker stimulates the ventricle at a fixed pace until a normal impulse inhibits the device.

DUAL-CHAMBER PACEMAKERS

For patients whose heart disease or life-style requires a more adaptable device, pacemakers have been developed that respond with different heart rates to varying demands on the heart. Called dual-chamber pacemakers, they stimulate the ventricles at the rate sensed in the atria and can enable even a patient with complete heart block (that is, a condition in which no impulses are getting through from the upper to the lower heart chamber) to enjoy fairly vigorous exercise. The most flexible dual-chamber device is the fully automatic or universal pacemaker, which senses and paces in both the right atrium and the right ventricle. In addition to compensating for failure of normal sinus rhythm and heart block, the universal pacemaker synchronizes the atrial and ventricular rates. This feature ensures that the atria always beat just before the ventricles, maintaining the atria's role as priming pumps that increase the volume of blood in the ventricles. Supplemental pumping can be especially important for patients whose own pumping function has fallen dangerously low because of heart disease, such as severe congestive heart failure.

Once implanted, most pacemakers can be reprogrammed from outside the body, using a wand that transmits signals to the pacemaker when held over it. Programmability enables a doctor to adjust the pacemaker's overall operation to changes in the patient's needs. Some pacemakers can also transmit information about heart rate and electrical activity that may be useful in diagnosis. Researchers are also working on alternative sensing devices to make pacemakers more responsive to changing demands on the heart. One such device employs a motion-sensor that vibrates in response to changes in the patient's motion. The device can be programmed for different degrees of sensitivity. Sensing devices have also been developed that respond to other physiological changes related to heart rate, such as blood temperature or acidity, cardiac output or pressure, or respiratory rate.

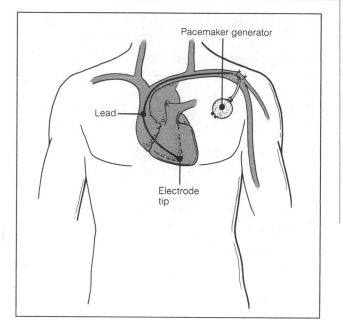

Figure 26.1
The pacemaker generator ("battery") is implanted under the skin on the upper portion of the chest, and the leads are threaded through a vein to the appropriate chambers of the right side of the heart. The model illustrated is one of a number in use.

PACEMAKER IMPLANTATION

Pacemaker implantation is a surgical procedure that is performed under local anesthesia and requires only a brief hospitalization. First, a catheter is inserted into the chest, usually through the subclavian vein, which is located below the collarbone and above the heart. The pacemaker's leads are then threaded through the catheter to the appropriate chamber or chambers of the heart. (See Figure 26.1.) The electrodes are maneuvered into contact with the inner surface of the atrium or ventricle. Finally the surgeon makes a small "pocket" in the pad of flesh (under the skin) on the upper portion of the chest wall to hold the power source. This pocket is then closed with stitches, leaving a small scar. The battery can usually be felt easily through the skin.

Complications related to implantation occur in only a few cases, and are typically those inherent in catheterization, such as bleeding, a punctured vein, infection, or a collapsed lung. Patients usually remain in the hospital for two or three days of evaluation to ensure that the pacemaker is working properly. Most people can resume a full schedule and return to work or school after two weeks. Accustomed sexual activity can also be resumed. A few activities will be restricted for about eight weeks.

All patients with pacemakers should have regular follow-up visits with their doctors to verify that the device is performing optimally. The increasing complexity of programmable pacemakers requires physicians to keep thorough and accurate records of the patient's pacemaker settings so that consistent follow-up is assured should the patient come under the care of a different doctor. Simple devices are available that allow the physician to test the function of the pacemaker battery. The lithium batteries typically last eight to ten years and can be replaced by reopening the pacemaker pouch under local anesthesia. This is a relatively minor surgical procedure that does not require hospitalization.

RARE COMPLICATIONS

Freed of their debilitating bradycardia symptoms, the vast majority of patients feel liberated by their pacemakers and remain satisfied with the devices. Nevertheless, anyone with a pacemaker should be alert to any symptoms or signs that might indicate malfunction. (See box, "Indications of Problems with Pacemakers.")

It is rare for a pacemaker to fail outright. In 1 to 2 percent of cases, leads may become dislodged and require reinsertion with a repeat catheterization.

Indications of Problems with Pacemakers

In the unlikely event that your pacemaker is not functioning properly you may experience any of the following signs and symptoms:

- Recurrence of original symptoms
- Shortness of breath or difficult breathing
- Dizziness or fainting
- Prolonged weakness or fatigue
- Chest pain
- Swelling of ankles, lower legs, wrists, or lower arms
- Muscle twitching
- Prolonged or excessive hiccupping
- Redness or drainage at the incision site
- Prolonged fever

If any of these symptoms occur, check your pulse and notify your physician as soon as possible.

Some patients exhibit "twiddler's syndrome," in which the patient tends to fiddle with the pacemaker in its pocket, which causes the device to rotate and sometimes dislodge or break the leads that go into the heart wall. For this reason, patients should consciously avoid "fiddling" with their pacemakers.

Pacemakers may occasionally sense and respond to outside signals that have nothing to do with demands on the heart, such as electrical activity in the muscles of the chest. Feelings of dizziness or lightheadedness may indicate that the device is not working properly and should be reported to the doctor.

Other complications that may arise include pacemaker pocket infection, the main symptom of which is reddening and tenderness at the site of the pocket. Such infection occurs in only about 2 percent of cases. Patients with single-chamber ventricular-pacing devices may experience a complication known as pacemaker syndrome, in which a lack of coordination between the upper and lower chambers reduces blood flow, resulting in fatigue and dizziness. Pacemaker syndrome can often be relieved by replacing the pacemaker with a dual-chamber device.

A problem sometimes found with dual-chamber pacemakers is an actual pacemaker-induced rapid heartbeat or tachycardia. The tachycardia results when the pacemaker stimulates the ventricle too early in the cardiac cycle (the sequence of events making up a complete heartbeat). The premature electrical impulse can flow backward over the AV node to the atria, triggering an atrial tachycardia in the same fashion as a premature ventricular contraction. Most new pacemakers have specific settings designed to prevent pacemaker-mediated tachycardia.

LIVING WITH A PACEMAKER

THE RECOVERY PERIOD

Most people adapt to their pacemakers quickly and soon find that they are hardly aware of them. For the first eight weeks, however, they need to take extra precautions. During this time, strenuous movement may dislodge a lead. Therefore the patient is advised to be careful moving the arm on the side in which the pacemaker has been implanted. The arm should not be raised above the head except to wash or dress. Sudden jerky actions should also be avoided. Activities that are prohibited for the first eight weeks include swimming, bowling, tennis, vacuum cleaning, carrying heavy laundry or trash, chopping wood, mowing or raking the lawn, and shoveling snow. After eight weeks, the lead becomes well set in the heart wall and the chance of dislodging it is decreased; the prohibited activities can then be gradually resumed.

CHECKING THE PULSE

Many physicians feel that checking the pulse regularly is not necessary. Other symptoms will serve as an alert if there is a problem. If an individual takes comfort in checking his or her pulse regularly, it should be taken for one full minute once a day at rest and at the end of any prolonged period of exercise. The pulse can be felt with the middle and index fingers on the inside of the wrist or on the carotid arteries on either side of the neck just under the jaw.

Each patient will have received from the physician an indication of his or her normal pulse rate range. If the pulse rate is five or more beats less than the lower end of the range and the individual is experiencing symptoms, the first step is to call the telephone monitoring clinic, if the patient is enrolled. Otherwise, the physician should be called, and if he or she is not available, the patient should be taken to the nearest hospital emergency room.

A pulse rate that is faster than the preset range is

not cause for alarm. On the contrary, it is a sign that the heart is probably beating on its own without using the pacemaker. However, if the pulse rate is consistently more than 100 beats a minute at rest, the physician should be notified.

CHECKING THE PACEMAKER SYSTEM

The entire pacemaker system—the battery and the leads—should be checked periodically. At Yale–New Haven Hospital, patients are scheduled for their first check approximately two weeks after implantation, followed by checks at three and six months. If they are to be enrolled in a telephone call-in service, office checks will be required only once a year; if not, checks will be scheduled every six months for the life of the pacemaker.

It is possible to check the pacemaker by telephone. Patients enrolled in a call-in service will receive a special transmitter that relays an electrocardiogram and the pacer rate over the telephone line. Although telephone service is not appropriate for some patients (such as infants and some elderly people), it is very convenient for those who can use it. According to current Medicare guidelines, pacemakers can be checked by phone every eight weeks for the first 37 months, then every four weeks for the life of the device. There is an expense involved in this approach, and some physicians do not believe that even a phone check is necessary more often than every four months or so during the first three to four years after the pacemaker is implanted.

USING ELECTRICAL APPLIANCES AND EQUIPMENT

Pacemakers being implanted now are well insulated and should not pose a problem around household appliances kept in good repair. The one exception may be older models of appliances or microwave ovens that are not well insulated. Even these can generally be used as long as the pacemaker patient avoids standing directly in front of one while it is operating. Just about any household appliance, from kitchen tools to hairdryers, radios, televisions, stereos, heating pads, and electric blankets, can be used without fear of problems. Office equipment, including copiers and computers, as well as woodworking and light metalworking shop tools, can also be used without concern. A few common-sense rules apply, however. All appliances should be kept in good working order to avoid electrical shock; repeatedly turning equipment on and off should be avoided. If electrical in-

terference is suspected, the individual should turn off the machine or move out of range.

ENVIRONMENTAL PRECAUTIONS

External sources of electrical signals such as antennas, high-voltage equipment, and heavy-duty electrical machinery can sometimes disrupt pacemaker functioning. The problem arises because a pacemaker may act as an antenna and pick up electrical signals from the environment. Unipolar pacemakers (in which pacemaker is the positive pole and the lead is the negative, forming a relatively larger antenna) are more likely to be affected. Most cardiologists therefore prescribe devices with bipolar sensing leads. Bipolar pacemakers have the negative and positive poles spaced closely together at the end of the lead, making them less likely to pick up the wrong signals. With the addition of improved insulation and shielding, the newer pacemakers are affected by only the strongest electrical fields, such as those around an industrial engine or a radio transmitter. Patients with pacemakers should also not be subjected to electrocautery during surgery if possible, since the large voltages involved can adversely affect their devices.

Magnetic fields may also pose problems. Passing through the magnetic field of an airport metal detector, for example, can reprogram the pacemaker and distort its ability to synchronize beats for the upper and lower chamber. In this state, the pacemaker will stop sensing properly, although it will continue to pace at a fixed rate sufficient to protect the patient until he or she can see a doctor. Nevertheless, *pacemaker patients should avoid metal detectors.* (Airport security personnel are accustomed to dealing with this problem and will perform a physical check instead.) In addition, pacemaker patients should not have magnetic resonance imaging (MRI) scans, because the exceedingly strong magnetic fields involved can dislodge pacemakers.

AUTOMATIC IMPLANTABLE CARDIOVERTER DEFIBRILLATORS

The use of electronic devices to treat life-threatening tachycardias is a relatively new and rapidly developing field. Although commonly called implantable defibrillators, these devices frequently supplement defibrillation with other modes of tachycardia termination. Since the first devices to counteract potentially lethal heart rhythm disorders were introduced in 1981, they have proved their ability to prevent sudden death caused by cardiac arrest. In patients at high risk for life-threatening arrhythmias, the rate of sudden death is only 1 to 4 percent among those who have had the device implanted, compared with 10 to 15 percent for those patients receiving drug treatment. Keep in mind, however, that these patients represent only a very small fraction of the population.

The technical name for the most common antitachycardia device is automatic implantable cardioverter defibrillator (AICD). Unlike pacemakers, which work to keep the patient's heart rate sufficiently high in one or both heart chambers, these implantable defibrillators slow down or halt excessively rapid heart rates that arise specifically in the ventricles. The aim is to prevent ventricular fibrillation, a state in which the ventricles contract in a completely unsynchronized, uncoordinated, or quivering manner that is insufficient to cause heart muscle contraction and the pumping of blood. This total lack of rhythm results in cardiac arrest, which can be fatal within minutes if there is no emergency intervention.

The typical candidate for an implantable defibrillator is a patient with a history of serious recurrent ventricular arrhythmias, indicating a high risk for sudden death. If drug therapy does not suppress the dangerous arrhythmias, then the patient may benefit from an implantable defibrillator. Often, patients who receive these devices are among the 20 percent of victims fortunate enough to have survived cardiac arrest.

Electrophysiology studies (EPS), in which electrodes are threaded via a catheter through veins to the heart and used to evaluate a patient's arrhythmia, are essential for anyone who might require an implantable defibrillator. Cardiologists use this diagnostic test to determine the types of arrhythmias to which the patient is susceptible and to localize any sites of poor conduction that may trigger a tachycardia. Electrophysiology studies are also used to evaluate medications and to test for any previously undetected heart problems. In rare instances, a patient undergoing electrophysiology studies to diagnose other arrhythmias may be found to be a good candidate for an implantable defibrillator, even though he or she has not experienced episodes of ventricular tachycardia that produced noticeable symptoms. Although patients may initially find the news that they need an implantable defibrillator upsetting, the overwhelming majority end up feeling thankful for their devices, which can help them to live free of the fear of sudden death.

HOW IMPLANTABLE DEFIBRILLATORS WORK

Implantable defibrillators use one or more of three basic modes of operation: antitachycardia pacing, low-energy cardioversion (a shock that restores normal heart rhythm), and defibrillation. Most devices in use today employ high-energy defibrillation for ventricular tachycardia or fibrillation. Experimental devices now undergoing clinical trials supplement this defense with antitachycardia pacing.

Antitachycardia pacing should not be confused with the pacing to treat bradycardia that is discussed earlier in this chapter. Rather, it short-circuits the rapid ventricular rhythms by sending brief bursts of impulses to the heart muscle at a pace faster than the already accelerated ventricular rate. The aim is to depolarize the heart muscle at the right moment, interrupting the abnormal rhythm and thereby halting the tachycardia. The tachycardia ceases within a few seconds, with no pain and little stress to the patient. A device can safely induce antitachycardia pacing hundreds of times per day if necessary, with little drain on its power source. This makes antitachycardia pacing especially attractive for patients who have frequent ventricular tachycardias that have not been controlled by medical therapy.

Low-energy cardioversion and defibrillation work differently from antitachycardia pacing. A device employing low-energy cardioversion to counteract ventricular tachycardia does so by delivering a mild shock to the heart muscle, in the range of 0.5 to 2 joules (a unit of energy). The shock depolarizes a small section of the ventricle, breaking the abnormal rhythm causing the tachycardia. Low-energy cardioversion is generally more reliable than antitachycardia pacing.

A low-energy shock, however, will not stop ventricular fibrillation, in which many currents flow through the heart muscle in a chaotic fashion. When an implantable defibrillator senses such a dangerous arrhythmia, it defibrillates just like the external electronic defibrillators used to revive patients in emergency care for cardiac arrest. Defibrillation requires a minimum 10-to-15-joule shock, but most devices deliver 30 joules to allow a margin of safety. Devices typically can give up to five shocks, pausing between each one to sense if the arrhythmia has been checked. This sequence can be repeated more than 100 times over the lifetime of the defibrillator.

Successful defibrillation will save the patient from sudden death, but there is no escaping the fact that the experience of receiving a shock can be distressing. Patients whose devices have fired often describe the shock as similar to a kick in the chest. Many patients lose consciousness from the arrhythmia in the 15 to 20 seconds required for the device to charge up and deliver the shock. Though some patients may be fearful of this experience, the vast majority find their devices reassuring. Currently, about half of patients with implantable defibrillators must also take antiarrhythmic drugs to cut down on extra ventricular contractions and suppress ventricular flutter and fibrillation, as well as other arrhythmias that might cause the device to fire too often or unnecessarily.

DEFIBRILLATOR IMPLANTATION

The defibrillation device is usually implanted using procedure called a thoracotomy (surgical opening of the chest), a more complicated operation than that required for pacemaker implantation. During the operation, two approximately 2-by-3-inch electrode patches are affixed to the outer wall of the ventricle. These patches, attached by guide wires to the device's

Figure 26.2
The power source (generator) of the defibrillator is implanted in a pocket underneath the skin on either side of the abdomen. Connected to the power source are leads, for heart rate monitoring and defibrillation, which are tunneled under the skin, up through the diaphragm to the heart. Electrode patches, affixed to the outer wall of the left ventricle, and the superior vena cava lead are used for defibrillation.

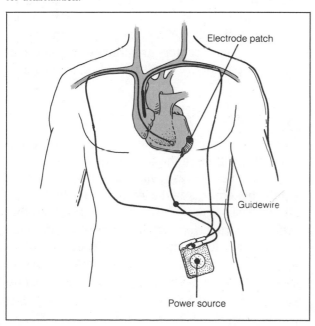

battery, will deliver the charge if the device is called on to defibrillate. The wires are then tunneled under the skin through the diaphragm to the abdomen. The power source and circuitry of the AICD are contained in a device a little larger than a deck of cards and weighing about 8 ounces; this is implanted in a pocket underneath the skin of the abdomen. This is easily felt through the skin. Some patients may find the power pack unsightly; future devices promise to be smaller and less obtrusive. (See Figure 26.2.)

Once the chest is opened for the defibrillator implantation, other desirable heart surgery, such as coronary arterial bypass, may be performed, because many candidates for an implantable defibrillator also suffer from coronary heart disease. After the defibrillator patches are in place, such operations become more difficult.

For some patients, a defibrillator may be implanted by using a sternotomy procedure, in which the main incision is made lengthwise over the breastbone, or a subxiphoid procedure, in which the main incision is made lengthwise below and slightly to the left of the breastbone. In both of these, a small incision near the collarbone may also be made.

After surgery, patients will usually spend a day or two in the coronary care unit, where they can be carefully monitored. Recovery will continue for another seven to ten days in the hospital (longer if other surgery is required), during which time activities are gradually resumed. The cardiologist may order a 24-hour ambulatory electrocardiogram (Holter monitor), electrophysiologic studies, exercise stress test, or a combination of several tests. (See Chapter 9.)

By the end of the week, the stitches are usually removed and, if all tests are completed, the patient is released to continue recuperating at home, generally for another six to eight weeks. The same general precautions recommended for pacemaker patients during the recovery period (see the earlier discussion of living with a pacemaker) are advised for patients with implantable defibrillators.

COMPLICATIONS

Implantable defibrillators save lives, but the devices carry some risks. Implantation thoracotomy is a major operation that has a significant, though small, mortality rate of 1 to 2 percent. Patients usually spend at least one week in the hospital (longer if other surgery is required) and another six to eight weeks recovering at home. In 4 to 5 percent of cases, infection requires removal of the device, an operation that often requires a repeat thoracotomy. A very few cases of scarring around the patch site that constricts the heart muscle have been reported as well. Although shocks delivered by the devices do not cause any apparent damage to the heart, inappropriate discharges will remain a potential problem until sensing capabilities are refined.

Implantable defibrillators may also impose lifestyle limitations. Because of the risk of fainting during defibrillation, patients with these devices may not be able to drive or operate heavy machinery. Regular follow-up exams must be performed at specialized clinics, which may mean travel over long distances. The power packs must be replaced every three to seven years, a procedure done under local anesthesia during a brief hospital stay or on an outpatient basis.

Most patients willingly trade these disadvantages for the reassurance that an implantable defibrillator can save them from fatal cardiac arrest. Patients typically express the hope that their device will never go off, but say they are glad to know it is there, just in case. Some 8,000 to 10,000 people in the United States now have implantable defibrillators. Of the 400,000 people who die each year from cardiac arrest, 30 percent of those at risk for sudden death can now be identified ahead of time, and may benefit from an implantable defibrillator. Those patients who still require antiarrhythmic drugs can take them in much lower doses, reducing side effects.

Future prospects for these devices are promising. Current devices requiring extensive surgery for implantation will eventually be replaced by defibrillators with leads that can be installed through the veins and electrode patches that are placed beneath the skin, making implantation no more invasive than pacemaker installation. Even so, today's implantable defibrillator represents a real triumph over life-threatening arrhythmias, enabling doctors to offer patients who might otherwise feel helpless before the risk of sudden death genuine assurance of enjoying a longer life.

LIVING WITH AN IMPLANTABLE DEFIBRILLATOR

ENVIRONMENTAL PRECAUTIONS

Patients with an implantable defibrillator should avoid strong electromagnetic fields, such as may be found surrounding heavy industrial equipment, arc welders, and transmitting antennas. In such an environment, the device may begin to generate beeping sounds as if it is being tested, or it may actually turn off. If this happens, the patient should move away from the equipment and call his or her physician for instructions as soon as possible.

INFORMING THE PHYSICIAN

The patient should inform his or her cardiologist each time a shock is received from the device. The physician should also be told about any symptoms of ventricular arrhythmias such as nausea, fainting, periods of unconsciousness, or an extremely rapid pulse rate. It is possible for the device to fire without the patient's experiencing symptoms of a rhythm disturbance. Conversely, the patient may experience symptoms of abnormal rhythm without the defibrillator issuing a shock. This may happen if the heart rate is too slow for the device to recognize.

ALERTING OTHERS

Patients with implantable defibrillators should always carry an identification card or, better yet, wear a Medic Alert identification (available from the non-profit Medic Alert Foundation as a bracelet or on a neck chain). Family and coworkers should be made aware of the condition and told what to expect if the device fires. For example, the shock, although mild, can be felt on the patient's skin on the chest and back. Other physicians, dentists, and any emergency care personnel (should the patient be transported to the hospital after a shock from the device) should be informed as well. Certain procedures such as diathermy (artificial raising of body temperature to high levels) and electrocautery treatments are contraindicated for patients with implantable defibrillators.

TESTING IMPLANTABLE DEFIBRILLATORS

In general, implantable defibrillators are tested every two months, although the cardiologist may set a different schedule. The test, which consists of checking the pulse generator and the leads, is done in the physician's office or clinic. A sensing device is used that discharges the pulse generator from outside the body to ensure that it is working properly. The patient does not feel a shock, however, since the shock stays inside the pulse generator. The test is usually not uncomfortable and the patient should report any discomfort to the physician.

CHAPTER 27

CARDIAC EMERGENCIES

MICHAEL REMETZ, M.D.

INTRODUCTION

One and a half million Americans will have a heart attack this year. Fortunately, two out of three will survive it, but that number could be much higher. Consider this: Of the 500,000 deaths that will occur, 300,000 will be within the first hour of the onset of symptoms. Most of these people will die before they reach a hospital. Almost three-quarters of these sudden deaths occur at home. A person who suffers a cardiac arrest outside a hospital has a 25 to 30 percent chance of surviving if cardiopulmonary resuscitation (CPR) is administered promptly; when CPR isn't started until an emergency medical team arrives, the survival rate is just 5 percent. Furthermore, the new clot-dissolving drugs used to treat heart attack, which can have a major impact on survival, must be administered promptly to be effective.

The conclusion is obvious: It is imperative for family members of cardiac patients (or of those at risk of developing coronary heart disease) to be able to recognize the warning signs of an impending heart attack, to know what to do in a cardiac emergency, and to learn the vital lifesaving skill of cardiopulmonary resuscitation.

During a heart attack, the heart is deprived of oxygen, but it may continue to function. A serious com-

plication of a heart attack is cardiac arrest, which occurs when the heart either stops beating or quivers (fibrillates) uncontrollably. When a person is in cardiac arrest, blood—and thus oxygen—is not pumped out of the heart to the rest of the body.

Cardiopulmonary resuscitation is a combination of breathing for the victim—to supply oxygen—and compressing the chest wall, which squeezes the heart and pushes blood out to vital organs. In this way, oxygen is delivered to the brain and to the arteries of the heart itself. Unless breathing and circulation are established within four to six minutes of a cardiac arrest, irreversible brain damage occurs, and eventually the individual dies. CPR cannot preserve life indefinitely, but it can keep a person alive until more effective medical intervention is available to restore normal heart function. For example, chest compression may help the heart muscle to pump blood, but it will not reverse fibrillation of the ventricles. The use of an electric shock to the heart may be necessary for this. CPR can, however, preserve functions until the patient goes to a facility with a machine that can defibrillate the heart muscle.

CPR is a valuable lifesaving skill that can be used not only to revive victims of a heart attack, but also in cases of drowning, suffocation, electric shock, severe allergic reaction, trauma, and drug overdose. An easy mnemonic for remembering its key components is *ABC*: opening and maintaining an *airway*; provid-

Quick Rundown of CPR Procedures for Cardiac Events

1. Tap person and shout, "Are you okay?" Call for help.

2. Position victim supine on floor.

3. Tilt head back to open airway.

4. Look, listen and feel for breathing.

5. Pinch nostrils, make a mouth-to-mouth seal and give two breaths.

6. Check pulse on side of neck.

7. If possible, have someone call 911 or the local emergency number, or do it yourself.

8. If pulse is present, give 12 breaths a minute. Recheck pulse.

9. If there is no pulse, give 15 chest compressions, then two breaths. Give three more sets of 15 and two. Check pulse. If there is still no pulse, continue sets of 15 and two until help arrives or until pulse returns and breathing resumes.

ing artificial respiration with mouth-to-mouth *breathing*; and applying external chest compressions to provide artificial *circulation*. (See box, "Quick Rundown of CPR Procedures for Cardiac Events.")

This chapter will describe basic life support skills, but it should not be considered a substitute for a hands-on CPR course that will allow you to learn under the supervision of an instructor and to practice your skills on a specially designed mannequin. Lives have been saved by rescuers without formal training who attempted CPR, and few would argue that it is better to try *something* while waiting for medical help than to stand by helplessly. Nonetheless, CPR done incorrectly may cause injury to the victim's chest and, worse, may be ineffective. For these reasons, you are urged to take a course.

CPR courses range from three-hour sessions teaching single-rescuer techniques for use on adults to longer (generally 9- and 12-hour) courses, teaching two-rescuer CPR and techniques for use on infants and children. To locate courses in your area, check with your local American Red Cross or American Heart Association. In addition, many hospitals and YMCAs provide CPR training. Finally, some large corporations sponsor on-site CPR courses periodically; if your employer does not have such a program, you may want to inquire about whether one can be initiated. The same organizations mentioned above may be able to provide teaching resources.

This chapter can, however, teach you how to assess an emergency and access the emergency medical care system, and you will develop some understanding of the techniques used in performing CPR. It will aid your comprehension if you visualize yourself performing each of the steps as you read about them. (You should never practice CPR on a person; instead, realistic dummies are used for practice sessions.)

WHO IS VULNERABLE TO A CARDIAC EMERGENCY?

A person who has already suffered a heart attack, or who has had episodes of angina pectoris (chest pain that lasts for several minutes triggered by exercise, emotional upset, or other causes), is particularly vulnerable to a cardiac emergency. This emergency need not be a cardiac arrest. It may be an episode of severe chest pain, a sudden episode of shortness of breath, or the sudden onset of a rapid heartbeat.

A number of factors are associated with increased risk of a heart attack or other cardiac emergency. Some are uncontrollable—family history of heart disease at an early age, for instance, remains an unalterable fact in a person's risk profile. Others are controllable—for example, the effect of obesity or high blood pressure on overall risk can be eliminated by maintaining an ideal body weight and keeping blood pressure at normal levels. The more risk factors a person has, the higher the odds that he or she will have a heart problem. It is important to familiarize yourself with these risk factors. Knowing them will also help you to identify family members who may be in danger of experiencing a cardiac emergency and to make the rapid decisions and assessments that will increase chances of survival. Not all of those stricken experience the classic symptoms, while others may deny that they are having a heart attack. (See Chapters 3, 5, and 11 for more complete information.)

If a family member is under the care of a cardiologist, discuss with the doctor ahead of time what you should do in case of an emergency. The doctor may help you develop an emergency plan or may prefer to be notified at the time of the emergency to give instructions about what, if any, medication to give and to which hospital the patient should be taken. Of course, if a cardiac arrest occurs, you may have to act on your own, even before calling the doctor.

TYPES OF CARDIAC EVENTS

In coronary heart disease (also known as coronary artery disease), fatty deposits called plaque build up on the walls of the arteries that feed the heart muscle. Eventually, blood flow to the heart is reduced to the point where the heart muscle cannot get enough oxygen, a condition known as *myocardial ischemia*, which may result in such symptoms as angina (chest pain) and shortness of breath on activity. In many cases, coronary artery disease leads to a heart attack, or myocardial infarction (which literally means "heart muscle death"). (See Chapter 11.)

Heart attacks often occur without warning, but they usually have classic symptoms. (See box, "Warning Signs of a Heart Attack.") Unlike angina, the pain associated with a heart attack does not diminish with rest and may last 30 minutes or longer. It may subside and return again (although it is never appropriate to delay getting help to see if it abates by itself). The pain may be experienced as a crushing pressure or a burning sensation in the middle of the chest. It may radiate to the shoulders or arms (typically on the left side, although either or both sides may be involved) or to the neck, jaw, or back. The individual may also feel dizzy, nauseated, or faint; he or she will feel clammy to the touch. A person having a heart attack may simply report an impending sense of doom or a vague feeling that "something isn't right." Often, a victim will deny that he or she is having a heart attack, attributing the symptoms to another cause, such as indigestion or a hiatal hernia.

Arrhythmias are abnormalities in the electrical activity controlling the rate or rhythm of the heartbeat. (See Chapter 16.) Some types of arrythmias may be life-threatening, as when the heart, rather than contracting forcefully, just quivers (a condition called fibrillation). Symptoms of an arrythmia include palpitations (an awareness of the heartbeat and, in some cases, the sensation that the heart is racing or "out of control"), shortness of breath, dizziness, fainting, and fatigue. Abnormalities of heart rhythm are quite common after a heart attack. The heart rate may become very slow (heart block), very rapid, or totally irregular.

Congestive heart failure is the inability of the heart to pump out all the blood that returns to it from the rest of the body. Symptoms will vary, depending on whether the left or right ventricle of the heart is most affected, but they may include shortness of breath, fatigue, cyanosis (blue tint to the skin), cough, swelling of the ankles, and sweating. Congestive heart failure is a chronic condition that usually develops slowly and can be managed with medication. One type, however, may come on suddenly and present a cardiac emergency. *Acute pulmonary edema* is a life-threatening situation in which the patient suffers extreme shortness of breath, cyanosis, pallor, fainting, restlessness, anxiety, a sense of suffocation, and, perhaps, wheezing or fainting. This situation may occur following a heart attack. Fortunately, it is reversible in most cases with proper treatment. Getting the patient to the hospital as soon as possible is a must.

GETTING EMERGENCY MEDICAL HELP

If symptoms of any of these cardiac events last longer than a few minutes or there is a medical history of heart disease, or several risk factors for heart disease exist, there is reason to suspect a cardiac emergency. Even in an apparently "healthy" person, if there is a pressing pain in the center of the chest, you should assume an emergency. In any case, prompt medical attention should be sought.

During a cardiac event, the victim may lose consciousness. If you have not witnessed the onset of symptoms, you must assume that immediate attention is necessary. It should be remembered, however, that shortness of breath or fainting can have several causes. If, for example, a person not known to have heart disease passes out in your presence in a warm

---

Warning Signs of a Heart Attack

- Steady, squeezing pressure or burning pain in the center of the chest that lasts two minutes or more
- Pain that radiates from the center of the chest down one (usually the left) or both arms and to the shoulders, neck, jaw, or back
- Sweating or clamminess
- Dizziness, light-headedness, or fainting
- Shortness of breath
- Nausea or vomiting
- A sense of anxiety or impending doom

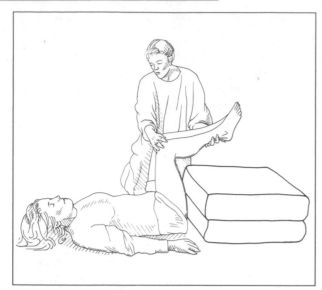

Figure 27.1
An unconscious person who has a pulse and is breathing has simply fainted. Placing him or her in a reclining position with legs slightly elevated in a cool environment is all that is needed.

room, or after a few drinks or a heavy meal, this is probably an instance of simple fainting. As long as the person is breathing, just letting him or her lie down for a few minutes may be all that is necessary. (See Figure 27.1.)

If a person experiencing cardiac symptoms is under the care of a cardiologist, call the doctor or follow your prearranged emergency plan. If the person does not have a cardiologist or if you cannot reach the doctor immediately, call the Emergency Medical Service (EMS)—accessible in all parts of the country by dialing 911. If possible, have someone else make the call while you stay with the patient.

Tell the EMS dispatcher that you suspect a heart attack. Give your exact location—street address with cross streets and, if applicable, floor and room or apartment number. Do whatever possible to make it easy for EMS technicians to get to the patient quickly. At night, turn on outside lights; if possible, have someone go to the edge of the driveway or to the lobby to keep the elevator free and to escort emergency personnel to the scene.

While you are waiting for medical help to arrive, keep the person calm and try to be reassuring. Make sure the individual is comfortable—for example, loosen tight clothing—but do not force him or her to lie down (unless he or she has fainted). It may be better in some instances for the person to be sitting up, because if vomiting occurs, the contents of the stomach may get into the lungs and cause an infection if the person is lying down. It is best not to allow the individual to drink anything, except for some water.

Hot or cold liquids or caffeine-containing beverages should probably be avoided, especially if heartbeat irregularities are present. If the individual is acutely short of breath but is not feeling faint or having severe chest pains, it may be useful to open a window (if the room is stuffy) and have him or her stand up. Standing may help shift the blood from the lungs to the abdomen and legs, and symptoms may ease somewhat.

BASIC LIFE SUPPORT/ ONE-RESCUER CPR

If you come upon an apparently unconscious individual or if the individual loses consciousness while you are waiting for the ambulance, you may need to start cardiopulmonary resuscitation. Be assured that it is natural to doubt your ability to perform CPR effectively or to fear that your strength will give out after only a few minutes. But when faced with a life-and-death medical emergency, chances are that you will not panic or faint and you will tap reserves of stamina you did not know you had. The important thing is that by knowing the warning signs of a heart attack or other serious cardiac event and by learning CPR, you may be able to give someone a second chance.

Following are the basic steps of CPR.

1. ESTABLISH UNRESPONSIVENESS AND CALL FOR HELP

First determine whether the victim is unresponsive. Kneel at right angles to the victim with your knees at about the level of his or her shoulder. Shake the victim gently by the shoulders while shouting, "Are you okay?" two or three times. (Whether or not they speak English, most people know what "Okay" means.) CPR is unnecessary if a person is conscious, so it is important to be sure that he or she is not just sleeping.

If you cannot arouse the individual, shout for help. If someone responds, and you have not already called EMS, have that person do so. If you are alone, continue your assessment. (See Figures 27.2A–B.)

2. POSITION THE VICTIM

Next you will need to position the individual properly in anticipation of having to perform CPR. The person must be lying on his or her back on a firm, flat surface

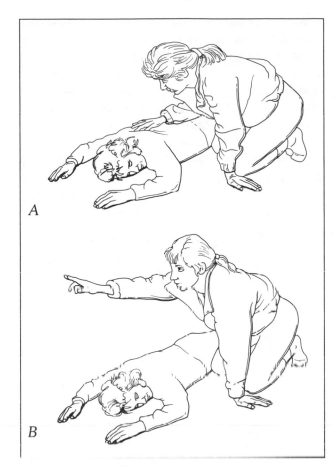

Figure 27.2A
Following the basic steps of cardiopulmonary resuscitation (CPR), first establish unresponsiveness. Gently tap or shake the victim and shout, "Are you okay?"

Figure 27.2B
If you cannot arouse the victim, shout for help.

in order for CPR to be effective. To turn over someone who is face down, first take the arm closest to you and stretch it out straight over his or her head. With one hand behind the victim's neck for support, grasp the other arm above the elbow and roll him or her toward you. Once the victim has been turned, place the arms alongside the body. (*Positioning the victim should take four to ten seconds.*)

3. OPEN THE AIRWAY

When a person loses consciousness, the tongue slackens, falling against the back of the throat, which cuts off the air supply from the mouth and nose to the lungs. To open the airway, place the hand that is closer to the top of the victim's head across the forehead and place the middle fingers of the other hand on the bony part of the jaw under the chin. Push down and back on the forehead while lifting the chin up. Since the tongue is attached to the lower jaw, this head-tilt/chin-lift maneuver lifts it away from the back

of the throat and will usually open the airway. (See Figures 27.2C–D.)

4. CHECK FOR BREATHING

Keeping the head tilted, check for signs of breathing. Place your ear over the victim's mouth and listen for the sounds of breathing; at the same time, look to see whether the victim's chest is rising and falling and check for the feel of exhaled air on your cheek. You must hear or feel air to know that the person is breathing; chest movement alone is not always a reliable indicator. Sometimes just opening the airway will allow the victim to resume breathing. If breathing does not start spontaneously and immediately, go to the next step. (*Checking for breathing should take three to five seconds.*)

Figure 27.2C
An individual who is not lying on his or her back must be repositioned. This is done by stretching the arm over the head. While supporting the victim's neck, gently roll him or her over. To open the airway, place one hand across the forehead and the middle fingers of the other hand on the bony part of the jaw under the chin.

Figure 27.2D
Push down and back on the forehead while lifting up the chin. Then check for breathing.

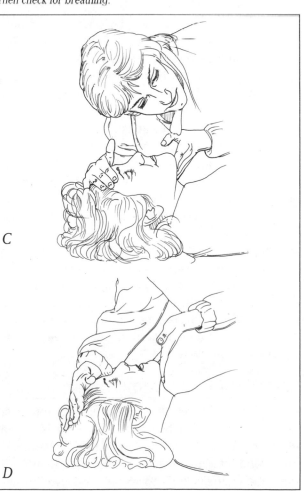

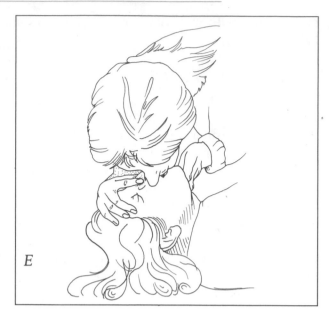

E

Figure 27.2E
Keeping the head tilted, pinch the victim's nostrils with your thumb and forefinger. Place your lips around the victim's mouth to make a tight seal. Give two forceful breaths, each taking 1 to 1½ seconds.

5. GIVE TWO RESCUE BREATHS

Maintaining the head tilt, use the thumb and forefinger of your hand that is on the victim's forehead to pinch off his or her nostrils to keep air from escaping from the nose. Breathe deeply, open your mouth wide, and place your lips around the outside of the victim's mouth to make an airtight seal. (If the victim wears dentures, leave them in so that you can get a tighter seal.) Exhale forcefully—but not too quickly —into the victim's mouth. Remove your mouth, take another deep breath, reestablish the seal, and exhale into the victim's mouth again. Each breath should take one to one and a half seconds. (See Figure 27.2E.) Watch for the chest to rise or expand as you blow air into the lungs. The victim's lungs should deflate between breaths. (When this happens, you will see the chest fall).

If you cannot feel the air going in as you blow and you do not see the victim's chest rise and fall, reposition the victim's head by attempting to open the airway again, and then repeat the two breaths. If you are still unsuccessful, assume the airway is obstructed and use the technique described later in the chapter for obstructed airways.

6. CHECK FOR CIRCULATION

To determine whether blood is circulating, you must check for a pulse. The best place to do this is on the carotid arteries, located on either side of the neck. While continuing to maintain the head tilt by keeping your hand on the victim's forehead, place two fingers

of your other hand on the voice box (Adam's apple). Then slide your fingers into the groove on the side of the neck nearest you and press gently. If you don't feel a pulse, move your fingers around a little. (See Figure 27.2F.) If you still cannot detect a pulse, your suspicions of cardiac arrest are confirmed, and you will need to initiate chest compressions to create artificial circulation of blood to the lungs, heart, brain, and other organs. (See box, "The Chest Thump.") If there is a pulse, performing chest compressions may result in serious medical complications. (*Checking for circulation should take five to ten seconds.*)

Figure 27.2F
1) While checking the pulse, maintain the open airway by keeping the head tilted with your hand on the forehead.
2) To check the pulse, place two fingers on the Adam's apple.
3) Then slide fingers into the groove on the side of the neck, and press gently to find the pulse. If the victim has no pulse, start chest compressions.

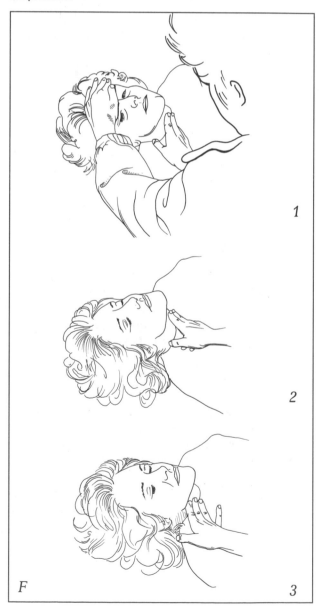

1

2

F

3

The Chest Thump

When a patient is in complete cardiac arrest, the heart is not pumping any blood. Sometimes a quick thump on the chest with the fist can restart the heart spontaneously, obviating the need for chest compressions. The chest thump should only be done in cases of a witnessed arrest—when you have actually seen the patient slump over and become unconscious.

When CPR was first taught to laypersons in the early 1970s, the chest thump was included as part of the procedure. In order to simplify instruction and because the chest thump was on occasion misused, the American Heart Association and other organizations have now dropped it from the curriculum. At Yale, however, we feel that it is a useful lifesaving technique. It only delays the start of chest compressions by a few seconds and may, in fact, make them unnecessary. We teach it to our personnel and we are recommending it here.

In the case of a witnessed arrest, make a fist with one hand, enclosing the thumb in the fingers. Hold your fist as if you were going to pound it on a table. Give a strong blow to the center of the chest across the bottom third of the breastbone. Check the pulse again. If the pulse does not return, begin chest compressions.

7. CALL 911 TO ACTIVATE THE EMERGENCY MEDICAL SERVICE (EMS) SYSTEM

If there is a pulse, but no breathing, continue rescue breathing. If there is no pulse, start compressions as well. In either case, if no one was around earlier to call EMS, the rescuer should stop now, call EMS, and return to the victim as quickly as possible.

8. PERFORM RESCUE BREATHING

If you detect a pulse but there is no breathing, start rescue breathing. Use the same technique as you did for the initial two breaths. Breathe for the victim at a rate of one breath every five seconds, or 12 breaths a minute. Although you will feel some resistance from the victim's lungs, you should be able to feel the air going in as you blow, and you should see the chest rise and fall. Continue until the victim resumes breathing on his or her own or emergency personnel arrive and are ready to take over.

After every 12 breaths, recheck for breathing and pulse. If the pulse disappears, start chest compressions.

9. BEGIN CHEST COMPRESSIONS

If the victim has no pulse, you must start chest compressions. (See also box, "The Chest Thump.") This is best done on a hard surface. If the victim is in bed and you have help or the victim is light enough for you to move, move him or her to the floor. Be sure to protect the head and neck while doing so. On the other hand, if the victim is very heavy and you are alone, it is better to attempt CPR on the bed than to try to move him or her and risk ending up in a position in which you cannot administer CPR at all. Quickly try to find something firm to slide under the victim's back. Is nothing is immediately available, attempt CPR anyway.

To begin chest compressions, kneel at right angles to the victim with your knees at about the victim's shoulder level. Reestablish the head tilt by once again pushing down and back on the forehead with the hand closest to the victim's head while using the middle fingers of the other hand to lift the chin up.

Now move your hand from the chin to the abdomen. With the middle and index fingers, locate the bottom margin of the rib cage (on either side and just above the waist) and follow the edge of the rib cage up toward the center of the chest. You will feel a notch where the ribs meet the breastbone; this is the sternum. Place your middle finger on this notch with your index finger next to it. (See Figure 27.2G.) Place the heel of your other hand on the sternum next to your index finger. Now place your first hand on top of the second (you can either extend the fingers of both hands or interlace them, but to avoid injury to the ribs, only the heel of your hand should come in contact with the chest). (See Figure 27.2H.)

Shift your weight forward on your knees until your shoulders are directly over your hands and your elbows are locked. Keeping your elbows locked, push down 1½ to 2 inches and come up again. To achieve the proper rate and rhythm for the compressions, count out loud: 1 and 2 and 3 and 4 and 5. The compression phase should be the same length as the time between compressions (about a half-second for each). Do not lift your hands from the victim's chest between compressions or you may lose the correct positioning. (See Figure 27.2I.)

After every 15 compressions (counting from 1 to 5 three times), give two breaths. Remove your hands from the chest, perform the head tilt as before, pinch the nostrils, make a tight seal over the victim's mouth with your lips, and give two quick breaths (remember to observe whether the chest is rising in response). Then reestablish the proper hand position for the chest compressions and do another set of 15.

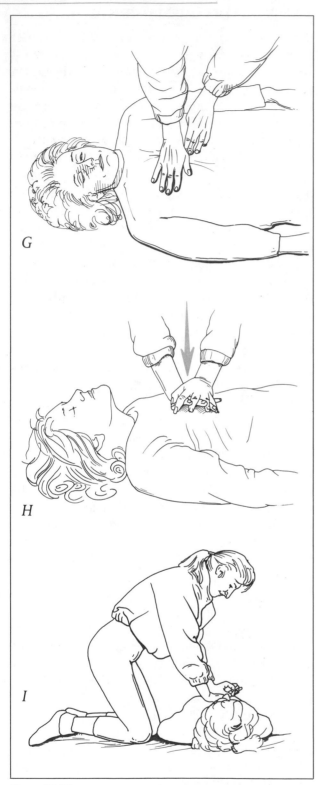

G

H

I

Figure 27.2G
To start chest compressions, position your hands by putting two fingers on the notch where the ribs meet the breast bone (sternum). Place the heel of your other hand next to your index finger.

Figure 27.2H
Now place your first hand on top of the second and either interlace fingers (as shown) or extend them to keep them off the chest.

Figure 27.2I
Shift your weight forward so that your shoulders are over your hands, keeping elbows locked. Push down 1½ to 2 inches with only the heel of your hand, and come up again.

Repeat this cycle of 15 compressions and two breaths four times (which should take about one minute), then reassess the victim for presence of pulse (which should take about five seconds).

If it is still absent, you must continue to perform CPR until:

- The victim regains consciousness (in which case he or she should be taken to the hospital immediately for evaluation and treatment).

- Another qualified lay rescuer or EMS personnel arrive to take over.

- You are too exhausted to continue your efforts.

OBSTRUCTED AIRWAY TECHNIQUES

Sometimes a person is unable to breathe because his or her airway is obstructed by foreign matter. (In adults, this is usually food.) This is not a cardiac emergency, but it may be interpreted as such because the individual may turn blue and may be gasping for air. At first the person is still conscious and may be clutching the throat. A simple way to determine if there is a blockage is to ask, "Are you choking?" If the person in distress cannot speak but can only nod, something is obstructing the windpipe, and you should perform the Heimlich maneuver. If the person can make sounds, then some air is getting through, and it may be better to let him or her clear the airway without your help by coughing or drinking liquids.

HEIMLICH MANEUVER

Stand behind the victim and encircle his or her waist with your arms. (See Figure 27.3A.) Make a fist with one hand, and place it, thumb side toward the victim, slightly above the navel. Grab your fist with your other hand and thrust your fist deliberately and forcefully inward and upward into the victim's abdomen. (See Figure 27.3B.) Air should be forced upward into the windpipe with enough pressure to expel the foreign matter. If it doesn't pop out, try again.

TECHNIQUE FOR UNCONSCIOUS PERSONS

If the person is unconscious and not breathing, and you have not already positioned him or her and attempted to open the airway and begin breathing, do

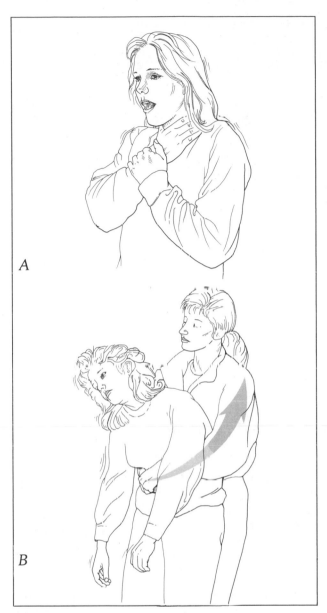

Figure 27.3A
A person who clutches the throat and cannot speak has an obstruction (usually food) in the windpipe. Performing the Heimlich maneuver will usually clear the airway.

Figure 27.3B
To perform the Heimlich maneuver, encircle the victim's waist with your arms from behind. Make a fist and place it slightly above the navel, thumbside toward the victim. Grasp the fist with your other hand and thrust forcefully inward and upward in the victim's abdomen to dislodge the foreign matter. Repeat if necessary.

so now. If you are unsuccessful, check for foreign objects by holding the tongue back and bottom jaw open with one hand while you use a hooked forefinger of your other hand to sweep the insides of the cheeks and throat. (Do not do this with a conscious person.)

Try rescue breathing again. If the airway remains blocked, use the Heimlich maneuver by straddling the victim on your knees and placing the heel of one hand on the person's abdomen just above the navel. With your second hand on top of your first, thrust both hands quickly upward into the abdomen. Give six to ten thrusts, then open the airway and attempt rescue breathing again. If the airway remains blocked, try the finger-sweep method again.

Keep repeating this sequence in rapid order: Heimlich maneuver, finger sweep, and rescue breathing. Without oxygen, the muscles relax; what was unsuccessful before may now work.

With pregnant or very obese persons, use the same technique but place your hands on the chest rather than the abdomen.

LEGAL ASPECTS OF CPR

Finally, a word about your legal obligations and liabilities. If you take a CPR course and become certified in basic life support, you may have a legal obligation to render assistance during a cardiac event or other medical emergency. However, "Good Samaritan" statutes will most likely protect you against legal action should the victim die, suffer irreversible brain damage before an EMS team arrives on the scene, or be injured as a result of the chest compressions or other lifesaving measures that may have been necessary. There are no known cases in which a layperson who performed CPR in good faith has been successfully sued.

CHAPTER 28

CARDIAC REHABILITATION

BARRY L. ZARET, M.D.

INTRODUCTION

All too often, general discussions of heart attacks or cardiac disease focus on risk factors and statistics, particularly on mortality. Of course, there is considerable justification for this emphasis—after all, cardiovascular disease remains the major cause of death in the United States and worldwide. Consequently, an overriding objective of cardiovascular medicine is to reduce risk and lower death rates. And there is no doubt that tremendous gains have been made in recent decades in lowering mortality from cardiovascular disease. But with this major emphasis on initially saving lives, many may overlook the short- and long-term prospects for the million or so people who survive heart attacks each year. Fortunately, this view has changed, and the change continues.

Rehabilitation initially focused primarily on patients who had had a heart attack. It is now clear that the rehabilitation process is equally important in patients who have undergone surgery or angioplasty, as well as in those who have stable coronary disease.

Obviously, simply surviving a heart attack or other major cardiovascular event is just the beginning of a long process. Physicians' objectives are to minimize the effects of the heart attack or other manifestation of cardiovascular disease and, as much as possible, to prevent future events in the setting of optimal quality of life. From a patient perspective, however, surviving the heart attack sets in motion a whole series of concerns and, at times, anxieties. After a heart attack, the big questions are: "How am I going to live the rest of my life?" and "What changes are going to be necessary?"

HISTORICAL PERSPECTIVE

Only a few decades ago, a heart attack often was viewed as the end to productive life—a harsh outlook for the typically middle-aged male patient. The heart attack survivor was told that from now on, he or she would have to "take it easy." Treatment usually consisted of weeks of bed rest. When the patient was finally allowed out of bed, he or she would feel extraordinarily weak. Often, this weakness was a result of the prolonged bedrest (a situation known as "deconditioning"). The patient would often misinterpret this state as a consequence of the heart attack, and become even more fearful of resuming former activities. In short, the person ran the risk of becoming a cardiac cripple, afraid to return to work or do anything that might provoke another heart attack.

The turning point came in the 1950s, as doctors

and patients alike came to realize that a heart attack was not necessarily the end of an active, productive life. The late Dr. Paul Dudley White and his most famous patient, President Dwight D. Eisenhower, did much to demonstrate this fact. After Eisenhower suffered a serious heart attack, Dr. White encouraged him to continue as President of the United States— perhaps one of the hardest, most tension-ridden jobs in the world—and to stay physically active. By fishing with his grandson, playing golf, or walking, President Eisenhower was setting an example for millions of fellow heart patients.

This is not meant to indicate that a heart attack is not serious. However, the patient can pick up and even enhance life afterward. Today, it is known that the majority of heart attack, surgical, and angioplasty patients can return to work, enjoy an active sex life, and resume other normal activities. For many, an acute event such as a heart attack can mark a vital turning point toward a more healthful life-style. As a result of cardiac rehabilitation, in recent years we have seen patients alter their diets, stop smoking, and change other detrimental habits. They have also become more physically active and have learned to cope better with stress. Along the way, many patients have gained a renewed sense of well-being and a better perspective of what is really important. Many of these patients actually enjoy better health after a heart attack than before! These results are the essence of successful cardiac rehabilitation.

Although rehabilitation must be tailored to each person's individual needs, virtually every heart attack patient can benefit from it. It can also benefit people with other forms of cardiovascular disease, including angina, heart failure, and impaired circulation, such as intermittent claudication. This chapter describes the basic principles of cardiac rehabilitation. Although virtually all heart attack patients can benefit from a rehabilitation program that includes physical activity, a word of caution is in order. Patients should not attempt to devise their own exercise program. Instead, a cardiologist or a specialist in cardiac rehabilitation should work with the individual to develop a program that takes into consideration particular circumstances. Furthermore, exercise is only one portion of the rehabilitation program. The process of rehabilitation involves the patient as a totality and also must include education, diet and nutrition consultation, stress modification and management, and emphasis on *permanent* modification of life-style. The patient on the program must always keep in mind the need for motivation and long-term maintenance of the program and its goals.

EMOTIONAL DOUBTS AND RESPONSES

People often assume that heart attack rehabilitation focuses mostly on physical activity. While exercise is an important part of cardiac rehabilitation, adjustment to the psychological impact of a heart attack may be the most important aspect affecting long-term goals.

A heart attack is a devastating event, not only for the patient, but also for the family and other loved ones. Often a heart attack strikes without prior symptoms and suddenly forces the patient to face his or her mortality. Because many heart attacks also occur with little or no warning, the typical patient is filled with denial and disbelief: "This couldn't be a heart attack—it must be a touch of indigestion or some other minor problem." (This type of denial could result in fatal delays in seeking emergency treatment.)

The real questions and doubts, however, come during the recovery period. The patient may ponder such questions as: "Am I going to be able to go back to work, and if so, when?" "How is this event going to change my life?" "What are my chances of having another heart attack?" Indeed, the fear of having another heart attack can paralyze the patient and hinder successful rehabilitation. Thus, many rehabilitation specialists recommend confronting underlying fears at the outset. In this regard, it should be noted that fear and worry are not confined to the patient; his or her spouse or companion is also likely to be fearful. Both the patient and spouse should consider appropriate professional counseling if these fears become dominant. Such counseling is often quite brief and extremely beneficial.

Many patients make the mistake of trying to suppress their fear and anxiety. They are reluctant to ask troubling questions, and thereby deny themselves opportunities for assurance. Remember, simply knowing what has happened and what to expect goes a long way toward allaying fear. This aspect of cardiac rehabilitation should start in the coronary care unit. Being hooked up to various monitors and undergoing high-tech lifesaving procedures can be frightening. With so much going on, doctors, nurses, and technicians don't always take the time to explain what is happening, and patients are often too frightened or ill to ask. When the immediate danger is past, however, the doctor should describe what has happened and what lies ahead. At this time, patients should begin to ask questions and express their concerns. Many persons are reluctant or embarrassed to do so, especially regarding subjects such as sex. (See box, "Sex After a Heart Attack.") The doctor or nurse may or may not anticipate unasked questions: "Are you concerned about whether this is going to affect your professional life, personal relationships, favorite pursuits?" Health care personnel should be able and available to discuss these issues, however, with little prompting from a patient. Today's approach to treating heart attacks helps put many of these fears to rest. They must at least begin to be addressed before discharge from the hospital.

THE HOSPITAL PHASE OF THE REHABILITATION PROCESS

Cardiac rehabilitation begins during hospitalization, not after discharge. Today's heart-attack patient who is free of complications is likely to be up and about in a day or two. At first, this activity may entail sitting up with feet dangling over the side of the bed or moving to a bedside chair while an aide remakes the bed. The patient may also be encouraged to do simple range-of-motion exercises, such as lifting and lowering the arms and legs. These exercises, which can be done sitting in bed, in a chair, or when standing, help prevent muscle and joint stiffness and the formation of blood clots, especially in the legs. Often a physical therapist will help with these exercises, at least initially. During this time, heart rate will also be monitored.

In a short time the patient will be encouraged to take a few steps around the hospital room, and then to take short walks in the hallway. A simple act like walking to the bathroom or strolling up and down the hall is reassuring. Early activity (ambulation) also prevents the muscle weakness and deconditioning that comes with prolonged bedrest.

Even though early ambulation is encouraged during the hospital stay, there will also be careful monitoring and, if needed, various interventions to treat or prevent complications. These interventions, varying from simple medication to angioplasty or bypass surgery, may be frightening; but it's important to know that they are now routine aspects of modern treatment and do not necessarily signal a turn for the worse. For example, disturbances in the heart's natural rhythm or pulse are common in the first few days or weeks after a heart attack. These rhythm disturb-

Sex After a Heart Attack

Despite society's increased openness regarding sex, this is one subject that is often neglected in planning rehabilitation after a heart attack. All too often, patients and spouses are embarrassed to ask their doctors about sex. Doctors are either equally embarrassed or mistakenly assume that if a patient doesn't ask, there is no problem.

Studies indicate that there is a decrease in sexual activity after a heart attack or coronary bypass operation. This decline is more often due to anxiety or fear on the part of the patient and partner than to any physical incapacity. Many people mistakenly assume that sexual intercourse is likely to precipitate another heart attack. This very rarely happens; in fact, a study by a team of Harvard researchers found that heart attack patients who were sexually active actually had a reduced risk of future heart attacks.

Just when is it safe to resume sexual activity? Although every situation must be individualized, we generally recommend that sexual intercourse may be resumed during the second week after hospital discharge. There are exceptions in both directions. Indeed, in the absence of actual intercourse, kissing, petting, and other expressions of physical closeness may begin immediately after hospital discharge, if the patient so desires.

Typically, intercourse raises the heart rate to about 130 beats per minute. (Studies show it may go somewhat higher in extramarital sex.) Blood pressure also rises, but only modestly. In general, sexual intercourse should be safe for any patient who can climb 20 stairs in 10 or 15 seconds without the heart rate going more than 20 to 30 beats per minute above the resting heart rate or provoking other symptoms, such as shortness of breath or chest pain. No one position for sexual intercourse is advantageous from a cardiovascular standpoint. In any case, severe fatigue or shortness of breath should be avoided. If intercourse provokes angina or other warning signs, the physician should be notified. Nitroglycerine can at times be taken beforehand as a preventive measure. Conversely, some medications used to treat angina, high blood pressure, and other forms of heart disease can interfere with sexual function. Any reduction in sexual desire or persistent dysfunction should be discussed with your doctor. If medication is the problem, an alternative drug may be prescribed.

Not uncommonly, it is a spouse who is reluctant to resume sexual activity out of fear of causing harm. These anxieties should be recognized and discussed with the doctor.

ances may be due to damage to the heart's electrical system, the natural pacemaker cells that control the rhythmic contractions of heart muscle. Continual electrocardiographic (ECG) monitoring can detect abnormal changes prior to development of a severe arrhythmia or can warn of another impending heart attack. Medication may be given to stabilize the heartbeat. Don't hesitate to ask your doctor or nurse what is going on—simply knowing what is being done and why can be reassuring, and can help in achieving the peace of mind that is essential to full recovery.

Increasingly, the hospital rehabilitation phase also includes patient education sessions regarding lifestyle, diet, and detrimental habits, such as smoking. If the patient has smoked, this is the ideal time to stop. Most hospitals now ban smoking, so there probably will be no choice but to forgo cigarettes during this time. Unfortunately, many patients return to smoking after leaving the hospital. Numerous studies show that continued cigarette use increases the risk of a subsequent heart attack. Thus if the temptation exists to resume a cigarette habit after discharge from the hospital, patients should be referred to a smoking cessation program. There are many approaches to smoking cessation—the self-quiz in Chapter 6 can help the individual focus on which one is most appropriate. If possible, smoking cessation should be incorporated into the initial phase of the rehabilitation program. It may well be one of the most important steps taken in preventing a future heart attack or another life-threatening disease.

While the patient is in the hospital, meals will be provided. There may be some menu choices, but on the whole, hospital food does not rate culinary stars. Often patients say they look forward to eating "real food" again, and for many, this means the typical American diet, high in fat and calories. While it is not necessary or appropriate for patients to adopt a lifelong hospital diet, returning to former faulty eating habits is absolutely contrary to the total approach to cardiac rehabilitation. Patient education sessions should also involve direct interaction with a dietitian, either in a group session or in an individual consultation. In either case, these sessions should also include the patient's spouse, or whoever is responsible for food shopping and meal preparation.

Before the patient leaves the hospital, a dietitian should consult with him or her to work out an exact eating program that can be followed at home. This program should take into account any nutrition-related health problems, such as obesity, osteoporosis, or diabetes, as well as individual preferences and religious or ethnic food restrictions. (See Chapter 5 for a more detailed discussion of diet and heart disease.)

Also before leaving the hospital, the patient, if sufficiently stable, should generally undergo a modified exercise tolerance (or stress) test. This test entails exercising on a treadmill or stationary cycle while the heart's electrical activity (ECG) and blood pressure are monitored. It differs from a standard exercise tolerance test in that the patient will not be allowed to exercise to his or her peak tolerance. Instead, the goal is to make sure the patient can safely engage in normal activities, such as walking up a flight of stairs, without provoking symptoms. In addition, this test may uncover patients who are at high risk for further heart attacks and therefore should be treated more aggressively. Other studies such as a thallium scan (see Chapter 10) are frequently done at this time in conjunction with the routine exercise stress testing.

Using a modified exercise test as a guideline, the doctor can prepare an exercise prescription to be followed initially at home and used in the next rehabilitation phase. Generally, following hospital discharge, the patient is referred to a supervised exercise program as part of the total cardiac rehabilitation plan. Such programs are widely available at facilities such as hospital outpatient units, clinics, or organizations such as the YMCA. (See box, "Criteria for Judging a Rehabilitation Program.")

GOALS OF EXERCISE TRAINING OR REHABILITATION

As stated previously, exercise, although important, is only one component of total rehabilitation. There are many misconceptions regarding what an exercise conditioning program can and cannot do. For example, several long-term medical studies have shown that groups of people who are physically active live longer than their more sedentary counterparts. But these statistics are for population groups, and thus there is no guarantee that any one person who undertakes an exercise program will enjoy increased longevity. Similarly, there is no guarantee that cardiovascular exercise conditioning will prevent a subsequent heart attack. Still, there are clear and well-documented benefits that generally enhance the quality of life for most people. These include:

Criteria for Judging a Rehabilitation Program

Questions patients should ask when considering a formal cardiac rehabilitation program include:

- *Who is in charge?* An organized cardiac rehabilitation program should be directed by a qualified physician. When the doctor is not present, a nurse or other health professional with training in rehabilitation and emergency cardiovascular procedures should be on hand.

- *What role will my own doctor play?* At the least, the program should require referral from your personal physician. The program should also require a medical examination before enrollment, and your medical record should be reviewed, especially if you have had a recent heart attack, coronary bypass surgery, or other significant cardiovascular event. A pre-enrollment exercise test may be performed under your physician's supervision or under one at the rehabilitation facility itself.

- *What sort of exercise facilities do you have?* There should be a track, either indoor or outdoor, where participants can walk or jog. Stationary bicycle machines and/or treadmills are part of the Phase II program. A track is usually part of the Phase III program. Otherwise, elaborate exercise machines and facilities are not necessary. The knowledge and guidance of the program leaders are more important than expensive gear.

- *How will my program be developed?* At the very least, it should be individualized to meet your particular needs. It may be based on your doctor's exercise and rehabilitation prescription, or on one that is developed by the program physician after you undergo a medical examination. This individualization is the major difference between a medically supervised cardiac

rehabilitation program and commercial fitness programs, which often assume all participants will follow the same regimen.

- *What provisions are there for handling emergencies?* In addition to trained medical personnel, emergency equipment such as a defibrillator should be on hand in the exercise area. This equipment should be inspected periodically to make sure that it is in good working order.

- *Who actually directs the exercise sessions and what sort of training does he or she have?* The exercise director should be trained to work with heart patients.

- *Are the participants monitored during exercise sessions?* For most participants, periodic checks of pulse rate and blood pressure are all that is needed. Most participants can quickly learn how to do these checks themselves. For high-risk patients, continuous ECG (Holter) monitoring may be advised for the first few sessions to determine whether exercise provokes changes in the heart's rhythm.

- *Do you concentrate solely on exercise, or do you address other life-style factors as well?* As emphasized throughout this chapter, exercise conditioning is only one aspect of the total approach to cardiac rehabilitation. Modification of other risk factors, including weight control, dietary changes, smoking cessation, and stress management, is also important. Some rehabilitation programs offer counseling sessions for both heart patients and family members, occupational therapy, behavior modification and/or stress-management training, and weight control programs.

- Improved endurance and strength
- Increased sense of well-being
- Improved weight control
- Enhanced self-image

In addition, the exercise component of a total approach to rehabilitation helps overcome the fears and anxieties that so many people experience after a heart attack. Simply knowing that you can walk or jog around a track or work out on an exercise cycle provides the confidence that you can safely undertake other normal activities, including going back to work, resuming sexual relations, or enjoying a family outing.

DESIGNING AN EXERCISE REHABILITATION PROGRAM

First and foremost, any exercise component of cardiac rehabilitation must be tailored to the individual participant. There are general guidelines, but no one program applies to all persons. (See box, "Typical Exercise Session.")

Ideally, cardiovascular exercise conditioning should be derived from a physician's prescription based on the following considerations:

- The results of a thorough physical examination

Typical Exercise Session

There is no one exercise program or session that is ideal for all persons who have had a heart attack, angioplasty, or coronary bypass surgery. Instead, there are many variations and levels of intensity. Your doctor is the best judge of what is the most appropriate for you. In general, however, each exercise session is divided into three parts:

- *Warm-up* (five to ten minutes). All exercise sessions should begin with a few minutes of warm-up or stretching calisthenics. These range-of-motion exercises, which are designed to tone and stretch muscles and manipulate joints, are important in preventing orthopedic injuries.

- *Aerobic conditioning* (up to 30 minutes or more depending upon the activity and exercise prescription). Walking, jogging, cycling, swimming, climbing stairs, and working out on a rowing or climbing machine are all excellent aerobic activities.

- *Cool-down* (five to seven minutes). These are transitional exercises, which may be similar to the warm-up routine or simply a slow-paced continuation of the aerobic activity. They are designed to help muscles readjust to a resting state and to prevent cramping and other problems that may follow a vigorous workout.

that includes an exercise stress, or tolerance, test and assessment of cardiovascular risk factors

- Overall state of health, including physical fitness and previous exercise history

- Individual preferences and physical limitations (For example, arthritis or previous stroke can limit capabilities in certain types of exercise.)

In general, for an exercise program to improve cardiovascular fitness, it should (1) be sufficiently intense to have a conditioning effect, and (2) be undertaken at least three times a week, with each session lasting at least 20 to 30 minutes. Of course, it may take time to achieve the objectives. For example, in the beginning, a previously sedentary person who is in poor physical condition may be able to exercise for only a few minutes at a relatively low level of intensity. But most patients find that after a few weeks of gradually increasing the intensity and duration of each exercise session, they begin to experience a marked improvement in endurance.

ORGANIZED VS. HOME EXERCISE PROGRAMS

In recent years, there has been a marked increase in the number of medically supervised exercise programs for heart patients. Many of these programs are offered by hospital or medical center outpatient departments or research laboratories; others are offered by fitness centers or organizations such as the YMCA. Still others are commercial programs. Some are covered by insurance and some are not. (See box, "Insurance Reimbursement.")

Some experts contend that there is no need for a formal cardiac rehabilitation program for the majority of low-risk persons, and that such patients can accomplish what needs to be done on their own after two or three instructional sessions with a physician or rehabilitation specialist. At these sessions, which may begin in the hospital before discharge or on an outpatient basis in the first few weeks of at-home recuperation, the person learns how to monitor his or her pulse rate and how to do the basic warm-up and cool-down exercises. (See box, "How to Take Your Pulse," and Figures 28.1 and 28.2.)

The person will be instructed to follow an exercise prescription for a graduated cardiovascular conditioning program that includes exercises for muscle toning and strength building as well as aerobic activity such as walking, swimming, cycling, or a combination of exercises. Pick an activity that is enjoyable—one is more apt to continue an exercise if it is fun and not drudgery. Also, pick one that is convenient. Figure 28.3 shows a stationary cycle that may be used at a health club or at home. Many people become overly preoccupied with taking their pulse rates, blood pressure, and other aspects of self-mon-

Insurance Reimbursement

Insurance coverage for medically supervised cardiac rehabilitation varies considerably from state to state and company to company. Some policies cover only a limited number of outpatient sessions; others will pick up the tab for an entire 12-week program. Check with your insurance carrier to determine precisely what is and is not covered.

How to Take Your Pulse

1. Place palm up.
2. Use first two fingers of opposite hand. Do not use thumb.
3. Place first two fingers of opposite hand on the wrist in line with the thumb and feel the pulsation. This is the radial artery.
4. Count the number of pulsations you feel in 15 seconds and multiply by four for the heart rate (pulse).

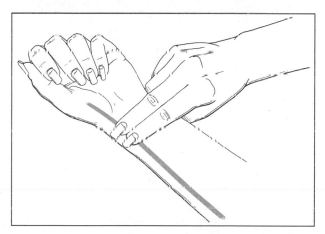

Figure 28.1
Taking the pulse using the radial artery.

itoring. After a few sessions, the individual should be able to judge without constantly stopping to take the pulse whether the exercise is vigorous enough or whether he or she is overdoing it. (See box, "Guidelines for Home Exercise Conditioning.")

The organized rehabilitation is more structured and more closely monitored. Proponents of organized programs point to a number of advantages that are lacking with home programs:

- *Exercise is done under direct medical supervision.* This is more important for high-risk patients, such as those who experience angina during physical activity or who have disturbances in cardiac rhythm or a drop in systolic blood pressure when exercising. Unsupervised exercise may also be risky for a survivor of a cardiac arrest. Since recurrent heart attacks are more common in the weeks or first few months after the initial one, medical supervision during exercise may be more important during this period than later. In addition, the presence of a

physician or other medical personnel helps overcome the fear that many patients experience in starting an exercise program.

- *There are psychological benefits in group activity.* Many participants in cardiac rehabilitation programs describe the importance of realizing that they are not alone, and that their fears are shared by others who have had similar experiences. Seeing the determination and progress of fellow patients, some of whom may be severely affected, provides extra encouragement. Also, the camaraderie of a group effort makes exercise more enjoyable.

- *An organized program may provide extra motivation to "stick with it."* All too often, a person leaves the hospital after a heart attack filled with determination to change his or her ways, to lose weight, stop smoking, start exercising, and so forth. Typically, the determination lasts for a few weeks, and then, as the fear recedes and life settles back into normal routine, the person begins to backslide into former habits. This is not as likely to happen if the person participates in an organized program. Also, if a person is paying to participate in a rehabilitation, he or she may be more compliant.

For these reasons, we generally favor organized rather than at-home rehabilitation programs. Since the strides taken at this time may influence the remainder of the patient's life, the most rigorous and careful monitoring and motivating are essential.

This latter point brings up the question of how long the rehabilitation program should last. There is no clear agreement among cardiologists and rehabilitation specialists. At Yale, we generally approach cardiac rehabilitation as a three-phase process.

- *The in-hospital phase* (Phase I). As soon as the patient is out of acute danger, he or she begins passive range-of-motion exercises, which progress over several days to early ambulation. The patient is expected to sit up and, as soon as possible, begin to walk and perform simple self-care tasks. Patient education is an important aspect of this phase, with input from physicians, nurses, dietitians, and other caregivers. By the time the patient leaves the hospital (typically five to nine days after the heart attack and a bit longer after coronary bypass surgery), he or she will have the basics of an at-home program for recuperation and rehabilitation.

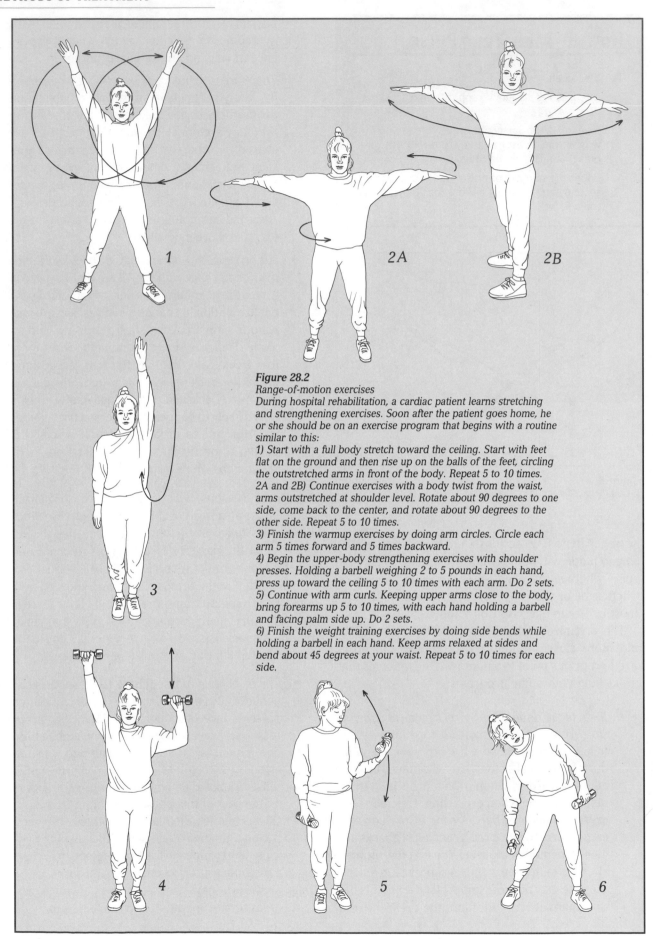

Figure 28.2

Range-of-motion exercises

During hospital rehabilitation, a cardiac patient learns stretching and strengthening exercises. Soon after the patient goes home, he or she should be on an exercise program that begins with a routine similar to this:

1) Start with a full body stretch toward the ceiling. Start with feet flat on the ground and then rise up on the balls of the feet, circling the outstretched arms in front of the body. Repeat 5 to 10 times.

2A and 2B) Continue exercises with a body twist from the waist, arms outstretched at shoulder level. Rotate about 90 degrees to one side, come back to the center, and rotate about 90 degrees to the other side. Repeat 5 to 10 times.

3) Finish the warmup exercises by doing arm circles. Circle each arm 5 times forward and 5 times backward.

4) Begin the upper-body strengthening exercises with shoulder presses. Holding a barbell weighing 2 to 5 pounds in each hand, press up toward the ceiling 5 to 10 times with each arm. Do 2 sets.

5) Continue with arm curls. Keeping upper arms close to the body, bring forearms up 5 to 10 times, with each hand holding a barbell and facing palm side up. Do 2 sets.

6) Finish the weight training exercises by doing side bends while holding a barbell in each hand. Keep arms relaxed at sides and bend about 45 degrees at your waist. Repeat 5 to 10 times for each side.

• *The outpatient phase* (Phase II). After two or three weeks of at-home recuperation, most patients have recovered sufficiently to be referred to an advanced rehabilitation program. These programs vary considerably. The ones offered at Yale generally call for three or four medically supervised group exercise sessions a week, each lasting 30 to 60 minutes. Depending upon the individual patient, there will also be extra sessions for smoking cessation, weight control, cholesterol control, stress modification, and special counseling. This outpatient program usually continues for an average of two months.

• *The community phase* (Phase III). By this time, the typical patient has recovered sufficiently to return to work or resume other normal day-to-day activities. Further rehabilitation is often needed to achieve the lasting life-style modifications that reduce the risk of subsequent heart attacks or other cardiovascular events. There may no longer be a need for a medically supervised program, but the person still can benefit from participating in a group effort. Appropriate programs are now available in most communities. Some are offered in a medical set-

Figure 28.3
Many cardiac patients find that a stationary cycle provides a convenient way to work out.

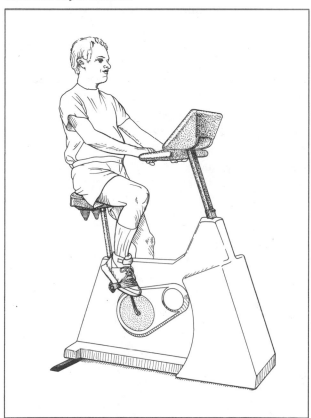

Guidelines for Home Exercise Conditioning

Almost anything that you do in an organized exercise or fitness program can be accomplished on your own at home. You don't need to invest in a home gym, although you may want to have a stationary cycle or treadmill that you can use indoors when the weather is not suited for outdoor exercise. Your doctor or rehabilitation therapist can work with you to draw up a specific regimen, but here are practical tips to get you started.

• Set aside a specific time to exercise three or four times a week and stick to it. Some people prefer to work out in the early morning; others find that a session at the end of the workday helps change gears and relax. The time of day is not as important as making it a part of your regular routine.

• Wear loose-fitting, comfortable clothing that is appropriate for the temperature and weather.

• Pay particular attention to your shoes. Invest in a good pair of exercise shoes that are designed specifically for your chosen activity (for example, walking or jogging).

• *Always* include warm-up and cool-down exercises in each session. These help prevent the orthopedic problems that put many exercisers on the sidelines.

• Do not exercise immediately after a meal; wait at least 30 to 60 minutes.

• When it is hot and humid, plan your exercise for the coolest part of the day, or exercise in an air-conditioned indoor area.

• Avoid exercising outdoors during periods of smog or heavy air pollution.

• Avoid exercising outdoors when temperatures fall below freezing or when there is excessive wind.

ting; organizations such as Mended Hearts, Inc. and the YMCA offer other programs. Some fitness clubs also have special programs for heart patients. Programs are also offered by some employee health departments. This phase generally lasts 6 to 12 months.

A large number of heart attack patients find that by this stage, they no longer need to participate in a group rehabilitation effort. Instead, they have modified their life-styles sufficiently to include all of the aspects offered in an organized program. If a patient falls into this category and is sufficiently motivated to follow through on his or her own, there may be no reason to join a group unless the patient truly enjoys the camaraderie or other benefits of a more organized effort. The aspect of group interaction and support should not be underemphasized and may be of great value to particular individuals.

Regardless of whether the rehabilitation is self-directed or carried out in a medically supervised setting, it is important that the individual learn to listen to his or her body in order to recognize possible warning signs. The majority of patients who survive a heart attack make a good recovery and are able to safely participate in a common-sense exercise program. But after a heart attack, there is always an increased risk of a recurrence; this risk exists in both sedentary and active patients. The patient should know when to stop and seek medical attention. (See box, "Important Warnings to Stop Exercising.")

Important Warnings to Stop Exercising

Stop exercising if you experience any of the following symptoms. Rest for a few minutes, and if the symptom persists, seek immediate medical attention.

- Chest pain
- Pain that spreads to the arms, ear, jaws, or back
- Light-headedness or dizziness
- Excessive fatigue
- Shortness of breath
- Excessive sweating
- Nausea or vomiting
- Irregular pulse
- Increased pulse rate that persists for more than five or six minutes after you stop exercising

In addition, stop exercising if you experience any unusual joint or muscle pain that may indicate an orthopedic injury.

GOING FORWARD

For most people, a heart attack or other major cardiovascular event marks an important turning point. Some emerge fearful and resigned to fate, convinced that it's too late to make any meaningful changes. Others regard the event as an opportunity to make a new beginning. Obviously, we would prefer that all our patients (as well as readers of this book) fall into this latter category. We are realistic enough to recognize that a heart attack *is* a life-threatening event. But for the majority of persons who have heart attacks each year, it is *not* the end to life. And it can mark a new beginning.

It's important to remember that no matter how determined one is to mend one's ways, one should not attempt to change 40 or 50 years of sedentary living and other possible detrimental habits overnight. A gradual, common sense program to modify life-style is more apt to succeed than a go-for-broke approach. The patient should work out a list of priorities with his or her doctor and then tackle the most important one or two at a time. It is neither realistic nor desirable to do everything at once. Expect an occasional lapse, forgive yourself, and go forward from there. Even though the patient is responsible for a comeback from a heart attack, it's important to remember that he or she does not function alone. The doctor, family, and loved ones must be considered a part of the individual's rehabilitation team.

CHAPTER 29

THE PATIENT AS A CONSUMER

MARVIN MOSER, M.D.

INTRODUCTION

Medical consumerism is a relatively new phenomenon that, along with the technological revolution, is changing the practice of medicine in this country. When I first began my medical practice some 40 years ago, medicine was still a cottage industry in which individual doctors provided almost total medical care for their patients. In those days, most of my patients wanted me to decide how and when they should undergo treatment, and they hesitated to question a medical decision. This attitude was by no means unique to my practice—that's simply the way medicine was practiced. All too often, patients would say: "Don't tell me what the options are—just do what you think is best."

Of course, this description no longer applies to the practice of medicine—at least not in the United States. Medicine is now a major industry in which technology has, in many instances, replaced the old standbys of observation, experience, and intuition (what we once called the "art of medicine"). It is certainly true that the advances in technology over the last few decades enable us to diagnose and treat many diseases that were once invariably fatal; the discovery of new drugs has certainly improved care. But along with technology, expansion, and testing has come a great deal of impersonalization and increased cost.

Unlike their parents and grandparents, today's patients *do* want to know about every aspect of their health care. Indeed, informed consent—which dictates that patients be fully informed before undergoing any major medical procedure—is now mandatory in most areas of medicine. More important, today's patient expects to participate in many of the decisions regarding his or her health care. Increased patient responsibility mandates that physicians take the time to explain the steps in diagnosis and treatment.

As a physician, I applaud this increased patient participation in areas that were once the exclusive domain of physicians. But if patients are to work with their physicians in a way that is truly in their best interest, it is essential that they become and remain well informed, and this may be difficult. Today's medical consumers are bombarded with information and advice. It's a rare newscast or newspaper that doesn't carry at least one news story about a medical advance or, just as often, a story refuting a previous pronouncement. Medical entrepreneurs' advertisements prevail on TV, in magazines and newspapers, and on bus and subway posters, often to the point of the ridiculous.

All too often, the messages and claims directed to health care consumers are conflicting or misleading; unfortunately, many are deceptive. Thus, the problem for today's medical consumers is not a lack of available information; instead, it's deciding what and whom to believe.

Lurking behind much of this so-called consumer health information is a blatant profit motive, for clearly there are huge profits to be made in delivering health care. As a nation, we spend far more for medical care than any other industrialized country. Health care now consumes about 11 to 12 percent of the nation's gross national product, and the health care industry is the fastest growing sector of the nation's economy.

Even so, billions of our health care dollars are being misspent each year. For example, Americans spend more than $25 billion a year on health quackery. Some economists estimate that we could reduce the nation's medical bills—which total more than $650 billion annually—by a third simply by eliminating waste, unnecessary procedures, and health fraud. In my opinion, achieving these goals should be the major focus of medical consumerism.

PROTECTING YOURSELF FROM HEALTH FRAUD

The late U.S. Representative Claude Pepper defined a quack as "anyone who promotes medical schemes or remedies known to be false, or which are unproven, for a profit." Many people think of medical quackery in terms of a sleazy, fast-talking huckster who goes from town to town peddling snake oil and other potions. They assume that because this type of charlatan is so easy to spot, they are in no danger of falling victim to a quack's sales pitch. Sadly, today's quack is a far cry from the turn-of-the-century medicine man, even though his or her remedies may be no more effective than snake oil. Dr. Victor Herbert, a nutrition scientist who has devoted much of his medical career to fighting health and nutrition fraud, writes in his *Mount Sinai School of Medicine Complete Book of Nutrition*: "The notion that it is easy to spot nutrition quackery and charlatans is false because today's quacks hide behind a cloak of science and respectability. They have impressive-looking certificates and degrees hanging on their walls; they use 'scientific' terms, appear on television talk shows, and write best-selling books touting their theories or products. They sound and look convincing, and their message is one that millions of people want to believe." (See box, "Tips on Avoiding Health Fraud.")

Because heart disease is still the leading cause of death in this country, it is understandable that heart

Tips on Avoiding Health Fraud

- Be wary of anyone with unfamiliar or strange-sounding degrees such as DN (Doctor of Naturopathy) or DM (Doctor of Metaphysics). To check a practitioner's credentials, check with your local medical society or look the name up in the *Directory of Medical Specialists* at your local library.

- Be wary of anyone who claims to offer an *exclusive* or new treatment that is unavailable elsewhere. Ask to see supporting evidence from *peer-reviewed* medical journals that describe the testing and efficacy of the treatment.

- Be wary of practitioners who ridicule traditional medicine and claim that their ideas and practices are rejected by the profession because of spite or greed.

- Be suspicious of any regimen or nutritional product that promises miraculous results, such as fast, painless weight loss; a cure for heart disease, cancer, or any other incurable or chronic disease; or a means of recapturing lost youth or sexual prowess. Remember the old adage, "If it sounds too good to be true, it probably is."

- Be wary of any treatment that requires you to travel to another country, such as an offshore island or a Mexican border town.

- Be wary of promises couched in medical jargon or pseudoscientific terms, such as regimens to "detoxify" your body or "correct chemical imbalances."

- Be wary of practitioners who sell an exclusive line of health remedies, such as high-potency vitamins or energy boosters.

patients are the targets of many questionable claims. Recent examples include:

Chelation therapy to "cure" atherosclerosis. Chelation entails administering a drug that binds with a substance, usually a mineral such as iron, lead, or copper, to remove it from the body. Practitioners of chelation therapy for atherosclerosis claim that because the fatty plaque that builds up in the arteries contains the mineral calcium, it can be removed from the body via chelation. There is no good evidence that this is of any benefit against atherosclerosis.

Biofeedback machines and other devices to lower blood pressure. While it is true that yoga, meditation, and biofeedback techniques may produce temporary reductions in blood pressure, there is no proof that over the long term they are effective in lowering blood pressure.

Herbal remedies for heart disease. Some of these can be highly dangerous. Tea brewed from foxglove (digitalis plant) can cause a digitalis overdose. Although folklore is full of herbal remedies, none of these should be used as a substitute for traditional drugs, which are subjected to testing and quality control.

In the *Yale Heart Book* we have tried to indicate which diagnostic procedures or treatments have proved effective and when they are indicated. These guidelines should help protect consumers from some of these questionable claims.

UNNECESSARY TESTS AND PROCEDURES

Americans probably spend more money on unnecessary tests and procedures than they do on quackery. The big problem in combating this problem is that the tests and procedures may be offered by highly respected and well-meaning physicians. Some doctors claim that a full battery of expensive tests is needed to protect themselves against later charges of malpractice if something is overlooked. While there is some validity to this defense, there are other reasons why testing is overdone. One is the demand of the public—people who are bombarded with TV and news items about the marvels of new technology. But a doctor's job is to resist doing a procedure if it is not going to help the patient.

For their part, consumers should review the legitimate reasons for special blood pressure tests, stress tests, and echocardiograms which are summarized in the various chapters of this book. Being informed helps to understand why certain tests are necessary.

It is understandably difficult for patients to determine whether a test or procedure is really needed. Thus, before undergoing any test or procedure, you should ask your doctor why it is being done and whether the results are likely to provide information that will alter the diagnosis or treatment. (See box, "Questions You Should Ask.")

WHAT IS IT GOING TO COST?

All too often, patients are reluctant to discuss costs with a doctor. This situation is changing somewhat

---

Questions You Should Ask

Before undergoing a test or procedure, always ask the following questions:

- What is the purpose of this test? Is it being done to screen for a possible asymptomatic disorder, such as high blood pressure, or is it needed to confirm a suspected diagnosis?

- Is it definitive or will additional tests be needed?

- What will it cost? Is there a less expensive alternative?

- How accurate is it?

- Does it cause discomfort?

- Are there possible complications or hazards? Does it require anesthesia or hospitalization?

- How will the information be used? Will it, for example, alter the recommended treatment?

- What is likely to happen if the test or procedure isn't done?

Much of the time the answer will be that the test is being used to provide baseline data or to confirm something picked up on a physical examination. This may not be a sufficient reason to justify the procedure. For example, the presence of a few extra or skipped beats in a patient without symptoms of coronary heart disease is not an indication for a 24-hour Holter monitor; even in patients with heart disease it may not be indicated. The presence of a heart murmur is not, by itself, an indication for an echocardiogram. Everyone who has a heart attack does not have to be catheterized. It is very difficult for a layperson to make a judgment about the necessity for a medical test, but by being informed, one can perhaps avoid at least some unnecessary inconvenience and expense.

---

as an increasing number of physicians ask for payment either in advance or before you leave their offices. Ask, too, about alternative therapies. For example, in treating high blood pressure, many doctors routinely prescribe some of the newer, more expensive drugs (such as calcium channel blockers or ACE inhibitors) instead of the older, less expensive ones (such as beta blockers and diuretics), which are usually just as effective. (See Chapter 23.) When receiving a prescription, ask the doctor if there is a generic drug that is as effective as the brand-name choice or if there is an equally effective, lower-priced alternative. (There may not be, but often doctors fail to consider price when they write prescriptions.) Of course, there are instances in which the newer or more expensive drugs are the best choice to treat certain heart diseases.

WHAT YOU CAN DO YOURSELF

No one should try to be his or her own physician, but there are a number of steps you can take to protect your health. As stressed in Chapter 6, the most im-portant is to abstain from cigarette smoking and other forms of tobacco use. Follow a prudent, com-monsense life-style that includes regular exercise and time for relaxation. Avoid food fads, crash diets, "6- or 8-week cholesterol cures," and self-medication with high-dose vitamins and other nonprescription drugs.

Above all, establish a good line of communication with your doctor. If you find it difficult to talk to him or her, you may do well to seek a physician with whom you have better rapport. (See box, "Finding a Doctor.")

Finding a Doctor

Although everyone should have a primary-care physician, studies show that a large number of people—perhaps 25 to 35 percent of all Americans—do not. Instead, they seek medical care only when they are sick or injured, relying on emergency rooms, walk-in clinics, or self-referrals to medical specialists. Even if you enroll in a health maintenance organization or other managed-care plan, you are likely to have a primary physician who oversees your care.

To get the name of a primary-care doctor, you can ask relatives, friends, or other people whose opinions you value if they have a doctor they would recommend. You can also get names from the local medical society or the department of medicine at a local hospital or medical center. Credentials can be checked with your local medical society or in the *Directory of Medical Specialists* at your local library.

Factors you should consider in choosing a doctor include:

- *Location and accessibility.* Is the doctor conveniently located and available for regular office hours and telephone consultation? What is his or her hospital affiliation?

- *Openness and rapport.* Are you able to discuss personal matters with him or her? Are questions answered thoughtfully or brushed off with comments such as "It's nothing to worry about" or "Why don't you leave that to me?"

- *Training, age, and experience.* Where did the doctor go to medical school? Take his or her training? In what field?

- *Type of practice and coverage.* Is the doctor in a solo or group practice? HMO or other managed care? Who provides care when the doctor is not available?

- *Costs and payment.* Does he or she accept insurance or Medicare assignments? If not, how does he or she expect to be paid? What are some typical charges?

Services you should expect of a primary-care doctor include:

- Providing basic health care, overseeing special care, and, if needed, coordinating the services of medical specialists

- Answering your questions in clear, understandable terms

- Giving you adequate time and instructions

- Providing information or forms necessary for insurance claims

Some of the same rules apply in picking a cardiologist, but many people may not need a cardiologist to guide them in treating high blood pressure or following an effective preventive cardiology program.

PART VII

ENCYCLOPEDIA OF COMMON HEART DISORDERS

INTRODUCTION

This "book within a book" is intended to provide a concise overview of common cardiovascular disorders and symptoms. It is set up in a consistent question-and-answer format to enable you to quickly find the information you seek. The various entries are cross-referenced to chapters that provide more detailed information.

CONTENTS

ANGINA PECTORIS

WHAT IS IT?

Angina pectoris is chest pain caused by myocardial ischemia, a condition in which the amount of oxygen the
heart muscle requires exceeds the amount it receives. It
usually occurs on exertion and is relieved by rest. Angina
generally is a symptom of coronary artery disease. In
more severe cases, it may occur with minimal effort or
at rest.

WHO GETS IT?

Angina affects both men and women, usually in middle
age. Men are much more likely than women to experience it before age 60. It may develop weeks, months, or
even years before a heart attack, or may be experienced
only after a heart attack has occurred.

WHAT ARE THE SYMPTOMS?

Angina itself is a symptom. The pain usually lasts only
a few minutes and may be felt in a number of ways,
although the characteristics are usually constant for any
given person. It may be experienced as only a vague ache
or mild discomfort, or it may be a burning, squeezing,
steady pressure, or fullness. The pain or discomfort most
commonly occurs in the center of the chest (under the
breastbone) but may also radiate down one (particularly
the left) or both arms, to the neck, shoulders, lower jaw,
or back. In its classic form, angina occurs with exertion
and is relieved by rest. It may be provoked as well by
mental stress and anxiety, or the combination of a heavy
meal and even mild exertion. In more advanced cases,
angina may occur at rest or even wake the individual
from sleep.

HOW IS IT DIAGNOSED?

The key to diagnosing angina is a careful history: the
patient's report that pain occurs on physical exertion or

mental or emotional stress and subsides when the activity is stopped. A resting electrocardiogram may show changes during the period of pain. An exercise stress test may be used to establish a diagnosis and to determine the level of exertion that produces symptoms. In some cases a thallium or other nuclear scan may be necessary to define how much of the heart is not receiving adequate oxygen when angina occurs.

HOW IS IT TREATED?

An episode of angina is treated by ceasing the activity that brought it on, and/or by taking medication, especially nitroglycerin.

WHAT ARE THE COMPLICATIONS?

In more severe cases, known as unstable angina, the episodes of pain may occur at rest and become quite frequent, more intense, and of longer duration. Untreated underlying coronary artery disease may lead to a heart attack or sudden death.

HOW CAN IT BE PREVENTED OR MINIMIZED?

Angina may be minimized by avoiding exertion or taking nitroglycerin before a stressful or strenuous activity known to produce pain. Several classes of drugs, sometimes used in combination with nitroglycerin, can reduce anginal episodes and increase the amount of activity that can be done before pain starts. Beta blockers reduce the heart rate, lower blood pressure, and diminish the force of the heart's contractions, thus reducing the heart's need for blood. Calcium channel blockers and long-acting nitrates lower blood pressure and help to dilate, or open up, the narrowed arteries. In more severe cases, coronary bypass, angioplasty, or a combination may be required. In all cases, some life-style changes—moderate exercise, weight loss if appropriate, smoking cessation, dietary changes, and stress modification—should be implemented as soon as possible.

See Chapter 11.

AORTIC ANEURYSM

WHAT IS IT?

An aneurysm is an outward bulge in the wall of a blood vessel. Aortic aneurysms occur in the aorta, the body's major artery. The aorta branches, to distribute blood throughout the body. The main branch travels down the body through the chest (thoracic) area and the abdominal area—the two primary sites for aortic aneurysms. Aneurysms may bulge on only one side of the aorta or around the full diameter in all directions. In a dissecting aneurysm (which also has a propensity for rupture), the inner and outer layers of the artery split apart and blood gets between the layers, causing swelling of the wall.

The blood supply to various organs (for example, the kidney) can be markedly reduced because the opening of the vessel has been narrowed.

WHO GETS IT?

Aneurysms develop in patients with atherosclerosis. An additional predisposing factor is hypertension. Patients with Marfan syndrome also develop dissecting aneurysms. Aneurysms may develop because of other congenital problems, but this is rare. Although aneurysms may develop in blood vessels in the limbs, this is rare and does not present the potentially life-threatening problems of those in the trunk.

WHAT ARE THE SYMPTOMS?

Aneurysms frequently produce no symptoms at all, and are detected only on physical examination. Rarely, thoracic aneurysms may cause chest pain. A dissecting aneurysm in the thoracic area can cause chest pain similar to that of a heart attack. In addition, a "tearing" sensation may be felt in the chest and back. Abdominal aneurysms often can be felt just beneath the skin as a small throbbing lump that is tender to the touch; when they begin to leak, they may cause pain that can radiate to the back and to the groin area. Dissecting aneurysms in the abdomen, which are rare, may cause severe pain and fainting.

HOW IS IT DIAGNOSED?

Aneurysms may be difficult to diagnose, because many produce no symptoms until they dissect or rupture. A routine chest X-ray may detect an aneurysm in that area. A physical examination and an X-ray of the abdomen may help to diagnose an aneurysm in the stomach. Echocardiography, CT scans, and MRI are also likely to be part of the diagnostic process for defining the size of an aneurysm. It is difficult to diagnose a blood vessel aneurysm in the brain except by special procedures.

HOW IS IT TREATED?

Drugs may be prescribed to lower blood pressure and reduce the risk of rupture. Abdominal aneurysms that are large or increasing in size should be treated surgically. Enlarging thoracic aneurysms should be considered for surgery. A dissecting or ruptured aneurysm requires emergency surgery.

WHAT ARE THE COMPLICATIONS?

Large aneurysms can apply pressure to and damage adjacent blood vessels or nerves. Aneurysms can also cause major disturbances in local blood flow and increase the risk of clot formation; if the clot breaks away, it can lodge elsewhere in the body and cause a stroke, or other organ damage. If an aneurysm bursts or ruptures, hemorrhage occurs and the supply of blood to tissues beyond the site is cut off. A major aortic rupture can cause circulatory collapse and death if not treated immediately.

HOW CAN IT BE PREVENTED OR MINIMIZED?

Congenital aneurysms cannot be prevented. A healthy life-style (a low-fat diet, regular exercise, and abstinence from smoking) can help prevent or slow down the course of atherosclerosis, a predisposing factor in the development of other aneurysms. Hypertension should be carefully controlled to prevent aneurysm formation or extension.

See Chapter 17.

AORTIC VALVE DISEASE

WHAT IS IT?

The aortic valve is one of four valves that control the flow of blood into and out of the heart. In particular, the aortic valve controls the flow of oxygenated blood pumped out of the heart from the left ventricle into the aorta, the main artery leading to the rest of the body. If the valve is abnormally narrow (stenosis), the heart must work harder for a sufficient amount of blood to be pumped out with each beat. On the other hand, if the valve does not close properly, it is called insufficient because some of the blood being pumped out into the aorta regurgitates, or leaks backward, into the left ventricle with each beat. In either case, the work of the ventricle increases. As a result, its muscular wall thickens (a condition known as hypertrophy) and the left ventricle may become larger (dilate).

WHO GETS IT?

A congenitally deformed valve and rheumatic fever are leading causes of aortic valve disease. Aortic regurgitation is occasionally but rarely associated with other types of rheumatoid (joint) disease, such as ankylosing spondylitis, Reiter's syndrome, rheumatoid or psoriatic arthritis, and systemic lupus erythematosus. Severe hypertension in the presence of other structural abnormalities of the valve also may cause aortic regurgitation.

WHAT ARE THE SYMPTOMS?

An aortic valve disorder usually does not cause any symptoms in its early stages. As the problem progresses, it may produce shortness of breath, angina, light-headedness, dizziness, and even fainting, especially upon exertion. Many elderly people with aortic stenosis remain free of symptoms.

HOW IS IT DIAGNOSED?

Most cases of aortic valve disease can be diagnosed by a physical examination, during which such signs as a

characteristic heart murmur can be detected. A chest X-ray, an electrocardiogram (to determine whether the heart is enlarged), and an echocardiogram may also be done. If enough significant symptoms are present to warrant possible surgery, cardiac catheterization may be necessary.

HOW IS IT TREATED?

Blood pressure and weight should be kept as normal as possible. Limitations on strenuous activity (especially lifting heavy objects) are recommended, particularly for those with stenosis. If symptoms are present with severe stenosis or regurgitation, surgery to replace the defective valve, either with a plastic or metal prosthetic device or with a pig valve, may be recommended. In general, individuals with aortic stenosis who are free of symptoms do not need surgery. Vasodilating drugs, used in treating hypertension, may be useful in aortic regurgitation but not in aortic stenosis.

WHAT ARE THE COMPLICATIONS?

In general, individuals with aortic valve disease are at risk for left-sided heart failure and for heart valve infections (infective endocarditis). Aortic stenosis also carries a risk of sudden death, but usually there are plenty of warning symptoms prior to a serious event.

HOW CAN IT BE PREVENTED OR MINIMIZED?

Avoidance of rheumatic fever, particularly by prompt treatment of a strep throat, is a major preventive measure. If aortic valve disease is present, the prophylactic use of antibiotics before any dental extractions or surgery is necessary to prevent infective endocarditis.

See Chapter 13.

ATHEROSCLEROSIS (ARTERIOSCLEROSIS)

WHAT IS IT?

Arteriosclerosis is a general term used to describe conditions in which the walls of arteries thicken and develop a buildup of fatty material on the inner surface and lose elasticity; its common name is "hardening of the arteries." Some hardening is a natural part of aging. More often, it is caused by atherosclerosis, a buildup of fatty deposits, fibrous tissue, and calcium, called plaque, on the interior of the artery walls. Lipids (fats), including cholesterol, are a major component of plaque. Arteriosclerosis can affect any artery. It is of major concern when it affects the arteries of the heart (coronaries), the neck and brain (carotid), and the legs and kidneys, as well as the aorta itself.

WHO GETS IT?

Although hereditary factors predispose people to arteriosclerosis, life-style plays a critical role in its development. Some degree of atherosclerosis is almost always present in middle-aged and elderly people in countries where the typical diet is high in saturated fat. Smokers and individuals who are obese or have hypertension, hyperlipidemia, or diabetes are at greater risk. It is also more common in men than in women, except after the age of 60, when the differences become less.

WHAT ARE THE SYMPTOMS?

Arteriosclerosis may cause no symptoms for many years. When an artery becomes significantly narrowed by plaque deposits, symptoms may occur and will vary according to the vessel involved. For example, when the coronary arteries are affected, symptoms of angina (chest pain) or a heart attack may occur. Narrowing of the carotid arteries may cause symptoms of stroke, such as weakness of an arm or leg, blurred vision, or slurred speech. Narrowing of the blood vessels in the legs may cause calf or thigh pain on walking (intermittent claudication).

HOW IS IT DIAGNOSED?

A certain degree of atherosclerosis may be presumed in all middle-aged and older adults. Feeling the carotid pulse in the neck or pulses in the feet may provide clues for vessel narrowing. Typical symptoms strongly suggest the diagnosis. The degree and location of narrowing can be diagnosed by angiography (studying the blood vessels after the injection of a dye) or, in the case of the carotid arteries, with certain types of echograms. A stress test may provide indirect evidence of atherosclerosis in the coronary blood vessels.

HOW IS IT TREATED?

There are limited, but encouraging, data to suggest that a major decrease in serum cholesterol level, accomplished through drugs and diet and other life-style changes, can slow and, in a few cases, reverse plaque buildup in the coronary arteries. Reducing elevated blood pressure and smoking cessation are also helpful. Depending on the degree of arterial narrowing and symptoms, medications may be prescribed to dilate blood vessels and help prevent the formation of blood clots. In severe cases, angioplasty may be advised to dilate the narrowed vessels with a balloon or surgery to bypass them with a section of vein or artery taken from elsewhere in the body.

WHAT ARE THE COMPLICATIONS?

Severe arteriosclerosis markedly narrows the artery, impeding the normal flow of blood, which can lead to pain in the legs or chest (angina), heart attack, or stroke, depending on the blood vessels involved. The disorder also increases the risk of thrombosis (the formation of blood clots); such clots may completely obstruct blood flow in the artery involved.

HOW CAN IT BE PREVENTED OR MINIMIZED?

Lifelong heart-healthy habits, such as eating a low-cholesterol, low-fat diet, exercising regularly, and avoiding smoking and obesity, may help prevent arteriosclerosis. If diabetes or hypertension is present, it should be carefully controlled through life-style changes and medical treatment.

See Chapters 2, 11, and 17.

ATHLETE'S HEART

WHAT IS IT?

Athlete's heart is a general term describing a series of changes often seen in the function and structure of the hearts of those who regularly participate in strenuous physical exercise and whose bodies are highly conditioned. These variations, which could suggest illness when seen in nonathletes, are considered normal physiological adaptations when seen in athletes. They enable the heart to deliver a higher than normal level of blood and oxygen to peripheral tissues in the arms and legs in order to sustain athletic performance.

WHO GETS IT?

Highly trained professional athletes, as well as recreational athletes who pursue extended exercise regimens, such as those who train for marathons, are most likely to develop athlete's heart.

WHAT ARE THE SYMPTOMS?

The hallmarks of athlete's heart are bradycardia (a slower than normal heartbeat—usually around 45 to 60 beats per minute), cardiomegaly (overall enlarged heart), and cardiac hypertrophy (thickening of the muscular wall of the heart, usually of the left ventricle). These changes usually occur in the absence of symptoms (such as shortness of breath, excessive fatigue, or chest pain) that would suggest heart disease. The physiological stress of dynamic exercise conditioning causes the heart to enlarge to meet the physical challenges encountered. Because the heart becomes more effective in its pumping ability, it does not need to beat as often to meet these challenges.

HOW IS IT DIAGNOSED?

Simply measuring the pulse indicates the presence of bradycardia. The enlarged heart sometimes may be observed by physical examination, but is more likely to be detected by X-ray or an ECG. Listening to the heart with a stethoscope may reveal a quiet murmur, indicative of the larger volume of blood being pumped with each beat. An echocardiogram may help to rule out any additional structural heart disease.

HOW IS IT TREATED?

Abnormalities in heart rate, size, and function that derive solely from exercise conditioning normally need not be treated, because they do not represent disease.

WHAT ARE THE COMPLICATIONS?

When such presumed abnormalities are detected in an athlete, it is important to assure that the abnormalities are indeed due solely to exercise conditioning and not to some concurrent cardiac disorder. In particular, special attention must be given to differentiate athlete's heart from various conditions that might cause a slow heartbeat (heart block) or heart enlargement secondary to high blood pressure or a heart valve defect. Because these cardiac disorders may occur in athletes as well as in nonathletes, care must be taken to avoid overlooking them. The greatest complication is misdiagnosis.

HOW CAN IT BE PREVENTED OR MINIMIZED?

Because athlete's heart is not pathological, no steps to prevent or minimize its development are necessary. Indeed, the changes in the heart appear to indicate that it may be more efficient than the heart of the nonathlete.

See Chapter 2.

ATRIAL FIBRILLATION

WHAT IS IT?

Atrial fibrillation is a form of tachycardia or rapid heartbeat. The heart normally beats at a rate of about 60 to 80 beats per minute at rest. In atrial fibrillation, the atria (the upper chambers of the heart) beat very rapidly and totally irregularly at more than 300 beats per minute. Blood is not pumped efficiently to the ventricles. The ventricles (the lower chambers of the heart) usually respond irregularly at rates that range from 100 to 200 beats per minute. As a result, the actions of the two chambers of the heart are completely uncoordinated. The ventricles do not get enough time to fill properly and the atria don't push out enough blood with each beat. The disorder may initially be intermittent, with periods of atrial fibrillation lasting a few minutes, hours, or days alternating with even longer periods of normal heart rhythm. However, atrial fibrillation may also become chronic.

WHO GETS IT?

Atrial fibrillation may occur in the absence of underlying anatomic heart disease. More commonly, however, it occurs in individuals with some form of heart disease, especially in older people with atherosclerosis or hypertension, or in those with valvular heart disease. Less commonly, it may occur in those who have chronic obstructive lung disease, overactive thyroid function, or certain congenital heart defects.

WHAT ARE THE SYMPTOMS?

The most common symptom is awareness of a rapid irregular heartbeat. It may be described as palpitations, or a fluttering sensation in the chest. If the heart rate is very rapid, the individual may feel weak, light-headed, or nauseous, have shortness of breath, or, in unusual cases, even lose consciousness.

HOW IS IT DIAGNOSED?

The presence of a rapid irregular heartbeat can be diagnosed by taking the pulse, listening to the heart with a stethoscope, and testing with an electrocardiogram. Because atrial fibrillation may come and go, there may be no signs of it when the patient visits the physician's office. In this case a portable ECG (Holter monitor), which provides a continuous recording over a 24- or 48-hour period, may be used. This test will obviously miss cases that do not recur during the monitoring period.

HOW IS IT TREATED?

In most people, treatment with medication such as digitalis and/or a beta blocker improves the efficiency of the ventricular contractions by slowing the heart rate and may restore the rhythm to normal. If therapy does not restore normal heart rhythm, supplementary drugs such as quinidine sulfate or procainamide may be prescribed. In some cases, persistent atrial fibrillation may be treated by electrical cardioversion—the administration of an electric shock to the heart while the individual is sedated or anesthetized. Once normal heart rhythm is reestablished, further medication may be prescribed to prevent recurrences, especially if the underlying cause of the disorder is a chronic one that cannot be effectively treated. Anticoagulant medication is frequently employed to decrease the risk of blood clot formation. Correcting an overactive thyroid may prevent further episodes.

WHAT ARE THE COMPLICATIONS?

Those who suffer with atrial fibrillation are at increased risk of blood clots, a serious complication, and therefore may be given anticoagulant medication or chronic aspirin therapy. In those with severe underlying heart disease, the rhythm disturbance may lead to decreased heart function and increasing heart failure.

HOW CAN IT BE PREVENTED OR MINIMIZED?

Measures to prevent valvular and coronary heart disease will decrease the chances of atrial fibrillation. In many cases, however, little can be done to prevent it, but potential triggers should be avoided. These vary from patient to patient, but include cigarettes, caffeine, and alcohol. Medication may be the only way to prevent recurrence if one episode has occurred. Individuals with atrial fibrillation should be under a physician's care in order to receive optimal, regulated medication.

See Chapter 16.

BRADYCARDIA

WHAT IS IT?

The adult heart at rest normally beats at a rate of about 60 to 80 beats per minute. A rate below 55–60 beats per minute is considered slow and is called bradycardia. Infants have a much higher normal rate (110 to 130 beats per minute), and so bradycardia in infants is a rate below 100 beats per minute.

WHO GETS IT?

Slower than average heart rates are normal in people who are physically fit, and are probably normal in all individuals during sleep. Many athletes who train regularly have resting heart rates of 45–60 beats per minute. Bradycardia also may occur secondary to certain illnesses (such as decreased thyroid function, certain gastrointestinal disorders, and jaundice) or to abuse of certain drugs. People with known heart disease (including hypertension) who are being treated with medications that slow the heart, such as beta blockers and certain calcium channel blockers, may experience bradycardia. It may also be a temporary consequence of certain types of heart attack. Bradycardia is common in elderly people, whether or not they suffer from arteriosclerosis, and in infants with certain types of congenital heart disease.

WHAT ARE THE SYMPTOMS?

Bradycardia usually does not cause symptoms unless the heart rate is below 40–45. The condition becomes a concern only if it results in an inadequate output of blood from the heart, producing such symptoms as fatigue, shortness of breath, light-headedness, and fainting. Such symptoms are most likely to occur upon exertion, when the body's need for oxygenated blood increases, but can also occur at rest.

HOW IS IT DIAGNOSED?

A slower than normal heartbeat can be detected simply by taking the pulse. An electrocardiogram will help to define the type of bradycardia and determine whether heart block or another condition is present.

HOW IS IT TREATED?

If the bradycardia does not cause symptoms, no treatment is necessary. If there are symptoms, medications can be given to increase the rate of the heartbeat. If fainting or serious symptoms persist despite medication, a permanent pacemaker may need to be implanted. In specific instances, certain medications may have to be withdrawn because of their slowing effect.

WHAT ARE THE COMPLICATIONS?

Severe bradycardia (fewer than 30 beats per minute) can be an emergency situation, leading to brain oxygen deprivation and convulsions. Death may result unless immediate medical measures are taken to increase the heart rate.

HOW CAN IT BE PREVENTED OR MINIMIZED?

Dosage instructions for heart disease and hypertension medications should be followed carefully. Since the more serious form of bradycardia is due to heart block or damage to heart muscle from a heart attack, measures to slow the process of atherosclerosis (cessation of smoking, control of blood pressure and blood cholesterol, and regular exercise) can be helpful.

See Chapter 16.

CARDIAC ARREST (SUDDEN DEATH)

WHAT IS IT?

Cardiac arrest is the failure of the heart muscle to pump blood because of a severe rhythm disturbance or cessation of all beating activity. If the heart rhythm is not restored within a short time, the condition is fatal.

WHO GETS IT?

Cardiac arrest most commonly occurs in those who have heart disease and develop a severely abnormal heart rhythm known as ventricular fibrillation; this arrhythmia may occur independently or during a heart attack. Others who have problems with lesser arrhythmias, particularly those arising from the ventricles, also may be at risk. In addition, cardiac arrest is frequently the final event of death from many causes. People with non-heart-related problems may go into cardiac arrest following severe sudden blood loss, major burns, severe allergic reactions (anaphylaxis), hypothermia, drug overdose, drowning, or electric shock. Cardiac arrest may also be the result of a complete heart block, in which impulses fail to get through to the pumping chambers of the heart and the muscle fails to contract.

WHAT ARE THE SYMPTOMS?

The person suffering cardiac arrest immediately collapses, loses consciousness, and has no pulse. If breathing continues briefly, it is shallow.

HOW IS IT DIAGNOSED?

The symptoms of cardiac arrest are dramatic and easily observed, even by a layperson. No special diagnostic techniques are required. If pulse is unobtainable and breathing has stopped, the diagnosis is confirmed.

HOW IS IT TREATED?

Immediate resuscitation efforts are necessary to prevent death. If the arrest occurs outside the hospital, a trained layperson can initiate cardiopulmonary resuscitation (CPR) to restore circulation until medical personnel arrive. This procedure involves opening the airway, breathing into the victim's mouth, and compressing the chest at regular intervals. If the arrest occurs in a hospital, resuscitation will be supplemented by advanced life support techniques. Defibrillation with an electric current may be successful in restarting the heart. Intravenous medications may be given. When the victim has stabilized, further care will include diagnosis and treatment of the disorder that caused the cardiac arrest.

WHAT ARE THE COMPLICATIONS?

Even if an individual is resuscitated after cardiac arrest, complications may occur. If resuscitation did not begin promptly (within approximately five minutes), permanent brain damage may result from brain oxygen deprivation during the absence of circulation.

HOW CAN IT BE PREVENTED OR MINIMIZED?

Every effort should be made to prevent or treat any cardiovascular or respiratory disease. If chest pain or tightness suggestive of a possible heart attack develops, immediate care should be obtained in a hospital emergency room. In addition, those at risk for cardiac arrhythmias should be identified and their condition treated. Some individuals with severe heart disease and a history of severe arrhythmias may require an implantable defibrillator (an AICD).

See Chapter 27.

CARDIAC TUMOR

WHAT IS IT?

Abnormal growths known as tumors rarely arise in the heart. Nevertheless, they can develop in the myocardium (the heart muscle itself), the endocardium (its inner lining), or the epicardium (the outer covering of the heart). Primary malignant cardiac tumors are particularly rare and occur mostly in children; most are the type of tumor known as sarcomas. More than 75 percent of primary cardiac tumors, however, are benign. The most common type is a myxoma, a tumor composed of mucouslike tissue, which accounts for half of all primary benign cardiac tumors. Most myxomas arise in the left atrium, although they can occur in any heart chamber. Other benign tumors, made up of muscle or fatty tissue, and cysts of the pericardium (outer heart lining) are also found, but those are rare. When tumors occur in the heart, they are more apt to be secondary tumors—malignancies that originally developed elsewhere and metastasized to the heart.

WHO GETS IT?

Although myxomas can arise at any age, they tend to occur in individuals between the ages of 30 and 60, are more common in women than in men, and may run in families. Secondary cardiac tumors are most likely to be metastases in people who have lung or breast cancer, lymphoma, or malignant melanoma, although other types of cancer can also spread to the heart.

WHAT ARE THE SYMPTOMS?

Depending on the location and extent of the tumor in the heart, symptoms may include pain, palpitations, fever, and weight loss; symptoms of heart failure (shortness of breath, fatigue, and swollen ankles) may occasionally be noted. Some cardiac tumors may cause no symptoms.

HOW IS IT DIAGNOSED?

Accurate diagnosis is often difficult. Some signs of cardiac tumor, such as a heart murmur (particularly with a myxoma), may be detectable on physical examination. Other tumors that cause no symptoms may be suspected after a routine X-ray shows heart enlargement. An electrocardiogram and an echocardiogram will often help make the diagnosis. Sometimes cardiac catheterization may be necessary.

HOW IS IT TREATED?

Surgical removal can usually completely cure myxomas. Tumors of the pericardium also may require surgery. Surgical success is less likely, but often possible, for muscle tumors. Only palliative therapy is available for tumors of the heart that metastasize from elsewhere. This therapy may include radiation or chemotherapy to slow the growth of the tumor or reduce its size.

WHAT ARE THE COMPLICATIONS?

Tumors such as myxomas can obstruct normal blood flow in the heart (particularly at the mitral valve) and increase the risk of blood clot formation, leading to a stroke or fainting. Primary malignant tumors often lead to the development of congestive heart failure, fluid collection between the heart muscle and the membrane that surrounds it (pericardial effusion), heartbeat irregularities, or heart block. The prognosis for patients with malignant cardiac tumors is poor.

HOW CAN IT BE PREVENTED OR MINIMIZED?

There are no known measures to prevent the occurrence of cardiac tumors. Early detection through surveillance and routine examination may allow treatment of cancers before they metastasize to the heart.

CARDIOMYOPATHY

WHAT IS IT?

Cardiomyopathy is a general term describing disease of the heart muscle. Primary cardiomyopathy involves changes in the muscle's structure or function from unknown causes. Examples include *congestive cardiomyopathy*, in which the heart enlarges, weakens, and no longer pumps effectively, increasing the risk of heart failure and blood clots; *hypertrophic cardiomyopathy*, in which the heart muscle overgrows and thickens, possibly impeding the flow of blood through the heart; and *restrictive cardiomyopathy*, in which the heart muscle wall stiffens. *Secondary cardiomyopathy* may result from some other systemic disease, metabolic disorders, or infection. Examples include diffuse coronary disease with multiple heart attacks; *alcoholic cardiomyopathy*, in which the muscle is believed to be damaged directly by alcohol and secondary nutritional deficiencies; and *viral cardiomyopathy*, which is caused by a viral infection of heart muscle.

WHO GETS IT?

Although some types of cardiomyopathy are attributable to specific causes in groups of people, such as alcoholics, a common underlying problem appears to be diffuse coronary artery disease. In some cases, no cause can be diagnosed. Hypertrophic cardiomyopathy is rare, but tends to occur more often in young adults and more often in men than in women.

WHAT ARE THE SYMPTOMS?

Except for cardiomyopathy associated with an infection, these disorders—and thus their symptoms—usually develop slowly. The most common symptoms are those of congestive heart failure, such as fatigue, swelling, and shortness of breath. They may be chronic or acute. In some instances, irregularities of heart rhythm may be a prominent symptom.

HOW IS IT DIAGNOSED?

Physical examination may reveal an enlarged heart, a characteristic murmur, or changes in heart sounds. Symptoms may suggest the diagnosis. This plus an ECG, chest X-ray, and possibly an echocardiogram or radionuclide studies will usually provide the information needed for a diagnosis. In some cases, cardiac catheterization and, rarely, a biopsy may be necessary.

HOW IS IT TREATED?

If a treatable underlying cause, such as alcoholism, can be identified, it should be treated. Depending on the type of cardiomyopathy, certain drugs may be prescribed to decrease the heart's workload, regulate the heartbeat, help prevent blood clot formation, and help prevent fluid accumulation in the body; these drugs include vasodilators, digitalis, ACE inhibitors, anticoagulants, and diuretics. Congestive and dilated cardiomyopathies often respond well, at least initially, to medical therapy. Treatment of some cardiomyopathies that result from viral infections may not be too effective. Therapy for those with restrictive cardiomyopathy may be particularly limited. If end-stage heart failure develops, heart transplantation may be an option.

WHAT ARE THE COMPLICATIONS?

Unless a treatable cause is identified and therapy provided, the outlook for some patients with cardiomyopathy may be bleak. Outlook is, at least in part, dependent upon the degree of cardiac dysfunction. Congestive heart failure commonly occurs. Arrhythmias or a heart block may develop. Heart block may require implantation of a pacemaker. In severe cases of congestive cardiomyopathy, blood clots form in the heart and may travel to other parts of the body and cause a stroke. Sudden death can occur.

HOW CAN IT BE PREVENTED OR MINIMIZED?

It is important to seek medical care early and to embark on an appropriate medical regimen, which should include therapy for any treatable primary causes of cardiomyopathy. Potential causes such as alcohol should be avoided. Hypertrophic cardiomyopathy is most frequently a congenital defect and cannot be prevented.

See Chapters 14 and 15.

CONGENITAL HEART DISEASE— CYANOTIC

WHAT IS IT?

Any defect of the heart or the major blood vessels that is present at birth is called congenital heart disease. In the more severe types of disorders (which, fortunately, are not common), a major symptom is blueness of the infant's skin at birth. Called cyanosis, this blueness indicates that the supply of oxygenated blood in the baby's body is inadequate. The most common of such heart disorders include *tetralogy of Fallot* (four abnormalities in heart structure that impair the normal flow of blood); *transposition of the great vessels* (transposition of the aorta and pulmonary arteries in their attachment to the heart, so that oxygenated blood goes back to the lungs instead of out to the body through the aorta); *tricuspid atresia* (lack of a valve to allow blood flow between the right heart chambers); and *total anomalous venous return* (inability of oxygenated blood from the lungs to reach the left atrium directly). In each instance, the fundamental problem is an inability to oxygenate blood because of altered cardiac anatomy.

WHO GETS IT?

About one in every 120 babies has some congenital heart defect. The majority of defects, however, are minor and do not cause cyanosis. A defect may occur with an associated genetic abnormality (such as Down syndrome). In some cases an illness (such as rubella) afflicted the mother during fetal heart development, and in some cases medication taken by the mother during pregnancy may have caused the defect. There may be no identifiable cause.

WHAT ARE THE SYMPTOMS?

The primary symptom of cyanotic congenital heart disease is bluish skin. Children with tetralogy of Fallot and transposition of the great vessels also are born with a drumsticklike swelling of the ends of the fingers and toes (termed "clubbed") and will be underdeveloped. If heart failure is present, the baby may have difficulty eating because he or she lacks energy for vigorous sucking. Such an infant tends to cry less than normal and also may experience shortness of breath.

HOW IS IT DIAGNOSED?

Complete evaluation of a cyanotic infant or child will include a physical examination, chest X-ray, electrocardiogram, and echocardiogram. Cardiac catheterization is often required to define the anatomic problem.

HOW IS IT TREATED?

Surgery to partially correct transposition of the aorta and pulmonary blood vessels, so that oxygenated blood can flow into the general circulatory system from the heart, is usually done before the baby is 2 to 3 months old. Further surgery will probably be necessary before the child enters school to create artificial blood vessels and establish normal circulation. Tetralogy of Fallot also requires surgical correction before age 4 or 5, although earlier emergency surgery may be necessary. Supplemental oxygen and medication may be necessary to help tide the baby over until the surgery.

WHAT ARE THE COMPLICATIONS?

Cyanotic congenital heart disease is a severe condition. In the days before effective surgery was available, it resulted in failure to thrive, severe heart failure, or sudden death. Fortunately, today the prognosis with surgery is good, although long-term status into adulthood has not yet been defined after most types of surgery.

HOW CAN IT BE PREVENTED OR MINIMIZED?

If there is any family history of congenital heart disease, genetic counseling before pregnancy should be considered. Women who have not been vaccinated against ru-

bella (German measles) should be vaccinated before becoming pregnant. Unnecessary drugs should be avoided during pregnancy.

See Chapter 20.

CONGENITAL HEART DISEASE— NONCYANOTIC

WHAT IS IT?

Any defect of the heart or the major blood vessels that is present at birth is called congenital heart disease. In the more severe types of disorders, a major sign is blueness of the infant's skin at birth. Called cyanosis, this blueness indicates that the supply of oxygenated blood in the baby's body is inadequate. Congenital heart disease that does not cause bluish skin is called noncyanotic. It is more common and less serious than cyanotic disorders. Noncyanotic disorders include *congenital aortic or pulmonic stenosis* (a narrowing of one or the other of these heart valves), *ventricular or atrial septal defects* (small holes between the heart's lower or upper chambers, yielding an excess of blood circulation in the lungs), *coarctation of the aorta* (an abnormal narrowing that impairs blood flow to the lower part of the body), and *patent ductus arteriosus* (failure of an extra blood vessel between the aorta and pulmonary artery to close down as it should after birth, causing excessive blood flow to the lungs).

WHO GETS IT?

Congenital heart defects occur in about one of every 120 babies. Many defects are minor. They may be caused by an associated genetic abnormality (such as Down's syndrome), by an illness (such as rubella or diabetes) that afflicted the mother during fetal heart development, by some medication taken by the mother during pregnancy, or frequently by some unknown factor.

WHAT ARE THE SYMPTOMS?

Many cases of noncyanotic congenital heart disease do not exhibit symptoms. If mild heart failure is present, the baby may have difficulty eating because of lack of energy for vigorous sucking. Such an infant may not gain weight normally and tends to cry less than normal. With more severe problems, the baby's breathing may be rapid and distressed. If the heart problem is not diagnosed in infancy, symptoms may first arise in young children who probably are growing at a below-normal rate. They may become short of breath upon exertion and, eventually, even at rest.

HOW IS IT DIAGNOSED?

Noncyanotic congenital heart problems can usually be detected by the presence of a heart murmur heard with a stethoscope. Most heart murmurs heard in childhood are benign and need not cause worry; but other heart murmurs signal the existence of particular types of congenital heart disorders. Further evaluations are likely to include a chest X-ray, electrocardiogram, and echocardiogram. When surgery is contemplated, cardiac catheterization may be necessary.

HOW IS IT TREATED?

Treatment depends upon the type of defect. Initial treatment usually is not needed for congenital aortic or pulmonic stenosis, and surgical correction may be delayed until late childhood or early adulthood. A severe condition, however, may necessitate immediate surgery. Small holes in the heart (atrial or ventricular septal defect) may not require treatment, or they can be closed in the catheterization laboratory using new techniques; surgical correction of larger holes may be delayed until after age 4. In general, coarctation of the aorta necessitates surgical correction, usually between the ages of 4 and 8. Sometimes patent ductus arteriosus can be corrected with medication; if not, surgical correction is performed before the child starts school. The use of prophylactic antibiotics before dental work or surgery is recommended for most cases. Children with these defects need not limit their physical activity unless exercise results in excessive fatigue or shortness of breath.

WHAT ARE THE COMPLICATIONS?

Ventricular and atrial septal defects pose a risk of pulmonary hypertension and heart failure if the hole is large and is not repaired until adulthood. Stenosed valves and coarctation of the aorta also may increase the work of the heart and, over time, cause heart failure.

HOW CAN IT BE PREVENTED OR MINIMIZED?

If there is any family history of congenital heart disease, genetic counseling before pregnancy should be considered. Women who have not been vaccinated against rubella (German measles) should be vaccinated before becoming pregnant. Avoidance of illness and drugs during pregnancy is the only known preventive measure. Prior to surgical repair of the defect, symptoms can be minimized by the use of diuretics or digitalis.

See Chapter 20.

CONGESTIVE HEART FAILURE

WHAT IS IT?

In contrast to cardiac arrest, when the heart stops pumping completely, heart failure is a condition in which the heart keeps pumping, but inefficiently, generally because of inadequate heart muscle contraction. Because the heart does not pump a normal amount of blood forward,

pressure may build up in the venous system. This may cause congestion in various tissues in the body. The most common sites of such congestion are the lungs, liver, and ankles, which become swollen.

WHO GETS IT?

The underlying cause of heart failure is damage to heart muscle. The damage may be the result of a variety of factors, including atherosclerosis, a heart attack, valvular heart disease, hypertension, rheumatic fever, elevated blood pressure in the lungs because of lung disease, and, in unusual cases, a congenital heart defect.

WHAT ARE THE SYMPTOMS?

Congestive heart failure often develops slowly, and its most common symptoms are shortness of breath, swollen ankles (edema), and weight gain. Initially, respiratory symptoms may occur only when the individual is exercising or lying flat in bed. However, as heart failure becomes more severe, these symptoms tend to occur even at rest in any position. Some irregularities in heart rhythm may also occur, which can result in palpitations and, less commonly, dizziness or syncope (fainting). Acute pulmonary edema is a form of heart failure that develops suddenly, causing extreme shortness of breath and severe anxiety. Wheezing may develop and be accompanied by a cough that produces frothy, pink phlegm.

HOW IS IT DIAGNOSED?

Diagnosis of congestive heart failure or acute pulmonary edema is largely based on the history of characteristic symptoms and a physical examination. Extra heart sounds and crackling sounds in the lungs (rales) may be heard on examination. A chest X-ray may reveal evidence of congestion in the lungs and heart enlargement. Other diagnostic tests may include an electrocardiogram or an echocardiogram.

HOW IS IT TREATED?

Therapy involves rest, medications such as diuretics and vasodilators to decrease the heart's workload, and a low-sodium diet to help rid the body of excess fluid. Digitalis is the preferred medication to increase the force of the heart's pumping action. If blood pressure is very high, specific blood-pressure-lowering drugs will also be used. In some cases if a specific treatable cause of the heart failure is identified (e.g., extreme narrowing of a heart valve), surgery may be indicated. In rare cases, if the heart is irreversibly damaged and does not respond to therapy, heart transplantation also may be an option.

WHAT ARE THE COMPLICATIONS?

If acute heart failure is not treated, the patient may experience respiratory failure, literally drowning in bodily fluid. Fortunately, this is rare. Serious rhythm irregularities may also occur, but can be treated. In some instances, heart failure becomes chronic and does not respond to therapy. About 34,000 deaths from congestive heart failure occur annually. Many of these, however, occur during the course of a heart attack.

HOW CAN IT BE PREVENTED OR MINIMIZED?

Some causes of congestive heart failure are unavoidable. Other cases may be prevented by early treatment of hypertension and life-style modifications to reduce the risk factors for atherosclerosis. Most cases of congestive heart failure will respond, at least initially, to medical therapy. Rigorous medical care is required.

See Chapter 14.

COR PULMONALE

WHAT IS IT?

Cor pulmonale is a form of secondary heart disease that is the result of abnormally high blood pressure in the pulmonary or lung arteries, known as pulmonary hypertension. The process begins when severe lung disease prevents the individual from getting enough oxygen. In response to the lack of oxygen, the pulmonary arteries—which carry blood from the heart to the lungs—constrict, adding to the pressure. Ultimately they become thickened, further impairing the flow of blood. The heart must work harder to compensate for this poor circulation, and its right side becomes enlarged and thickened. The additional workload can eventually cause right-sided heart failure.

WHO GETS IT?

Cor pulmonale occurs most often in adults who have severe lung disease. These individuals are usually smokers. It can also develop in people with lung disease such as cystic fibrosis, which is not caused by smoking. Risk also may increase in those who are very obese or who live at high altitudes. The pulmonary hypertension that leads to cor pulmonale may be caused by any disorder that impairs the flow of blood through the lungs. More than half of all cases are caused by chronic bronchitis or emphysema or both. Other possible causes include congenital heart disease, pulmonary embolism, primary pulmonary hypertension, certain vascular diseases, and chronic infections, as well as extensive loss of lung tissue because of surgery or trauma.

WHAT ARE THE SYMPTOMS?

Almost all patients have shortness of breath because of the underlying lung disease. Swollen ankles are also common. Other symptoms may be vague or similar to those causing the underlying lung disorder—a chronic cough, various types of chest pain, and drowsiness. The first specific signs indicating a failure of the right side of the heart may not occur until the cor pulmonale is considerably advanced.

HOW IS IT DIAGNOSED?

A complete physical exam may provide important clues. An electrocardiogram and chest X-ray will also be very helpful. Pulmonary function tests and, in some cases, an echocardiogram, a nuclear scan of the heart or lungs or both, and right-sided cardiac catheterization may be necessary to pinpoint the diagnosis. Even under optimal circumstances, however, the diagnosis may be difficult to make.

HOW IS IT TREATED?

Therapy for cor pulmonale is likely to include modified bed rest, supplemental oxygen, and diuretics to help rid the body of excess fluid. If right ventricular failure occurs, digitalis and vasodilating medications may also help. Even after successful treatment, cor pulmonale may cause recurrent problems unless the underlying cause of the pulmonary hypertension is amenable to treatment, which is often not the case. Daily home treatment with oxygen may be necessary on a long-term basis. Ultimately, in very rare and carefully selected cases, combination lung and heart transplantation may be recommended.

WHAT ARE THE COMPLICATIONS?

Although the main risks are associated with the underlying lung disorder, cor pulmonale can lead to heart failure and chronic invalidism.

HOW CAN IT BE PREVENTED OR MINIMIZED?

Medical attention is important for any lung or heart disorder or for any new symptoms in the course of existing lung disorders. Eliminating cigarettes and exposure to smoke and other sources of air pollution is imperative. Some cases of cor pulmonale that result from congenital heart disease may be helped by surgery.

CORONARY ARTERY DISEASE (ISCHEMIC HEART DISEASE)

WHAT IS IT?

Coronary artery disease, coronary heart disease, and ischemic heart disease are various names given to a condition in which the coronary arteries—those that feed the heart muscle itself—are narrowed. As a result, the blood supply to the heart muscle is decreased. The narrowing is almost invariably due to atherosclerosis, the buildup of fatty plaques on the inner walls of the arteries.

WHO GETS IT?

Coronary artery disease affects more than 6 million Americans and is the leading cause of death in the United States. It occurs more frequently in individuals with a family history of premature (below age 60) heart disease, as well as in those who smoke or have high blood pressure, high blood cholesterol, or diabetes mellitus (each of which is also somewhat influenced by heredity). Obesity, physical inactivity, and stress also play a role in the development of atherosclerosis. Risk rises with age, and men are at greater risk than women, although the female risk rises dramatically within five to ten years after menopause. Life-style changes, medication, or both can modify these risk factors, with the exception of heredity, age, and gender.

WHAT ARE THE SYMPTOMS?

Coronary artery disease may exist for many years without causing any symptoms. The most common symptom is chest pain (angina). In most instances, symptoms are not noticed until artery narrowing has progressed. These may not be symptoms, however, until one of the complications of coronary artery disease, a heart attack, occurs.

HOW IS IT DIAGNOSED?

In the absence of symptoms, coronary artery disease may be diagnosed as a result of positive findings during an exercise stress test (possibly including a nuclear imaging study), or it may be documented by a coronary angiogram. When chest pain on exertion is present, coronary artery disease should usually be considered; tests will be used to confirm the diagnosis or to determine its extent.

HOW IS IT TREATED?

Treatment is complex and must be individualized. It can include the following (ranging from simplest to most complex): life-style modifications; medications, including daily aspirin, cholesterol- or blood-pressure-lowering agents, beta blockers, nitroglycerin derivatives, and calcium channel blockers; coronary angioplasty; and bypass surgery.

WHAT ARE THE COMPLICATIONS?

The most common and serious complications of coronary artery disease are myocardial infarction (heart attack) and sudden cardiac death. These events are most often precipitated by the formation of a blood clot that obstructs a coronary artery already narrowed by atherosclerosis. Other complications may include various heart rhythm disturbances and heart failure.

HOW CAN IT BE PREVENTED OR MINIMIZED?

The same life-style measures applied for treatment are pivotal in helping prevent or minimize the impact of coronary artery disease. Maintaining ideal weight, exercising regularly, keeping blood pressure within a normal range, eating a low-fat, low-cholesterol diet, and avoiding cigarette smoking are the key elements of coronary artery disease prevention.

See Chapters 2 and 11.

ENDOCARDITIS

WHAT IS IT?

Endocarditis is an inflammation or infection of the endocardium, which is the inner lining of the heart muscle and, most commonly, the heart valves. It is usually caused by a bacterial infection. The bacteria cluster on and around the heart valves; this may impair their ability to function properly. The acute form of endocarditis may cause more severe symptoms, while symptoms of the chronic form may be milder, making it more difficult to diagnose.

WHO GETS IT?

Although bacterial endocarditis may occur in anyone at any time, it is unusual in persons who do not have valvular heart disease. Valves deformed by a previous attack of rheumatic fever were once a major predisposing factor, but this is less so today since rheumatic fever has become much less common. Other predisposing factors include artificial heart valves, some congenital heart disorders, and, infrequently, mitral valve prolapse. People with such risk factors are more likely to develop endocarditis when exposed to an infection from any source. Dental surgery, urologic or gynecologic surgery, colonoscopy, and skin infections increase the risk of endocarditis. Intravenous drug users are at particular risk for development of endocarditis, even if there is no preexisting anatomic valve deformity.

WHAT ARE THE SYMPTOMS?

The symptoms of bacterial endocarditis include a low-grade fever, fatigue, loss of appetite, night sweats, chills, headaches, joint discomfort, and tiny pinpoint-sized hemorrhages on the chest and back, fingers, or toes. Upon examination, the physician also may detect a new heart murmur and small hemorrhages in the mucous membranes of the eyes.

HOW IS IT DIAGNOSED?

Diagnosis is usually suspected based on the patient's history, symptoms, and findings such as a new murmur. It is confirmed by a blood test ("culture") to identify an infecting organism. An echocardiogram may occasionally be helpful in identifying a clump of bacteria on the heart valve.

HOW IS IT TREATED?

Bacterial endocarditis almost always requires hospitalization for antibiotic therapy, generally given intravenously, at least at the outset. Occasionally, therapy with oral antibiotics at home will be successful. Antibiotic therapy usually must continue for at least a month. In unusual cases, surgery may be necessary to eliminate areas of infection or to repair or replace a damaged heart valve.

WHAT ARE THE COMPLICATIONS?

If bacterial endocarditis is not adequately treated, it may be fatal. This is dependent upon the infecting organism. Even when treated, further damage to a heart valve may lead to heart failure. In addition, blood clots may form and travel through the bloodstream to the brain or lungs.

HOW CAN IT BE PREVENTED OR MINIMIZED?

Those who have any predisposing factors for bacterial endocarditis should be given antibiotics before any medical or dental surgery and whenever any significant skin infection occurs. Such prophylactic therapy will help prevent the spread of bacteria to the bloodstream. Those with a prior history of endocarditis must be monitored for at least a year because of the possibility of a relapse or reinfection of a heart valve.

See Chapter 13.

HEART BLOCK

WHAT IS IT?

The heart's electrical system normally sends impulses from the two atria (the upper chambers) to the two ventricles (the lower chambers) in a pattern that causes the coordinated contraction called the heartbeat. If these electrical messages are slowed or interrupted along their normal paths, the heart rate or rhythm can be impaired. There are various degrees of heart block. First-degree heart block is generally of no consequence to the individual and is detected only by an electrocardiogram. In second-degree heart block, occasional beats are not conducted and the pulse becomes a bit slower and somewhat irregular. In third-degree (or complete) heart block, the electrical messages don't get through to the ventricles at all and the atria and ventricles beat independently. Heart rate is usually slow and irregular. Complete heart block can produce symptoms such as syncope (fainting).

WHO GETS IT?

Heart block is most likely to occur in the elderly and those with atherosclerosis or primary myocardial disease (cardiomyopathy). It can also be seen in individuals with an enlarged heart as a result of untreated hypertension or rheumatic heart disease. An uncommon form is seen in infants (congenital heart block). Alternatively, it can develop as a side effect of certain cardiac drugs that can impair the normal electrical patterns. In some cases of heart block, the cause is never found.

WHAT ARE THE SYMPTOMS?

First- and second-degree heart block generally do not cause symptoms, because the heart rate and rhythm may remain quite normal. In third-degree heart block, there may be fatigue, light-headedness, fainting, or symptoms of heart failure. Very severe cases may result in sudden death.

HOW IS IT DIAGNOSED?

A slower than normal or irregular heartbeat can be detected simply by feeling the pulse. However, an electrocardiogram will show electrical patterns characteristic of the different degrees of heart block. (Many cases of slow or irregular heartbeat, however, are not a result of a heart block.) If there are symptoms but the heart block is intermittent and not detected on physical examination, the physician may recommend continuous monitoring of the heartbeat with a Holter monitor, a portable device that the patient wears while going about his or her usual daily activities.

HOW IS IT TREATED?

Most cases of first-degree and even second-degree heart block require no treatment, especially if there are no symptoms. If cardiac medications are being used for other purposes, reducing or changing them may occasionally eliminate or reduce the heart block. Chronic complete heart block *with symptoms* requires implantation of an artificial pacemaker to take over the job of providing regular electrical heart stimulation through the power of a very small, long-lasting battery. Depending on the type of heart block and the type of pacemaker used, it may simply send one regular signal, or may respond only when the heart's own pacemaker fails to function properly. In some cases, it may be programmed to vary the heart rate according to different needs—such as faster for exercise and slower for sleep. Transient third-degree heart block that occurs during a heart attack may require a temporary pacemaker, which can be removed when spontaneous heart rhythm returns to normal.

WHAT ARE THE COMPLICATIONS?

Most people with first- and second-degree heart block can go about their lives without difficulty. In some cases of second-degree heart block and in most cases of complete heart block, there is a danger of fainting, possible convulsions, and, in some cases, death. The risk for persons with first- and second-degree heart block is related more to the underlying disorder—coronary or hypertensive heart disease, etc.

HOW CAN IT BE PREVENTED OR MINIMIZED?

Prevention of atherosclerosis and early treatment of hypertension may help to prevent heart block. Routine evaluation, particularly of the elderly, may uncover heart block before it is symptomatic. If the individual is taking cardiac medication, it may be altered, or, if appropriate, a pacemaker may be considered. Since many cases of heart block are related to narrowing of the coronary arteries, a healthy life-style that includes a low-fat diet, regular exercise, and avoidance of smoking may help lower the risk.

See Chapters 16 and 26.

HYPERLIPIDEMIA

WHAT IS IT?

Hyperlipidemia is an excess of fatty substances called lipids, largely cholesterol and triglycerides, in the blood. It is also called hyperlipoproteinemia, because these fatty substances travel in the blood attached to proteins; the fat-protein complexes are called lipoproteins. The best-known lipoproteins are low-density lipoprotein (LDL) and high-density lipoprotein (HDL); another is very-low-density lipoprotein (VLDL). LDL, which carries most of the body's cholesterol in the blood, is known as the "bad" lipoprotein, because it tends to carry serum cholesterol from the liver to the arteries, where it forms plaques on arterial walls. HDL is known as the "good" lipid, because it tends to carry cholesterol away from arterial walls and back to the liver. A subcategory of hyperlipidemia is hypercholesterolemia, in which there is a high level of total cholesterol. (VLDL largely contains triglycerides).

WHO GETS IT?

Some types of hyperlipidemia, such as familial hypercholesterolemia, are hereditary. Others may occur secondary to diseases such as diabetes, nephrosis, hypothyroidism, and alcoholism. The most common type of hypercholesterolemia is believed to be due largely to an interaction between genetic factors and excess cholesterol and fat, especially saturated fat in the diet.

WHAT ARE THE SYMPTOMS?

Hyperlipidemia usually has no overt symptoms and tends to be discovered during routine examination or evaluation for atherosclerotic cardiovascular disease. Pinkish-yellow deposits of fat (known as xanthomas) may develop under the skin (especially around the eyes) in individuals with familial forms of the disorder or in those with very high levels of cholesterol in the blood.

HOW IS IT DIAGNOSED?

Diagnosis is made by evaluating laboratory analyses of blood samples, which provide information on total blood fat levels, as well as its fractions. Cholesterol and triglyceride levels tend to rise with age. A total serum cholesterol level under 200 mg/dl, with LDL below 130 mg/dl and HDL above 35–40 mg/dl, is considered normal for adults. If HDL levels are particularly high, a higher total serum cholesterol level may be acceptable. This is more common among women, who may have HDL levels of 60–70 mg/dl. While their total cholesterol level may be above 220–240 mg/dl, their risk for heart disease is not high. Triglyceride levels above 250 mg/dl are considered abnormal.

HOW IS IT TREATED?

A low-cholesterol, low-fat diet is the first line of therapy for hypercholesterolemia. A low-carbohydrate diet, eliminating alcohol, is recommended for hypertriglyceridemia. Maintaining ideal weight and increasing exercise may help both conditions. If life-style measures do not provide sufficient benefit, drug therapy may be necessary. A number of classes of cholesterol-lowering drugs are available.

WHAT ARE THE COMPLICATIONS?

Hyperlipidemia predisposes the individual to coronary heart disease and other vascular diseases. The risk tends to rise in direct correlation with increased levels of blood lipids and becomes substantially greater if other risk factors, such as cigarette smoking and high blood pressure, are present. Those with familial types of severe hypercholesterolemia are at risk of coronary heart disease early in life if the disorder is not diagnosed and treated.

HOW CAN IT BE PREVENTED OR MINIMIZED?

A healthy life-style, including a low-fat, low-cholesterol diet, regular exercise, and maintenance of desirable weight, can often prevent or minimize hyperlipidemias. Treatment of diabetes, if present, may also help to lower certain of the fats in the blood.

See Chapters 3, 4, and 5.

HYPERTENSION (HIGH BLOOD PRESSURE)

WHAT IS IT?

As blood circulates in the body, pressure is exerted against the inner walls of arteries. The level of that pressure is reported in two numbers: The systolic (the higher number) is the pressure of the blood on the artery walls when the heart beats (the pumping pressure); the diastolic (the lower number) is the pressure in the arteries between heartbeats (the resting pressure). A normal blood pressure in adults is between 110/70 and 140/90 mm Hg. Although blood pressure tends to fluctuate within this normal range, a persistent elevation of blood pressure above 140/90, regardless of age, is considered hypertension.

WHO GETS IT?

Essential, or primary, hypertension (for which the cause remains unknown) is more common in those over 40. It accounts for over 90 percent of cases. It tends to run in families and afflicts men and women equally, but it is more common in blacks than in whites. The far less common secondary hypertension is more likely to occur in younger people. When the underlying disorder is treated, the hypertension usually disappears. The use of oral contraceptives may result in high blood pressure, but this is rare. Elevated blood pressure occurs in about 5–10 percent of pregnancies, but it usually disappears afterward.

WHAT ARE THE SYMPTOMS?

Hypertension usually causes no symptoms unless it is severe. Contrary to popular belief, headaches are not common, although an early-morning headache in the back of the head may signal an elevated pressure. Dizziness may also be noted.

HOW IS IT DIAGNOSED?

Blood pressure is easily measured with an inflatable cuff attached to a sphygmomanometer. Because a variety of everyday circumstances (including anxiety in the doctor's office) can temporarily affect blood pressure, the diagnosis of hypertension should be made only after repeated readings. The exception is a very high pressure (150/105 to 170/110 mm Hg or higher). In this case, a diagnosis can be made on the basis of the first one or two recordings.

HOW IS IT TREATED?

Mild or borderline hypertension (140/90 to 160/100 mm Hg) usually is treated first with life-style modification, including reducing weight to ideal levels, stopping smoking, reducing salt and fat in the diet, exercising regularly, avoiding excessive alcohol and caffeine, and learning relaxation and stress reduction techniques. If these measures prove ineffective in reducing pressure to a normal level, drug therapy is usually recommended. Moderate to severe pressure (above 160/100) is more likely to be treated early on with medication in addition to life-style modification. Drugs that may be used alone or in combination include beta blockers, diuretics, angiotensin-converting enzyme (ACE) inhibitors, and calcium channel blockers.

WHAT ARE THE COMPLICATIONS?

The complications of prolonged untreated hypertension include stroke, heart attack, heart failure, retinal hemorrhages, and kidney failure. Untreated hypertension can dramatically decrease life expectancy.

HOW CAN IT BE PREVENTED OR MINIMIZED?

Even individuals with a family history of hypertension may be able to prevent it by maintaining ideal weight and eating a low-salt diet. Blood pressure should be checked in adolescence and early adulthood. If the reading is normal, testing should be repeated every three years. If there is a family history of hypertension, initial testing should begin earlier, and, in adulthood, should be repeated annually. Women who are pregnant or who use oral contraceptives should have more frequent checks. Life-style modification and drug therapy have greatly reduced the risks of complications associated with hypertension.

See Chapter 12.

KAWASAKI DISEASE

WHAT IS IT?

Also known as mucocutaneous lymph node syndrome, Kawasaki disease is a very rare disease of children that can affect the skin, mucous membranes, lymph glands, joints, heart, and coronary arteries. In the coronary arteries, the condition can cause dilation of the blood vessels and coronary artery aneurysm. The initial illness usually lasts only 2 to 12 weeks, but relapses may occur and damage to coronary arteries may be permanent.

WHO GETS IT?

Kawasaki disease occurs primarily in children under age 10, with 80 percent of those stricken under age 5. It is more common in boys than in girls and much more common in Asians (especially Japanese) than other races. Although the cause is unknown, Kawasaki disease does not appear to be hereditary or contagious. A virus is the likely cause.

WHAT ARE THE SYMPTOMS?

Kawasaki disease begins with a high fever, irritability, lethargy, swollen lymph glands in the neck, and, in some cases, colicky abdominal pain. Within a day or two a red rash appears on the trunk. In the next few days, the lips, tongue, and other mucous membranes take on a reddish color. Hands and feet swell, and skin on the palms and soles becomes red and then scaly, and then peels. Some patients also develop muscle or joint pain, diarrhea, pneumonia, or meningitis. When heart-related problems occur, they usually develop around the tenth day of illness when other symptoms are disappearing. The most common cardiac problem is inflammation of the coronary arteries, which occurs in about 20 percent of all cases; others include inflammation of heart muscle (myocarditis) or the lining around the heart (pericarditis), arrhythmias, and heart valve dysfunction. Most heart problems disappear within six weeks, but permanent coronary artery damage can result.

HOW IS IT DIAGNOSED?

Because there is no one test to reveal Kawasaki disease, the diagnosis is based on the presence of the critical symptoms and the exclusion of other possible disorders. Cardiac problems are diagnosed using an electrocardiogram and an echocardiogram.

HOW IS IT TREATED?

There is no specific treatment for the disease. Aspirin, given to reduce fever and pain and to help prevent blood clots, also may help reduce the risk of damage to coronary arteries.

WHAT ARE THE COMPLICATIONS?

As a result of inflammation, aneurysms (bulges or blisters) can form in the coronary arteries; if a blood clot forms in that area, myocardial infarction (heart attack) may occur. Less commonly, the aneurysm may burst. In about 1 percent of cases, death occurs, usually related to heart complications.

HOW CAN IT BE PREVENTED OR MINIMIZED?

Since the cause is unknown, Kawasaki disease cannot be prevented. Some research has suggested that intravenous gamma globulin, if administered early in the course of illness, may be effective in preventing coronary artery problems. Those who have developed heart-related problems because of Kawasaki disease should have regular medical check-ups. Aspirin therapy should be continued as long as a coronary aneurysm is present.

See Chapter 20.

LEFT VENTRICULAR ANEURYSM

WHAT IS IT?

The term *aneurysm* generally refers to an outward bulge in the wall of a blood vessel. Although aneurysms are more common in arteries, they sometimes arise in the left ventricle, or lower (pumping) chamber, of the heart. The portion of the ventricle bulges outward, deforming the shape of the heart, as well as not contracting well when the heart normally squeezes blood out to the body.

WHO GETS IT?

Left ventricular aneurysms usually arise as a result of a severe heart attack. In about 10–20 percent of heart attacks in which a substantial amount of the heart wall muscle dies, an aneurysm may form in the ventricle within a few days. It is often not detected until later on, when complications might occur.

WHAT ARE THE SYMPTOMS?

Ventricular aneurysms usually do not cause pain or specific symptoms. They set the stage, however, for the development of ventricular arrhythmia (tachycardia), heart failure, and the formation of thrombi (blood clots) in the heart, which may break loose and travel to other parts of the body. The symptoms of heart failure, especially shortness of breath, or an arrhythmia may indicate that a ventricular aneurysm is present after a heart attack.

HOW IS IT DIAGNOSED?

Aneurysms may be difficult to diagnose, because many produce no symptoms. A chest X-ray, echocardiogram, and radionuclide scan may be used, in addition to physical examination, to diagnose the aneurysm and define its size. Cardiac catheterization and angiography is most helpful and definitive in making a diagnosis.

HOW IS IT TREATED?

Treatment is generally focused on specific problems associated with aneurysm, such as heart failure, cardiac arrhythmia, and blood clots. Ventricular aneurysms may require surgical removal if heart failure or arrhythmias cannot be effectively treated with drugs. In the case of arrhythmias an implantable defibrillator (AICD) may be placed at the time of heart surgery.

WHAT ARE THE COMPLICATIONS?

Unlike other aneurysms, left ventricular aneurysms are not usually at risk of rupture. Because of the thinned and damaged heart muscle, however, arrhythmias and congestive heart failure are potential complications. A blood clot may form in the aneurysm. This presents a risk of embolization to other parts of the body and can cause additional complications such as stroke. Many people may live for years with a ventricular aneurysm.

HOW CAN IT BE PREVENTED OR MINIMIZED?

Measures to reduce the risk of a heart attack—low-fat diet, regular exercise, smoking avoidance, and careful control of high blood pressure and diabetes, if present —can help lower the risk of a ventricular aneurysm. Effective, early treatment of a heart attack may also be helpful.

See Chapter 11.

MARFAN SYNDROME

WHAT IS IT?

The Marfan syndrome is an inherited disorder of connective tissue that affects the heart, blood vessels, lungs, eyes, bones, and ligaments. When the heart is affected, the heart valves may be oversized and may function improperly, permitting a partial backward flow of blood (aortic, mitral, or tricuspid regurgitation) and resulting in a heart murmur. When the aorta (the body's main artery, which carries all blood exiting the heart) is affected, it may enlarge and/or split in one or more places, leaking blood into the chest or abdomen. This is known as a dissecting aortic aneurysm.

WHO GETS IT?

The Marfan syndrome is caused by an abnormal gene, inherited from one parent, that is believed to produce a defect in one of the proteins that make up connective tissue. Although the Marfan syndrome usually runs in families, the abnormal gene can result from a mutation. A rare disorder, the Marfan syndrome affects only about 25,000 Americans.

WHAT ARE THE SYMPTOMS?

Symptoms may be present at birth, may not appear until later in life, even in adulthood, or may never be experienced. All the possible signs of the Marfan syndrome (which may range from mild to severe) are rarely present in one person, nor are they limited to those with this syndrome. However, people with the Marfan syndrome usually are tall and slender, with long, thin arms and legs, loose joints, and long, thin fingers and toes. Other skeletal manifestations may include flat feet, a spinal curvature, a deformed breastbone, and a highly arched palate. Eye symptoms may include nearsightedness and an off-center lens. Cardiovascular symptoms depend upon the cardiovascular abnormalities involved; they may not be present or may include breathlessness, fatigue, palpitations, and fainting. If aortic dissection occurs, there may be a sudden onset of severe chest pain or cardiac collapse.

HOW IS IT DIAGNOSED?

No single test can diagnose the Marfan syndrome, but often the individual's appearance is quite typical. A complete examination will search for all possible signs of the disorder. Because eye lens dislocation rarely occurs in other disorders, even a subtle dislocation is an important diagnostic feature. It is detectable only by dilating the pupils for ophthalmologic examination. An electrocardiogram or other tests to detect cardiovascular abnormalities may also help confirm the diagnosis.

HOW IS IT TREATED?

The Marfan syndrome cannot be cured, but its symptoms can be treated. Treatment depends upon how the individual is affected. For cardiovascular problems, beta blockers or other drugs may be prescribed to regulate blood pressure and heart rhythms. In some cases a heart valve or a part of the aorta may be replaced surgically.

WHAT ARE THE COMPLICATIONS?

The greatest threat is the possibility of a sudden split (dissection) of the aorta, which can cause death if not identified and treated immediately with surgery.

HOW CAN IT BE PREVENTED OR MINIMIZED?

No test is yet available to determine if an unborn child has the Marfan gene. Genetic counseling can help affected families understand their risks. Regular medical checkups, at least yearly, are advised to monitor progression of the disorder so that appropriate treatment can be initiated. Antibiotics must be taken before dental or medical surgery to reduce the risk of endocarditis. Daily activities should be tailored to reduce heart strain; heavy exercise, contact sports, and lifting heavy objects should be avoided. Individuals who show early signs of the Marfan syndrome involving the first part of the aorta should be evaluated regularly by X-ray and echocardiography.

See Chapters 13 and 17.

MITRAL VALVE DISEASE— PROLAPSE

WHAT IS IT?

The mitral valve is one of four valves that control the flow of blood into and out of the heart. In particular, the mitral valve controls the flow of freshly oxygenated blood from the left atrium (upper heart chamber) into the left ventricle (lower heart chamber), from where it is pumped out into the body. If the valve is deformed, one or both of the leaflets—the flaps that open and close to form the valve—may bulge (prolapse) into the atrium during each heartbeat. In addition, a small amount of the blood that is supposed to enter the ventricle may regurgitate, or leak backward into the atrium. A characteristic clicking sound and/or murmur can be heard when listening to the heart with a stethoscope. Depending on the extent of the regurgitation, the heart may have to work harder to assure that an adequate amount of blood is circulated to all the body tissues.

WHO GETS IT?

Mitral valve prolapse is almost invariably congenital and present at birth but not usually detected until later. This common disorder occurs much more frequently in women and is particularly common in those who have a narrow, concave chest cavity and other skeletal abnormalities. The syndrome frequently is detected in teenage girls or women in their 20s and 30s, and it has been estimated that as many as 10 to 15 percent of the young female population may have this condition.

WHAT ARE THE SYMPTOMS?

Most people with mitral valve prolapse have no symptoms. When symptoms do occur, they are most likely to include palpitations, shortness of breath, and atypical, sticking chest pains that may occur at rest. In cases of significant regurgitation, heart failure may develop, but is rare.

HOW IS IT DIAGNOSED?

Some signs of mitral valve prolapse, such as the characteristic clicking sound and a heart murmur heard with a stethoscope, are detectable during a physical examination. An evaluation is likely to include a chest X-ray, an electrocardiogram, and an echocardiogram. Most of the time, however, the diagnosis can be made without specific tests.

HOW IS IT TREATED?

Most often, treatment for mitral valve prolapse is not necessary. If symptoms develop and interfere with the enjoyment of life, beta-blocking drugs may be helpful in relieving palpitations or chest discomfort. Individuals with signs of severe mitral valve prolapse may be advised to avoid strenuous competitive sports. Prophylactic antibiotics may be recommended prior to dental or surgical procedures to prevent endocarditis.

WHAT ARE THE COMPLICATIONS?

Serious complications are rare among those with mitral valve prolapse, but may include a greater risk of blood clot formation, and, very rarely, sudden death. Individuals with mitral valve prolapse also are at greater risk of infective endocarditis (inflammation of the lining of the heart) and problems associated with mitral regurgitation, including heart failure.

HOW CAN IT BE PREVENTED OR MINIMIZED?

There are no known methods of preventing mitral valve prolapse. It is a fairly widespread but benign condition, except in extremely unusual circumstances.

See Chapters 2 and 13.

MITRAL VALVE DISEASE—STENOSIS AND REGURGITATION

WHAT IS IT?

The mitral valve controls the flow of freshly oxygenated blood from the left atrium (an upper heart chamber) into the left ventricle (a major lower heart chamber), from where it is pumped out into the body. If the valve is stenosed (narrowed), the amount of blood that is pushed into the left ventricle is diminished. On the other hand, if the valve does not close properly, it is called incompetent (regurgitant or insufficient), because some of the blood that is pushed through the valve into the left ventricle regurgitates, or leaks backward, into the atrium

with each beat. In either case, the heart must work harder to try to pump an adequate amount of blood to the brain, kidneys, and other parts of the body. In response to regurgitation, the left ventricle and the chamber dilate. This can result in elevated pressure in the heart and, ultimately, heart failure. In mitral stenosis, pressure builds within the left atrium and is passed back through the pulmonary veins, leading to congestion in the lungs and, in severe cases, pulmonary edema.

WHO GETS IT?

Mitral stenosis is almost invariably caused by rheumatic fever, although a very small number of cases are congenital. Although mitral regurgitation also is frequently due to rheumatic fever, it also may be associated with various heart muscle disorders, as well as conditions such as mitral prolapse. Mitral regurgitation may follow a heart attack if the part of the heart muscle to which the valve structures are attached is damaged by the attack.

WHAT ARE THE SYMPTOMS?

Mitral valve disorders may not cause symptoms for many years. In the meantime, however, the burden on various chambers of the heart may result in a diminution of heart function. Lung congestion may result in shortness of breath, especially after exercise or when lying flat in bed. Pressure on the bronchial tree by the enlarged atrium may cause chronic coughing. Both stenosis and regurgitation can cause swollen ankles and marked fatigue. Sometimes easy fatigue is the only symptom suggesting that the valve disorder is resulting in poor heart function.

HOW IS IT DIAGNOSED?

Mitral valve disease may be diagnosed during a physical examination when signs such as specific types of heart murmur are detected. A chest X-ray, an electrocardiogram, and an echocardiogram will help confirm the diagnosis, delineate heart size, and help define the exact extent of the valve abnormality. For advanced cases, cardiac catheterization is usually indicated.

HOW IS IT TREATED?

No treatment is necessary for patients who remain free of symptoms. Prophylactic use of antibiotics prior to dental work or surgery is necessary to prevent endocarditis (infection of the lining of the heart valves). If an irregular heart rhythm like atrial fibrillation is also present, anticoagulant drugs may be prescribed to help prevent blood clot formation. Beta-blocking drugs and digitalis or quinidine may be used to slow the heart rate or to restore a normal rhythm in those subjects with mitral stenosis who develop atrial fibrillation. Breathlessness may be treated with diuretics to decrease fluid buildup. Drugs called "afterload reducers" that decrease the heart's work may be effective in alleviating some of the symptoms that may be noted with mitral regurgitation. If symptoms persist in cases of mitral stenosis, a surgical procedure called valvulotomy may be used to widen the valve, or surgery to replace the valve may be advised.

WHAT ARE THE COMPLICATIONS?

Individuals with mitral valve disease are at risk for heart failure and endocarditis. The long-term complications of both stenosis and regurgitation include atrial fibrillation, a rhythm disturbance that may be associated with the formation of blood clots within the atria. This arrhythmia increases the risk of a stroke, because a blood clot may break loose and travel through the bloodstream to lodge in various arteries.

HOW CAN IT BE PREVENTED OR MINIMIZED?

Avoidance of rheumatic fever by prompt treatment of a strep throat is the major preventive measure. If mitral valve disease is present, the prophylactic use of antibiotics before dental extractions or surgery can help prevent infective endocarditis.

See Chapters 2 and 13.

MYOCARDIAL INFARCTION

WHAT IS IT?

Myocardial infarction is the medical term for a heart attack. An infarct (an area of dead or dying tissue) occurs in the myocardium (heart muscle) when there is a marked decrease in the oxygen supply to an area of the muscle. In more than 90 percent of cases, this decrease is caused by an obstruction or closure of one of the coronary arteries, caused by a blood clot blocking an artery narrowed by atherosclerosis. Less commonly, the obstruction may be caused by an arterial spasm, which also closes off the blood flow.

WHO GETS IT?

The highest incidence of myocardial infarction is in middle-aged and elderly men. The incidence in women rises about five to ten years after menopause. About 45 percent of all individuals who experience a heart attack are under age 65; 5 percent are under 40. Heart attacks are more common in those who smoke, are obese, or have high blood cholesterol levels, high blood pressure, diabetes, or a family history of arteriosclerosis at an early age (before age 65). A small number of heart attacks occur in people who have none of these risk factors.

WHAT ARE THE SYMPTOMS?

The most common symptoms of a heart attack are a feeling of pressure, tightness, squeezing, or pain in the center of the chest, lasting at least 5–15 minutes and less commonly for more than an hour. The discomfort may spread to the shoulders, neck, jaw, or arms, particularly radiating down the left arm. Pain may or may not be accompanied by sweating, nausea, light-headedness, or shortness of breath. In many people, the symptoms of heart attack are mistaken for indigestion. Further, in about 20 percent of heart attacks, there are no noticeable symptoms ("silent" heart attacks).

HOW IS IT DIAGNOSED?

Heart attack should be suspected and medical attention sought whenever an adult experiences unexplained chest pain or pressure. Heart attacks are usually diagnosed based on the patient's symptoms and an evaluation of heart function by examination with a stethoscope, as well as measurements of blood pressure and pulse. An electrocardiogram and blood tests (cardiac enzymes) will usually, but not invariably, confirm the diagnosis. Initial therapy is usually based on these evaluations. Follow-up examination to assess the extent of the heart attack and heart damage may include echocardiography, a stress test, nuclear scans, and coronary angiography.

HOW IS IT TREATED?

All heart attacks require urgent medical treatment. Many can be aborted and heart muscle damage minimized if the individual immediately seeks emergency care and is treated with drugs (such as tissue plasminogen activator, streptokinase, APSAC, or urokinase) that may dissolve the blood clot. To be maximally effective, these "thrombolytic" drugs must be started within two to four hours from onset of symptoms. Other treatment may include medications to alleviate pain, to stabilize abnormal heart rhythms, to dilate blood vessels, to lower the heart's workload, and to decrease the risk of further blood clot development. Follow-up care may include angioplasty to open narrowed vessels or cardiac surgery to provide adequate blood supply. In addition, life-style changes (cessation of smoking, regular exercise, and diet modifications) may be recommended as appropriate.

WHAT ARE THE COMPLICATIONS?

Severe arrhythmias, heart failure, shock, and cardiac arrest are potentially life-threatening complications of a heart attack. With improved early treatment, these complications are becoming much less frequent. Rarely, the heart muscle may rupture, requiring immediate surgery.

HOW CAN IT BE PREVENTED OR MINIMIZED?

Appropriate life-style changes that reduce the risk of atherosclerosis may help prevent a heart attack. These include stopping smoking, eating a low-fat diet, losing excess weight, and controlling blood pressure and diabetes. For individuals who have had a heart attack, routine use of aspirin is generally advised. The need to recognize symptoms of a heart attack and seek immediate treatment cannot be overemphasized. It may be lifesaving.

See Chapter 11.

MYOCARDITIS

WHAT IS IT?

Myocarditis is an inflammation of heart muscle—the muscle that contracts to pump blood out of the heart and relaxes to allow its return. This inflammation can seriously impair both the pumping action and the electrical activity of the heart. Consequently, myocarditis can result in congestive heart failure and arrythmias.

WHO GETS IT?

Myocarditis is uncommon, but can occur in virtually anyone. The inflammation is a complication of a variety of infectious diseases, most commonly the Coxsackie Type B virus. It also can arise as a result of infection with other viruses, bacteria, parasites, or fungi. Less commonly, myocarditis develops after exposure to certain drugs, arsenic, or other toxic chemicals, or as a complication of some metabolic, granulomatous, or connective tissue disorders.

WHAT ARE THE SYMPTOMS?

Symptoms of myocarditis vary widely. In adults, they can sometimes mimic those of a heart attack—mild to severe pain in the center of the chest, which may radiate to the neck, shoulders, and upper arms. In severe cases, symptoms include breathlessness, rapid pulse, and heart arrhythmias. In infants, symptoms also may include bluish skin, heart murmurs, and a poor appetite.

HOW IS IT DIAGNOSED?

Myocarditis may be suspected whenever chest pain or arrhythmia symptoms suggestive of congestive heart failure occur during the course of an infectious illness, especially a viral one. It should also be suspected when such symptoms occur in the absence of an obvious diagnosis. Diagnosis may require blood tests, a chest X-ray, electrocardiogram, echocardiogram or radionuclide angiocardiogram, and, in rare cases, biopsy of a tissue sample from the heart muscle.

HOW IS IT TREATED?

Mild, viral-related myocarditis in adults often cures itself with little or no direct treatment. Similarly, mild cases caused by other types of infection often require only taking antibiotics or other drugs to treat the underlying disease. More severe myocarditis may cause marked heart arrhythmias and heart failure if inflammation sufficiently damages the heart muscle or myocardium. In such cases, medications to stabilize heart function may be necessary. These may include vasodilators, digitalis, diuretics, ACE inhibitors, and other drugs. In certain severe types of myocarditis, steroids may be prescribed. Sometimes even after myocarditis is resolved, the heart muscle remains permanently damaged. If a heart block or marked slowing of the heart rate occurs, a pacemaker may be required. In advanced, severe cases, cardiac transplantation may be the only alternative.

WHAT ARE THE COMPLICATIONS?

In severe cases, myocarditis can lead to heart failure and even death.

HOW CAN IT BE PREVENTED OR MINIMIZED?

There are only a few known measures to reduce the occurrence of this rare disease. Avoiding exposure to infectious diseases and having any such illness treated promptly may help. Should myocarditis occur, bed rest is usually required until the inflammation subsides. During this time, alcohol, salt, and any other substances that may increase the heart's work or irritate it further should be avoided.

See Chapter 15.

PERICARDITIS

WHAT IS IT?

The heart is wrapped in a cellophane-like bag or membrane called the pericardium. Pericarditis is an inflammation of this membrane. There are two major types: acute and chronic constrictive pericarditis.

WHO GETS IT?

Acute pericarditis comes on suddenly and may be caused by a bacterial, viral, or fungal infection, or it may occur in association with certain diseases, such as rheumatic fever, rheumatoid arthritis, systemic lupus erythematosus, scleroderma, chronic kidney failure, and tumors. It may also be precipitated by a heart attack or a serious chest injury. A form of pericarditis may also be noted within several weeks after heart surgery. Chronic pericarditis, which is uncommon, develops slowly and may be caused by a chronic infection, such as tuberculosis.

WHAT ARE THE SYMPTOMS?

Acute pericarditis usually causes pain in the center of the chest, which may radiate to the neck or left shoulder. Unlike angina or heart attack, this pain may be "sticking" in nature and worsens with deep breathing, coughing, or twisting of the upper body. Nevertheless, the pain at times may mimic that of a heart attack. When acute pericarditis is triggered by an infection, fever, chills, and weakness also tend to occur. Chronic pericarditis may not cause any symptoms until the long-term inflammation of the pericardium causes it to thicken and contract to the point where it interferes with normal heart filling. (This condition is known as *constrictive pericarditis*.) Pain may not be a prominent symptom, but symptoms that mimic heart failure may develop, including shortness of breath and edema (accumulation of fluid in the legs and abdomen), swelling in the abdomen because of fluid (ascites), and swelling of the liver.

HOW IS IT DIAGNOSED?

The patient's history may be sufficient to make a diagnosis. Characteristic sounds heard through the stethoscope (a rubbing sound), an electrocardiogram, a chest X-ray, and an echocardiogram may be necessary to confirm the diagnosis of acute pericarditis. Additional tests to identify the cause of the pericarditis may include blood cultures, skin tests, and, depending on the individual case, sampling of the fluid in the sac surrounding the heart, or (rarely) a biopsy of the pericardium itself. Diagnosis of chronic obstructive pericarditis generally requires cardiac catheterization.

HOW IS IT TREATED?

Analgesics, ranging from aspirin to morphine, as well as anti-inflammatory drugs may be given to ease the pain or reduce the inflammatory reaction of acute pericarditis. No further treatment may be necessary for pericarditis caused by a viral infection, which tends to clear by itself within a few weeks. If an underlying treatable cause for the pericarditis can be identified, further treatment will be directed toward its alleviation. Antibiotics may be given for a bacterial infection, while steroids such as cortisone may be given in other cases, and nonsteroidal anti-inflammatory agents such as indomethacin in still other cases. Steroid drugs may also be prescribed to reduce the inflammation in pericarditis resulting from a heart attack. Diuretics and a salt-restricted diet are also recommended for constrictive pericarditis. In severe cases, surgery may be necessary to remove the thickened pericardium.

WHAT ARE THE COMPLICATIONS?

The major complication of acute pericarditis is pericardial effusion, in which fluid collects in the sack between the pericardium and the heart. If a large amount of fluid collects, the result may be *cardiac tamponade*, in which the return of blood to the heart from the veins is severely impaired, resulting in a fall in blood pressure. In such cases, the pericardial fluid must be removed by needle aspiration. This is usually a relatively easy and safe procedure. The major problems with *chronic* pericarditis include congestive heart failure with symptoms that mimic liver or kidney failure. Such complications may require surgical intervention to remove the pericardium.

HOW CAN IT BE PREVENTED OR MINIMIZED?

Prompt treatment of any infection or other condition affecting the lining of the heart or other organs may help prevent this disorder. In many cases it cannot be prevented; on the other hand, the majority of cases are uncomplicated and of short duration. Prompt diagnosis and therapy with anti-inflammatory agents can help minimize the symptoms of pericarditis.

PERIPHERAL VASCULAR DISEASE

WHAT IS IT?

Peripheral vascular disease is a disorder in which the blood supply to the legs or arms is impaired; when normal blood flow is limited, pain may occur. This pain, called intermittent claudication, occurs most often with walking or similar exercise of the legs and is akin to angina, the chest pain that occurs when the heart muscles do not receive enough blood. Peripheral vascular disease is caused by the build-up of fatty deposits, known as atherosclerotic plaque, on the interior surface of the large arteries of the extremities (especially the legs), thus narrowing the channel through which blood can circulate. It is also known as arteriosclerotic obliterans, peripheral atherosclerotic disease, and angina of the leg.

WHO GETS IT?

Peripheral vascular disease primarily occurs in those who are middle-aged or elderly. At greater risk are individuals who already have atherosclerosis elsewhere, or who are at high risk of developing it: those who smoke, have diabetes, high blood cholesterol, hypertension, and a family history of cardiovascular disease and are overweight.

WHAT ARE THE SYMPTOMS?

Pain that occurs upon exercise and ceases with rest is the classic symptom. The discomfort can range from mild aching to cramps to severe pain. Pain is usually centered in the calf, but also can arise in the thigh, hip, or buttocks. In severe cases, pain occurs with minimal exercise or at rest, and there may be ulceration of the skin. In some circumstances, impotence may occur in males, and the legs may feel cool to the touch. In unusual cases, peripheral vascular disease can cause pain in the arms during exercise.

HOW IS IT DIAGNOSED?

Physicians often diagnose the condition solely on the description of symptoms and by finding a reduced or absent pulse on examination of the leg arteries. Ultrasound can also be valuable in making the diagnosis. If surgery is being considered, arteriography may be recommended to confirm the precise location and severity of the arterial narrowing.

HOW IS IT TREATED?

Various medications may be prescribed to dilate blood vessels and help prevent blood clots. Unfortunately, drug treatment is ineffective in many cases. The best treatment is walking, which helps develop additional (collateral) blood vessels, allowing blood flow to bypass the affected arteries. If in some cases symptoms are disabling, several procedures are available to widen the narrowed artery: balloon angioplasty, to compress the plaque against the inner arterial walls; surgical endarterectomy, to remove plaque from the walls; or surgery to bypass the blocked artery, using a vein taken from elsewhere in the leg or a synthetic artery.

WHAT ARE THE COMPLICATIONS?

The foot on the affected leg may become cold and numb, with dry skin and limited nail growth. Skin ulcers may develop, even after only slight injury. A blood clot may form in a narrowed artery, cutting off circulation to the lower leg or foot and causing acute pain. In severe cases, which are not too frequent, impaired blood flow can be disabling and may increase the risk of gangrene. Urgent surgery may be required to save the limb in these cases.

HOW CAN IT BE PREVENTED OR MINIMIZED?

Avoiding smoking and adopting a low-fat, low-cholesterol diet and a regular exercise regimen can help prevent peripheral vascular disease. Diabetes and hypertension should be treated at an early stage. If peripheral vascular disease does occur, weight reduction can reduce the burden on the legs and daily exercise can assist the body in its efforts to increase the size and distribution of the smaller blood vessels in the area (known as collateral circulation). Scrupulous foot care should include keeping the feet warm and dry and avoiding constricting garters and tight shoes or socks as well as prompt professional treatment for calluses, corns, ulcers, or foot injuries.

See Chapter 17.

PREMATURE BEATS—ATRIAL AND VENTRICULAR

WHAT IS IT?

The heart's beating rhythm is controlled by a natural pacemaker in an area called the sinoatrial node, located toward the top of the heart. It sends out electrical stimuli in rhythmic waves that normally follow prescribed pathways from the atria (the upper chambers) to the ventricles (the lower chambers), producing sequential and coordinated contractions. If erratic electrical stimuli originate elsewhere in the heart muscle, the normal rhythm is disturbed and becomes irregular. The result is called extra or premature beats. The stimulus for such premature beats may arise in the atria, in the ventricles, or (less commonly) in the AV node—the area that separates the upper and lower parts of the heart. Although the heart chamber where the stimulus arises beats prematurely, the following beat usually occurs after a "compensatory" pause and is generally a stronger contraction. Nevertheless, the following beat arises in a normal fashion.

WHO GETS IT?

The occasional occurrence of premature beats is quite common and often is noted in people with a completely normal heart. Atrial or ventricular premature beats may be triggered by the use of tobacco, alcohol, caffeine, and certain drugs or can be provoked by factors such as anxiety, which causes excess release of adrenalinelike substances. Ventricular premature beats (VPBs) are also frequently seen in those who have heart disease. Even in these patients, however, an occasional atrial premature beat (APB) or ventricular premature beat is not of great significance. Premature beats may be noticed in subjects with rheumatic or atherosclerotic heart disease, mitral prolapse, myocarditis, cardiomyopathy, and heart failure and during attacks of angina. VPBs occur to some extent in more than 90 percent of individuals who have a heart attack.

WHAT ARE THE SYMPTOMS?

Premature beats often may not even be noticed, or may be experienced as a sensation of a skipped or extra heartbeat, palpitation, or heart flutter. If these occur in runs of more than five to ten, there may be some light-headedness or a feeling of weakness.

HOW IS IT DIAGNOSED?

Premature beats are identifiable by listening to the heart with a stethoscope or taking the pulse at the wrist. Premature beats usually are easily recognizable on an electrocardiogram. Once the premature beats have been identified, further diagnostic procedures are usually not necessary. If the beats are very frequent, arise from different parts of the heart, or cause symptoms, further studies may be necessary to determine whether they are harbingers of a more serious rhythm disturbance or whether they indicate underlying heart disease. These tests may include an exercise stress test, nuclear imaging studies of the heart, Holter monitoring, and an echocardiogram.

HOW IS IT TREATED?

Occasional premature beats that cause no symptoms in a healthy person are of no concern and need not be treated. Eliminating the use of caffeine or nicotine and reducing alcohol intake (if appropriate) may control both APBs and VPBs. If premature beats occur as part of heart failure or following a heart attack, correcting or treating the basic problem may eliminate the extra beats. *Medications should be used only if symptoms are annoying or runs of extra beats occur.* More harm than good may often be done by treating people with premature beats. Reassurances that the "extra beats" are not life-threatening are an important element of treatment.

WHAT ARE THE COMPLICATIONS?

Premature beats may be the forerunners of more severe heart arrhythmias, such as ventricular tachycardia or fibrillation, especially following a heart attack. Usually they are not.

HOW CAN IT BE PREVENTED OR MINIMIZED?

Excessive use of caffeine should be avoided. Smoking cessation and limiting the intake of alcohol can help reduce the occurrence of this type of heart rhythm abnormality.

See Chapter 16.

PULMONARY EDEMA

WHAT IS IT?

Pulmonary edema is a condition that is usually secondary to heart disease, most commonly to heart failure. When the left side of the heart is not pumping effectively, pressure builds up in the heart. Blood in the pulmonary veins (the pathway from the lungs to the heart) gets backed up. Accumulation of excess fluid raises pressure in the pulmonary veins and eventually in the lung tissue. As a result of the backup and increased pressure, fluid passes out of the blood vessels into the little sacs of the lungs (alveoli) that are the normal sites of oxygen and carbon dioxide exchange. As fluid builds up, the lung tissue becomes waterlogged; this condition is called pulmonary edema. Acute pulmonary edema is a potentially life-threatening event.

WHO GETS IT?

Pulmonary edema is a severe symptom of heart failure and may have such diverse causes as heart attack, heart valve disorders, cardiomyopathy, cardiac arrhythmias, and severe hypertension. It may be the first sign of a heart problem that has gone undiagnosed and untreated for an extended period. It also may occur in people who suffer from "mountain sickness" at very high altitudes.

WHAT ARE THE SYMPTOMS?

Shortness of breath develops and worsens over the course of minutes to several hours. Sometimes it is so acute that the individual gasps for breath and has a sense of suffocation. It may be accompanied by a cough, which is at first dry but eventually produces blood-tinged sputum. Sometimes wheezing occurs. A severe attack also can produce pale skin, sweating, anxiety, and low blood pressure. Symptoms may develop slowly or rapidly, presenting an acute crisis. Pulmonary edema may begin with an acute attack at night, when blood pools in the lungs as the individual lies in bed. Those with chronic pulmonary edema will experience fatigue and shortness of breath, especially after exertion.

HOW IS IT DIAGNOSED?

The symptoms listed above and characteristic signs, such as the sound of rales (a sound like the wrinkling of paper) heard in the chest with a stethoscope, indicate pulmonary edema. A physical examination, blood tests (particularly to evaluate gases in the blood), and a chest X-ray may confirm the diagnosis.

HOW IS IT TREATED?

Acute pulmonary edema is an emergency that usually requires hospitalization and oxygen support. If an acute attack occurs, emergency medical personnel should be called immediately. Until help arrives, the individual should sit upright. If nitroglycerin tablets are available, one should be placed under the tongue to dilate blood vessels and help distribute blood away from the lungs. Once the patient is stabilized, various medications will be given, such as a diuretic to help drain excess fluid from the lungs, digitalis to improve heart function, and morphine to slow and deepen breathing. Sometimes a phlebotomy—the removal of a certain volume of blood from the body—may be necessary. Additional therapy will depend upon the underlying cause of the heart failure. Chronic pulmonary edema is a form of chronic heart failure and is treated accordingly.

WHAT ARE THE COMPLICATIONS?

If not treated promptly, acute pulmonary edema can be fatal. Effective treatment usually enables restoration of heart function. With proper therapy, individuals who have survived an episode of acute pulmonary edema can lead a reasonably normal life, although they may have to restrict some activity.

HOW CAN IT BE PREVENTED OR MINIMIZED?

Proper treatment of cardiac problems can help prevent pulmonary edema. Patients with heart failure must strictly adhere to a low-salt diet. A significant amount of sodium ingested over a short period can precipitate pulmonary edema.

See Chapters 14 and 27.

PULMONARY HYPERTENSION

WHAT IS IT?

Pulmonary hypertension is a condition in which the pressure in the vessels that carry blood from the heart to the lungs (the pulmonary blood vessels) is abnormally high. Primary pulmonary hypertension is a rare disorder of unknown cause in which the small and medium pulmonary arteries become narrowed and the pressure elevated. Secondary pulmonary hypertension is a more common disorder that occurs as a result of some other lung or heart disease. Both tend to be chronic conditions, although the primary condition is more serious.

WHO GETS IT?

Primary pulmonary hypertension is very uncommon but is three times more common in women than in men, and the average age at diagnosis is 35. Secondary pulmonary hypertension may be caused by almost any chronic lung disorder, but its association with chronic bronchitis and emphysema is especially common. It is also associated with certain types of congenital heart disease in which there is increased flow to the lungs, as well as with scleroderma, a disorder characterized by excessive buildup of fibrous connective tissue, and some neuromuscular diseases that affect the respiratory muscles.

WHAT ARE THE SYMPTOMS?

Pulmonary hypertension may result in shortness of breath, chest pain, and occasional dizziness upon exertion. In addition, there also may be wheezing, coughing, and swollen ankles because of water retention. In secondary pulmonary hypertension, the symptoms may be primarily those of the underlying condition.

HOW IS IT DIAGNOSED?

Often pulmonary hypertension will be suspected on the basis of the patient's report of symptoms and the findings of characteristic heart or breathing sounds during a complete physical examination. Tests to confirm the diagnosis may include a chest X-ray, electrocardiogram, echocardiogram, and tests to monitor the level of oxygen in the blood.

HOW IS IT TREATED?

Primary pulmonary hypertension is largely untreatable medically, although some patients may be helped by drugs that dilate the blood vessels. The effect of such drugs must first be evaluated during cardiac catheterization, because in some patients they may cause serious problems. In secondary pulmonary hypertension, treatment of the underlying condition (such as heart failure) may help alleviate the lung problem. If it is the result of congenital heart disease, surgery may be advised. Medications such as diuretics to relieve fluid retention or digitalis to improve heart muscle contraction may be prescribed, as well as a period of bed rest, perhaps with supplemental oxygen. If all other treatments fail, a lung or heart/lung transplant may be recommended.

WHAT ARE THE COMPLICATIONS?

Primary pulmonary hypertension can be fatal within two to five years after the initial diagnosis, although many people survive for years with the condition and without any specific treatment. Secondary pulmonary hypertension usually can be treated, but it also can have grave complications. The outcome for the patient depends on the condition causing it. If the condition is chronic heart failure or severe emphysema, the prognosis is not good. If pulmonary hypertension causes the right ventricle of the heart to enlarge, the condition is then called cor pulmonale.

HOW CAN IT BE PREVENTED OR MINIMIZED?

Primary pulmonary hypertension cannot be prevented. Prompt treatment of conditions that may be associated with secondary pulmonary hypertension may prevent or minimize it. Since chronic lung disease—most commonly caused by smoking—is a major cause of secondary pulmonary hypertension, stopping smoking is an important preventive measure. Prompt treatment for infection and regular treatment for any heart or lung disorder or scleroderma are also important. If secondary pulmonary hypertension becomes chronic, prophylactic antibiotics and annual influenza immunization may be recommended to help protect against respiratory infections.

See Chapter 25.

PULMONIC VALVE DISEASE

WHAT IS IT?

The pulmonic valve controls the flow of blood from the right ventricle (lower chamber) of the heart into the pulmonary artery, through which it travels to the lungs for oxygenation. If the valve is stenosed (narrowed), its opening is abnormally small and the heart must work harder to overcome the resulting resistance in order to pump a sufficient quantity of blood. In severe cases, it cannot accomplish this and an insufficient amount of blood moves out of the ventricle with each heartbeat. On the other hand, a pulmonary valve that does not close properly is called regurgitant (incompetent or insufficient), because with each beat, some of the blood that should be pumped from the heart into the pulmonary artery regurgitates, or leaks backward, into the ventricle. In either case, the heart must work harder to pump adequate amounts of blood. The right ventricle may compensate for this either by enlargement (dilation) or an increase in muscle thickness (hypertrophy).

WHO GETS IT?

Pulmonic valve disease is extremely rare and is almost invariably congenital. In severe cases, it can cause a life-threatening emergency in infants. Rarely, the condition may go unrecognized until adulthood.

WHAT ARE THE SYMPTOMS?

In newborns, pulmonic valve stenosis often occurs in conjunction with other heart abnormalities, and symptoms may arise from the combination of anomalies. The main signs and symptoms are shortness of breath and cyanosis (bluish skin), indicating that the baby's blood is not being sufficiently oxygenated. In older children and adults, the only symptoms may be pale skin, shortness of breath on exertion, and easy fatigability. Frequently there will be no symptoms.

HOW IS IT DIAGNOSED?

Some signs of pulmonic valve disease, such as a heart murmur, are detectable during a physical examination. A chest X-ray, an electrocardiogram, and an echocardiogram will usually confirm the diagnosis. Cardiac catheterization is necessary if surgery is planned to correct the valve abnormality.

HOW IS IT TREATED?

Mild pulmonic valve disorders may not require treatment. However, severe stenosis in a newborn requires immediate surgery to establish more normal blood flow. In older children and adults who develop symptoms that impair quality of life, surgery to replace the defective valve may be warranted.

WHAT ARE THE COMPLICATIONS?

As in other types of valve disease, pulmonary valve deformities increase the risk of infective endocarditis, an infection on the valve surface. In severe pulmonic valve disease, right-sided congestive heart failure may develop.

HOW CAN IT BE PREVENTED OR MINIMIZED?

Congenital heart disease cannot be avoided, but fortunately it is rare. In patients with pulmonary valve disease, prophylactic use of antibiotics before dental extractions and surgery can help prevent the development of infective endocarditis.

See Chapters 13 and 20.

RHEUMATIC HEART DISEASE

WHAT IS IT?

The term *rheumatic heart disease* does not refer to a single disorder, but rather to the various types of acute and chronic heart disorders that may occur as a result of rheumatic fever. Every part of the heart, including the pericardium (the outer covering) and the endocardium (the inner lining), may be damaged by inflammation caused by rheumatic fever. However, the most common form of rheumatic heart disease relates to the heart valves, particularly the mitral valve. If the heart has been involved in an attack of acute rheumatic fever, it may take several years for valve damage to develop.

WHO GETS IT?

Rheumatic fever is no longer common in the United States. When it does occur, it usually affects children between the ages of 5 and 15, following a sore throat caused by streptococcal bacteria (strep throat). If the sore throat is not treated promptly with antibiotics, the infection may affect other parts of the body, including the heart.

WHAT ARE THE SYMPTOMS?

Symptoms vary depending upon the type of heart damage caused by the rheumatic fever. In milder cases, there are usually no symptoms. In cases of advanced valve abnormalities, breathlessness, palpitations, heart arrhythmias, fever, swollen feet, dizziness, and chest pain may be experienced.

HOW IS IT DIAGNOSED?

In some cases, a heart murmur (which can be heard with a stethoscope) develops during or after a bout of rheumatic fever, signaling the development of minor to major heart valve changes. In others, more severe problems become immediately apparent. In the majority of cases, symptoms of heart disease develop slowly after an initial attack of rheumatic fever and do not appear until young adulthood or middle age. Diagnosis of heart involvement usually requires a chest X-ray, electrocardiogram, or echocardiogram.

HOW IS IT TREATED?

If heart damage from rheumatic fever is identified in childhood or young adulthood, prophylactic antibiotics may be recommended daily until about the age of 25–30 to prevent recurrence of rheumatic fever and to help avoid the development of endocarditis. Further therapy depends on the type of heart damage present. Medications may be prescribed to help slow a rapid heartbeat, while anticoagulant drugs may be recommended to help prevent the development of blood clots. In advanced cases, surgery may be needed to replace the damaged heart valves.

WHAT ARE THE COMPLICATIONS?

The most common long-term heart problems involve an abnormal flow of blood in the heart because of damaged heart valves. Generally the mitral or aortic valve is involved and does not open fully (stenosis) or close properly (insufficiency). Individuals with rheumatic heart disease also have a greater risk of developing bacterial endocarditis.

HOW CAN IT BE PREVENTED OR MINIMIZED?

Rheumatic fever and subsequent heart disease have become fairly rare in the United States since the development of antibiotics. Any child with a persistent sore throat should have a throat culture to check for strep. Penicillin or another antibiotic will usually prevent the development of rheumatic fever from such an infection. About 60 percent of those afflicted with rheumatic fever develop some degree of subsequent heart disease. Individuals who have had rheumatic fever should receive prophylactic antibiotics before any medical or dental surgery to help prevent infection and subsequent bacterial endocarditis.

See Chapters 2, 13, and 20.

SHOCK

WHAT IS IT?

Shock occurs when blood pressure falls to a severely low level (about 50 to 60 mm Hg for the upper reading, or systolic pressure) for a period of time, causing the flow of blood to the body to become inadequate. Because the flow of oxygenated blood to vital tissues and organs is impaired, they may cease to function adequately. If this lasts for a short period of time, the effects will be transient. If shock becomes prolonged, it will result in permanent impairment of certain organ systems and can ultimately lead to death. Major types of shock are *cardiogenic* (from a cardiac source such as a heart attack), *hypovolemic* (after severe loss of blood or fluids), *anaphylactic* (from an allergic reaction), and *septic* (as a result of overwhelming infection).

WHO GETS IT?

Shock occurs in a wide variety of circumstances and affects various individuals, as defined by the type of shock. Cardiogenic shock occurs when the heart fails to pump adequately; it may result from a heart attack, a severe, sustained arrhythmia, cardiomyopathy, or pulmonary embolism. Hypovolemic shock is caused by acute blood or fluid loss, which might result from external bleeding because of severe injury or internal bleeding from a peptic ulcer, ruptured ectopic pregnancy, or other disorder, or it may arise from fluid loss caused by prolonged severe diarrhea or vomiting, heat exhaustion, or severe burns. Anaphylactic shock is the result of an intense allergic reaction that causes blood vessels to dilate dramatically, leading to a relative shortage of blood volume. Septic shock occurs in the course of a severe infection and is also associated with profound blood vessel dilation.

WHAT ARE THE SYMPTOMS?

Fatigue, faintness, nausea, and a feeling of panic are often the major symptoms of shock. Other symptoms may include chills, cold hands and feet, pale and clammy skin, palpitations, sweating, and thirst. Breathing is rapid but shallow, and the pulse is rapid but weak. In septic or anaphylactic shock there may also be fever. If the condition is not treated promptly, lethargy, drowsiness, confusion, and loss of consciousness may occur.

HOW IS IT DIAGNOSED?

Low blood pressure alone does not constitute shock. Someone can faint from low blood pressure and *not* be in shock! If the skin is warm and dry and few symptoms other than low blood pressure are present, the patient has hypotension but not shock. Shock is diagnosed based on the overt symptoms and appearance of the individual, the presence of one of the diseases that may cause it, a very low blood pressure, and a weak pulse that is usually greater than 100 beats per minute. While laboratory tests and other diagnostic measures such as an electrocardiogram can aid in reaching a precise diagnosis, such measures should only be considered after appropriate emergency treatment has been employed.

HOW IS IT TREATED?

Emergency treatment is essential for survival. The patient is placed flat on his or her back with legs raised to provide maximum blood flow to the heart and brain. An exception might be the patient who is breathing rapidly with gurgling sounds in the chest. This suggests congestion in the lungs secondary to cardiogenic shock. In this case the patient should be kept in a semi-sitting position. If blood or fluid loss is believed to be the cause of the shock, intravenous fluids should be given, or if there has been blood loss, blood transfusions. Drugs may be injected to strengthen the heartbeat, slow a runaway heartbeat, and raise blood pressure. Oxygen support may be provided. After blood pressure has stabilized at a level sufficient to relieve symptoms and return more normal function to organs such as the kidneys, therapy for the underlying cause of the shock can be instituted.

WHAT ARE THE COMPLICATIONS?

If not treated promptly, shock may be fatal. If the brain and kidneys are deprived of adequate blood and oxygen, severe damage may occur. Kidney failure may result if shock is not reversed within a few hours.

HOW CAN IT BE PREVENTED OR MINIMIZED?

Immediate first aid should be provided until emergency medical personnel arrive. This includes keeping the victim warm and lying down with legs slightly raised (about a foot)—except in certain circumstances (see above). As noted, if breathing worsens in this position, heart failure may be part of the shock syndrome and the person should be kept in a sitting position. If breathing or heartbeat stops, cardiopulmonary resuscitation should be undertaken. In the case of trauma, if bleeding is observed, the flow should be stemmed by applying direct pressure to the site of the bleeding or using a tourniquet above the bleeding site (if possible). In the case of an anaphylactic shock, the immediate injection of an antihistamine or adrenaline may be lifesaving. Many people with a history of severe allergic reactions carry these medications (in injectable form) with them. Most important, get the person to a hospital emergency room at once.

See Chapter 27.

STROKE AND TIA

WHAT IS IT?

A stroke, sometimes called a cerebrovascular accident, is a form of cardiovascular disease affecting the blood supply to the brain. The most common types (cerebral thrombosis and cerebral embolism) are caused by blood clots that interfere with the delivery of oxygen to various parts of the brain. Cerebral thrombosis is similar to a heart attack, in that a blood clot forms in an artery (already narrowed by atherosclerosis) in the brain or one in the neck leading to the brain. In a transient ischemic attack (TIA or ministroke), the interruption of blood flow, and thus the occurrence of symptoms, is only temporary or intermittent. In a cerebral embolism, a blood clot formed elsewhere (usually in the heart) travels in the bloodstream to block blood flow in or to the brain. Less common, but usually more serious, are hemorrhagic strokes (cerebral hemorrhage and subarachnoid hemorrhage), which occur when a blood vessel in the brain bursts, interrupting the normal flow of oxygen to the brain.

WHO GETS IT?

Cerebral thrombosis most commonly occurs in older people with long-established atherosclerosis and untreated high blood pressure. Cerebral emboli are more frequent in those who have irregular heart rhythms such as atrial fibrillation, heart attacks, or heart failure. Hemorrhagic strokes are more common in those with uncontrolled high blood pressure. They may also arise as a result of a head injury or a burst congenital aneurysm (weakened arterial wall in the brain).

WHAT ARE THE SYMPTOMS?

The symptoms of a stroke may include sudden weakness or numbness of the face, arm, and leg on one side of the body; difficulty in speaking or understanding others; dimness or impaired vision in one eye; unexplained dizziness or unsteadiness; and sudden falls. TIA symptoms are similar but milder, such as temporary weakness, visual disturbances, or loss of feeling on one side of the body, or other stroke symptoms that last only a few minutes. TIAs themselves are a significant warning sign of a future stroke.

HOW IS IT DIAGNOSED?

A complete history and physical and neurological examination form the basis for diagnosing most strokes and TIAs. Observation of the patient's symptoms can reveal much about the stroke's location to a neurologist. A CT scan of the brain will usually pinpoint the area of the stroke. An evaluation of brain blood flow, such as by Doppler ultrasound scan of the carotid arteries (arteries in the neck that bring oxygenated blood to the brain), may be performed to help determine prognosis and design optimal therapy.

HOW IS IT TREATED?

Blood clots cause at least 70 percent of all strokes; if such strokes are treated within a few hours of onset with anticoagulants (blood-thinning drugs), some stroke damage may be avoided. Such drugs can even be hazardous, however, with hemorrhagic strokes. After the acute phase, treatment focuses on rehabilitation and therapy to prevent a stroke recurrence. The therapy includes treatment or modification of risk factors (high blood pressure, exposure to cigarette smoke, high cholesterol, etc.). It may involve antiplatelet drugs, including aspirin, and anticoagulants. For some patients, an endarterectomy—surgery to remove atherosclerotic plaque in a neck artery—may be advised.

WHAT ARE THE COMPLICATIONS?

When areas of the brain are deprived of oxygen, nerve cells in the area die in a matter of minutes. As a result, near and distant body parts controlled by these brain centers can no longer function properly. Depending on the extent of the stroke, impairment of movement, speech, memory, vision, behavior, or other functions may occur. In some cases the impairment may be permanent; in others, recovery may range from partial to complete. Hemorrhagic strokes generally are more life-threatening, because extensive bleeding can cause pressure within the brain and damage to areas around the bleeding site.

HOW CAN IT BE PREVENTED OR MINIMIZED?

Stroke prevention is aimed at controlling or eliminating key risk factors, such as high blood pressure, heart disease, diabetes, high serum cholesterol levels, cigarette smoking, obesity, and physical inactivity.

See Chapters 2 and 18.

SYNCOPE (FAINTING)

WHAT IS IT?

Syncope, or fainting, is simply a loss of consciousness.

WHO GETS IT?

Fainting is usually the result of decreased blood flow to the brain. The most common cause is vasovagal syncope, a nerve response in which the heartbeat slows and blood vessels in the abdomen and lower limbs dilate. The blood then pools in these areas, and less is available to the brain. This type of fainting occurs following an emotional upset, such as viewing an accident or having blood drawn. A similar mechanism operates when someone faints after a few drinks or a large dinner, or after standing still for a long time on a hot day. Fainting also may be caused by a very slow heartbeat (below 40–45 beats a minute) or a very rapid one (more than 140–150 beats a minute). It can occur as a result of heart failure, a heart attack, or severe stenosis (narrowing) of the aortic valve. Some antihypertensive medications may briefly lower blood pressure too much when the patient stands up (orthostatic hypotension). Other causes of syncope include severe low blood sugar, heat exhaustion, hyperventilation (rapid breathing), severe anemia, and stroke.

WHAT ARE THE SYMPTOMS?

The onset of fainting may be heralded by a feeling of weakness, unsteadiness, light-headedness, or, in some cases, palpitations or a feeling of emptiness in the chest. Numbness, tingling, loss of movement on one side of the body, blurred vision, confusion, or difficulty speaking may infrequently follow the fainting episode.

HOW IS IT DIAGNOSED?

A medical history and physical examination most often will reveal a simple explanation for syncope—e.g., a vagal episode, orthostatic hypotension after extended bed rest and getting up suddenly, or an emotional upset that causes hyperventilation. In some cases, a complete diagnostic evaluation to identify the underlying cause of the syncope may require blood tests, an electrocardiogram, Holter monitoring, or other, more complicated studies.

HOW IS IT TREATED?

Someone who faints should be kept in a reclining position with feet slightly raised in as cool an environment as possible. An upright position should not be resumed until the person regains consciousness, and then only slowly. The choice of further treatment is totally dependent upon the cause of the syncope. Occasional benign syncope usually warrants none. Frequently a simple fainting episode is overtreated. Drug-related fainting may require a change in medication. Sometimes lifestyle modification, such as dietary measures for low blood sugar (more frequent meals), may be indicated. In unusual cases, medical or surgical therapy may be needed to control or correct the underlying disorder. For example, severe changes in heart rates or rhythms may warrant drug therapy or implantation of a pacemaker; an aortic valve stenosis may warrant surgery to replace the valve.

WHAT ARE THE COMPLICATIONS?

A single fainting episode in an otherwise healthy person may not present a problem, assuming there was no fall resulting in injury. However, some medical evaluation should be undertaken to exclude a specific medical cause of syncope. If the fainting was caused by a serious cardiac disorder or stroke, specific treatment is obviously necessary.

HOW CAN IT BE PREVENTED OR MINIMIZED?

People who have a tendency to faint when blood is drawn, or in emotional situations, should sit down or lie down immediately if they begin to feel light-headed. If dizziness occurs after taking medication, the doctor should be notified. Recurring rapid or slow heart rate or heart valve disease requires specific medical treatment. Older men who might have a tendency to feel dizzy or actually faint after urinating at night should probably sit rather than stand. (Fainting can occur after the sudden emptying of the bladder.)

See Chapter 2.

TACHYCARDIA

WHAT IS IT?

The heart normally beats at a rate of about 60 to 80 beats per minute at rest. A rate faster than 100 beats a minute in an adult is called a tachycardia. Most people experience transient rapid heartbeats, called sinus tachycardia, as a normal response to excitement, anxiety, stress, or exercise. If tachycardias occur at rest or without a logical cause, however, they are considered abnormal. The two main types of tachycardias are: abnormal *supraventricular tachycardias* (which originate in the upper chambers of the heart, the atria) and *ventricular tachycardias* (which originate in the lower chambers of the heart, the ventricles). The most common forms of tachycardia are *paroxysmal supraventricular tachycardia*, which generally has a rate of 140 to 200 beats per minute, develops spontaneously, and stops and starts suddenly, but may recur; *atrial flutter*, in which the atria beat at 240 to 300 beats per minute, although the actual pulse rate is much slower, because not all of these impulses are translated into contractions of the ventricles; *ventricular tachycardia*, a very serious arrhythmia initiated in the ventricles, in which the heart rate is usually between 150 and 250; and *atrial fibrillation* (see separate entry).

WHO GETS IT?

Sinus tachycardias are most likely to occur in those who are easily excitable, suffer anxiety, or drink a lot of caffeine-containing beverages. They may also be seen in people with thyroid disease with fevers or with certain drugs (especially asthma or allergy medications and those containing adrenaline). The occurrence of tachycardia under any of these circumstances does not necessarily imply underlying heart disease. More severe types of tachycardia tend to occur in those who have underlying heart disease. They may be caused by an electrical disturbance within the heart without an anatomic deformity, or by congenital defects, coronary artery disease, chronic disease of the heart valves, or chronic lung disease. Tachycardias may also occur in the course of a heart attack.

WHAT ARE THE SYMPTOMS?

The main symptom is awareness of a rapid heartbeat, commonly called "palpitations." Depending on the cause and extent of the tachycardia, other symptoms may include shortness of breath, dizziness, actual syncope (fainting), chest pain, and severe anxiety.

HOW IS IT DIAGNOSED?

The type of tachycardia usually can be diagnosed by measuring the pulse and taking an electrocardiogram. In unusual instances, more complex electrophysiologic evaluation may be necessary.

HOW IS IT TREATED?

Medical treatment depends on the cause and type of the tachycardia. Sinus tachycardias usually do not require treatment other than therapy for the underlying cause, if any. A supraventricular paroxysmal tachycardia may respond to certain simple maneuvers. This may involve holding one's breath for a minute, bathing the face in cold water, or massaging the carotid artery in the neck. In other cases, medication may be prescribed to slow the heartbeat on a continual basis. If tachycardia is severe, or arises from the ventricle, immediate injectable medication or electric shock (electroconversion) may be required to stimulate the heart to return to a normal rate. In rare severe and resistant cases of ventricular tachycardias, a defibrillation device (AICD) something like a pacemaker may be implanted surgically to help maintain a normal heart rhythm. In elderly people or those with underlying heart disease, it is important to stop even the less severe types of tachycardias within a few hours, if at all possible, because a prolonged rapid rate may result in decreased heart function.

WHAT ARE THE COMPLICATIONS?

In persistent cases of a ventricular tachycardia, the rapid rate continues, the heart cannot pump blood effectively, and ventricular fibrillation, in which normal heart muscle contraction fails and the heart quivers, may occur. If fibrillation is not stopped with an electrical shock and normal rhythm restored within a few minutes, it will be fatal.

HOW CAN IT BE PREVENTED OR MINIMIZED?

Complete medical evaluation is mandatory in order to identify any serious arrhythmias. Most cases of palpitations will be benign. In certain instances, medication must be taken regularly. Environmental factors such as caffeine and smoking should be eliminated.

See Chapters 16 and 26.

TRICUSPID VALVE DISEASE

WHAT IS IT?

The tricuspid valve is one of four valves that control the flow and direction of blood in and out of the heart. Blood enters the right atrium (upper heart chamber) and passes through the tricuspid valve into the right ventricle (lower pumping chamber), from where it is pumped out through the pulmonary artery to the lungs. If the valve is narrowed (stenosed), it becomes difficult for a sufficient amount of blood to move through the right heart chambers with each beat. If the valve does not close properly, some blood flowing into the ventricle leaks back into the atrium with each beat. This condition is known as regurgitation or insufficiency. In both cases, the heart must work harder to pump an adequate amount of blood. In stenosis, the right atrium becomes enlarged, while the right ventricle does not fill completely and remains small. In regurgitation, both right chambers enlarge substantially.

WHO GETS IT?

Tricuspid valve disorders, *which are rare*, often occur in conjunction with other heart valve problems, particularly with mitral valve disorders. Tricuspid valve stenosis is usually caused by rheumatic heart disease, although it is occasionally due to a congenital condition. Tricuspid valve regurgitation is often secondary to high pressure within the heart's chambers, usually caused by pulmonary hypertension. Rheumatic heart disease can also cause it. Isolated tricuspid regurgitation may be the result of endocarditis, particularly in intravenous drug abusers.

WHAT ARE THE SYMPTOMS?

Tricuspid regurgitation and stenosis may be present for years without symptoms. When symptoms do occur, they may include an uncomfortable fluttering sensation in the neck or chest because of heart rhythm irregularities. Both conditions can produce the symptoms of right-sided heart failure, including discomfort in the upper abdomen because of an enlarged liver, fatigue, and swelling.

HOW IS IT DIAGNOSED?

Signs of tricuspid valve disease, such as a heart murmur and an abnormal pulse in the jugular vein in the neck, may be detectable during a physical examination. A chest X-ray, an electrocardiogram, and an echocardiogram are helpful in reaching the diagnosis. Cardiac catheterization may be performed if surgery is being considered.

HOW IS IT TREATED?

Tricuspid valve disorders usually require no treatment in and of themselves, although related heart valve problems may require specific treatment. If atrial fibrillation is present, it can be treated with oral antiarrhythmic drugs. In the case of severe stenosis or regurgitation, surgery to replace or repair the defective valve may be recommended.

WHAT ARE THE COMPLICATIONS?

Individuals with tricuspid valve disease are at risk for heart failure and for atrial fibrillation (which in turn increases the risk of blood clot formation). As in other types of valve disease, tricuspid disorders also increase the risk of infective endocarditis.

HOW CAN IT BE PREVENTED OR MINIMIZED?

Limiting the risk of rheumatic fever, particularly by prompt treatment of strep throat, is the major preventive measure for tricuspid disease. Prophylactic use of antibiotics before dental extractions and surgery can help prevent the development of infective endocarditis.

See Chapter 13.

VENOUS DISEASE

WHAT IS IT?

Veins are vessels that carry blood from arms, legs, the head, etc., back to the right side of the heart. The most common venous diseases are phlebitis and varicose veins. Phlebitis is an inflammation of a vein that may be caused by an injury, infection, or chemical irritation. Often a clot is formed in the inflamed vein; this condition is called thrombophlebitis. There are two types of phlebitis. Superficial phlebitis, which is not serious, is the inflammation of a surface vein that may occur after an intravenous infusion or a bruise. The other type is deep thrombophlebitis, which refers to a clot forming in an inflamed vein below the skin surface. In deep thrombophlebitis, there may be some danger of a clot being thrown off to another part of the body. Repeated phlebitis can lead to poor venous drainage or venous insufficiency with chronic swelling. Varicose or swollen and twisted veins may result from poor function of the internal valves that normally help to push blood upward from the legs to the heart.

WHO GETS IT?

Women develop these venous diseases more often than men, and a hereditary predisposition may underlie them. Obesity, hypertension, pregnancy, a family history with genetic predisposition, and the use of garters around the thighs may contribute to the development of varicose veins. Those at greater risk of phlebitis include smokers, people who have varicose veins or other evidence of venous insufficiency, those who are bedridden for long periods of time, especially after surgery or a fracture, and those having intravenous therapy. People who are overweight or who have heart disease are also susceptible. The risk of thrombus (clot) formation is greater in those who are aged, inactive, have heart disease, or use oral contraceptives or after long airplane or car trips.

WHAT ARE THE SYMPTOMS?

Swollen veins just under the skin surface are likely to be varicose. The legs also may be achy, painful, warm to the touch, and easily fatigued. In phlebitis, the leg may be swollen, tender, and red and may feel achy and heavy. As phlebitis progresses, the skin may become painful and bluish. The only symptom of superficial phlebitis may be slight tenderness.

HOW IS IT DIAGNOSED?

Venous diseases usually are easily diagnosed by simple observation. The major symptom of superficial phlebitis may be a hard, clothesline-like area in the arm or leg. In some cases of suspected thrombophlebitis, it may be necessary to inject a dye into the vein to visualize its interior surface (venography).

HOW IS IT TREATED?

Therapy for an acute, deep phlebitis may include bed rest and elevation of the leg, a nonsteroidal anti-inflammatory drug to reduce inflammation, warm soaks, bed rest, and an anticoagulant to help prevent blood clots. If an embolism is identified, a fibrinolytic drug to dissolve the clot may be prescribed; in rare cases, surgical removal of the clot may be needed. Superficial phlebitis may merely require warm wet soaks and aspirin. The use of specially fitted elastic stockings will help ease the symptoms of varicosities (varicose veins). If varicosities cause skin ulcers or pain or are particularly unsightly, injections of drugs to obliterate the vein or surgery to remove it may be advised.

WHAT ARE THE COMPLICATIONS?

Severe varicosities may predispose the patient to skin ulcers and thrombophlebitis. The major complication of phlebitis is dislodging of a blood clot, which may travel to the lungs (pulmonary embolism). This can have serious consequences and may be fatal.

HOW CAN IT BE PREVENTED OR MINIMIZED?

Avoidance of overweight and of garter usage can help prevent varicose veins. If they occur, the use of support hose and the avoidance of long periods of standing can help alleviate symptoms. Elastic stockings and, in some, medical therapy can help prevent phlebitis in those at risk after surgery or during periods of mandatory bed rest. The chances of repeated attacks of phlebitis may be decreased by avoiding inactivity. Physical therapy with an active exercise plan after surgery can decrease risk of phlebitis. For certain individuals, anticoagulants may be necessary.

See Chapter 17.

WOLFF-PARKINSON-WHITE SYNDROME

WHAT IS IT?

Wolff-Parkinson-White (WPW) syndrome represents a congenital abnormality involving the heart's electrical function. Although many people with this abnormality exhibit no symptoms, the syndrome can result in episodes of rapid heartbeat called paroxysmal supraventricular tachycardia (PSVT). In contrast to a normal 60 to 80 beats per minute, the rate rises, generally to 180 to 240 per minute. WPW is caused by abnormal conduction of electrical signals in the heart. Electrical signals arrive at the ventricles prematurely, because they travel through a shortcut (bypass tract) between the atria and the ventricles. This condition makes the heart susceptible to rhythm abnormalities.

WHO GETS IT?

Although the congenital anomaly that causes Wolff-Parkinson-White syndrome is present at birth and symptoms may arise in infancy or childhood, tachycardias are more likely to develop later in life. WPW may be associated with other congenital malformations, but generally it occurs alone.

WHAT ARE THE SYMPTOMS?

People who have WPW may have no symptoms at all or may experience palpitations and, possibly, chest pain, shortness of breath, and fainting. Fainting indicates that the heart is beating so rapidly that it is unable to pump adequate amounts of blood to the brain. The palpitations may be described as skips, thumps, butterflies, fluttering, or racing of the heart.

HOW IS IT DIAGNOSED?

In the presence of WPW, an electrocardiogram shows characteristic changes indicating the existence of an abnormal pathway from the atria to the ventricles. If attacks of tachycardia are frequent, special studies of the electrical activity of the heart (electrophysiologic tests) may be done to determine the location of the shortcut pathway and its response to different drugs.

HOW IS IT TREATED?

In the absence of tachycardias, often no treatment is necessary. When it is, it is best individualized and dependent upon the extent and frequency of the tachycardia and based upon electrophysiologic studies. Sometimes, simple avoidance of stress and dietary sources of caffeine may be helpful in preventing episodes of tachycardia. In other cases, the physician will prescribe medication to stabilize heart rhythm. This medication may be taken only at the time of an attack or, more likely, on a continuing basis to prevent the development of supraventricular tachycardia. If an attack cannot be controlled by medication, treatment with a brief electrical shock may be necessary to restore normal rhythm. If medication is insufficient to control the repeated episodes of rapid rhythm, open-heart surgery may be necessary to eliminate the abnormal pathway. A new technique uses radiofrequency current, delivered via a catheter, to eliminate the abnormal pathway without surgery.

WHAT ARE THE COMPLICATIONS?

The paroxysmal supraventricular tachycardias of WPW can be disconcerting but, by themselves, are not usually life-threatening. In some people, however, the tachycardia may be so rapid that it causes fainting. Certain individuals with this disorder are at greater risk of ventricular tachycardia or fibrillation, a much more serious irregular rhythm that can be fatal.

HOW CAN IT BE PREVENTED OR MINIMIZED?

Beyond taking medication, the patient should learn nonmedical techniques to decrease the risk of tachycardia (such as avoidance of caffeine and of excessive alcohol) and mechanical methods to help slow down the heart or terminate an episode of tachycardia. One such method is straining by closing the nose and mouth and trying to exhale.

See Chapters 16 and 26.

PART VIII

APPENDIX

Glossary

Directory of Resources

Selected Bibliography

Index

GLOSSARY

adrenal glands Hormone-producing (endocrine) glands that rest atop each kidney and secrete several hormones, including adrenaline (which increases heart rate and raises blood pressure) and aldosterone (which regulates the levels of potassium and sodium).

adrenaline (epinephrine) Hormone produced by the adrenal glands that increases heart rate and blood pressure by narrowing (constricting) blood vessels. An important hormone secreted in stressful situations as part of the body's fight-or-flight response.

aldosterone Hormone secreted by cortex or outer portion of the adrenal glands; regulates potassium secretion and the retention of salt and water by the kidneys.

anemia A reduction in the normal amount of hemoglobin or the number of red blood cells in the circulation. Anemia may be a symptom of iron deficiency, chronic bleeding, or some other underlying disorder.

aneurysm A bulging out (protrusion) or blistering in a major blood vessel at a point where there is a weakness in the vessel wall.

angina A pressure or an intense chest pain resulting from a reduced oxygen supply to the heart muscle.

angiogram An X-ray of blood vessels or other part of the cardiovascular system.

angiography A diagnostic procedure in which a contrasting dye is injected into the bloodstream to make blood vessels or heart chambers visible on an X-ray image.

angioplasty Therapeutic procedure in which a catheter with a deflated balloon at the tip is inserted into a narrowed artery. The balloon is then inflated at the site of narrowing to widen it.

angiotensin A blood chemical that constricts blood vessels, thereby raising blood pressure.

angiotensin-converting enzyme (ACE) inhibitors Drugs that inhibit the action of angiotensin and that are used to treat high blood pressure or congestive heart failure.

anorexia The medical term for loss of appetite.

antiarrhythmics A group of drugs used to treat irregular heartbeats (arrhythmias).

anticoagulants Drugs that suppress the blood-clotting process.

anticonvulsants Drugs used to treat seizures.

antihypertensives Drugs used to lower high blood pressure.

anxiety Feelings of apprehension and uneasiness.

aorta The largest artery in the body. It receives blood from the left ventricle of the heart; the blood is then distributed through a branching system of arteries to all parts of the body.

aortic regurgitation (insufficiency) Failure of the aortic valve to close properly, allowing some blood to flow back into the left ventricle with each heartbeat instead of forward into the circulation.

aortic stenosis A narrowing or stiffness of the aortic valve causing an obstruction to blood flow; this results in an increased workload for the heart.

aortic valve The valve that controls the flow of blood between the aorta and the left ventricle, the heart's major pumping chamber.

aphasia Loss of the ability to speak, usually as a result of injury or disease of the brain.

arrhythmia Deviation from the normal heartbeat rhythm because of a disturbance in the electrical impulses to the heart.

arterial lumen The channel of an artery through which blood flows.

arteries Blood vessels that carry oxygenated blood away from the heart to all parts of the body.

arterioles The smallest arteries, which distribute blood to the capillaries.

arteriosclerosis A condition in which the walls of arteries thicken and lose elasticity; commonly called "hardening of the arteries." See atherosclerosis.

arteriovenous malformation A tangle of arteries and veins without the capillaries that normally connect the two.

ascites A collection of excess fluids in the abdominal cavity.

atheroma A collection of fatty plaque. It is a common pathologic event of atherosclerosis.

atherosclerosis A form of arteriosclerosis resulting from the buildup of fatty substances called plaque on the walls of the arteries, causing a reduction in blood flow.

atresia The absence of a normal body passage or opening (orifice) from an organ or other part of the body.

atrial fibrillation An abnormal heart rhythm (arrhythmia) in which the heart's atria contract at an excessive and irregular rate.

atrial septal defects Abnormal congenital openings in the wall dividing the heart's upper chambers.

atrial septum A thin wall dividing the heart's left and right atria or upper chamber.

atrioventricular (AV) node It is the small mass of conduction tissue, located between the upper and lower chambers of the heart, through which electrical impulses pass, controlling heart rhythm pass.

atrium (plural: atria) One of the two upper chambers of the heart. The left atrium receives newly oxygenated blood from the lungs. The right atrium receives deoxygenated blood from various parts of the body.

autonomic nervous system The involuntary nervous system that controls unconscious body functions such as heart rate and blood pressure.

balloon angioplasty See angioplasty.

balloon-tipped catheter A type of catheter with a balloon at the end that can be inflated under pressure to clear a blocked or occluded blood vessel. Used in angioplasty or valvuloplasty.

balloon valvuloplasty See valvotomy or valvuloplasty.

beta-adrenergic receptors Nerve receptors that receive and act on nerve impulses that increase the heart rate, dilate blood vessels, and regulate certain metabolic functions.

beta blockers A group of medications used to treat angina, hypertension, and cardiac arrhythmia by blocking (beta-adrenergic) nerve receptors, thereby reducing the force and rate of the heartbeat. Also effective in angina by reducing the total work of the heart.

blood pressure The force that blood exerts on the walls of the arteries as it is pumped throughout the body. It is stated in two numbers, such as 120/80. The 120 represents the systolic pressure, which is the pressure recorded each time the heart pumps or contracts; the 80 represents the diastolic pressure, which is the residual pressure in the vessels recorded when the heart relaxes between beats.

bradycardia An abnormally slow heart rate, generally defined as less than 60 beats per minute in adults.

bruit A murmur arising in a blood vessel because of narrowing.

Buerger's disease A rare condition in which blood vessels in the legs and arms become inflamed, causing a narrowing of the arteries in these extremities that may lead to gangrene.

bundle of His A bundle of conduction fibers that runs from the heart's atrioventricular (AV) node and conducts electrical impulses between the lower chambers of the heart.

calcium channel blockers A group of drugs used in the treatment of angina, hypertension, and cardiac arrhythmias. They work by inhibiting the effect of calcium on the muscles of arteries, thereby reducing the degree of contraction. This results in a decrease in the workload of the heart, a decrease in blood pressure, and improved circulation of blood.

capillaries Tiny, thin-walled blood vessels through which the exchange of oxygen, nutrients, and wastes takes place.

carbon dioxide An odorless, colorless gas present in the air; also a by-product of metabolism. In the body, it is carried by the blood to the lungs and is then expelled from the body through exhaling.

cardiac arrest Incident during which the heart stops beating and loss of consciousness occurs because of cutoff of blood flow to the brain. It is usually the result of ventricular fibrillation, in which the heart's ventricles twitch randomly and ineffectively rather than beating in a rhythmic fashion to pump blood from the heart. A complete cessation of all heartbeats can also cause a cardiac arrest.

cardiac catheterization Insertion of a catheter through the blood vessels into the chambers of the heart to measure pressure or to inject a dye to visualize the coronary arteries.

cardiac cycle The cycle of activities associated with one heartbeat.

cardiologist A physician specializing in the diagnosis and treatment of disorders of the heart.

cardiology The branch of medicine dealing with the functions of the heart and blood vessels.

cardiomyopathy A term denoting any disease of the heart muscle.

cardiopulmonary bypass machine (heart-lung machine) The machine that takes over the body's heart and lung functions during open heart surgery.

cardiopulmonary resuscitation (CPR) Administration of lifesaving procedures such as compression of the heart muscle and mouth-to-mouth breathing for a person suffering cardiac arrest. This is done in order to restore blood circulation to the brain as quickly as possible to prevent possible brain damage.

cardiovascular Of or pertaining to the heart and blood vessels.

cardioversion Use of an electrical shock to restore normal heart rhythm. (See also defibrillation.)

carotid arteries The principal arteries of the head and neck, each of which has two main branches, the external carotid artery and the internal carotid artery.

carotid sinus A small nerve center located at the point where the internal carotid artery branches off from the main or common carotid artery.

catheter A flexible tube that is inserted into a blood vessel or cavity for the purpose of examination, drainage of fluid, or other procedures.

cerebellum The region of the brain that coordinates movement and maintains posture and balance.

cerebrovascular accident The sudden blockage of a blood vessel in the brain caused by an embolus, or thrombosis, and resulting in decreased blood circulation in the brain. Also may result from a ruptured blood vessel that causes a cerebral hemorrhage.

cerebrum The largest portion of the brain. It consists of two hemispheres and an outer covering (the cortex); it controls mental functions and sensory activities.

cholesterol A fatty substance necessary for hormone production, cell metabolism, and other vital processes. It is also a component of cell membranes in all animals. Cholesterol is manufactured in the body and is also consumed in the diet. Dietary cholesterol is found *only* in animal products. High levels of blood cholesterol are a contributing factor to coronary heart disease.

circulatory system The system that is made up of the heart and blood vessels and is responsible for circulating blood throughout the body, providing the tissues with oxygen and nutrients, and removing waste products.

circumflex Name of one of the three major coronary arteries.

coarctation of the aorta Also referred to as aortic coarctation; a congenital defect characterized by narrowing of the main artery (aorta) of the upper body, resulting in a reduced blood supply to the lower body and legs. As a result, blood pressure is increased in the upper portion of the body and decreased in the lower portion.

collateral circulation Blood vessels that sometimes gradually take over the blood circulation when a main vessel is partially or completely blocked. They go around the narrowed area.

computerized tomography (CT) scan A diagnostic technique involving the use of computers and multiple X-ray images to produce cross-sectional images of body tissue. This technique provides more clearly detailed images than traditional X-rays.

congenital heart defects Abnormalities of the heart existing at birth.

congestive heart failure Inability of the heart to pump sufficient blood, resulting in an accumulation of fluids in the lungs, abdomen, and legs. This condition usually develops over a period of years, but may also result from a heart attack that damages a large portion of heart muscle.

contrast venography A diagnostic procedure in which a contrasting medium is injected into the veins to make them visible on X-ray film.

coronary artery disease Diseases of the arteries that supply blood to the heart muscle.

coronary bypass surgery Surgery to improve blood flow to the heart muscle in the presence of severe coronary artery disease. The procedure involves creating bypass routes for blood flow from the aorta to various areas of the heart muscle. The bypass grafts are usually portions of veins taken from the legs or a repositioned artery on the chest wall, which lies near the heart (the internal mammary artery).

coronary care unit (CCU) An intensive care unit for patients who have had a heart attack or other acute emergent cardiac problem.

coronary heart disease Diseases of the heart caused by narrowing of the coronary arteries, resulting in reduced blood flow to the heart. Also known as coronary artery disease and ischemic heart disease.

cyanosis A bluish discoloration of the skin caused by an abnormally high level of deoxygenated hemoglobin in the blood. It is noted in heart failure, some types of congestive heart disease, etc.

defibrillation An electric shock administered to the heart to stabilize an irregular heartbeat or restore a normal heartbeat after cardiac arrest.

diabetes A disorder characterized by problems in glucose (blood sugar) metabolism. There are two forms of diabetes: Type I (also called juvenile-onset or insulin-dependent diabetes), in which the body ceases to produce insulin (the hormone essential for glucose metabolism); and Type II (also called adult-onset or insulin-resistant diabetes), in which the body fails to utilize insulin effectively.

diastolic The lower of the two numbers recorded when a person's blood pressure is taken. It represents the arterial pressure when the heart's pumping chambers (ventricles) are relaxed between beats and refilling with blood.

dietitian A health professional trained in the field of dietetics, the science dealing with nutrition and health.

digitalis A drug derived from the foxglove plant and used in the treatment of heart failure and abnormal heart rhythms. Digitalis works by strengthening the pumping action of the heart, thereby improving blood circulation, or by slowing down some of the electrical impulses from the atria to the ventricles. The most commonly used form of this drug is digoxin.

dilated cardiomyopathy A disorder in which muscle cells in the walls of the heart do not function normally; the walls enlarge and dilate, and heart failure develops.

dissecting aneurysm A condition in which blood is forced through a fissure or tear in an artery's inner wall and remains between the layers of its lining, causing the vessel to bulge.

diuretics Medications used to treat fluid retention by increasing the kidney's output of urine and the excretion of sodium from the body. Effective in the treatment of hypertension and heart failure.

dyspepsia The medical term for indigestion.

dyspnea Shortness of breath or difficulty breathing.

echocardiogram See echocardiography.

echocardiography/echography A diagnostic procedure that uses high-frequency (ultrasound) waves to visualize structures within the heart. The picture produced is called an echocardiogram.

eclampsia A rare disorder in pregnancy characterized by seizures, coma, and sometimes death. It is marked by hypertension, the excretion of protein in the urine, and swelling (edema).

edema A swelling of parts of the body because of fluid retention.

electrocardiogram (ECG or EKG) A visual record of the heart's electrical activity.

electrocardiography A diagnostic procedure that records the electrical activity of the heart muscle.

embolism, embolus, emboli A clot or other substance carried in the bloodstream from one site to another, causing the blockage of an artery. Emboli is the plural.

endarterectomy A surgical procedure to remove the interior lining of an artery that has been narrowed by fatty deposits.

endocarditis Inflammation of the interior lining of the heart (the endocardium) and heart valves; generally occurs because of bacterial infection or rheumatic fever.

endocardium The interior lining of the heart.

epinephrine One of the hormones produced by the adrenal glands. It is secreted in stressful situations and dilates blood vessels and increases heart rate. Also known as adrenaline.

estrogen The female sex hormone produced by the ovaries. It is instrumental in reproduction. The ovaries cease to produce estrogen after menopause, and this lack of estrogen is believed to make older women more vulnerable to heart disease.

exercise stress test An electrocardiogram that is done while a person exercises, usually on a treadmill (often called a treadmill test) or a stationary bicycle.

fibrin A stringy protein that is instrumental in blood clotting.

fibrinogen A component of blood that is necessary for clotting. It is converted by enzymes in the blood into fibrin.

fluoroscope An X-ray device that helps to visualize moving images of internal organs such as the heart. X-rays are passed through the body onto a screen on which an organ can be observed in action.

Foley catheter A catheter used to drain the bladder of urine.

Fontan operation A surgical procedure for certain types of congenital heart disease, in which blood from the atrium is shunted through a conduit to the pulmonary artery.

foramen ovale An opening between the two atria that normally closes after birth. In individual cases, it may remain open and/or be one site of an atrial septal defect.

Friedreich's ataxia A rare inherited genetic disease in which the nerve fibers break down, resulting in a loss of coordination and balance (ataxia).

fusiform aneurysm A weakening of an area of an artery that goes around its circumference. Blood pools there, causing a bulge that tapers at each end.

gamma globulin A circulatory protein containing antibodies.

heart failure A condition resulting from the heart's inability to pump sufficient blood to maintain normal circulation. This often leads to congestive heart failure, in which blood and fluids back up in the lungs, causing congestion in the abdomen or legs.

heart murmur An abnormal sound caused by turbulent blood flow as a result of a defective heart valve or certain forms of congenital heart disease. It can also be of no medical importance.

heart transplant Replacement of a damaged or diseased heart with a healthy heart taken from a donor.

Heimlich maneuver A first-aid maneuver for choking victims.

hematoma A swelling in an organ or tissue containing blood; caused by a tear or break in a blood vessel wall.

hemochromatosis An inherited disorder characterized by the overabsorption of iron. It can result in liver damage, cardiac arrhythmias, and other heart disorders.

hemoglobin The red pigment in the blood that carries oxygen.

hepatomegaly Enlargement of the liver.

high-density lipoprotein (HDL) A lipid-carrying protein that transports the so-called *good* cholesterol in the bloodstream. HDL is responsible for carrying excess cholesterol away from the artery walls and to the liver, where it is metabolized.

Holter monitor A portable electrocardiographic device worn for a 24-hour period or longer to monitor irregular heart rhythms and other cardiac abnormalities.

hormones Chemicals produced by various endocrine glands or tissues, and released into the blood. Hormones are instrumental in controlling metabolism, reproduction, and virtually every body function.

hyperglycemia Abnormally high levels of blood sugar (glucose). It occurs mostly in patients with diabetes.

hyperlipidemia Excessive amount of fats (lipids) in the blood.

hyperplasia A noncancerous enlargement of an organ or a portion of an organ because of increases in its component cells.

hypertension The medical term for high blood pressure.

hyperthyroidism A condition in which an overactive thyroid gland secretes excessive thyroid hormones, resulting in a rapid heartbeat and other manifestations of speeded-up metabolism.

hypertrophic cardiomyopathy An abnormal increase in the thickness of the walls of the heart, usually because of an inherited heart muscle disorder.

hypertrophy Enlargement of muscle tissue resulting from an increased workload.

hypoglycemia Abnormally low levels of blood sugar (glucose), often a result of an insulin overdose in the treatment of diabetes.

hypothyroidism Reduced production of thyroid hormones because of a goiter or other thyroid disorder.

hypoxia Insufficient level of oxygen in the tissues of the body.

inferior vena cava A major vein that carries deoxygenated blood from the lower part of the body (abdomen and legs) back to the heart.

intermittent claudication Exercise-induced, sporadic pain in the muscles of a limb, resulting from reduced blood flow.

invasive techniques Medical procedures that involve a surgical incision, needle puncture, or passage of a tube (catheter) into an artery.

ischemia A deficiency in oxygen in parts of the body because of an obstructed blood vessel. For example, ischemic heart disease is the result of narrowing of the coronary arteries that supply blood to the heart muscle.

Kawasaki disease A rare childhood disease that affects the heart (coronary arteries) and other body systems. It was originally observed in Japan during the 1960s.

laser A device that produces a concentrated beam of light radiation. The term is an acronym, standing for *l*ight *a*mplification by *s*timulated *e*mission of *r*adiation. It is used in a variety of medical procedures.

low-density lipoprotein (LDL) The lipid-carrying protein that transports the so-called *bad* cholesterol in the bloodstream. High levels of LDL cholesterol are significant risk factors in the development of atherosclerosis.

lumen The cavity or opening in tubelike organs, such as arteries.

magnetic resonance imaging (MRI) A diagnostic technique that uses the response of atoms to a magnetic field to produce cross-sectional images of the body's internal structures.

Marfan syndrome A rare inherited disease of the connective tissues that produces abnormalities in the skeleton, heart, and blood vessels.

metabolism The physical and chemical processes necessary to sustain life.

micturition The medical term for urination.

mitral insufficiency (regurgitation) Failure of the mitral valve to close properly, allowing some blood to flow back into the left atrium rather than moving forward into the left ventricle.

mitral valve The valve that controls the flow of oxygenated blood from the left atrium into the left ventricle.

mitral valve prolapse A congenital abnormality in which the leaflets, or flaps, of tissue that make up the mitral valve are larger than normal.

monounsaturated fats Fatty acids that are capable of absorbing more hydrogen. They are soft at room temperature and have little effect on the amount of cholesterol in the blood. Examples include olive oil and chicken fat.

multigated acquisition (MUGA) scan A radioisotope test used to measure heart function and performance.

multivessel disease Blood vessel disease in which more than one vessel (usually coronary) is blocked or otherwise impaired.

murmur See heart murmur.

muscular dystrophy An inherited childhood disease characterized by progressive muscle wasting and weakness. The disease affects male children, who inherit the defective gene from their mothers.

myocardial infarction Medical term for a heart attack, denoting damage of the heart muscle as a result of a reduction in blood flow.

myocarditis Inflammation of the heart muscle.

myocardium The heart muscle.

myxomatous degeneration A metabolic process in which valve tissue loses elasticity and becomes redundant.

neuron A nerve cell.

nitroglycerin A drug used to treat angina. It dilates coronary arteries.

noninvasive techniques Medical procedures that do not involve surgery, a needle puncture, or entering an artery.

norepinephrine A hormone secreted by nerve endings and the adrenal glands that helps to maintain constant blood pressure by constricting certain blood vessels when blood pressure drops.

Norwood procedure An operation to treat pulmonary insufficiency in which a shunt is created to provide blood flow from the heart to the lungs.

obesity A body weight 20 percent or more above the accepted standard for a person's age, sex, and body type.

occipital lobes The back part of the brain.

occlusion Blockage of an opening or vessel in the body.

open-heart surgery A major surgical procedure on the heart during which circulatory functions are temporarily taken over by a heart-lung machine.

orthopnea Shortness of breath that occurs when lying down, usually a symptom of heart failure.

orthostatic hypotension A sudden drop in blood pressure that occurs when a person stands up. Can cause fainting.

ostium primum In the heart of a fetus, an opening that serves as a link between the two developing atria. It closes as the septum fully develops.

ostium secundum In the heart of a fetus, an opening that develops as the ostium primum closes, continuing communication between the atria.

pacemaker The center of electrical activity in the heart that regulates the heartbeat. The term is also used for an artificial device implanted in the heart to provide an adequate heart rate.

palliative therapy Treatment that is aimed at relieving the symptoms rather than curing the ailment.

palpitations A feeling that the heart is pounding against the chest, caused by an irregular, strong, or rapid heartbeat.

parietal lobes The top middle part of the brain.

paroxysmal nocturnal dyspnea Difficulty in breathing that comes on intermittently and suddenly when the affected person is lying down, often waking him or her from sleep.

paroxysmal tachycardia A sudden increase in heart rate up to 130 to 260 beats per minute from the normal 60 to 80 beats per minute. This condition may last for from a few minutes to several days.

patent ductus arteriosus A heart defect in which the fetal opening between the aorta and pulmonary artery fails to close at birth. As a result, oxygenated blood from the aorta goes into the lungs, through the left side of the heart, and then out through the aorta.

percutaneous transluminal coronary angioplasty (PTCA) The technical name for balloon angioplasty of the coronary arteries.

perfusion imaging A test using radionuclide scanning that shows the pattern of the flow of blood in the heart.

pericarditis An inflammation of the sac around the heart (pericardium).

pericardium The membranous sac around the heart.

peripheral vascular disease (PVD) Disease that affects the outlying blood vessels (arteries) such as those in the limbs.

phlebitis Inflammation of a vein or veins, occurring most often in the legs.

plaque Fatty deposits that form raised patches in the inner lining of the arteries. Denotes atherosclerosis.

plasma The pale yellow fluid portion of the blood.

platelets The smallest of the blood cells, also called thrombocytes; responsible for clotting.

platelet scintigraphy A radionuclide scan studying the behavior of the platelets, the prime components in the blood-clotting process.

pleural effusion Accumulation of excessive fluid between the layers of the membrane (pleura) that lines the lungs and chest cavity.

polyunsaturated fats Fatty acids that carry the least amount of hydrogen. They are soft at room temperature and can produce a lowering of blood cholesterol. Sources include canola, corn, safflower, and sunflower oils.

positron emission tomography (PET) scanning A nuclear diagnostic test that employs special radioisotopes that emit positrons and produce unique three-dimensional isotope pictures (scans) of heart blood flow and metabolism.

potassium A mineral (electrolyte) that is essential in maintaining the body's proper biochemical balance.

pre-eclampsia A condition that can occur during the last three months of pregnancy. Also called toxemia, its symptoms include high blood pressure, fluid buildup, and headaches.

prophylactic antibiotics (prophylaxis) Antibiotics administered to prevent infection, usually for patients with endocarditis or rheumatic heart disease.

prostaglandins Hormonelike chemicals that are secreted by many body tissues and are instrumental in many body functions, including blood clotting, control of blood vessel size, and muscle function.

pulmonary embolism A blocking of the pulmonary artery or one of its branches by a blood clot (embolus).

pulmonary hypertension Abnormally high blood pressure in the arteries that supply the lungs.

pulmonary regurgitation (insufficiency) A defect in the pulmonary valve, allowing a backflow of blood into the right ventricle.

pulmonary stenosis A narrowing or obstruction of the pulmonary valve or artery, impeding the flow of blood to the lungs.

pulmonary valve The valve between the right ventricle and the pulmonary artery.

pulse The expansion and contraction of a blood vessel, especially an artery, that corresponds to the beating of the heart.

Purkinje fibers Conduction fibers that form a network in the lower chambers of the heart and that carry electrical impulses to the walls of the ventricles.

radioisotope or radionuclide scanning A test in which a radioactive substance (isotope) is injected and tracked by a gamma camera (scintillation camera).

rales Chest sounds that can be heard with a stethoscope when a person with excessive lung fluid (pulmonary edema) breathes. Caused by air passing through the fluid.

Raynaud's disease A circulatory disorder characterized by episodes of reduced circulation to the fingers and toes. Small vessels contract suddenly in response to cold or emotional upset, cutting off the blood supply.

Raynaud's phenomenon A term used when the symptoms of Raynaud's disease are secondary to another condition.

red blood cells (erythrocytes) Disk-shaped blood cells whose primary function is to carry oxygen. Hemoglobin, the red pigment contained in red blood cells, enables the cells to pick up oxygen molecules from the lungs.

regurgitation In heart disease, the backflow of blood through a valve that has not closed properly (insufficiency).

renin An enzyme that is secreted mainly by the kidney and is important in regulating blood pressure.

restenosis Recurrent narrowing or blockage of a blood vessel after treatment such as balloon angioplasty.

restrictive cardiomyopathy A heart muscle disease that results in increased stiffness of the heart, causing it to have difficulty filling adequately.

rheumatic fever A childhood disease that can damage the heart, joints, and other organs. It usually develops after a strep throat infection, and is now uncommon in the United States thanks to early treatment of strep infections.

risk factor A condition or behavior that increases the likelihood of a disease or injury. Major cardiovascular risk factors include high blood pressure or elevated blood cholesterol levels and a history of smoking. A family history of early heart attacks, diabetes, a sedentary existence, male sex, and age also increase the risk.

rubella A viral infection, also called German measles, that can cause congenital heart disease and other defects in infants born to women who contracted the disease during pregnancy.

saccular aneurysm A round, protruding distention in a weak part of an artery.

saphenous vein The vein in the legs that is often removed and used to bypass a blocked vessel in coronary bypass surgery.

sarcoidosis A rare disease that can cause inflammation of the heart muscle or heart muscle dysfunction (cardiomyopathy), as well as inflammation of the lymph nodes and tissues in other parts of the body.

saturated fats Fatty acids that contain the maximum possible amount of hydrogen. They are hard at room temperature and include most animal fats as well as palm, palm kernel, and coconut oils.

semilunar valves Heart valves that are composed of cusps in the shape of a half-moon (crescent-shaped), such as the aortic and pulmonary valves.

septal defect A congenital abnormality in which there is an opening in the dividing wall (septum) between the left and right sides of the heart. This can occur between either the atria or the ventricles.

shock A condition characterized by insufficient blood supply to vital parts of the body, which deprives them of oxygen and causes them to temporarily cease functioning. If not treated immediately, shock can lead to brain damage and even death.

single photon emission computed tomography (SPECT) A diagnostic test that is a type of radionuclide scanning. It produces a three-dimensional image through the use of a camera that rotates around the subject.

sinoatrial node The natural pacemaker in the heart, consisting of a group of specialized muscle cells on the wall of the right atrium. It controls the heart's electrical activity.

sphygmomanometer A device used to measure blood pressure. It consists of an inflatable rubber cuff, an air pump, and a column of mercury or a dial that registers air pressure. Readings are expressed in millimeters of mercury (mm Hg).

stasis Reduced or discontinued flow; for example, a slowing of the flow of blood.

stenosis Narrowing of a blood vessel, heart valve, or other bodily passage.

stents Tiny metal "scaffolds" that support tubular structures such as arteries. A stent may be used to keep a collapsed artery open until surgery can take place, it may hold a vessel open while a physician works on it, or it may provide a permanent opening in a blocked artery, placed during percutaneous transluminal coronary angioplasty (PTCA).

stethoscope The instrument used to amplify and listen to the sounds made by the heart, blood vessels, and lungs.

stroke A disruption of blood flow to the brain, usually caused by a clot or rupture of a blood vessel.

stroke volume The amount of blood the heart pumps out at each contraction.

subarachnoid hemorrhage Bleeding beneath the membrane covering the brain's surface, which can compress the brain tissue.

superior vena cava The major vein that carries deoxygenated blood from the upper portion of the body (head, neck, and chest) back to the heart.

supraventricular tachycardia A too-rapid heartbeat (140 to 180 beats per minute). It can persist for several minutes to hours or days. It occurs when the tissue above the ventricles generates impulses at a faster rate than the usual pacemaker of the heart, the sinoatrial node.

sympathetic nervous system The part of the autonomic nervous system that controls heart rate, size of blood vessels, and numerous other body functions.

syncope The medical term for fainting.

systolic blood pressure The part of the blood pressure reading that corresponds to the heart's contraction or heartbeat. This is the greater of the two numbers in a blood pressure reading.

tachycardia Rapid heartbeat (more than 100 beats per minute in an adult).

temporal lobes The lower side of each half of the main part of the brain (the cerebrum).

tetralogy of Fallot A four-part congenital heart defect including a displaced aorta, a narrowed pulmonary valve, a hole in the ventricular septum, and a thickened wall in the right ventricle.

thallium stress test A radioisotope diagnostic stress test for defining areas of the heart with decreased blood flow. It can be done either with exercise or with a drug, dipyridamole (Persantine), that causes the heart blood flow to increase as it would during exercise. The electrocardiogram (ECG) is taken with the nuclear scans.

thrombus A blood clot inside a blood vessel.

tissue plasminogen activator (TPA) Clot-dissolving substance that can be produced in the body or through genetic engineering techniques. Such substances have become important in the treatment of heart attack victims. (Other commonly used clot-dissolving substances include streptokinase and APSAC.)

transdermal Delivered through the skin.

transient ischemic attack (TIA) Also called ministroke; temporary symptoms resembling those of a stroke (transient paralysis, speech problems, blindness in one eye, etc.), which result from a disruption in blood flow to the brain. TIAs are usually of short duration (a few minutes), but may be warning signs of an impending permanent stroke.

tricuspid regurgitation (insufficiency) The inability of the tricuspid valve to close properly, thereby allowing blood to leak back into the right atrium.

tricuspid stenosis Narrowing or stiffness of the valve between the right atrium and the right ventricle. A rare disorder that usually affects people who have had rheumatic fever.

tricuspid valve A valve consisting of three cusps located between the upper and lower chambers (atrium and ventricle) of the right side of the heart.

triglyceride A fatty substance (lipid) found in the body's fatty (adipose) tissues. High levels are found in diabetics and may play a role in atherosclerosis.

Type A behavior pattern Characterized by a deeply ingrained struggle to overcome real and imagined obstacles imposed by events, by other people, and especially by time. Resulting traits may be impatience, competitiveness, irritability, anger, suspicion, and hostility. People who display this behavior may be at greater risk for heart disease.

Type B behavior pattern Denoted by the lack of Type A traits. Type B people are less driven, less competitive, and more easygoing than Type A people.

ultrasound High-frequency sound waves used for diagnostic and treatment purposes. See echocardiography.

vagus nerve The major nerve of the parasympathetic nervous system that slows the heart rate when stimulated. It is involved in gastrointestinal function.

valvotomy/valvulotomy An open-heart operation to correct a blocked heart valve. A newer, less invasive technique known as balloon valvulotomy employs a balloon-tipped catheter to open up the valve.

valvuloplasty Reconstructive open-heart surgery to repair a defective heart valve. Balloon valvuloplasty uses a balloon-tipped catheter. When inflated, the balloon can separate any narrowed or stiffened leaflets of the valve.

varicose veins Swollen, twisted veins found mostly in the legs. They swell because blood drains back down into the legs and pools, the result of defective valves in the veins.

vasoconstriction Constriction of the blood vessels.

vasodilator A substance that causes blood vessels to relax or dilate.

vasospasm Spasm (an abnormal, sudden, and involuntary contraction) of the blood vessels.

vasovagal response Temporary light-headedness or loss of consciousness because of a sudden reduction in heartbeat and blood pressure. People who faint at the sight of blood typically have an extreme vasovagal response.

vein A blood vessel that conveys blood from various parts of the body back to the heart.

venous thrombosis The medical term for blood clots in the veins.

ventricles The two lower or main pumping chambers of the heart. They receive blood from the atria and pump it to the lungs and the various parts of the body.

ventricular fibrillation Rapid, uncoordinated, and ineffective contractions of the heart initiated by electrical impulses from the ventricles. Can be fatal if it is not reversed.

VEST scan One of the newest radionuclide diagnostic tests; it uses a miniaturized radionuclide detector (VEST) that can be worn for ambulatory monitoring.

white blood cells (leukocytes) Any of several types of blood cells whose function is to destroy foreign substances in the body, such as bacteria.

Wolff-Parkinson-White syndrome A congenital cardiac syndrome characterized by episodes of rapid heartbeats, from 120 to 200 beats per minute. It is caused by abnormal conduction of electrical signals in the heart.

DIRECTORY OF RESOURCES

The following organizations can provide further information on the topics indicated, as well as free or low-cost pamphlets in some cases. They can also offer help in locating local groups or local chapters of national organizations.

Aging
American Association of Retired Persons (AARP)
601 E Street, NW
Washington, DC 20049
(202) 434-2277

National Council on the Aging
409 Third Street, SW, 2nd Floor
Washington, DC 20024
(202) 479-1200

Alcohol Resources
1-800-ALCOHOL
(This hotline is available 24 hours a day, seven days a week, to offer counseling and assistance in finding local treatment centers.)

Alcoholics Anonymous, Inc.
15 East 26th Street, Room 1817
New York, NY 10010
(212) 683-3900

National Clearinghouse for Alcohol and Drug Information
P.O. Box 2345
11426 Rockville Pike
Rockville, MD 20852
(301) 468-2600

Birth Defects
March of Dimes Birth Defects Foundation
1275 Mamaroneck Avenue
White Plains, NY 10605
(914) 428-7100

Cardiovascular
American Heart Association
7320 Greenville Avenue
Dallas, TX 75231
(214) 373-6300

Mended Hearts, Inc.
7320 Greenville Avenue
Dallas, TX 75231
(214) 706-1442

National Heart, Lung and Blood Institute
National Institutes of Health
7200 Wisconsin Avenue, Suite 500
Bethesda, MD 20814
(301) 951-3260

National High Blood Pressure Education Program
Information Center
National Institutes of Health
7200 Wisconsin Avenue, Suite 500
Bethesda, MD 20814
(301) 951-3260

Consumer Information
The Council for Better Business Bureaus
4200 Wilson Boulevard
Arlington, VA 22203
(703) 276-0100
Att: Standards and Practices
(For brochures, including *Tips on Medical Quackery*, send a self-addressed stamped legal-size envelope and $1.)

Diabetes
American Diabetes Association, Inc.
1660 Duke Street
Alexandria, VA 22314
(800) 232-3472

National Diabetes Information Clearinghouse
National Institutes of Health
Box NDIC
9000 Rockville Pike
Bethesda, MD 20892
(301) 468-2162

Drug Abuse

Drug Abuse and Narcotic Addiction
Cocaine Abuse Hotline
1-800-COCAINE

Drug Abuse Clearinghouse
P.O. Box 2345
11426 Rockville Pike
Rockville, MD 20852
(301) 443-6500

Drug Crisis Hotline
(800) 522-5353

Health Information

American Red Cross
431 18th Street, NW
Washington, DC 20006
(202) 737-8300

Office of Disease Prevention and Health Promotion
National Health Information Center
P.O. Box 1133
Washington, DC 20013-1133
(800) 336-4797

Home Care

National Association for Home Care
519 C Street, NE, Stanton Park
Washington, DC 20002
(202) 547-7424

Medical Emergencies

American Trauma Society
8903 Presidential Parkway
Suite 512
Upper Marlboro, MD 20772
(800) 556-7890

Medic Alert Foundation International
P.O. Box 1009
Turlock, CA 95381
(800) ID-ALERT
(209) 668-3333

Nutrition

American Dietetic Association
216 West Jackson
Chicago, IL 60606
(312) 899-0040

National Cholesterol Education Program
National Institutes of Health
7200 Wisconsin Avenue
Bethesda, MD 20814

Rehabilitation

National Rehabilitation Association
1910 Association Drive
Reston, VA 22091
(703) 715-9090

National Rehabilitation Information Center
8455 Colesville Road
Silver Spring, MD 20910
(800) 346-2742
(301) 588-9284

Smoking

American Cancer Society
1599 Clifton Road NE
Atlanta, GA 30329
(404) 320-3333

American Lung Association
1740 Broadway
New York, NY 10019
(212) 315-8700

1-800-4-CANCER for all areas of the U.S. except:
Alaska (800) 638-6070
Oahu, HI (800) 524-1234

National Center for Health Promotion
Smoker Stoppers Program
3920 Varsity Drive
Ann Arbor, MI 48108
(313) 971-6077

Seventh Day Adventists
Community Health Services
P.O. Box 1029
Manhasset, NY 11030
(Send for free pamphlet *How to Stop Smoking*, or consult the telephone book for the nearest Seventh Day Adventist church. Smoking cessation programs are offered on a community-demand basis.)

Smokenders
1430 East Indian School Road, Suite 102
Phoenix, AZ 85014
(800) 828-4357

Stroke
Courage Center
Courage Stroke Network
3915 Golden Valley Road
Golden Valley, MN 55422
(800) 553-6321
(612) 520-0466 in Minnesota

National Stroke Association
300 East Hampden Avenue
Suite 240
Englewood, CO 80110-2654
(303) 839-1992

Stroke Clubs
These support groups are primarily independent, although some are affiliated with local chapters of the Easter Seal Society or the American Heart Association. For the nearest Stroke Club, contact the Courage Center (see listing above).

SELECTED BIBLIOGRAPHY

TEXTBOOKS
These are the primary cardiology textbooks that were used as references for this book.

Beamish, R. E., P. K. Signal, and N. S. Dhalia. *Stress and Heart Disease*. Boston: Martinus Nijhoff Publishers, 1984.

Braunwald, E. *Heart Disease*. 4th ed. Vols 1–2. Philadelphia: W. B. Saunders/Harcourt Brace Jovanovich, 1991.

Eagle, K. A., E. Haber, R. W. DeSanctis, et al., eds. *Principles of Cardiology*. 2nd ed. Boston: Little, Brown, 1989.

Hurst, J. Willis, et al. *The Heart*. 7th ed. New York: McGraw-Hill, 1990.

Liberthson, R. R. *Congenital Heart Disease: Diagnosis and Management in Children and Adults*. Boston: Little, Brown, 1989.

ADDITIONAL BOOKS

Frohlich, Edward D., and Genell Subak-Sharpe. *Take Heart*. New York: Crown, 1990.

Herbert, Victor, and Genell Subak-Sharpe, eds. *The Mount Sinai School of Medicine Complete Book of Nutrition*. New York: St. Martin's Press, 1990.

Kwiterovich, Peter. *Beyond Cholesterol: The Johns Hopkins Complete Guide for Avoiding Heart Disease*. Baltimore: Johns Hopkins Press, 1989.

Moser, Marvin. *Lower Your Blood Pressure and Live Longer*. New York: Berkley Books, 1989.

INDEX

(Page numbers in *italics* refer to illustrations.)

Minnesota Heart Survey, 242
minoxidil (Loniten), 303
mitral annular calcification, 267
mitral regurgitation, 16, 173, 384–385
mitral stenosis, 15–16, *168,* 173, 310, 384–385
mitral valve, 4, 5, 15, 167–168, 191, 250, 254, 318–319
mitral valve prolapse, 16, 172–173, 243–244, 383–384
mitral valvuloplasty, 310
monoamine oxidase inhibitors (MAOIs), 287
monounsaturated fats, 47, 55, 56, 59
moricizine (Ethmozine), 202–203
morphine, 146
Moser, Marvin, 149–166, 283–304, 359–362
Mount Sinai School of Medicine Complete Book of Nutrition (Herbert), 360
MUGA scan (multigated acquisition scan; equilibrium radionuclide angiocardiogram), 123–124, 138, 190, 193
Multiple-Risk Factor Intervention Trial (MRFIT), 42
multivariate analysis, 25
muscular dystrophy, 189–190
myocardial infarction, *see* heart attack
myocardial ischemia, 134–135, 185, 194, 210, 213, 214, 341
    diagnosis of, 118, 121
    silent, 98, 118, 121, 134, 136, 137
    stress and, 97–98
myocarditis (heart muscle inflammation), 19, 178, 187–188, 386
    causes of, 19, 187–188, 386
    treatment of, 19, 188, 386
myocardium, 3, 5, 181
myxomatous degeneration, 171, 172

N

nadolol (Corgard), 293
National Cancer Institute, 52, 77
National Center for Health Promotion, 74, 77
National Center for Health Statistics, 23, 134
National Cholesterol Education Program, 37, 44
National Heart, Lung, and Blood Institute, 44, 52, 142, 149, 242
National High Blood Pressure Education Program, 149
National High Blood Pressure Information Center, 164

National Institutes of Health (NIH), 237, 273
nausea, 12, 260
nephritis, 155
nephrotic syndrome (kidney disease), 19, 29, 31, 52, 239, 285
    edema and, 112
nervous system, 9, 14
    autonomic, 164, 165, 172, 196
    "hyperpneic" children and, 256
    parasympathetic, 196
    sympathetic, 97, 100, 172, 196
neurotransmitters, 9
New England Journal of Medicine, 53, 61
New Haven, Conn., obesity survey in, 276
New York Heart Association, 178
niacin (nicotinic acid; Nia-Bid, Niacels; Niacor; Niaplus; Nicolar; Nicobid; Slo-Niacin), 43, 49, 61, 297
nicardipine (Cardene), 294
nicotine, 30, 72, 73, 74, 77
nicotinic acid, *see* niacin
nifedipine (Procardia; Procardia XL), 294
nimodipine (Nimotop), 224, 294
nitrates, 140–141, 245, 286, 301–302
nitroglycerin, 136, 140–141, 144, 146, 174, 194, 301
NMDA-receptor blockers, 233
nonsteroidal anti-inflammatory drugs (NSAIDs), 19
norepinephrine (noradrenaline), 9, 82, 165, 286, 292
Norwood procedure, 258
nuclear cardiology, 122–125
    major uses of, 122–123
    MUGA scan, 123–124, 138, 190, 193
    perfusion (blood flow) imaging, 124, 125
    thallium stress test (thallium scan), 125, 138
    VEST scan, 124
Nurses' Health Study, 239, 240
nutritional deficiency, 80, 114
    cardiomyopathy and, 187, 189
nuts, 61

O

oat bran, 53
obesity, 29, 47, 72, 240–241
    android (male-pattern), 31, 63, 241, 242
    diet and, 51, 52
    in elderly, 270
    exercise and, 85, 92
    peripheral vascular disease and, 211
    race and, 276
    stroke and, 31, 218–219
    see also overweight

occipital lobes, 217
occupational therapy, after stroke, 229
oils, 55–56, 59, 64
    tropical, 55, 62
olive oil, 55, 56
omega-3 fatty acids, 53, 61
omega-6 fatty acids, 61
oophorectomy, 239
ophthalmoscope, 153
oral contraceptives, 72, 156, 219, 239–240
orthopnea, 178, 180
orthostatic hypotension, 165, 265, 284
Oslo Diet and Antismoking Study, 43
osteoporosis, 32, 61, 285, 299
Ostfeld, Adrian, 273–280
ostium secundum defect, 252, 254
outpatient phase, 357
overweight:
    hypertension and, 157, 161–162
    overfat vs., 63
    tests for, 63
    see also obesity
oxygen:
    "blue babies" and, 17
    brain's use of, 216
    in capillaries, 7, 150
    decrease in, 9
    delivery of, 3, 4, 7, 8, 9, 134, 150
    deprivation of, *see* myocardial ischemia
    fainting and, 111, 112
    hemoglobin and, 8, 87
    hypoxia, 180
    increased need for, 5, 109–110
    in lungs, 178, *179*
    stenosis and, 15
    training effect and, 87
    see also cyanotic conditions

P

pacemakers, 18, 198, 203, 267, 331–335
    alphabet for, 332
    complications of, 333–334
    demand, 332
    dual-chamber, 332–333
    implantation of, 333, *333*
    living with, 334–335
    natural, 116, 267, 331
Paffenbarger, Ralph, 93
pain, 13
    in calves, 13
    in chest, *see* chest pain
    in joints, 16
    in legs, 13, 23, 157, 207–208, 210, 211, 212
    peripheral vascular disease and, 208, 209
    in thighs, 13
Palmaz-Shatz stent, 309